Lyme Borreliosis

nova
Medicine & Health
New York

Infectious Diseases and Microbiology Series

Dietary Polyphenols for Infectious Diseases
Md. Faiyazuddin and Sumel Ashique (Editors)
ISBN: 979-8-89530-750-2
eBook ISBN: 979-8-89530-841-7

The Encyclopedia of COVID (18 Volume Set)
Sue Ng-Lau (Editor)
eBook ISBN: 978-1-68507-653-5

Malaria: Mechanisms of Infection and Disease Progression. Prospects for Diagnosis, Treatment and Prevention
Huseynov Elchin Mammad
ISBN: 979-8-89113-906-0
eBook ISBN: 979-8-89113-940-4

Critical Care and COVID-19
Salim Surani, Syed Anjum Khan, MD and Reena Shah (Editors)
ISBN: 979-8-88697-940-4
eBook ISBN: 979-8-88697-969-5

Infectious Diseases: From Prevention to Control
Yvette S. Brewer (Editor)
ISBN: 979-8-88697-657-1
eBook ISBN: 979-8-88697-664-9

Psychological Consequences of the COVID-19 Pandemic on Children, Teenagers and Adults
Jean-Pascal Assailly, PhD
ISBN: 978-1-68507-963-5
eBook ISBN: 979-8-88697-072-2

Data Science Applications of Post-COVID-19 Psychological Disorders
Vijayalakshmi Kakulapati, PhD (Editor)
ISBN: 979-8-88697-165-1
eBook ISBN: 979-8-88697-316-7

Interdisciplinary Approaches on Opportunistic Infections and Future Prospects
Jayapradha Ramakrishnan, PhD and Ganesh Babu Malli Mohan, PhD (Editors)
ISBN: 978-1-68507-984-0
eBook ISBN: 979-8-88697-342-6

More information about this series can be found at
https://novapublishers.com/product-category/series/infectious-diseases-and-microbiology/

Mykhaylo Andreychyn
Mykhaylo Korda
Maria Shkilna
Oleh Ivakhiv
Editors

Lyme Borreliosis

nova
Medicine & Health
New York

DOI: https://doi.org/10.52305/CCXD5454

Library of Congress Cataloging-in-Publication Data

Library of Congress Control Number: 2025945992
ISBN: 979-8-89530-657-4 (Hardcover)
ISBN: 979-8-89530-847-9 (eBook)

Published by Nova Science Publishers, Inc. † New York

Contents

Preface

Lyme borreliosis is one of the insufficiently studied zoonotic diseases with a natural focus and is characterized by the continuous expansion of geographically affected areas and increasing incidence worldwide. Experts suggest that it is gradually acquiring the characteristics of a pandemic infection, making it an increasing concern in various countries.

These circumstances highlight the need for in-depth research. As a result, the number of publications on Lyme borreliosis is growing each year, particularly in North America and Europe. In the past 10 to 15 years, Ukraine has also started paying more attention to this issue.

Researchers at Ivan Horbachevsky Ternopil National Medical University began studying Lyme borreliosis over ten years ago. In 2017, in agreement with the Ministry of Health of Ukraine, the Centre for Lyme Borreliosis and Other Tick-Borne Diseases Research was established at the University. In a short time, the Centre's laboratory was equipped with the necessary apparatus, and research methods were developed in accordance with global standards. This progress was greatly facilitated by collaboration with scientists from the State Higher School of the Pope John Paul II (Biała Podlaska, Poland), the Institute of Rural Medicine (Lublin, Poland), IGeneX Inc. (Milpitas, California, USA), and researchers from Finland, France, and Spain. In 2019, our university received the Seeding Labs grant (Boston, USA), which enabled the acquisition of modern equipment for the laboratory.

The main research was conducted as part of comprehensive research projects of the Department of Infectious Diseases, Epidemiology, Skin and Venereal Diseases of Ivan Horbachevsky Ternopil National Medical University. These projects were titled: "Study of epidemiology, pathogenesis and clinic manifestations of Lyme borreliosis in endemic regions of Ukraine, including Ternopil region, and improvement of its diagnostics, therapy, rehabilitation measures and prevention" (state registration number 0118U000357) and "Mono- and mixed tick-borne infections, improvement of treatment and diagnostic technologies and biosafety measures" (state registration number 0120U104348). Over fifty scientists and support staff participated in these projects.

The data obtained have been presented at numerous national and international scientific events, partially published in periodicals, and received positive feedback. Several dissertation papers have been completed as well.

It is worth noting that foreign scientists have published several monographs on the problem of Lyme borreliosis, presenting the results of their own research. However, to date, no monographs on this topic have been published in Ukraine. As a result, our team of authors decided to partially address this gap by preparing a book that summarizes the latest global achievements and the key findings from our own research.

We hope that our monograph will not only contribute to the dissemination of knowledge among scientists interested in this issue, but also assist practitioners in improving the diagnosis of Lyme disease, treatment of patients and anti-epidemic measures. These include epidemiologists, infectious disease specialists, cardiologists, rheumatologists, acarologists, neurologists, entomologists, molecular biologists, and laboratory physicians. We would be grateful for any suggestions from our readers that aim to stimulate further research and facilitate the sharing of experiences in this critical area of biology and medicine.

List of Abbreviations

ACA	acrodermatitis chronica atrophicans
AVDL	adequate vitamin D level
CBEM	chronic borrelial encephalomyelitis
CEBVI	chronic Epstein-Barr virus infection
CI	confidence interval
CICs	circulating immune complexes
CNS	central nervous system
CRP	C-reactive protein
CSF	cerebrospinal fluid
CT	computer tomography
DAS	disease activity score
DEET	N,N-diethyl-meta-toluamide
DM	dermatomyositis
EBV	Epstein-Barr virus
ECG	electrocardiography
ELISA	enzyme-linked immunosorbent assay
EM	erythema migrans
EM LB	erythema migrans form of Lyme borreliosis
EP	encephalopathy
FM	fibromyalgia
GIS	geographic information system
HGA	human granulocytic anaplasmosis
IFN	interferon
IgM, IgG	immunoglobulins of M and G classes
IIFR	indirect immunofluorescence reaction
IL	interleukin
LB	Lyme borreliosis
LD	Lyme disease
Lq	lower quartile
LVDD	left ventricular diastolic dysfunction
Me	median
MIC	minimum inhibitory concentration
MEM	multiple erythema migrans
MMP	matrix metalloproteinases
MRI	magnetic resonance imaging
MS	multiple sclerosis
NDPT	newly diagnosed pulmonary tuberculosis

NEM LB	non-erythema migrans form of Lyme borreliosis
NS	nervous system
NSAIDs	nonsteroidal anti-inflammatory drugs
OR	odds ratio
PCR	polymerase chain reaction
PLD	post-Lyme disease
PNP	polyneuropathy
RA	rheumatoid arthritis
RP	radiculopathy
SVDL	safe vitamin D level
TBRF	tick-borne relapsing fever
TNF-α	tumour necrosis factor-α
Uq	upper quartile
USI	ultrasound imaging
VAS	visual analogue scale
VDD	vitamin D deficiency
VDI	vitamin D insufficiency
ΔT	temperature difference between compared areas of the body on the thermogram

Chapter 1

The Relevance of Lyme Borreliosis and Scientific Tasks

Mykhaylo Andreychyn[1]
and Mykhaylo Korda[2]

[1]Academician of the National Academy of Medical Sciences of Ukraine,
Honoured Master of Sciences and Technologies of Ukraine, DSc in Medicine, Professor,
Head of the Department of Infectious Diseases with Epidemiology,
Dermatology and Venerology, I. Horbachevsky Ternopil National Medical University, Ternopil, Ukraine
[2]Corresponding Member of the National Academy of Medical Sciences of Ukraine,
Honoured Master of Sciences and Technologies of Ukraine, DSc in Medicine, Professor,
Department of Medical Biochemistry, I. Horbachevsky Ternopil National Medical University,
Ternopil, Ukraine

Lyme borreliosis (LB) or Lyme disease (LD) is a naturally occurring infection belonging to the group of bacterial zoonoses caused by Borrelia, transmitted by ticks, and characterized by damage to the skin (in the form of erythema migrans (EM)), musculoskeletal, cardiovascular and nervous systems.

The first mention of this ailment dates back to 1909, when the Swedish botanist Adam Afzelius showed the scientists of the Swedish Society of Dermatology a patient with ring-shaped erythema that spread from the site of a tick bite [1–3]. However, significant progress in the study of the disease occurred only in 1975-1976, when American researchers A. C. Steere et al., analysed a group outbreak of infection in the city of Lyme, Connecticut (USA), which took the form of juvenile rheumatoid arthritis occurring after tick bite and was often combined with ring-shaped erythema migrans. Treatment success was achieved with penicillin [4–7]. The new ailment was named "Lyme disease." In 1982, the American entomologist and microbiologist Willy (Wilhelm) Burgdorfer and his colleagues, while examining the contents of the intestines of the Ixodes tick, discovered the causative agent of LB, i.e., a spirochete and suspected its involvement in the clinical manifestations of this disease [8]. Subsequently, the bacterium received the official name "*Borrelia burgdorferi*" [6, 9], and the disease was defined by the more precise term "Lyme borreliosis" [10].

LD is the most common tick-borne infection in the United States and Europe. About 300,000 patients are registered annually in the USA alone [11], up to 85,000 in Europe [12]. The incidence rate in different European countries ranges from 9–10 cases per 100,000 population (Poland, Belarus) to 35 (Lithuania), 100 or more (Slovenia) [13, 14]. However, WHO experts believe that the number of registered cases is at least 5 times lower than the actual

In: Lyme Borreliosis
Editors: Mykhaylo Andreychyn, Mykhaylo Korda, Maria Shkilna and Oleh Ivakhiv
ISBN: 979-8-89530-657-4

number. Tick-borne pathogens are already diagnosed in more than 80 countries, and by 2050 they may affect 35% of the world's population [15].

LB in Ukraine is officially included in the group of particularly dangerous infectious diseases [16]. Its registration began in 2000. Its incidence tends to increase in all regions, with the largest number of patients registered in the forest-steppe landscape-geographic zone, namely: Vinnytsia, Kyiv, Lviv, Sumy, Ternopil, Cherkasy and Chernihiv regions [17, 18]. The number of registered patients increased from 58 in 2000 to 5,418 in 2019. In particular, in Ternopil region during this period, the incidence increased from 4 to 125. In 2019, the incidence of LB was 10.62 per 100 thousand population in comparison with 3.77 in 2014 [18, 19]. However, there are reasons to believe that modern official statistics do not reflect the actual epidemic situation regarding LB, as they are significantly underestimated. One of the reasons for underreporting is the lack of vigilance of doctors regarding LB and frequent false diagnoses.

Ternopil region is an endemic centre of LB, as it is located in an area with fertile soils, a moderate continental climate, forest landscapes (the total area of the forests in the region is 199.3 thousand ha with broad-leaved and mixed-broad-leaved tree species), which contributes to the preservation in nature of the main reservoir of Borrelia – Ixodes ticks. Ixodes tick-borne borreliosis was detected in 57 settlements in 14 districts of the region and in the city of Ternopil [19].

There are obviously no isolated natural foci of individual blood infections. In Europe, there are associated regions containing up to seven pathogens that can be transmitted during the sucking of ixodid ticks. It has been established that in 84.4% of cases, LB occurs as a mixed infection with tick-borne encephalitis, human granulocytic anaplasmosis, and monocytic ehrlichiosis [20].

Infection of ticks with Borrelia, selected from different natural regions, ranges from 1.5 to 75.0% [21–24]; with anaplasmas in the USA – from 7.6 to 53.0%, in European countries – from 0.8 to 24.4% [25]; with *B. miyamotoi* (the causative agent of tick-borne fever) – from 0.4 to 4.8% [26–28]. However, there is very little data on the infection of *B. burgdorferi*, *A. phagocytophilum*, *B. miyamotoi*, and *Babesia sp.* ticks collected from humans [29, 30], and such studies were conducted only abroad.

B. miyamotoi is known to cause the disease in the population of Europe [31, 32] and the USA [33], including foresters [34]. However, there has been no data on the involvement of this Borrelia genotype in diseases among residents of Ukraine, including forestry workers.

Numerous evidence of the etiological role of – Borrelia in the development of diseases of various organs and systems have been published. In 18.3% of patients with LB, damage of the musculoskeletal system was detected, in 10.7% – those of the cardiovascular system [35], in 5–64.0% – of the nervous system [36]. Polysystem damage complicates clinical diagnosis, which is why LB got the name "great imitator" of various human diseases [37]. The propensity for a long asymptomatic course of the disease, the development in a third of patients of difficult-to-diagnose erythematous forms, and the possibility of repeated diseases make the problem of LB extremely relevant [35, 38].

Lyme borreliosis negatively affects the course of pregnancy. The chronic form of the disease can lead to irreversible changes in the skin, joints, cardiovascular and nervous systems, a decrease in the quality of life, partial or complete loss of working capacity, to disability and even death [10, 39, 40].

An important feature of LB is significant differences in the course of the disease not only due to infection with +different types of the pathogen, but also in different stages of the disease [41, 42].

Foresters belong to professional population groups with a high risk of Borrelia infection [34, 43]. Awareness of different groups of the population regarding LB, in particular students [44–46] and forestry workers [13, 47], and their infecting with *B. burgdorferi* was studied in a number of European countries [48, 49]. In Ukraine, similar studies were conducted only among a small number of forestry workers in the Lviv region [35] and further studies are needed both in Ternopil region and in other regions. Diagnosis of LB and treatment of patients require improvement [50, 51], especially regarding detection of erythematous forms of the disease and rational use of antibiotics. However, there is currently no unified approach to antibacterial therapy, and there are no final recommendations regarding the choice of a specific etiotropic agent and the scheme of its administration [52, 53]. Preventive measures in endemic areas of LB require significant optimization.

References

[1] Thyresson, N. Historical notes on skin manifestations of Lyme borreliosis. *Scand J Infect Dis* [Internet]. 1991 [cited 1 Feb 2025];23(Suppl 77):9-13. Available from: https://www.tandfonline.com/doi/epdf/10.3109/inf.1991.23.suppl-77.01?needAccess=true.

[2] Radolf, J. D., Strle, K., Lemieux, J. E., Strle, F. Lyme Disease in Humans. *Curr Issues Mol Biol.* 2021;42:333-384. DOI: 10.21775/cimb.042.333.

[3] Popovych, O. Lyme borreliosis: current problem of infectiology (Clinical Lecture). *Actual Infectology.* 2022;(3.12):114-22. doi: 10.22141/2312-413x.3.12.2016.81725. [in Ukrainian].

[4] Steere, A. C., Malawista, S. E., Snydman, D. R., Shope, R. E., Andiman, W. A., Ross, M. R., Steele, F. M. Lyme arthritis: an epidemic of oligoarticular arthritis in children and adults in three connecticut communities. *Arthritis Rheum.* 1977;20(1):7-17. doi: 10.1002/art.1780200102.

[5] Steere, A. C., Malawista, S. E., Hardin, J. A., Ruddy, S., Askenase, W., Andiman, W. A. Erythema chronicum migrans and Lyme arthritis. The enlarging clinical spectrum. *Ann Intern Med.* 1977;86(6):685-98. doi: 10.7326/0003-4819-86-6-685.

[6] Berndtson, K. Review of evidence for immune evasion and persistent infection in Lyme disease. *Int J Gen Med.* 2013;6:291-306. doi: 10.2147/IJGM.S44114.

[7] Schotthoefer, A. M., Frost, H. M. Ecology and epidemiology of Lyme borreliosis. *Clin Lab Med.* 2015;35(4):723-43. doi: 10.1016/j.cll.2015.08.003.

[8] Burgdorfer, W., Barbour, A. G., Hayes, S. F., Benach, J. L., Grunwaldt, E., Davis, J. P. Lyme disease-a tick-borne spirochetosis? *Science.* 1982;216(4552):1317-9. doi: 10.1126/science.7043737.

[9] Smoleńska, Ż., Masiak, A., Strzelecki, A., Zdrojewski, Z. The role of Borrelia burgdorferi infection in scleroderma. *Reumatologia.* 2014;52(5):326-31. doi: 10.5114/reum.2014.46671.

[10] Chemych, M., Lutai, I. Lyme disease. Modern issue condition. *East Ukr Med J.* 2020;8(2):230-41. doi: 10.21272/eumj.2020;8(2):230-41. [in Ukrainian].

[11] Mead, P. S. Epidemiology of Lyme disease. *Infect Dis Clin North Am.* 2015;29(2):187-210. doi: 10.1016/j.idc.2015.02.010.

[12] Raileanu, C., Moutailler, S., Pavel, I., Porea, D., Mihalca, A. D., Savuta, G., Vayssier-Taussat, M. Borrelia Diversity and Co-infection with Other Tick Borne Pathogens in Ticks. *Front Cell Infect Microbiol.* 2017;7:36. DOI:10.3389/fcimb.2017.00036.

[13] Lewandowska, A., Kruba, Z., Filip, R. Epidemiology of Lyme disease among workers of forest inspectorates in Poland. *Ann Agric Environ Med* [Internet]. 2013 [cited 1 Feb 2025];20(2):329-31. Available from: https://www.aaem.pl/pdf-71937-9164?filename=9164.pdf.

[14] Reye, A. L., Stegniy, V., Mishaeva, N. P., Velhin, S., Hübschen, J. M., Ignatyev, G., Muller, C. P. Prevalence of tick-borne pathogens in Ixodes ricinus and Dermacentor reticulatus ticks from different geographical locations in Belarus. *PLoS One.* 2013;8(1):e54476. doi: 10.1371/journal.pone.0054476.

[15] Davidsson, M. The Financial Implications of a Well-Hidden and Ignored Chronic Lyme Disease Pandemic. *Healthcare (Basel).* 2018;6(1):16. doi: 10.3390/healthcare6010016.

[16] Kundiiev, Y. I., Andreychyn, M. A., Nahorna, A. M., Varyvonchyk, D. V. *Professional Infectious Diseases. Zoonoses.* Kyiv: Avitsena; 2014. p. 360-522 (406-19) pp. [in Ukrainian].

[17] Zadorozhna, V. I., Rudenko, A. O., Klius, V. Yu. Lyme-borreliosis is a particularly dangerous infection. Threats and risks. *Veterynarna medytsyna* [Internet]. 2017 [cited 1 Feb 2025];103:30-2. Available at: https://www.jvm.kharkov.ua/sbornik/103/1_5.pdf. [in Ukrainian].

[18] Nebogatkin, I., Shulhan, A. Epidemiological and epizootic features of Lyme disease in 2019 in Ukraine. *Actual Infectology.* 2020;8(5-6):44-8. doi: 10.22141/2312-413x.8.5-6.2020.217959. [in Ukrainian].

[19] Vasilyeva, N. A., Ivakhiv, O. L., Kachor, V. O., Avsyukevych, O. E., Voloshyn, S. B., Prodan, A. M., Gerasymenko, O. A., Velychko, S. V., Biletska, G. V., Semenyshyn, O. B. Lyme Disease in the Ternopil Region. *Infectious Diseases.* 2011;(20):50–53. doi: 10.11603/1681-2727.2011.2.577 [in Ukrainian].

[20] Malyi, V. P., Shepileva, N. V. Tick-borne Infections (Lyme Disease, Granulocytic Anaplasmosis, and Monocytic Ehrlichiosis) in the Kharkiv Region. *Clinical Immunology. Allergy. Infectology* [Internet]. 2013 [cited 1 Feb 2025];(2):49-52. Available at: https://kiai.com.ua/en/archive/2013/2%2861%29/pages-49-52/klishchovi-infekciyi-hvoroba-layma-granulocitarniy-anaplazmoz-i-monocitarniy-erlihioz-u-harkivskiy-oblasti [in Ukrainian].

[21] Zakovska, A., Kucerova, H., Nejezchlebova, H., Bartonkova, N., Rasovska, T., Norek, A. Monitoring the prevalence of pathogenic Borrelia burgdorferi sensu lato in ticks in two Brno locations. *Klin Mikrobiol Infekc Lek* [Internet]. 2011 [cited 1 Feb 2025];17(5):179-83. Available at: https://is.muni.cz/publication/963692/klistata_hanka_011.pdf. [in Czech].

[22] Cisak, E., Zając, V., Wójcik-Fatla, A., Dutkiewicz, J. Risk of tick-borne diseases in various categories of employment among forestry workers in eastern Poland. *Ann Agric Environ Med* [Internet]. 2012 [cited 1 Feb 2025];19(3):469-74. Available at: https://www.aaem.pl/pdf-71805-9031?filename=9031.pdf.

[23] Mavrutenkov, V. V. Lyme Disease. General Issues (Part I). *Child Health.* 2014;(2):106-10. doi: 10.22141/2224-0551.2.53.2014.75955 [in Russian].

[24] Crowder, C. D., Carolan, H. E., Rounds, M. A., Honig, V., Mothes, B., Haag, H., Nolte, O., Luft, B. J., Grubhoffer, L., Ecker, D. J., Schutzer, S. E., Eshoo, M. W. Prevalence of Borrelia miyamotoi in Ixodes ticks in Europe and the United States. *Emerg Infect Dis.* 2014;20(10):1678-82. doi: 10.3201/eid2010.131583.

[25] Klymnyuk, S. I., Romanyuk, L. B., Shkilna, M. I. Modern views about the granulocytic anaplasmosis of a man. *Infectious Diseases.* 2017;(3):4-9. doi: 10.11603/1681-2727.2017.3.8220. [in Ukrainian].

[26] Geller, J., Nazarova, L., Katargina, O., Järvekülg, L., Fomenko, N., Golovljova, I. Detection and genetic characterization of relapsing fever spirochete Borrelia miyamotoi in Estonian ticks. *PLoS One.* 2012;7(12):e51914. doi: 10.1371/journal.pone.0051914.

[27] Cochez, C., Heyman, P., Heylen, D., Fonville, M., Hengeveld, P., Takken, W., Simons, L., Sprong, H. The Presence of Borrelia miyamotoi, A Relapsing Fever Spirochaete, in Questing Ixodes ricinus in Belgium and in The Netherlands. *Zoonoses Public Health.* 2015;62(5):331-3. doi: 10.1111/zph.12154.

[28] Venczel, R., Knoke, L., Pavlovic, M., Dzaferovic, E., Vaculova, T., Silaghi, C., Overzier, E., Konrad, R., Kolenčík, S., Derdakova, M., Sing, A., Schaub, G. A., Margos, G., Fingerle, V. A novel duplex real-time PCR permits simultaneous detection and differentiation of Borrelia miyamotoi and Borrelia burgdorferi sensu lato. *Infection.* 2016;44(1):47-55. doi: 10.1007/s15010-015-0820-8.

[29] Gałęziowska, E., Rzymowska, J., Najda, N., Kołodziej, P., Domżał-Drzewicka, R., Rząca, M., Muraczyńska, B., Charzyńska-Gula, M., Szadowska-Szlachetka, Z., Ślusarska, B., Guty, E. Prevalence of Borrelia burgdorferi in ticks removed from skin of people and circumstances of being bitten – research from the area of Poland, 2012-2014. *Ann Agric Environ Med.* 2018;25(1):31-5. doi: 10.5604/12321966.1233906.

[30] Lernout, T., De Regge, N., Tersago, K., Fonville, M., Suin, V., Sprong, H. Prevalence of pathogens in ticks collected from humans through citizen science in Belgium. *Parasit Vectors.* 2019;12(1):550. doi: 10.1186/s13071-019-3806-z.

[31] Komarenko, N. S., Vynohrad, N. O. Species varietion of borrelia and theirimportance for regional pathology. *Annals of Mechnikov Institute* [Internet]. 2011 [cited 1 Feb 2025]; (3):20-22. Available at: https://www.imiamn.org.ua/journal/3_2011/PDF/6.pdf. [in Ukrainian].

[32] Szekeres, S., Coipan, E. C., Rigó, K., Majoros, G., Jahfari, S., Sprong, H., Földvári, G. Eco-epidemiology of Borrelia miyamotoi and Lyme borreliosis spirochetes in a popular hunting and recreational forest area in Hungary. *Parasit Vectors.* 2015;8:309. doi: 10.1186/s13071-015-0922-2.

[33] Jobe, D. A., Lovrich, S. D., Oldenburg, D. G., Kowalski, T. J., Callister, S. M. Borrelia miyamotoi Infection in Patients from Upper Midwestern United States, 2014-2015. *Emerg Infect Dis.* 2016;22(8):1471-3. doi: 10.3201/eid2208.151878.

[34] Jahfari, S., Herremans, T., Platonov, A. E., Kuiper, H., Karan, L. S., Vasilieva, O., Koopmans, M. P., Hovius, J. W., Sprong, H. High seroprevalence of Borrelia miyamotoi antibodies in forestry workers and individuals suspected of human granulocytic anaplasmosis in the Netherlands. *New Microbes New Infect.* 2014;2(5):144-9. doi: 10.1002/nmi2.59.

[35] Zinchuk, O. M. Lyme Borreliosis: Clinical-Immunopathogenetic Features and Emergency Preventive Treatment [Author's Abstract]. Kyiv; 2010. 41 c. [in Ukrainian].

[36] Antonenko, K. V., Cherenko, T. M., Turchina, N. S., Vakulenko, L. O., Sirota, N. V. Huntington's disease in training with Lyme borreliosis: analysis of clinical experience. *Ukrainian neurological journal* [Internet]. 2016 [cited 1 Feb 2025];(1):93-97. Available at: https://ukrneuroj.vitapol.com.ua/svizhij_nomer.php?nid=38. [in Ukrainian].

[37] Cochat Costa Rodrigues, M. C., Moreira, I., Peixoto, M. J., Silveira, C. The New Great Imitator – Neuropsychiatric Symptoms of Lyme Disease. *European Psychiatry.* 2017;41(S1):S232-S232. doi: 10.1016/j.eurpsy.2017.01.2242.

[38] Bamm, V. V., Ko, J. T., Mainprize, I. L., Sanderson, V. P., Wills, M. K. B. Lyme Disease Frontiers: Reconciling Borrelia Biology and Clinical Conundrums. *Pathogens.* 2019;8(4):299. doi: 10.3390/pathogens8040299.

[39] Malyi, V. P., Kratenko, I. S. *Systemic Tick-Borne Borreliosis (Lyme Disease):* A Teaching Aid. Kharkiv: Folio; 2006. 127 p. [in Russian].

[40] Zinchuk, O. M. Lyme Borreliosis. In: Malyi V. P., Andreychyn M. A. (Ed.). *Infectious Diseases: Textbook in 2 vol.* Vol 2. Lviv: Magnolia-2006; 2018. c. 400-5. [in Ukrainian].

[41] Kugeler, K. J., Farley, G. M., Forrester, J. D., Mead, P. S. Geographic Distribution and Expansion of Human Lyme Disease, United States. *Emerg Infect Dis.* 2015;21(8):1455-7. doi: 10.3201/eid2108.141878.

[42] van den Wijngaard, C. C., Hofhuis, A., Simões, M., Rood, E., van Pelt, W., Zeller, H., Van Bortel, W. Surveillance perspective on Lyme borreliosis across the European Union and European Economic Area. *Euro Surveill.* 2017;22(27):30569. doi: 10.2807/1560-7917.ES.2017.22.27.30569.

[43] Jovanovic, D., Atanasievska, S., Protic-Djokic, V., Rakic, U., Lukac-Radoncic, E., Ristanovic, E. Seroprevalence of Borrelia burgdorferi in occupationally exposed persons in the Belgrade area, Serbia. *Braz J Microbiol.* 2015;46(3):807-14. doi: 10.1590/S1517-838246320140698.

[44] Nejezchlebova, H., Kiewra, D., Žákovská, A., Ovesná, P. Students' attitudes to tick risks. *Ann Agric Environ Med.* 2016;23(3):437-41. doi: 10.5604/12321966.1219183.

[45] Pańczuk, A., Tokarska-Rodak, M., Tarelkina, I., Voita, D. Prevention of Lyme borreliosis among students from Poland and Latvia. Hygeia. *Public Health.* [Internet]. 2018 [cited 1 Feb 2025];53(3):307-12. Available at: http://www.h-ph.pl/hyg.php?opc=AR&lng=pl&art=719.

[46] Pańczuk, A., Tokarska-Rodak, M., Mikuľáková, W., Kendrová, L., Magurová, D. Exposure to ticks and undertaking Lyme borreliosis prevention activities among students from Poland and Slovakia. *Ann Agric Environ Med.* 2019;26(2):217-221. doi: 10.26444/aaem/99089.

[47] Pańczuk, A., Tokarska-Rodak, M., Plewik, D., Paszkiewicz, J. Tick exposure and prevalence of Borrelia burgdorferi antibodies among hunters and other individuals exposed to vector ticks in eastern Poland. *Rocz Panstw Zakl Hig.* 2019;70(2):161-168. doi: 10.32394/rpzh.2019.0066.

[48] Chmielewska-Badora, J., Moniuszko, A., Żukiewicz-Sobczak, W., Zwoliński, J., Piątek, J., Pancewicz, S. Serological survey in persons occupationally exposed to tick-borne pathogens in cases of co-infections with Borrelia burgdorferi, Anaplasma phagocytophilum, Bartonella spp. and Babesia microti. *Ann Agric Environ Med* [Internet]. 2012 [cited 1 Feb 2025];19(2):271-4. Available at: https://www.aaem.pl/pdf-71773-8999?filename=8999.pdf.

[49] Tokarska-Rodak, M., Plewik, D., Kozioł-Montewka, M., Szepeluk, A., Paszkiewicz, J. Risk of occupational infections caused by Borrelia burgdorferi among forestry workers and farmers. *Med Pr Work Health Saf.* 2014;65(1):109-17. doi: 10.13075/mp.5893.2014.017. [in Polish].

[50] Chandra, A., Wormser, G. P., Marques, A. R., Latov, N., Alaedini, A. Anti-Borrelia burgdorferi antibody profile in post-Lyme disease syndrome. *Clin Vaccine Immunol.* 2011;18(5):767-71. doi: 10.1128/CVI.00002-11.

[51] Pancewicz, S. A., Garlicki, A. M., Moniuszko-Malinowska, A., Zajkowska, J., Kondrusik, M., Grygorczuk, S., Czupryna, P., Dunaj, J. Polish Society of Epidemiology and Infectious Diseases. Diagnosis and treatment of tick-borne diseases recommendations of the Polish Society of Epidemiology and Infectious Diseases. *Przegl Epidemiol* [Internet]. 2015 [cited 1 Feb 2025];69(2):309-16, 421-8. Available at: https://www.przeglepidemiol.pzh.gov.pl/pdf-180534-101094?filename=Diagnosis%20and%20treatment.pdf [in English, Polish].

[52] Tseng, Y. J., Cami, A., Goldmann, D. A., DeMaria, A. Jr., Mandl, K. D. Incidence and Patterns of Extended-Course Antibiotic Therapy in Patients Evaluated for Lyme Disease. *Clin Infect Dis.* 2015;61(10):1536-42. doi: 10.1093/cid/civ636.

[53] Moore, A., Nelson, C., Molins, C., Mead, P., Schriefer, M. Current Guidelines, Common Clinical Pitfalls, and Future Directions for Laboratory Diagnosis of Lyme Disease, United States. *Emerg Infect Dis.* 2016;22(7):1169–77. doi: 10.3201/eid2207.151694.

Chapter 2

The Etiology and Epidemiology of Lyme Borreliosis

Mykhaylo Andreychyn[1]
Mykhaylo Korda[2]
Mariia Shkilna[3]
Oleh Ivakhiv[4]
Larysa Fedoniuk[5]
Mykola Kashuba[6]
Svitlana Nykytiuk[7]
Volodymyr Panychev[8]
Alina Petruk[9]
Stepan Podobivskyi[10]
Lidia Romanyuk[11]
Kateryna Shtokailo[12]
Andrii Sverstyuk[13]
and Stepan Zaporozhan[14]

[1]Academician of the National Academy of Medical Sciences of Ukraine, Honoured Master of Sciences and Technologies of Ukraine, DSc in Medicine, Professor, Head of the Department of Infectious Diseases with Epidemiology, Dermatology and Venerology, I. Horbachevsky Ternopil National Medical University, Ternopil, Ukraine
[2]Corresponding Member of the National Academy of Medical Sciences of Ukraine, Honoured Master of Sciences and Technologies of Ukraine, DSc in Medicine, Professor, Department of Medical Biochemistry, I. Horbachevsky Ternopil National Medical University, Ternopil, Ukraine
[3]DSc in Medicine, Professor, Department of Infectious Diseases with Epidemiology, Dermatology and Venerology, I. Horbachevsky Ternopil National Medical University, Ternopil, Ukraine
[4]Honoured Doctor of Ukraine, PhD in Medicine, Associate Professor, Department of Infectious Diseases with Epidemiology, Dermatology and Venerology, I. Horbachevsky Ternopil National Medical University, Ternopil, Ukraine
[5]DSc in Medicine, Professor, Head of the Department of Medical Biology, I. Horbachevsky Ternopil National Medical University, Ternopil, Ukraine
[6]DSc in Medicine, Professor, Head of the Department of General Hygiene and Ecology, I. Horbachevsky Ternopil National Medical University, Ternopil, Ukraine

In: Lyme Borreliosis
Editors: Mykhaylo Andreychyn, Mykhaylo Korda, Maria Shkilna and Oleh Ivakhiv
ISBN: 979-8-89530-657-4

[7]DSc in Medicine, Associate Professor,
Department of Children's Diseases and Paediatric Surgery,
I. Horbachevsky Ternopil National Medical University, Ternopil, Ukraine
[8]PhD in Medicine, Deputy Director General for Research of Biological Factors,
State Institution "Ternopil Regional Centre for Disease Control and Prevention of the Ministry of Health of Ukraine", Ternopil, Ukraine
[9]PhD in Medicine, Dermatovenerologist at the Krasyliv Multidisciplinary Hospital, Krasyliv, Khmelnytskyi Oblast, Krasyliv, Khmelnytskyi Oblast, Ukraine
[10]PhD in Biology, Associate Professor, Department of Medical Biology, I. Horbachevsky Ternopil National Medical University, Ternopil, Ukraine
[11]PhD in Medicine, Associate Professor, Department of Microbiology,
Virology and Immunology, I. Horbachevsky Ternopil National Medical University, Ternopil, Ukraine
[12]PhD in Medicine, Assistant Professor,
Department of Infectious Diseases with Epidemiology, Dermatology and Venerology,
I. Horbachevsky Ternopil National Medical University, Ternopil, Ukraine
[13]DSc in Technology, Professor, Department of Medical Informatics,
I. Horbachevsky Ternopil National Medical University, Ternopil, Ukraine
[14]Honoured Health Worker of Ukraine, DSc in Medicine, Professor,
Department of General Surgery, I. Horbachevsky Ternopil National Medical University, Ternopil, Ukraine

Abstract

This chapter presents a comprehensive overview of the morphological and biological properties of *Borrelia* microorganisms, including the structural features of their genome, ecology, and geographic distribution. It also describes the characteristics of ixodid ticks, the primary reservoirs and vectors of *Borrelia*, highlighting their feeding behaviour, reproductive biology, and developmental cycle. The chapter provides detailed acarological studies conducted across various locations in the investigated region, including objective criteria for standardizing tick population metrics and infection rates with *Borrelia* and other microorganisms. It further analyses the awareness levels among at-risk groups and the general population regarding this pathogen. Epidemiological features of both erythema migrans and non-erythema migrans forms of Lyme borreliosis are discussed. Special attention is given to tick attack patterns, timing and techniques of tick removal in different locations of Western Ukraine, and organ/system involvement depending on the clinical form of the disease. The chapter also presents the development and application of a medical geographic information system (GIS) for collecting, storing, analysing, and visualizing data on the distribution of ticks and tick-borne infections in the western regions of Ukraine.

Keywords: Lyme borreliosis, etiology, epidemiology, ixodid ticks, erythema migrans and non-erythema migrans forms of Lyme borreliosis, medical geographic information system

1. Introduction

To date, Lyme borreliosis (LB), along with the natural reservoirs and transmission mechanisms of its causative agents in endemic areas of Ukraine, remains insufficiently studied. There is a pressing need to investigate the prevalence of pathogens in ticks, taking into account their genus and species, as well as transmission dynamics to humans based on professional activity and lifestyle. Particular attention should be given to assessing public awareness across various population groups, understanding the epidemiological features of both the erythema migrans and non-erythema migrans forms of LB, and developing a medical geographic information system to monitor the spread of the infection.

2. Etiology of Lyme Borreliosis

Lidia Romanyuk
and Kateryna Shtokailo

LB is caused by a heterogeneous population of various species of bacteria belonging to the genus Borrelia. The general list of borreliae includes not only bacteria pathogenic to humans, such as agents of LD, relapsing fever caused by ticks, and epidemic louse-borne typhus, but also a large group of spirochetes of this genus whose role in human pathology is either proven only in specific territories or not yet fully understood. Non-pathogenic microbes belong to this group, too.

2.1. Morphology of Borreliae

Borreliae form a distinct group of microorganisms classified within the class *Spirochaetes*, order *Spirochaetales*, family *Spirochaetaceae*, and genus *Borrelia*. They were named after the French microbiologist A. Borrel, who studied this type of spirochete at the beginning of the 20th century. Apart from the genus Borrelia, according to Bergey's classification, there are other genera of spirochetes: *Brevinema*, *Clevelandina*, *Cristispira*, *Diplocalix*, *Pillotina*, *Serpulina*, *Spirochaeta*, and *Treponema*. The genera Borrelia and Treponema include representatives pathogenic to humans [1, 2].

Borreliae are generally spiral-shaped microorganisms with a diameter of 0.2–0.5 μm and a length of 3–20 μm. They have 3–10 irregular turns that spiral either to the right or left, and 15–20 periplasmic flagella (Figures 1, 2) [3, 4].

The sizes of representatives of the genus *Borrelia* vary widely: the length varies from 8 μm (*B. coriaceae*) to 20–30 μm (*B. burgdorferi*), width – from 0.20 μm (*B. burgdorferi*) to 0.50 μm (*B. recurrentis*). They also differ in the density of coils, their regularity and the number of periplasmic fibres. They can change in different hosts and depend on the age of the culture (as a rule, cells are elongated in the stationary phase) and the composition of the nutrient medium. In terms of shape, Borrelia are a winding, left- or right-handed spiral. With dark field or phase contrast microscopy, the spiral shape of bacteria, which is characterized by significant instability, is well defined. At vital observation, their slow rotational movements are noted. Under an electronic microscope, structural elements of borrelia can be distinguished: a thick amorphous mucoid layer known as the "S-layer" is situated on the surface, followed by the cytoplasmic membrane, periplasm, endoflagellar complex, and protoplasmic cylinder (Figure 3) [5].

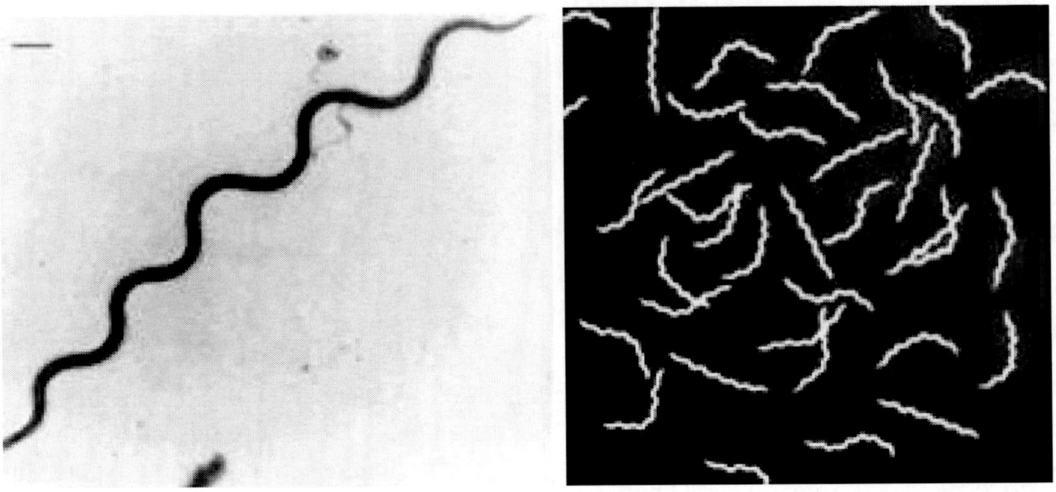

Figure 1. Morphological features of *Borrelia recurrentis* (left); Borrelia stained with silver nitrate in the dark field (right) [3].

The outer membrane contains proteins, lipids and carbohydrates, there is practically no lipopolysaccharide, but there are glycolipids that occupy half of all lipids. It also contains transmembrane-binding proteins of low density. This variant of the structure contributes to the survival of bacteria and the avoidance of the action of the immune system. Borrelia of the Argas tick-borne borreliosis group are able to produce lipoproteins that stimulate the formation of tumour necrosis factor-α (TNF-α), which, in turn, contributes to their recognition by vertebrate receptors [6].

In addition to the typical form of borrelia, other morphologically altered variants have been described, known as "forms of unbalanced growth." Some cells may elongate into cylindrical shapes, or adopt filamentous, looped forms, or spheroplasts, disc-shaped, or granular forms, and occasionally cysts surrounded by a protective mucoid envelope [7]. It is known that morphologically altered forms of borrelia, such as cystic and granular forms, retain the ability to reproduce and under certain conditions can revert to typical spiral-shaped forms while maintaining their pathogenic properties [8].

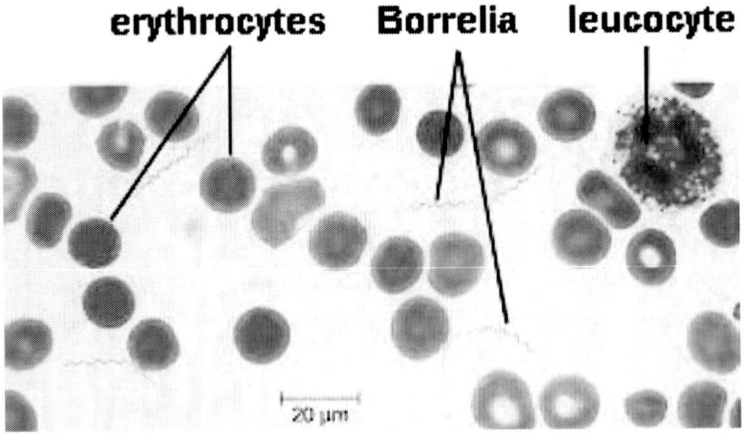

Figure 2. Borrelia in a smear from peripheral blood drop. Romanowsky-Giemsa staining [4].

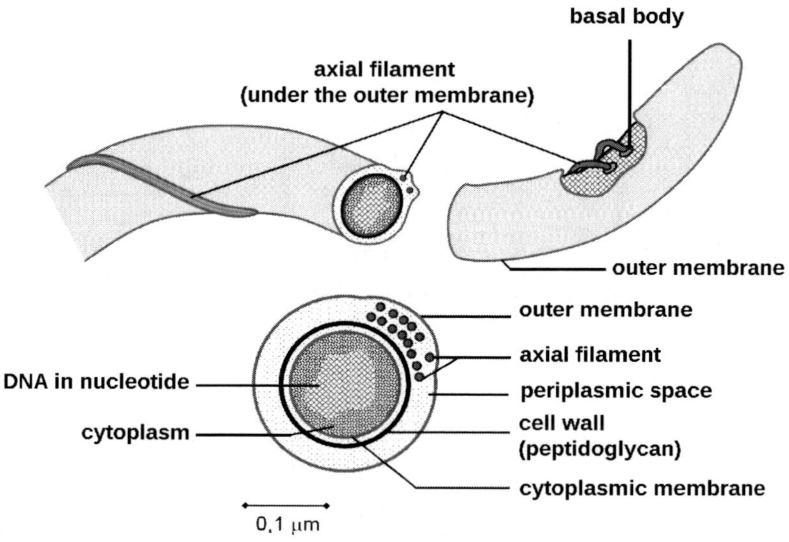

Figure 3. Borrelia structure [5].

Borrelia are sensitive to desiccation, as well as to hyper- and hypotonic conditions, the effects of various detergents, and temperatures above 40°C. They are easily inactivated by formalin, phenol, ethanol, and other disinfectants, as well as ultraviolet radiation. In the case of cultivation in a nutrient medium, they reproduce poorly at a temperature lower than 30–31°C and higher than 35°C, they are very sensitive to the pH level of the medium. Cultures that have already grown are able to maintain their viability for 30–45 days at a temperature of +4°C, they can be stored in glycerol for a long time at -70°C [6].

The causative agents of borreliosis are sensitive to tetracyclines, macrolides, cephalosporins of the III generation. They are characterized by low values of the minimum inhibitory concentration (MIC_{90}) –< 0.04 μg/mL and average values of the minimum bactericidal concentration –<1 μg/mL. However, they are resistant to high concentrations of fosfomycin, rifampicin, which can be used in the creation of selective media. It should also be noted that the sensitivity of Borrelia to different antibiotics varies significantly. In particular, the MIC of penicillin G for *B. afzelii* isolates is 10 times higher than for B. burgdorferi, B. bisettii, and 100 times higher than for *B. garinii* strains. The most sensitive to erythromycin are B. burgdorferi with MIC ≤0.15 μg/mL, ampicillin and mezlocillin are more active than penicillin G [9].

Other experiments studied *in vitro* and *in vivo* activity of some antibiotics for 10 human-derived *B. burgdorferi* isolates. These borrelia showed the greatest sensitivity to erythromycin, ceftriaxone and cefotaxime (MIC_{90} was 0.06, 0.06, 0.12 μg/mL, respectively). The activity of tetracycline, amoxicillin and lincomycin (MIC_{90} 0.50 μg/mL), imipenem and augmentin (MIC_{90} 0.25 μg/mL), oxacillin (MIC_{90} 1 μg/mL), ciprofloxacin (MIC_{90} 2 μg/mL), ofloxacin (MIC_{90} 4 μg/mL). Penicillin G, which is commonly used to treat patients with LB, showed MIC_{90} 4 μg/mL. With the exception of erythromycin, *in vitro* activity was consistent with *in vivo* activity. erythromycin was less active *in vivo*, and penicillin G showed weak activity both *in vitro* and *in vivo* [10].

Table 1. Some species of the Borrelia genus that are associated with ticks

Group	Pathogen species	
Argas tick borreliosis	*B. anserina*	*B. latyschewii*
	B. baltazardii	*B. mazzottii*
	B. brasiliensis	*B. merionesi*
	B. caucasica	*B. microti*
	B. coriaceae	*B. queenslandica*
	B. crocidurae	*B. parkeri*
	B. dugesii	*B. persica*
	B. duttonii	*B. recurrentis*
	B. graingeri	*B. tillae*
	B. harveyi	*B. turcica*
	B. hermsii	*B. turicatae*
	B. hispanica	*B. venezuelensis*
Ixodes tick borreliosis	*B. afzelii*	*B. japonica*
	B. americana	*B. lusitaniae*
	B. andersonii	*B. sinica*
	B. bavariensis	*B. spielmanii*
	B. bissettii	*B. tanukii*
	B. burgdorferi	*B. texasensis*
	B. californiensis	*B. theileri*
	B. carolinensis	*B. turdi*
	B. garinii	*B. valaisiana*
	B. kurtenbachii	
	B. lonestari	
	B. miyamotoi	

Further numerous randomized clinical trials demonstrated the effectiveness of antibiotic therapy in patients with EM, which is one of the clinical manifestations of LB [9]. According to the results of these studies, such antibacterial drugs as doxycycline, amoxicillin and cefuroxime, are characterized by equivalent effectiveness in the early stage of LB [11].

Doxycycline is one of the antibiotics most often used to treat patients with LB. It is also effective in the treatment of infections caused by other potential co-infectious agents (*A. phagocytophilum* and *B. miyamotoi*). Among the oral antibacterial agents that are commonly used in the management of LB, doxycycline is characterized by the best ability to penetrate the central nervous system (CNS) [11].

The optimal duration of therapy for EM was also studied in Europe, where most cases of LB are caused by the pathogen B. afzelii (as opposed to B. burgdorferi, which dominates in the United States of America). Research results by D. Stupica et al., [12] demonstrated that 10 days of doxycycline was as effective as 15 days.

In the USA, macrolides (azithromycin, clarithromycin, erythromycin) are not recommended for use as first-line therapy in early EM, because these drugs are less effective than amoxicillin [13, 14] and probably other first-line preparations. Resistance to macrolides has been identified in some strains of B. burgdorferi [14]. The use of macrolides is justified in patients who cannot take amoxicillin, doxycycline, and cefuroxime [9, 13].

In the papers by V. Preac-Mursic et al., it was shown that *B. burgdorferi* is very sensitive to erythromycin (MIC ≤ 0.15 μg/ml). Ampicillin and mezlocillin are more active than penicillin G. The authors recommended using tetracycline hydrochloride because of its low MIC *in vitro* and high extracellular and intracellular efficiency [5].

Table 2. Ecological and geographical characteristics of the *B. burgdorferi s. l.* species

Species, year of discovery	Area	Carriers of the diseases	Reservoir hosts
B. burgdorferi s. s., 1984	North America, Europe, North Africa, China, Taiwan	*Ixodes scapularis*, *I. ricinus*, *I. pacificus*	Small mammals, birds, reptiles
B. garinii, 1992	Europe, Russia, China, Japan, Canada, Korea, Mongolia, North Africa	*I. ricinus*, *I. persulcatus*, *I. nipponensis*, *I. trianguliceps*	Birds, hedgehogs, small mammals
B. afzelii, 1993	Europe, Russia, China, Japan, Korea, Mongolia	*I. ricinus*, *I. persulcatus*, *I. granulatus* and others	Small mammals, birds
B. japonica, 1993	Japan	*I. ovatus*	Small mammals
B. lusitaniae, 1997	Europe, North Africa, Turkey	*I. ricinus*, *I. hexagonus*, *I. uriae*	Small mammals, birds, reptiles
B. valaisiana, 1997	Europe, China, Japan, Korea	*I. ricinus*, *I. hexagonus*, *I. persulcatus*, *I. nipponensis*	Birds, reptiles
B. bussetti, 2007	Central Europe, North Africa	*I. scapularis*, *I. ricinus*, *I. pacificus*	Small mammals, reptiles
B. spielmanii	Central Europe, Hungary, Ukraine	*I. ricinus*, *I. hexagonus*	Hedgehogs
B. bavariensis	Central and Eastern Europe, Russia, Central Asia, China, Japan	*I. ricinus*, *I. persulcatus*, *I. trianguliceps*	Small mammals
B. kurtenbachii	North America, Europe	*I. pacificus*, *I. scapularis*	Small mammals
B. miyamotoi, 1995	Japan, Europe, Russia, North America	*I. persulcatus*, *I. ricinus*, *I. pacificus*, *I. scapularis*	Small mammals

Many borrelia, such as *B. recurrentis*, *B. duttoni*, *B. hermsii*, etc, cause infectious diseases in humans, for example, tick-borne relapsing fever. One of the Borrelia, *B. burgdorferi*, is named after the American entomologist and microbiologist Willy (Wilhelm) Burgdorfer, who together with A. Barbour in 1982 isolated these microorganisms from a patient with LB. In 1984, R. Johnson identified the spirochete isolated by W. Burgdorfer, and showed that it is a previously unknown species of the genus Borrelia, and named it *B. burgdorferi sp. nov.*, thus establishing the aaetiology of a long-known disease [15]. Further study of many Borrelia isolates obtained from ticks and from patients at different points of the nosological range of this infection demonstrated that there are significant intraspecies differences in the group of Borrelia belonging to the same species.

Currently, several tens of Borrelia species are distinguished, which are grouped into 3 unsystematized groups: 1) LB group (more than 50 bacteria), whose representatives, due to their high phenotypic and genotypic similarity, form a complex *B. burgdorferi sensu lato* (*s. l.*); 2) a group of tick-borne relapsing fever (TBRF) (*B. duttoni*, *B. hermsii*, *B. parkeri*, *B. turicatae*, etc.), which are mainly transmitted by argas ticks, but this group also includes *B. recurrentis*, which is carried by lice Pediculus vestimenti (louse relapsing typhus), and 3 species of microorganisms detected in Ixodes ticks (*B. miyamotoi*, *B. lonestari*, *B. theileri*) (Table 1); 3) a group of Borrelia related to reptiles, that has recently been described, including B. turcica and a number of unspecified species [16-18].

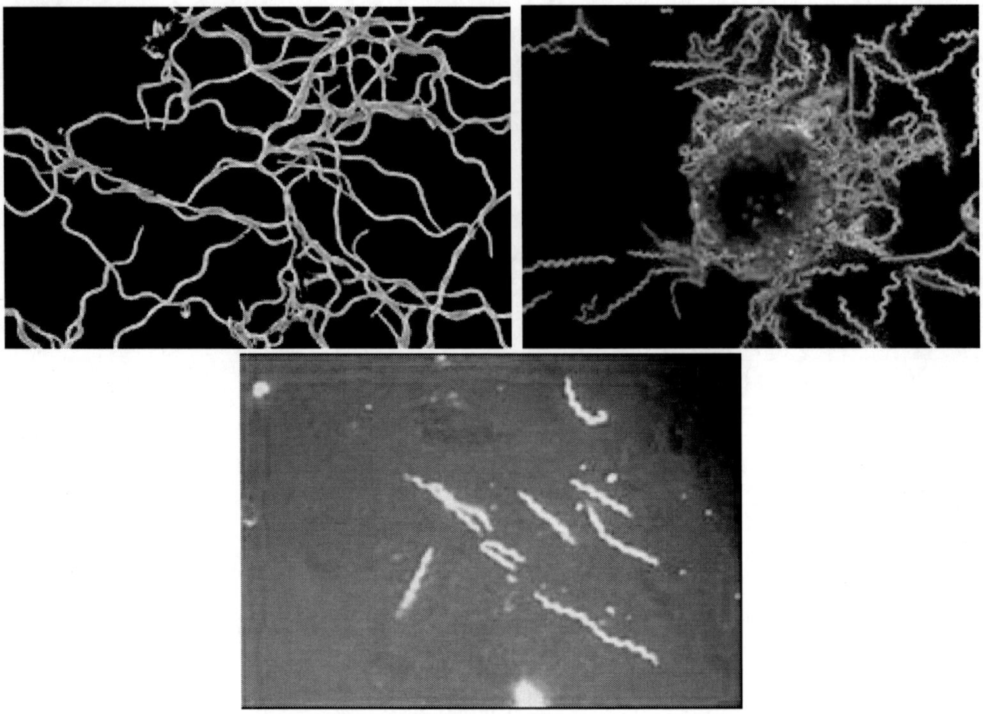

Figure 4. Morphological features of *B. burgdorferi* [33].

All known species of the genus Borrelia are morphologically very similar, so the taxonomy of Borrelia at the level of species is often refined, as a result, the list of species is supplemented with new ones. Now, based on differences in DNA nucleotide sequences within the *B. burgdorferi s. l.* complex, at least 19 species are distinguished, 9 of them were described after 2005. All of them are unevenly distributed within the nosological area of LB (Table 2).

Not all borrelia of this complex are pathogenic for humans. In Europe, the pathogenicity of 5 genospecies has been proven – *B. burgdorferi sensu stricto* (*s. s.*), *B. garinii*, *B. afzelii*, *B. spielmanii* and *B. bavariensis* [19–21]. A number of scientists note that in the western regions of Ukraine there are 5 species of Borrelia that are pathogenic for humans: *B. burgdorferi s. s.*, *B. garinii*, *B. afzelii*, *B. lusitaniae* and *B. valaisiana* [22]. Another group of scientists considers *B. burgdorferi s. s.*, *B. garinii*, *B. afzelii*, *B. valaisiana* and *B. spielmanii* to be pathogenic in Ukraine [23]. The prevalence of these genospecies in different geographical regions of the world is also not the same as that of other representatives of the *B. burgdorferi s. l.* complex. Variability in the composition of surface proteins, especially OspA and OspC, is observed even in the same Borrelia genospecies. Their greatest heterogeneity is found in *B. garinii* (for OspC – 13 variants, for OspA – 7 variants) and *B. afzelii* (for OspC – 8, for OspA – 2 variants). *B. burgdorferi s. s.* differs from others in the relative constancy of the spectrum of surface proteins, and the most conservative in this regard are North American strains [24].

It was established that *B. spielmanii*, which was discovered in Germany, Hungary and Slovenia, is the etiological agent of EM [25]. *B. miyamotoi*, which belongs to the group of causative agents of tick-borne relapsing fever [26], was first isolated in Japan in 1995 from ticks of the *I. persulcatus* species, as well as from Apodemus argenteus mice [27]. Subsequently, this Borrelia species was found in ticks of the *I. ricinus* species in a number of

European countries [20, 28, 29]. Currently, 3 types of *B. miyamotoi* are distinguished: Asian or Siberian (transmitted mainly by ticks of the *I. persulcatus* species), European (by ticks of the *I. ricinus* species) and American (by ticks of the *I. scapularis* and *I. pacificus species*) [30–32].

B. burgdorferi are mobile spiral-shaped microaerophile bacteria that have an inner and outer membrane, a cell wall with a tendency to bend. They are stained with aniline dyes. Cells of different Borrelia species vary in length, diameter, density of coils, their regularity, and the number of periplasmic fibrils. As a rule, the diameter of the cell is up to 1 μm, the length is 10–25 μm. *B. burgdorferi* is not classified as a gram-positive or gram-negative bacterium, although it is weakly negative by Gram staining and has some features of gram-negative bacteria, but at the same time there are differences (Figure 4) [33].

In the composition of the outer membrane of *B. burgdorferi*, lipopolysaccharides are not detected. In addition, the outer membrane of *Borrelia spp.* is characterized by greater lability, has a lower density of transport proteins and easily dissolves in weak solutions of surface-active substances. Such outer membrane proteins as Osp (outer surface protein), in particular OspA and OspB, encoded by linear plasmids lp 54 and OspC, which, in turn, is encoded by the circular plasmid sr 26 are the most studied [6].

Borrelia's S-layer is extremely unstable, it is very easily separated from the outer membrane and is often absent. The mucoid layer is sometimes an obstacle for electron microscopy due to its very intense staining and shading of the microbial cell structures [34].

The next structural element is a very flexible bilipid cytoplasmic membrane, between the layers of which there is an endoflagellar complex, which snake-like intertwines with the protoplasmic cylinder along the length of the microorganism. Each endoflagellar complex consists of flagellar filaments, a flagellar hook, and a main disk. It is the shortening of the threads linked together and attached to the ends of the microbial cell, as well as their spiral-like arrangement along the entire length, that provide rotational and translational movements of Borrelia [34].

The number of endoflagella in different isolates of Borrelia is variable – from 3 to 20, which depends on the physiological state of the bacterial cell and the cultivation conditions (pH of the medium, nutritional supplements, etc.) [34].

The protoplasmic cylinder is located behind the inner layer of the cytoplasmic membrane and contains the nucleoid, ribosomes, DNA-associated molecules and other cellular components. Sometimes on the surface of Borrelia, protrusions are visible, which can be of two types. First, protrusions of the outer layer of the cytoplasmic membrane are often formed closer to the terminal areas of Borrelia on its lateral surfaces. Such changes are characteristic of dying cells. Similar protrusions are also often observed in Borrelia culture *in vitro* as a result of their long-term incubation. Secondly, they are formed as spherical bulges at the ends of Borrelia and are formed by the actual cytoplasmic membrane and protoplasm, which contains plasmid DNA [34].

Borrelia are chemoorganotrophs, the main source of energy for which is glucose, and the end product of metabolism is lactic acid. Microorganisms can also use glycerol, fructose, and maltose as an alternative source of carbon. In addition, Borrelia are able to utilize N-acetylglucosamine and, accordingly, chitin, which allows them to exist for a long time in the tick's digestive tract between its feeding cycles. Like many other parasitic microorganisms, Borrelia have lost the genes for a number of enzymes of the main metabolism, namely: Krebs cycle, oxidative phosphorylation, electron transport chain, fatty acid oxidation, synthesis of many enzymes, and, accordingly, have a low level of metabolism, which causes low growth rates (generation time) and high demand for nutrient medium [35].

Many years of attempts to obtain cultures *in vitro* have led to the creation of complex cell-free media for cultivation. These bacteria belong to microaerophiles. This fact is taken into account during their cultivation. Today, liquid media enriched with amino acids, other nutrients, and vitamins are used for the cultivation of borrelia. Some Borrelia, in particular *B. hermsii*, grow on Kelly medium, to which N-acetyl-glucosamine is added, that is necessary for the construction of the cell wall and as a source of energy. Later, the Barbour-Stoenner-Kelly (BSK) medium and its selective variant, BSK II were created, which differ from the previous one by adding to their composition bovine albumin, rabbit serum, agarose, yeast extract, gelatin (to provide collagen-like viscosity), as well as other components with an optimal pH of 7.6. At a cultivation temperature of 32–34°C, such an environment can primarily support the growth of *B. burgdorferi* and *B. hermsii*. The generation time of cells is 8–24 and even 24–48 h, so they grow long enough, although the concentration of Borrelia adapted to the environment can reach 10^8 cells per 1 ml. The normal pink colour of the medium changes to yellow during the growth of Borrelia. Sharp yellowing and turbidity usually indicate contamination of the environment with other bacteria, and redness indicates the presence of mould fungi. However, some Borrelia species (in particular, *B. miyamotoi*) could not be cultured on BSK II medium. In 2014, there were reports of modifications of BSK medium and modified Kelly-Pettenkofer (MKP) medium capable of supporting growth of *B. miyamotoi* [36]. The growth of microorganisms can be detected after 2–3 weeks of incubation in the dark at a temperature of 34-37°C using dark field microscopy, then confirmed by immunofluorescence microscopy. Some Borrelia species can be cultivated in tick cell cultures [6].

2.2. Peculiarities of the Organization of the Borrelia Genome

The size of the chromosome in different Borrelia ranges from 0.91 to 4.3 Mb. The low content of guanine and cytosine, along with low DNA homology, distinguishes the genus Borrelia from other spirochetes. The genome of microorganisms of the genus Borrelia consists of one linear chromosome with covalently closed ends 910,725 nucleotide pairs long and numerous plasmids, both circular and linear, ranging in size from 5 to 200 thousand nucleotide pairs. So far, whole-genome sequences have been obtained for 7 species of *B. burgdorferi s. l.* and 11 – groups of ixodid tick-borne borreliosis. The chromosome of the typical strain of *B. burgdorferi* B31 consists of 860 genes, 797 of which encode proteins, and 26 pseudogenes. Chromosomes, which carry most of the genes of their own apparatus, are relatively stable in terms of composition and location of genes within the genus, while the genetic information localized in plasmids is significantly more variable. The genome of *B. burgdorferi B31* includes 12 linear and 9 circular plasmids, but their number varies depending on the species and may decrease during cultivation. The functions of most plasmid genes have not yet been studied, but it is known that some of them cause the synthesis of various lipoproteins, porins, decorin-fixing proteins, etc. [6].

The organization of Borrelia rRNA genes deserves special attention. Borrelia complex *B. burgdorferi s. l.* have one copy of 16S rRNA and 2 copies of each of the 23S rRNA and 5S rRNA genes, and all genes are located inside a chromosome section about 10,000 nucleotide pairs long. Individual copies of 23S-5S repeats are separated by spacers about 180 nucleotide pairs long. Within the 23S-5S repeat, the 23S and 5S rRNA sequences are separated by spacers 22 nucleotide pairs long. There is only one copy of each rRNA gene in the Borrelia genome of the Ixodes tick-borne borreliosis group [37].

The absence of genes encoding the synthesis of amino acids, fatty acids, cofactors and nucleotides in Borrelia explains such high requirements for the conditions of their cultivation with the use of serum supplements. In addition, since Borrelia are chemoorganotrophic anaerobes, they must obtain energy for ATP synthesis from the phosphorylation substrate, which is present only in the cytoplasm of other cells, therefore, Borrelia do not have genes encoding the respiratory chain of phosphorylation. Pyruvate, which is one of the most important intermediate links of metabolism and allows the cell to use energy for anabolism, is probably formed from glucose in the process of glycolysis. Borrelia also lack other enzymes required for the tricarboxylic acid cycle and phosphorylation. Thus, the ability of their own metabolic components is so limited that for their existence they must have a host organism that guarantees a supply of ready-made nutrients. In other words, Borrelia demonstrate a clearly expressed phenomenon of parasitism, which arose at the genetic level [38].

The presence of extrachromosomal coding of certain features is not an exclusive property of Borrelia. The same is observed in some other representatives of prokaryotes (for example, gram-negative microorganisms). However, the fact that Borrelia can have quite a large number of linear and circular plasmids distinguishes them from other microorganisms. It should be noted that even individual isolates of the same Borrelia genotype can have pronounced differences in plasmids in terms of their number (from 5 to 20) and size (from 9 to 70 kb). Another feature of Borrelia is that plasmids are detected mainly during the initial isolation of strains in culture. Subsequent transplants lead to a decrease in their number and even their complete loss. This changes the antigenic profile of the pathogen, up to the complete loss of invasiveness. This circumstance allows us to assume that plasmids contain information about specific proteins (antigens) that determine the pathogenicity of a microorganism [39].

Only 16 of the decoded DNA sequences of the chromosome and plasmids of the reference strain *B. burgdorferi B31* can be compared with known Borrelia proteins, including: various lipoproteins (OspA-D), porins, decorin-fixing proteins, enzymes for porin synthesis, various antigens. Many membrane lipoproteins of Borrelia are immunogenic, and therefore have great importance in the formation of an immune response from the host's body.

The circulation of pathogens in a natural environment is accompanied by dynamic changes in the system "microorganism –microorganism –environment." In view of this, Borrelia should have such adaptation mechanisms that would allow them to adapt to biochemical features of the new host in a very short time. and ensure the possibility of surviving in this organism. In many ways, these mechanisms are associated with dynamic changes at the level of the functioning of the genome (regulation of gene expression) of the microorganism, which are manifested by the transformation of the composition of the surface proteins of Borrelia when they are found in different hosts, which ultimately leads to a significant change in the initially genetic, and then their antigenic profile. Thus, the composition of surface proteins in Borrelia is dynamic and largely determined by the spatial and temporal conditions of their existence [2].

The study of the protein composition of Borrelia using electrophoresis made it possible to identify more than 30 proteins with different electrophoretic mobility, that is, molecular weight. Thus, the protein spectrum of Borrelia is highly variable and different not only among microbes of different genotypes, but also among isolates of the same genotype. However, it should be noted that, regardless of species affiliation, Borrelia contain 2 main protein components with a molecular weight of 41 kDa (p41, or flagellin) and 60 kDa (HSP60). Flagellin has separate specific areas that are characteristic of certain Borrelia species. The HSP60 protein is not specific, but is present in many species of bacteria.

In Borrelia, the mechanisms of temperature-dependent regulation of gene expression, which carry information about 2 proteins of the outer membrane – OspA and OspC, have been studied in the most detail. When the microorganism penetrates the body of the mite (the temperature is lower than +24 °C), the genes responsible for the synthesis of surface proteins are at different levels of activity. this is reflected in the protein composition of the cell's outer membrane, where the OspA protein is always present, and the OspC protein is extremely rare. An increase in the temperature of the environment or entry of Borrelia into the body of a warm-blooded animal or human leads to the activation of the gene responsible for the synthesis of OspC, and the corresponding protein is detected on the membrane of Borrelia. Regarding OspA, an inverse relationship is observed. this can explain the weak immune response of the human body to OspA and the distinct reaction to the membrane protein OspC. Some other proteins, such as EppA, are detected only when Borrelia are present in the human body, while they are absent in cultured Borrelia. Such a vivid surface-protein variability of the microorganism can be caused both by the defect of some organic substances under the conditions of "depleted nutrient medium," and by the interaction of Borrelia with endothelial cells or the effects of the complement system factors [2].

Protein profile of North American strains of *B. burgdorferi s. s.* is homogenous in terms of OspA and OspC (the latter is found much less often), and is more variable by OspB presence. Thus, 2 membrane proteins OspA and OspC are considered by many researchers as the main candidates for the creation of recombinant vaccines against LB.

To date, some other Borrelia membrane antigens have been established and are quite well studied: p83/100, Oms66 (p66), BmpA (p39), HSP60 (p60), p18, OspD, OspE, OspF. The genetic information of most of them is located in plasmids, therefore the loss of individual plasmids, for example, in the case of long-term persistence of Borrelia in the human body, necessarily leads to a change in the structure of surface antigens, and therefore to a change in the immune response [37].

2.3. Ecological Features of Borrelia

Borrelia are the only spirochetes that require arthropod vectors (mostly ticks) for maintenance and transmission. The necessity for reproduction both in the bodies of cold-blooded hosts (ticks) and warm-blooded hosts (birds, mammals) has led to the evolutionary development of a range of ecological adaptations that are absent in other spirochetes.

Infected ticks transmit Borrelia to animals through saliva during feeding, while uninfected vectors acquire the pathogens from animals whose blood circulates Borrelia. Populations of vertebrate animals acting as reservoir hosts for Borrelia encompass around 100 species of small mammals (such as field mice, rats, squirrels, rabbits, hedgehogs, etc.) and over 170 species of birds (mostly ground-nesting birds). Despite the significant number of warm-blooded hosts, only some of them can effectively support the reproduction and survival of Borrelia, as well as facilitate their transmission to ticks during feeding [40].

Susceptibility of hosts to Borrelia is mostly determined by the presence in their blood of specific proteins-components of the complement system, which have bactericidal activity.

Since the activation of the complement system of the vertebrate host can significantly affect the circulation of Borrelia in natural habitats, it can determine the circle of potential hosts. It was proved that *B. afzelii* and 4 serotypes of *B. garinii* are sensitive to blood serum of birds, while other serotypes of *B. garinii* are resistant to it, but die under the influence of rodent serum, which contains complement components that are activated upon exposure to pathogen. However, such associations with vectors, although experimentally proven, cannot be considered as indisputable, since in some cases it is possible to detect Borrelia in "atypical" hosts. Migratory birds probably play a more significant role in the spread of Borrelia, because they are not only reservoir hosts for species such as *B. burgdorferi*, *B. garinii*, *B. valaisiana*, but also carry infected ticks over long distances. It has been proven that in the body of some species of birds, a latent infection can be activated when their immune system is weakened, which explains the spread of spirochetes in the case when the flight time of birds exceeds the time of tick feeding [41].

Borrelia of *B. burgdorferi s. l.* complex are used as carriers of hard ticks of the genus Ixodes, while the main role is played by 4 types of ticks: *I. ricinus*: *I. ricinus L* (Europe), *I. persulcatus Schulze* (Asia), *I. scapularis Say* (Atlantic coast of the USA) and *I. pacificus Cooley & Kohls* (Pacific coast of the USA). It has been demonstrated that Ixodes pavlovskyi (also known as Ixodes persulcatus or the taiga tick), found in the Altai and Far East regions, are competent vectors of Borrelia and may play a significant role in maintaining the population of Borrelia within their range [42].

Due to the mobility of ticks, the spread of pathogens that they carry is primarily related to the movement of reservoir hosts (pathogens can be found both in the tissues of the host and in the ticks that feed on them). To understand the processes of microorganism spread, particularly Borrelia, it is essential to consider the contribution of various pathways of transmission between components of the parasitic system (such as transmissive, transstadial, etc.). Infection of vertebrates with Borrelia occurs through the tick's saliva during its feeding. Since the tick's intestines are the main environment for the reproduction of bacteria, it takes a certain amount of time for them to move to the salivary glands and then enter the blood. In the experiment, it was determined that for the effective transmission of Borrelia by ticks of the *I. scapularis* and *I. pacificus species*, it takes time for them to feed, which is more than 36 hours. For *I. persulcatus*, this time is much shorter and is less than 24 h, and the proportion of hungry ticks with generalized infection and, accordingly, the number of Borrelia in the salivary glands is much higher than in *I. scapularis* [43].

Infecting an uninfected tick occurs when blood containing Borrelia is absorbed, that is, such transmission is possible only in the presence of a systemic infection in the host's body, accompanied by bacteraemia. However, it has been proven that ticks can be infected by sharing food: infected and uninfected ticks from the same inflammation without systemic infection of the host. However, the role of this transmission route has not been determined to date [44].

Transovarial transmission of *B. burgdorferi s. l.* (from infected female to eggs) has been shown in a number of experiments, but it is a rare phenomenon and, apparently, does not play a major role in maintaining the Borrelia population. But this type of transmission is probably important for Borrelia of the tick-borne relapsing fever group, in particular *B. miyamotoi*. Unlike transovarial transmission, transstadial transmission, for example to subsequent life stages of the tick during molting, is effective and allows Borrelia to persist in the tick throughout its lifespan [45, 46].

Mature ticks feed mainly on large wild animals, and nymphs and larvae feed on small ones. After infection of non-immune animals, mainly small rodents, the causative agent multiplies in their body. Since the infection of susceptible animals does not occur simultaneously, but during the entire seasonal period of tick activity, they play a significant role as reservoirs of infection in nature. Data about the importance of vertebrates in the circulation of the pathogen expands if we take into account the longer storage of Borrelia in the body of hibernating animals (during hibernation) [47].

In settled areas with developed animal husbandry, domestic animals (large and small ruminants) are the predominant hosts for the adult forms of ticks. However, their significance as reservoirs of infection is low because there are practically no LB pathogens in the peripheral blood of these animals [45].

Humans are infected in natural and anthropogenic foci of LB [48]. The infection is transmitted by a transmissible way during a tick bite, as well as when its faeces fall on the skin, followed by their rubbing when scratching [49]. If the tick breaks during its improper removal, the causative agent may enter the wound [50]. Infection is possible when consuming raw goat or cow's milk of infected animals [51]. Thus, in terms of morbidity, borreliosis ranks first among tick-borne infections and one of the leading places among all naturally occurring diseases. In recent decades, incidence rates have increased in all countries where they are common.

3. Source of Pathogen, Transmission Mechanism, Susceptible Organism

Mariia Shkilna
and Oleh Ivakhiv

The sources and reservoirs of LB pathogens are rodents, wild and domestic animals, and certain bird species [52–55]. Borrelia are transmitted to humans during the feeding of ixodid ticks, which not only act as vectors but also serve as primary reservoirs since they maintain Borrelia throughout their entire lives and can transmit them transovarially to their offspring [56–58]. Ticks can acquire Borrelia at any stage of their development through transstadial, transovarial, and transmissive transmission, and they can maintain the pathogens for over 4 years through seasonal changes [59].

It has been established that a single tick of the *I. ricinus* species can concurrently harbour up to 7 pathogens of viral and bacterial origin. Coinfection often leads to atypical disease progression, complicates diagnosis, and consequently treatment [60–63]. Literature reports indicate that tick infection rates with multiple pathogens simultaneously range from 3.2% to 45.0% across different European countries [64–66].

Ticks commonly attach in areas with thin skin and intense blood supply such as the neck, chest, armpits, and folds, making these locations prone to infestation [67]. Initially, ticks transmit borreliae located in their salivary glands. If borreliae are only present in the tick's gut, transmission occurs during the second feeding phase (1–2 days after attachment) [68]. Thus, early tick removal prevents infection in many cases, a crucial consideration in decisions regarding prophylactic treatment. There is potential for transmission via tick faeces if they enter micro-cracks in the skin or come into contact with mucous membranes through rubbing [69]. Cases of mechanical transmission of borreliae occur when ticks are inadvertently crushed during removal from animals (dogs, cats), and their gut contents enter microskin abrasions or the conjunctiva of the eyes [70]. The alimentary route of infection (by consuming raw goat milk or dairy products without prior thermal processing) has not been definitively proven [71, 72]. Borreliae can also be transmitted transplacentally from mother to foetus during pregnancy [73, 74].

The seasonality of Lyme disease correlates with the spring-summer period due to tick activity and human presence in forested park areas and woodland regions [75]. Natural foci of tick-borne borrelioses in Europe, including Ukraine, are typically found in forested landscapes. The majority of Ukraine is endemic for this zoonosis, with the highest incidence of LB recorded in western regions [76].

Currently, 1811 settlements in Ukraine are identified as affected by ixodid borrelioses. However, the lack of adequate laboratory infrastructure in public health practice prevents a proper assessment of the epidemiological situation regarding LB in the country [77]. The susceptibility to LB is high, affecting predominantly individuals of active working age, especially those in occupational risk groups such as forestry workers, shepherds, and hunters.

Literature data indicate that the overall infection rate of ticks with spirochetes of the *B. burgdorferi s. l.* complex in North America (USA and Canada) ranges from 27.0% to 47.0% [78], and in Europe (Poland, Czech Republic, and Serbia) from 5.6% to 25.1% [79, 80]. Genotyping of *B. garinii* among infected ticks revealed prevalence rates ranging from 1.4% to 64.0%, *B. burgdorferi s. s.* from 2.2% to 61.4%, *B. afzelii* from 7.0% to 22.9%, *B. luisitaniae* up to 11.3%, and *B. valaisiana* up to 1.4% [81, 82].

In Ukraine, spontaneous infection rates of ticks collected from the environment with spirochetes of the *B. burgdorferi s. l.* complex range from 7.0% to 25.0%, with an average of 17.2% [70]. However, information regarding tick infection rates collected from humans in Ukraine, including in Ternopil region, is not readily available in the literature.

Multiple genovariants of borreliae have been diagnosed in 69.4–70.0% of infected ticks from the environment in the USA and Southern Canada, 24.7% in Poland, and 1.5–19.0% in the Ural and Northwest Russia [83, 84].

It has been established that *B. burgdorferi s. s.* is associated predominantly with joint involvement, *B. garinii* and *B. bavariensis* with the development of meningoradiculitis, and *B. afzelii* with skin manifestations [58, 85–89].

4. Ticks as the Main Reservoir and Vectors of Borrelia spp.

Larysa Fedoniuk
Stepan Podobivskyi
and Mariia Shkilna

Ticks are vectors or reservoirs for many zoonotic diseases. These diseases include Lyme borreliosis, tularaemia, tick-borne viral and spring-summer encephalitis, Crimean-Congo haemorrhagic fever, certain rickettsioses, granulocytic anaplasmosis, babesiosis, ehrlichiosis, Q fever, and others. Tick-borne infectious diseases are naturally focal, and their foci are often interconnected. Pathogens are integral to complex parasitic systems. Diseases can be caused simultaneously by several pathogens. In recent years, the epidemiological situation has been complicated by an increase in tick attacks in urban areas. The formation of urban foci is a recognized problem.

4.1. History of Tick Research

The sheep tick of the species Ixodes ricinus was first described in 18th century (Linnaeus, 1758). However, Europe became interested in it only in the 30s and 50s of the 20th century. So, in the UK, it began to be studied in connection with the breeding of sheep on mountain farms. A number of scientists studied the issue of the distribution of Ixodes ticks on the territory of Eurasia. The spread of ticks in Europe was studied by G. Karbowiak [90], and one of the foundational works on ticks in Central Europe is the monograph by a team of Austrian researchers [9]. Much later, the species composition of ticks in the Palaearctic was compiled by Agustín Estrada-Peña and co-authors [92].

Jose de la Fuente and his co-authors [95] made an important contribution to the study of the biology and medical significance of ticks. In his monograph, he focused on the distribution, life cycles, trophic relationships and importance of Ixodes ticks as carriers of pathogens of many human infectious diseases.

Until now, many researchers have focused their attention on ticks from the position of considering them as the main reservoirs and carriers of pathogens of numerous infections that they transmit to humans and animals, and the consequences of these ailments in the absence of adequate prevention and treatment. At the same time, the impact of environmental changes on ticks is being studied less and less.

Ixodes ticks mostly belong to species from forest biocenoses, as well as meadow-steppe and even steppe biocenoses. They are everywhere, where there are suitable conditions.

James E. Keirans [96] was one of the acarologists who studied the worldwide distribution of Ixodes ticks and summarized the already available information on many genera of ticks. According to his data, ticks of the genus *Dermacentor Koch.*, which includes about 30 species in the world fauna, belong to the family *Ixodidae*, which unites 9 genera distributed on all continents in most natural and geographical zones [91]. It is assumed that the *Ixodidae* family includes 14 genera [96]. All these genera are combined into 4 subfamilies: *Ambliomminae Banks*, *Haemaphisalinae Banks*, *Hyalomminae Schulze* and *Rhipiciphalinae Banks* [97]. The total number of Ixodes ticks in the world fauna can reach about 644 species [92] and even 700 species [97].

On the territory of Ukraine, ticks were studied in the most detail by Ye. M. Yemchuk [98]. In Ukraine, the author singles out 3 main ecological and faunal complexes: forest, steppe and Crimean mountain-forest. The territory of Western Ukraine lies within several landscape-geographical zones: Eastern Carpathians, Carpathians, Polissia and forest-steppe. Polissia is represented by Small Polissia, which includes Volyn and Rivne regions. The forest-steppe represents Western Podilia, namely Ternopil, partly Lviv and Khmelnytskyi regions. The Eastern Carpathians cover part of Lviv, Chernivtsi, Ivano-Frankivsk, and Transcarpathian regions. The Carpathian and Transcarpathian lowlands constitute a special landscape zone.

Ye. M. Yemchuk [98] states that there are possibly 26 species of Ixodes ticks of 6 genera in Ukraine: *Ixodes L.*, *Haemophysalis Koch.*, *Boophilus Cur.*, *Dermacentor Koch.*, *Rhipicephalus Koch.*, *Hyalomma Koch.*

About 15 species of Ixodes ticks of 5 genera are common in the western regions of Ukraine [99]. *I. ricinus*, *D. reticulatus*, *D. marginatus* are the species that are widely found in Polissia. *I. crenulatus*, *I. trianguliceps*, *I. vespertilionis* occur much less often. The number of *D. marginatus* increases from north to south. In the Eastern Carpathians, the same species as in Polissia are common, but the *I. pospelovae* species is still present here. The southwestern slopes of the Carpathians and the Transcarpathian lowland are characterized by the richest species diversity and abundance. In the highlands, mainly *I. ricinus*, *I. trianguliceps*, and *I. pospelovae* are common. Species of the genus *Dermacentor* are distributed in small numbers mainly in the foothills of the southern and northern slopes of the Carpathians. The forest-steppe is rich in species of both forest and steppe biocenoses. *I. ricinus*, *I. trianguliceps*, *I. crenulatus*, *I. lividus*, *D. marginatus* are the species that are often found here. The following species enter the forest-steppe zone from the steppe: *I. laguri laguri*, *H. punctata*, *H. sulcata*, *H. otophila*, *R. rossicus*, *H. scupense*, *H. plumbeum plumbeum*.

4.2. General Characteristics of Ticks of the Genus *Ixodes Latr*

Ixodes ticks have a flattened body in the dorsoventral direction and are composed of two main parts – the gnathosoma and the idiosoma. The proboscis, or gnathosoma, results from the fusion of the chelicerae and pedipalps. Ticks also possess palps and a hypostome, the primary function of which is blood feeding. The proboscis is covered with chitinous backward-facing hooks that expand to help the tick grip onto the host during feeding.

The body of ticks is variably chitinized and covered with a dorsal shield. In females, nymphs, and larvae, it covers only a third of the body and can take various shapes such as heart-shaped, round, rhomboid, and others. In males, the entire body is covered with a dorsal shield, which forms festoons at the rear. Species of the genus Ixodes lack eyes. In addition to the dorsal shield, males also have ventral shields, which restrict abdominal expansion and allow ticks to consume only minimal amounts of blood. Males of the genus Ixodes have 7 abdominal shields, and on the abdomen, closer to the front edge, males and females have a genital opening in the form of a transverse slit. Larvae and nymphs do not have a genital opening. Closer to the rear end of the abdomen there is the anus surrounded by a groove. In ticks of the genus Ixodes, the groove is closed above the genital opening, in ticks of all other genera – below it. On each side of the abdomen in males, females and nymphs there is spiracles, or peritreme. The chitin ring, which borders the peritreme, can have an oval, round or retort-like shape. There are no peritremes in the larvae.

Adult ticks and their nymphs have 4 pairs of legs, while larvae have 3. The limb is six-jointed and has a coxa, trochanter, femur, tibia and tarsus. Coxae, as a rule, have 2 spines: external and internal. Ticks of the genus Ixodes have solid spines, ticks of all other genera have bifurcated spines. The foot of ticks has suckers and 2 claws.

The colour of the body of ticks is yellowish or brownish and changes depending on the degree of their saturation with the blood of the host. Larvae and nymphs are mostly white or dirty grey. The intestine is visible through their coverings.

The sizes of hungry ticks range from 1.5 to 4.2 mm, their nymphs – from 0.8 to 1.5-2.0 mm, larvae – from 0.4 to 0.8 mm.

As already mentioned, out of 26 species of Ixodes ticks common on the territory of Ukraine, only 15 are found in its western regions. Of these, only 6-7 species are capable of attacking humans and possibly transmitting pathogens of infectious diseases to them.

The common or dog tick (*Ixodes ricinus Latr.*) belongs to the European-Mediterranean fauna and is the most common species not only in Ukraine, but also in Europe, the European part of Russia, the Caucasus, Turkey, and North Africa. Data on the distribution of this tick species are shown in Figure 5, where the current known distribution of the species I. ricinus in Europe is at the "regional" administrative level (NUTS3) as of January 2019. In Ukraine, the dog tick is widespread in all western, northern and central regions. The biotopes in which it is most often found are sparse mixed and coniferous forests, forest edges, protective forest strips, parks, squares, gardens. often ticks found on the sides of roads and paths where people and animals pass.

The dog tick is active from the end of March until November. the frequency of its detection decreases significantly in July and August, when the air temperature is 28–30°C and more, and the humidity drops to 80% and less.

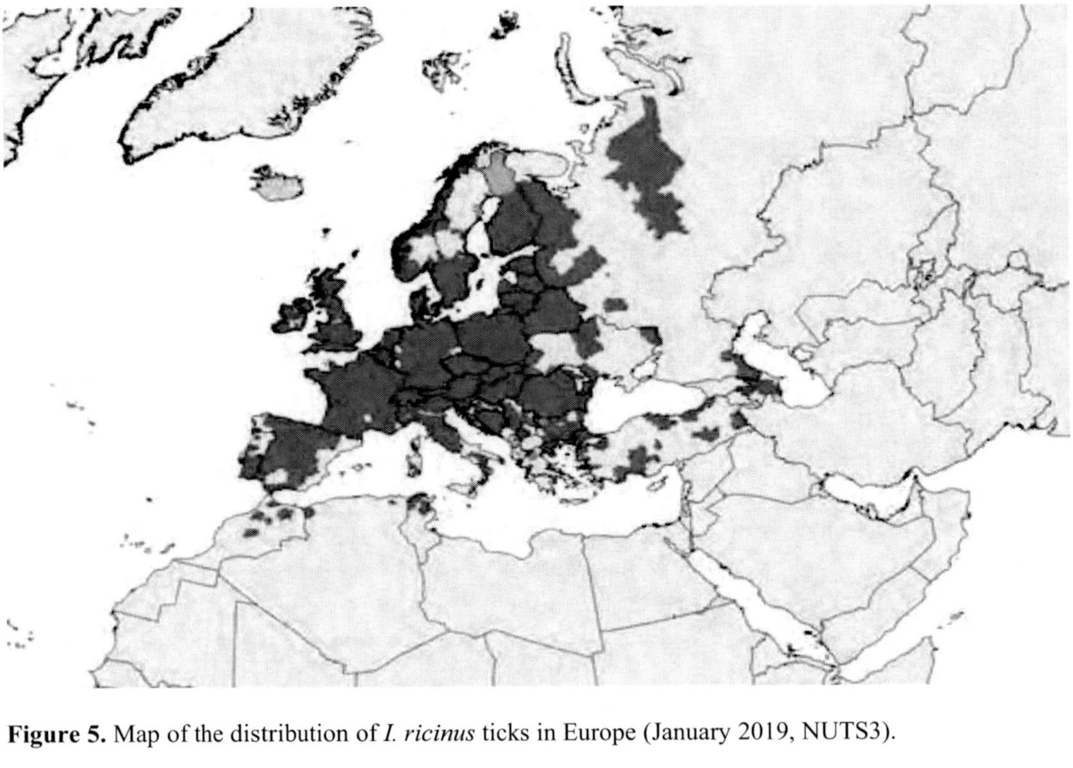

Figure 5. Map of the distribution of *I. ricinus* ticks in Europe (January 2019, NUTS3).

Male dog ticks are small in size, brownish or dark brown in colour (Figure 6). In male ticks of the species *I. ricinus*, stabilizing selection acts on the width and length of the palps, and the length increases due to a decrease in width, while disruptive selection acts on the scutum and the length of the gnathosoma. Morphological examinations have shown that the total body length of males is 2.4–2.5 mm, the length of their gnathosomas is 0.3–0.4 mm, and the width of the abdomen is 0.3–0.4 mm [100]. The dorsal shield is slightly darker than the body and completely covers it from above. The hypostome is short, wide and covered with rows of strong prongs, pointed downwards. The width of the abdomen of a hungry tick is about 1.3 mm, it depends very much on the degree of saturation with the host's blood. The coxae of the forelimbs have a long, unforked spine. The anus has the form of a transverse slit. Peritremes are small, transversely elongated.

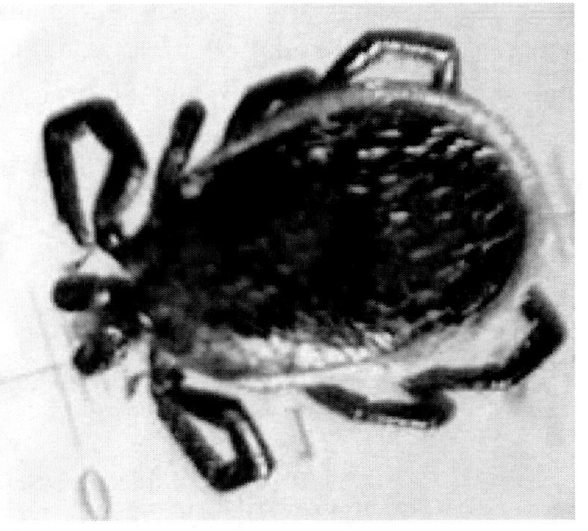

Figure 6. Male dog tick.

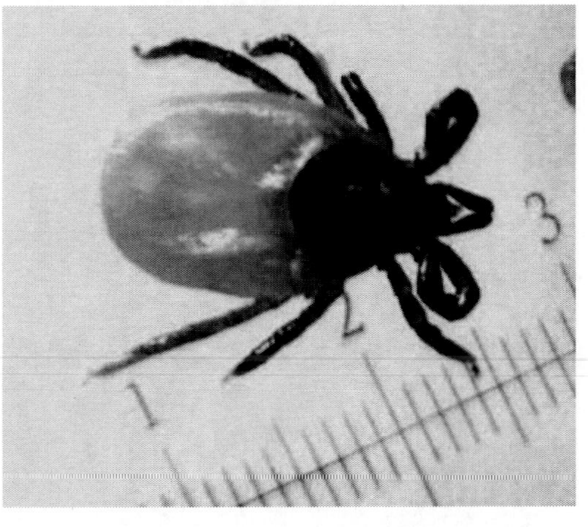

Figure 7. Female dog tick.

In hungry females, the abdomen is yellow-red (Figure 7), and in blood-saturated females, it is yellow-grey. The shield is dark brown, covering only a third of the female's body. Examination of a large number of females of this species showed that their morphological indicators proportionally depend on the degree of blood saturation of the host. Thus, the total length of females caught in nature did not exceed 3.2–3.4 mm, the length of the gnathosoma was about 0.8 mm, the length of the shield was 0.6 mm, and the width of the abdomen is about 2 mm. In the case of average blood saturation in females, a constriction appears on the abdomen, while the width of the front fragment is slightly larger than the back. On the contrary, at their maximum saturation with blood, the width of the back fragment is slightly greater than the width of the front. The palps are long and tapering towards the front, resembling a blade. The hypostome is elongated and has 4 rows of stout teeth directed laterally. External spurs are present on all coxae. The internal spur on the first pair of coxae is long and undivided. Peritremes are small and transversely elongated.

Hungry nymphs are white, translucent (Figure 8), the dark branched intestine shines through their integuments. The shape of the body is elongated-oval. When saturated with blood, it becomes egg-shaped with a dark brown colour. Body sizes range from 1.2 to 1.4 mm. their shield is oval, much darker, about 0.6-0.8 mm long. Gnathosoma is elongated, 0.5-0.7 mm long. The hypostome is spear-shaped, pointed, has 3 longitudinal rows of teeth.

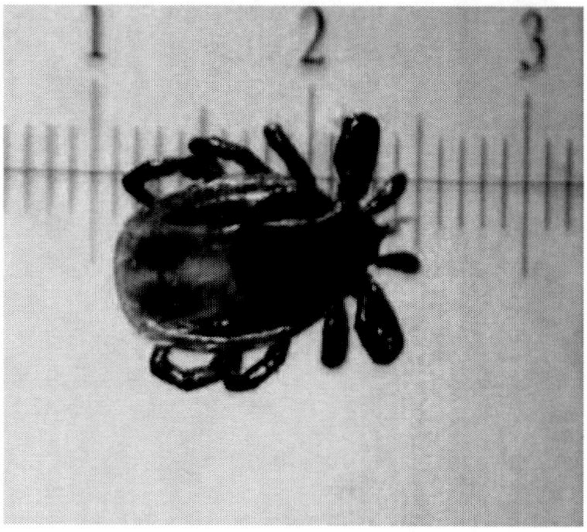

Figure 8. Dog tick nymph.

Larvae are very small (0.4-0.7 mm in size), the width of their abdomen is 0.4 mm. The body is rounded, with 3 pairs of limbs (Figure 9). The covers are translucent, the dark branched intestine is visible through them. The length of the gnathosoma is about 0.2 mm. The hypostome is long, with 4 rows of teeth. There is no peritremes.

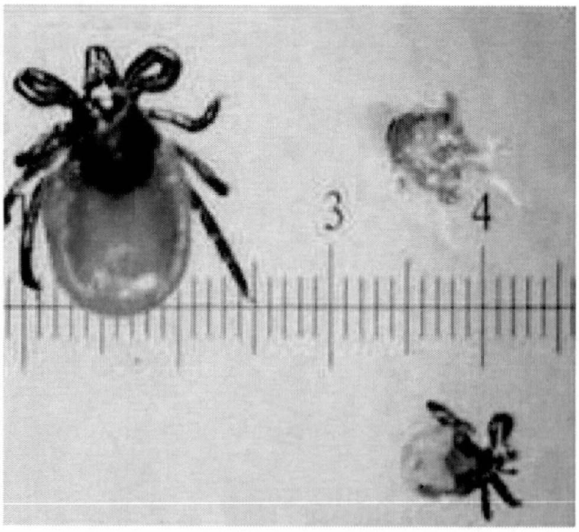

Figure 9. Dog tick female and larvae.

4.3. Nutrition

In general, the dog tick, being at different stages of development, can use about 300 species of terrestrial vertebrates for its nutrition [101]. Larvae of the tick species Ixodes ricinus most commonly parasitize on rodent-like rodents, such as the wood mouse (*Apodemus sylvaticus*), striped field mouse (*A. agrarius*), yellow-necked mouse (*A. flavicollis*), house mouse (*Mus musculus*), harvest mouse (*Micromys minutus*), common vole (*Microtus arvalis*), and European bank vole (*Clethionomys glareolus*). In addition to rodent-like rodents, insectivorous animals often serve as hosts for the larvae of this tick: European hedgehog (*Erinaceus europaeus*), common shrew (*Sorex araneus*), pygmy shrew (*Sorex minutus*), forest dormouse (*Dryomys nitedula*), edible dormouse (*Myoxus glis*), mole (*Talpa europaea*), and lesser water shrew (*Neomys anomalus*). Larvae are also found on the common squirrel (*Sciurus vulgaris*) and European hare (*Lepus europaeus*). Birds play a significant role in the feeding and especially in the distribution of tick larvae across habitats. They are most often found on the bodies of species such as the tree pipit (*Anthus trivialis*), chaffinch (*Fringilla coelebs*), European robin (*Erithacus rubecula*), crested tit (*Parus cristatus*), and hazel grouse (*Bonasa bonasia*) [102-104].

Our studies have shown that the dog tick attacks humans at practically all stages of development. In the larval stage, it is rarely detected in humans. Thus, during the year, there are 7–10 larvae per 300–400 instances of ticks. Morphological characteristics of larvae, nymphs and adults, in particular, the total length of their body and the width of the abdomen, are determined by the degree of their saturation with the blood of the host. Accordingly, 4 degrees of saturation are distinguished: unsaturated, partially saturated, saturated and very saturated (Figure 10).

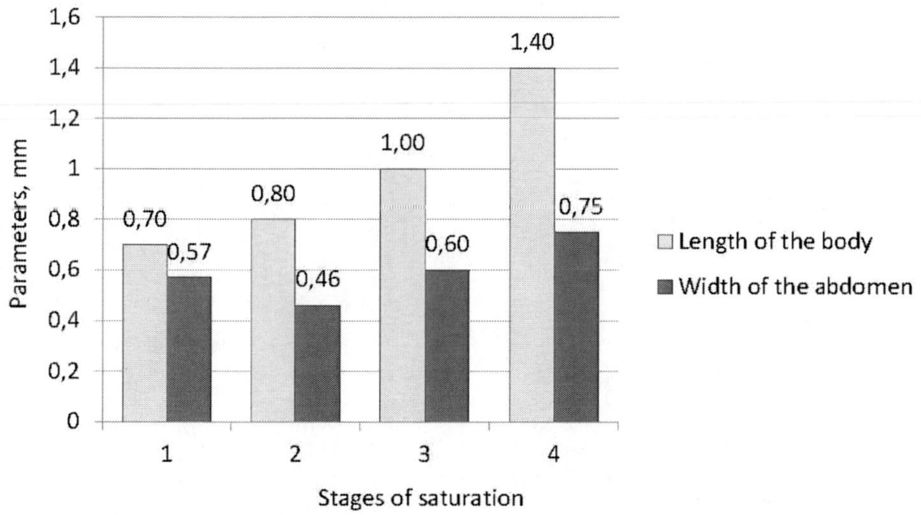

Figure 10. Changes in morphological parameters of *I. ricinus* tick larvae depending on the degree of saturation of their host's blood.

As we can see, the body length of very saturated larvae increases by 2 times compared to hungry ones, while the width of the abdomen is only 1.3 times.

The dependence of the morphological parameters of the body and its individual parts on the degree of blood saturation of the host in nymphs is shown in Figure 11.

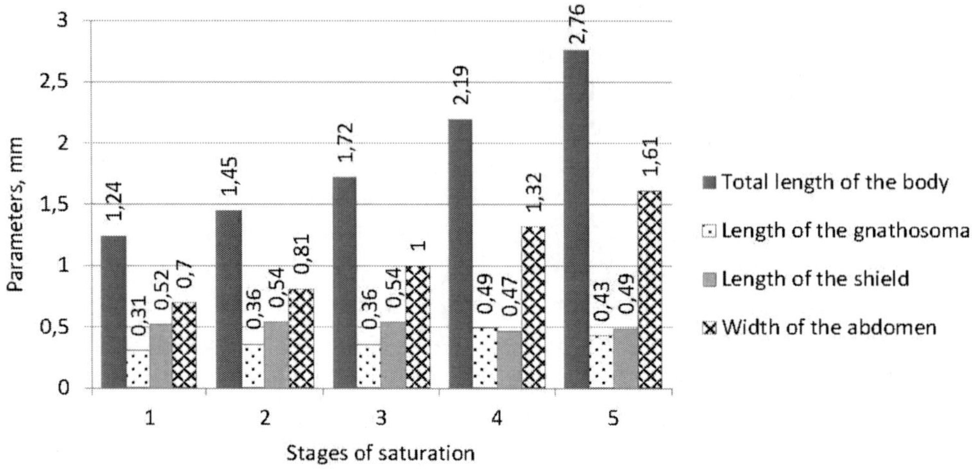

Figure 11. Changes in the morphological parameters of nymphs of the *I. ricinus* ticks depending on the degree of saturation of their host's blood.

Thanks to the analysis of morphological indicators in nymphs, certain regularities were found in the ratio of the total body length to the width of the abdomen at different degrees of saturation: 1:0.56; 1:0.58; 1:0.6 [105]. The average ratio of the largest body length to the smallest is 2.2 times, and the width of the abdomen is 2.3 times. The width of the abdomen increases very slowly and mainly its length increases.

The analysis of the morphological parameters of the body and its individual parts in females also shows a complete dependence on the degree of saturation of their host's blood. The obtained results are shown in Figure 12.

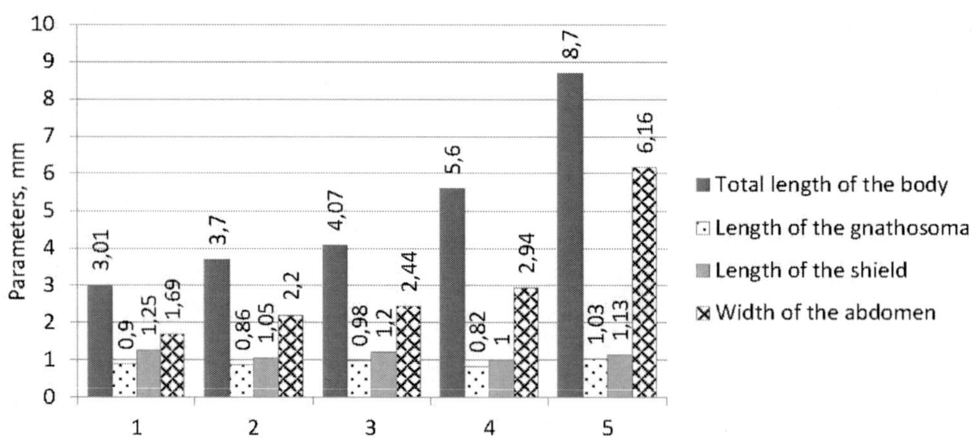

Figure 12. Changes in the morphological parameters of female ticks of the *I. ricinus* species depending on the degree of saturation of their host's blood.

In females, there is a corresponding correlation between the total length of the body and the width of the abdomen: 1:0.56; 1:0.59; 1:0.53; 1:0.6; 1:0.7. The average ratio of the largest body length to the smallest is 2.8 times, and the width of the abdomen is 3.6 times.

Changes in body parameters depending on the degree of blood saturation of males are insignificant and occur in the average range of 1.7–2.0 times (Figure 13). This is due to the presence of dorsal and abdominal chitinous shields, which block excessive stretching of the abdomen.

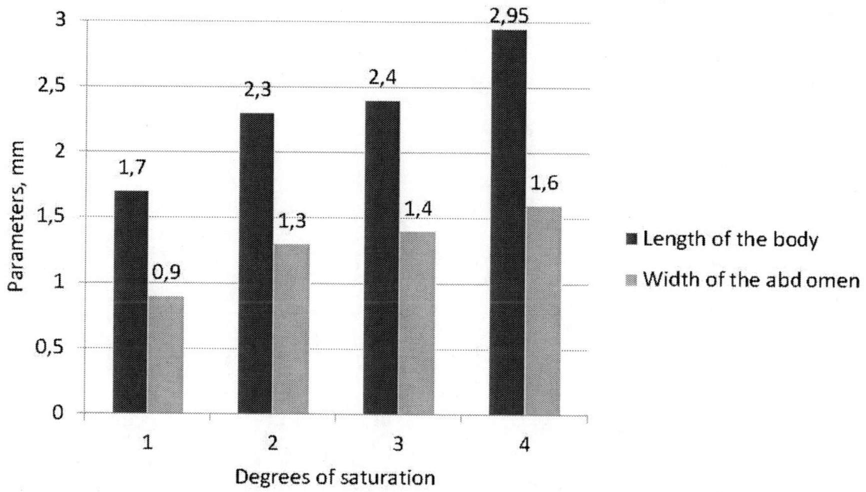

Figure 13. Changes in body parameters of male ticks of the *I. ricinus* species depending on the degree of saturation of their host's blood.

Thus, only male *I. ricinus* ticks have limited ability to consume large amounts of blood, and consequently, their feeding time on the host is also limited.

4.4. Reproduction and Development of the Dog Tick, Frequency of Attacks on Humans

The activity of ticks, including the dog tick, is determined by the environmental temperature and humidity. Accordingly, once temperatures rise above 12-15°C and humidity exceeds 75%, ticks emerge from their shelters and begin to hunt for hosts. Observations over several years have shown that the first ticks appear in nature and start attacking humans and domestic animals by late March to early April, continuing until October. However, recent years have shown a trend towards extending tick activity into November.

For example, in 2018, the annual activity of ticks at different stages of development was analysed. Ticks, which were brought by residents of Ternopil and Ternopil region to the laboratory of the Centre for Lyme Borreliosis and Other Tick-Borne Diseases Research, which operates at I. Horbachevsky Ternopil National Medical University (TNMU), were thoroughly studied (Figure 14).

Thus, during the spring-autumn period, 468 instances of ticks were identified. It was not possible to identify 21 specimens due to their excessive damage. In April, the identification of ticks started from the second decade. A total of 25 specimens were examined this month, including 12 adults and 13 nymphs. In May, 150 ticks were processed, of which 52 adults, 84 nymphs and 4 larvae were found. In June, the number of ticks that attacked people decreased to 138 specimens, including 56 adults, 78 nymphs and 4 larvae. In July, it decreased by almost 2 times – up to 75 specimens, of which there were 28 adults, 47 nymphs. During August, September and October, the number of removed ticks gradually decreased. So, in August, 42 specimens were obtained, of which 14 were adults, 16 were nymphs, and 6 were larvae. In September, 22 specimens were examined, including 12 adults, 6 nymphs, and 3 larvae, and in October – 16 ticks, including 10 adults and 6 nymphs.

An analysis of the frequency of dog tick larvae's attacks on people in the spring-autumn time period shows that they appear in late April – early May, and the peak of their development and attacks on people occurs in May – June and August – September (Figure 15).

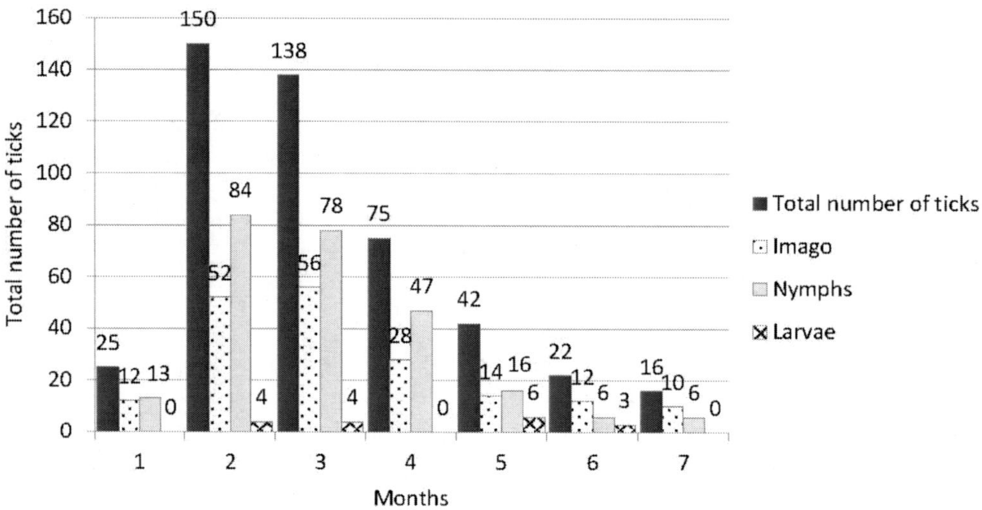

Figure 14. The frequency of attacks by *I. ricinus* ticks on humans in April – October 2018.

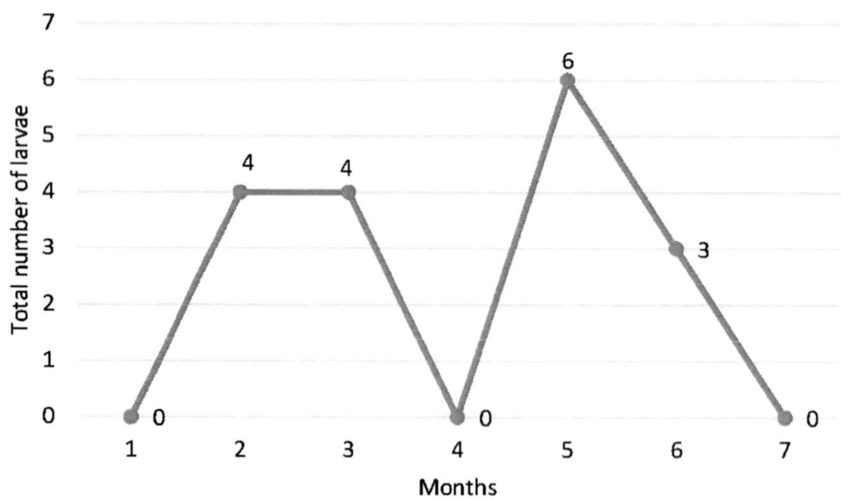

Figure 15. Seasonal activity of *I. ricinus* tick larvae in 2018.

Our data in general correlate with the results of many researchers, including M. Stanko [105], according to which the largest number of larvae can be observed in the third decade of June, at the end of July and at the beginning of August. The development of larvae from eggs takes 15–20 days, their transformation into nymphs takes approximately one month [103, 107].

Changes in larval activity are caused by the temperature regimen observed in Ukraine in recent years, which is defined by a maximum temperature above 27–30°C and a decrease in humidity below 70%. During this period, ticks at almost all stages of development fell into a state of diapause.

4.5. Epidemiological and Epizootological Significance of the Dog Tick

There are numerous publications discussing the role of these ticks as vectors and reservoirs of pathogens causing many infectious diseases in humans and animals. Ukrainian acarologist Ye. M. Yemchuk [98] highlighted the significance of Ixodid ticks in transmitting and maintaining pathogens such as piroplasmosis and nuttalliosis in horses, babesiosis and theileriosis in cattle, relapsing fever caused by ticks, and tick-borne encephalitis in humans, among others. In recent years, the role of these ticks in transmitting pathogens of certain infectious diseases from animals to humans and from humans to humans has sharply increased.

In the USA in the 1980s there appeared a problem of infecting people with pathogens of borreliosis, in particular LB. The main role in this was played by ticks of the genus Ixodes. A little later, this problem also appeared in Europe, in particular in Sweden, the UK, the Czech Republic and many other countries [108, 109]. Since 2000, LB diseases have also been diagnosed in Ukraine.

Another very common tick-borne disease is human granulocytic anaplasmosis (HGA). Tick fever caused by A. phagocytophilum was first described in the USA in 1969 in horses [110].

Research on HGA in Europe began in 1995, when antibodies against *A. phagocytophilum* were found in the blood of people who had experienced tick attacks. The dog tick was recognized as a vector in the transmission of this pathogen [111].

In Italy, a group of scientists investigated the genotypes of *A. phagocytophilum* in wild ungulates and in the dog tick. Using PCR, they detected the agent of anaplasmosis in nearly half of the spleen samples from deer, roe deer, and chamois, as well as in ticks collected from these animals [112].

Many scientists are studying *A. phagocytophilum* and the role of the dog tick in its transmission in different regions of Ukraine. For example, the results of research on LB, anaplasmosis, and ehrlichiosis in the Sumy region were published by T. O. Boletska, M. D. Chemych [113], tick infections in the eastern regions of Ukraine by V. P. Malyi, N. V. Shepyleva, L. V. Tkachenko [114], tick infections in the territories of Ukraine bordering Belarus and in Belarus itself were studied by H. V. Biletska, I. M. Lozynskyi, and R. S. Morochkovskyi [115], manifestations of anaplasmosis in the western region of Ukraine were studied by I. I. Ben, H. V. Biletska, and O. V. Korolyuk [116]. The causative agents of aplasmosis and ehrlichiosis in dog ticks and pasture ticks in the Zaporizhzhia region was studied by O. V. Zelenukhina, N. Ya. Kovryha, and Ye. M. Chebotok [117].

Since 2017, in the laboratory of TNMU Centre for Lyme Borreliosis and Other Tick-Borne Diseases Research, using real-time PCR analysis, the DNA of tick-borne pathogens is isolated in the suspension of ticks. The ROTOR Gene-6000 amplifier is used. So, in 2021, out of 296 ticks, 119 females, 174 nymphs and 3 larvae were examined. Of all females, 46 (38%) individuals were carriers of infectious agents, including 34 (74%) females considered to be vectors of *B. burgdorferi s. l.*, 10 (22%) – *A. phagocytophilum* and 2 (4%) – *B. miyamotoi*. Out of 174 nymphs, 54 (31%) individuals were carriers of pathogens, of which 29 (54%) nymphs were considered to be *B. burgdorferi s. l.*, 13 (24%) – *A. phagocytophilum*, 5 (9%) – *B. miyamotoi*.

In 2018, 494 ticks were examined in the laboratory of TNMU Centre for Lyme Borreliosis and Other Tick-Borne Diseases Research: 489 – *I. ricinus*, 4 – *D. reticulatus*, 1 – *R. sanguineus* [118]. Out of the ticks of the *I. ricinus* species, 171 (35%) females, 22 unidentified ticks (4.5%), 273 (55.8%) nymphs, 19 (3.8%) larvae, and 4 (0.8%) males were examined. The total number of infected ticks was 205 (41.5%) individuals. Among all infected ticks, there were 100 (48.8%) nymphs, 2 (1.0%) larvae, 98 (47.8%) females and 5 (2.4%) unidentified ticks.

In 2019, 482 ticks were identified [119]. *I. ricinus* was represented by 477 specimens, *D. reticulatus* – 5. Among the ticks of the *I. ricinus* species, 152 (31.6%) females, 8 (1.4%) males, 299 (62.8%) nymphs and 10 (2.3%) larvae were examined. It was not possible to establish the stage of development and sex for 8 (1.9%) ticks.

The analysis of tick contamination using the PCR method showed that 167 (35.0%) individuals were carriers of infectious disease agents. Among them, there were 70 (42.0%) adults, 93 (55.6%) nymphs. 4 (2.4%) ticks were unidentified in terms of developmental stage and sex.

Ticks were infected with *B. burgdorferi s. l.*, *B. miyamotoi*, *A. phagocytophilum* and *Babesia species*. Summarized data on the infection of ticks at various stages of development (according to PCR data), studied during 2017–2019 [120] in the laboratory of Centre for Lyme Borreliosis and Other Tick-Borne Diseases Research, are given in Table 3.

Table 3. Infection rate of ticks of the *I. ricinus* species at different stages of development, studied in 2017–2019

Causative agent	Adult individuals				Nymphs				Larvae				Not identified				Total number of examined ticks
	2017	2018	2019	Total	2017	2018	2019	Total	2017	2018	2019	Total	2017	2018	2019	Total	
B. burgdorferi s. l.	22	57	38	117	8	42	50	100	0	2	0	2	9	4	2	15	234
B. miyamotoi	1	5	3	9	1	1	9	11	0	0	0	0	1	0	0	1	21
A. phagocytophilum	9	34	25	68	10	57	34	101	1	2	0	3	4	1	2	7	179
Babesia sp.	0	0	4	4	0	0	0	0	0	0	0	0	0	0	0	0	4
Total	32	96	70	198	19	100	93	212	1	4	0	5	14	5	4	23	438

According to the obtained results, during 3 years in the laboratory of TNMU Centre for Lyme Borreliosis and Other Tick-Borne Diseases Research, 1267 ticks of the *I. ricinus* species were studied, of which 438 (almost 34%) were carriers of infectious disease pathogens. Apparently, spirochetes *B. burgdorferi s. l.* (234, or 53%) prevailed. The *A. phagocytophilum* species (179, or 41%) is the next most frequent tick infection. 21 (5%) ticks were carriers of *B. miyamotoi*. 4 (1%) ticks were considered to be carriers of *Babesia sp.*

The infection rate of Ixodes ricinus ticks is actively studied in various urban ecosystems, including recreational areas in large cities. Ukrainian acarologists I. A. Akimov and I. V.

Nebohatkin have researched the infection rates of ticks within the green zones of Kyiv. [121]. According to their research conducted in 1989–2009 and 2012–2014, 28.38% ticks were carriers of *B. burgdorferi s. l.* In 1997, 100% of ticks examined by dark field microscopy were carriers of spirochetes [122]. Czech scientists conducted similar studies in natural and urban biocenoses of Ostrava [108]. Thus, in the city park "Belsky Forest," the general infestation of ticks with spirochetes *B. burgdorferi s. l.* was 13.8%, of which the infection rate of females was within 17.8%, males – 17.6%, nymphs – 11.7%. Accordingly, in the natural biocenosis of Proskovice, the minimum infection rate of ticks was 15%, of which this parameter was about 20% in females, 12.5% in males, and 14.9% in nymphs. A number of European scientists [123], based on studied literature sources, provide data on the infestation of ticks of the *I. ricinus* species at various life stages in the landscape conditions of a number of European cities. For example, the parameters of tick infestation with *B. burgdorferi s. l.* in the city of Brno is as follows: nymphs – 14.7%, females – 29.7%, males – 30.7%, in Paris – nymphs 10%, females – 32%, males – 20%, in Berlin – nymphs 2.4%, females – 9.1%, males – 6.1%. In Budapest in 2013, the total infestation of ticks in parks and cemeteries was 40.8%, in Vilnius – 25%, in Warsaw – from 19.2 to 31%, in Belgrade – 21.9%, in Bratislava – 7.8%, in Basel – 16.4%, in London – 7.7%.

A. phagocytophilum in ticks of the *I. ricinus* species was detected in 30 European countries. Prevalence varied, for example, in Norway – from 0.4 to 17.1%, in Estonia – from 3 to 6.5%, in Slovakia – from 1.1 to 8.3%, in Germany – from 1.0 to 17.4%. Data on dog tick infection with B. miyamotoi spirochetes in Europe are almost absent at the present moment. It is known that this pathogen was first discovered in 1994 in Japan. For a long time, it was considered non-pathogenic [124].

4.6. General Characteristics of Ticks of the *Dermacentor Koch* Genus

Ticks of the *Dermacentor* genus differ from ticks of the Ixodes genus by the presence of an enamel pattern on the dorsal shield. The body is relatively large, expanded to the rear end, dark brown. In females, the shield covers a third of the abdomen, and in males – the entire abdomen. The hypostome is relatively short and wide. Pedipalps are short and wide. On the sides of the dorsal shield, slightly convex eyes stand out. The legs are short and strong, with a white pattern. The first coxae have a bifurcated tooth. The anal groove closes under the anus.

In the western regions of Ukraine, there are 2 types of ticks of this genus: *D. reticulatus Koch* and *D. marginatus Sulz.* The latter is much less common and can be found further south, in the forest-steppe, closer to the steppe.

4.7. Dermacentor Reticulatus Koch

D. reticulatus is found in the European part of Russia, in Western Siberia, in the Caucasus, in Central Asia. In Europe, the species is widespread in Poland, Romania, England, Germany, and Hungary. One of the first data on the ranges of *D. reticulatus* within Ukraine was given in a monograph by Ye. M. Yemchuk [98]. According to this information, the specified species of ticks is distributed in 10 regions of Ukraine (Lviv, Ternopil, Volyn, Rivne, Khmelnytskyi, Vinnytsia, Kyiv, Sumy, Zhytomyr, Chernihiv), and it mainly occupies forest biotopes.

Issues related to the biology and distribution of ticks of the *Dermacentor* genus in the territory of the Carpathians and Transcarpathia were studied by I. I. Turianyn [125–127]. In particular, he pointed to the detection of ticks of this genus in Transcarpathia, Ivano-Frankivsk, Lviv and Chernivtsi regions.

There are individual works on the distribution of the *D. reticulatus* species in urbocenoses. Thus, the monograph and scientific articles of I. A. Akimov [121] and I. V. Nebohatkin [128] provide data on the distribution of the species in the biotopes of Kyiv. According to the results of research conducted by scientists in 1988, 1991–1992, and 2008–2009, the southern ranges of *D. reticulatus* were established, in particular in the Autonomous Republic of Crimea. The papers also revealed the reasons of the inclination to inhabit in populated areas, including cities.

In May 2017 – November 2019, the laboratory of TNMU Centre for Lyme Borreliosis and Other Tick-Borne Diseases Research studied 447 specimens of *D. reticulatus* ticks, of which 287 were females and 160 were males. The ticks were collected in 74 locations of 67 settlements in 10 regions of Ukraine: Transcarpathia (2 locations), Ivano-Frankivsk (3), Lviv (8), Ternopil (21), Volyn (9), Rivne (10), Khmelnytskyi (8), Vinnytsia (2), Zhytomyr (3), Chernihiv (1) [129]. The main animals on which adult ticks of both sexes fed were dogs (34 cases), cows (16), cats (4), horses (3), and humans (15).

In 2000–2018, researchers of the Department of Acarology of I. I. Schmalhausen Institute of Zoology of the National Academy of Sciences of Ukraine conducted field studies of ticks of the *I. ricinus* and *D. reticulatus* species in the southern regions of Ukraine, in particular in the Crimea [128]. *D. reticulatus* ticks were found in 311 locations in 79 settlements of Odesa, 45 – Mykolaiv, 44 – Kherson, 60 – Zaporizhia, 57 – Donetsk regions and in 26 sites of Crimea. They were collected on the flag, taken from small mammals, domestic and wild animals and people.

According to the summarized results of our research and the data of the Department of Acarology of I. I. Schmalhausen Institute of Zoology of the National Academy of Sciences of Ukraine, *D. reticulatus* was found in 385 locations of 351 settlements in 15 regions of Ukraine and in the Autonomous Republic of Crimea.

The body of the males has a somewhat pear-shaped form, narrowed at the front and widened at the back (Figure 16). The tick is dark brown with a white enamelled pattern covering the entire surface of the dorsal shield, which has 11 festoons on the posterior edge. Along the sides of the dorsal shield, closer to the head, there are weakly convex small eyes. The hypostome is short, covered with 4 rows of teeth. Palps are short and broad, protruding beyond the edges of the gnathosoma. The scutum is quadrangular from the dorsal side. Legs are long and thick, with coxae of the first pair of legs bifurcated. The internal spur is broad, the external one is long and cylindrical. The genital aperture is located at the level of the second pair of coxae, and the anal aperture at the fourth. Peritremes are elongated, with a short, stub-like projection. The body size of the unfed tick ranges from 2.4–2.7 to 3.8–4.2 mm.

Females have an elongated-oval, more flattened body (Figure 17). The dorsal shield covers a third of the body and has a distinct white enamelled pattern, more pronounced in the anterior part. The hypostome is short, covered with 4 rows of teeth. Palps are short and broad, protruding beyond the edges of the gnathosoma. The scutum is quadrangular from the dorsal side. Peritremes are rounded-oval, with a broad dorsal projection. The body size of the female averages 2.7–3.2 mm.

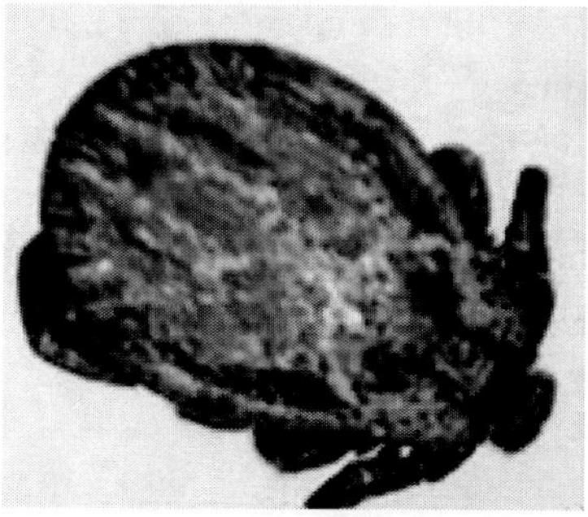

Figure 16. A male tick of the *D. reticulatus* species.

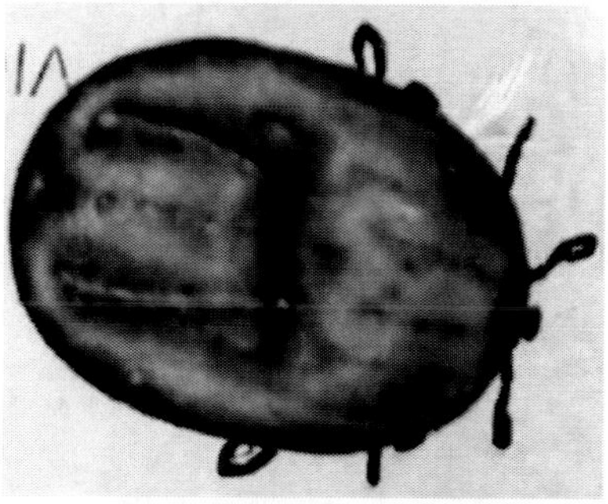

Figure 17. A female tick of the *D. reticulatus* species.

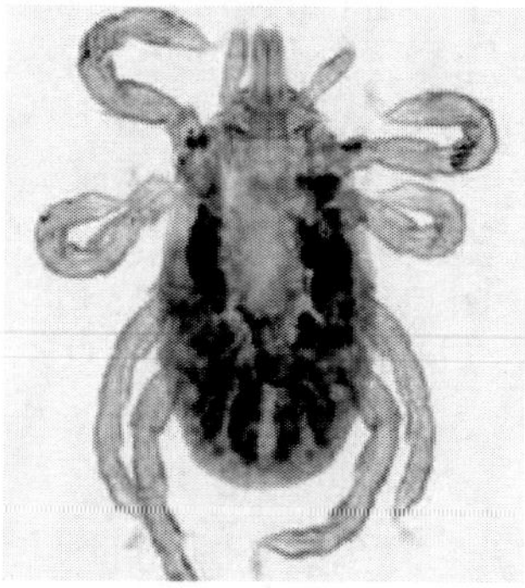

Figure 18. A tick nymph of the *D. reticulatus* species.

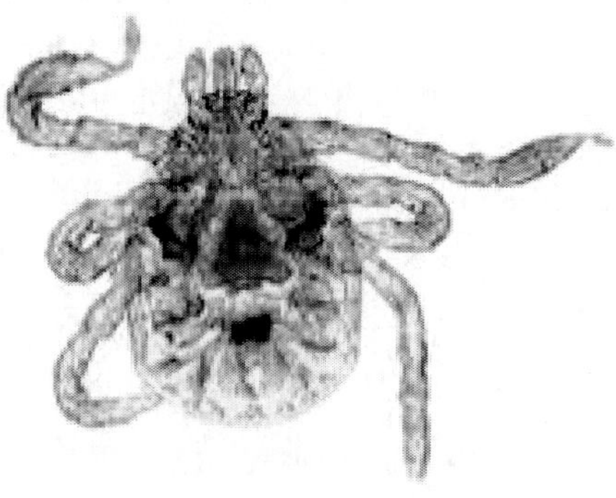

Figure 19. A tick larva of the *D. reticulatus* species [133].

Nymphs have an elongated-oval body ending with 11 festoons (Figure 18). The shield is also elongated-oval, with parallel lateral edges relative to the body and a rounded posterior edge. The length of the shield is 0.52–0.55 mm [125]. The hypostome is thin and long, approximately 0.35 mm in length. There are external spurs on all coxae, and an additional internal spur on the first pair. The peritremes are small and elongated.

Larvae are small, their body is elongated and ends with 9 festoons (Figure 19). The sides of the body are almost parallel. The dorsal shield is small, shiny, slightly wider than it is longer (0.322 and 0.210 mm, respectively) [60]. The hypostome is short and wide, the palps are broad and four-segmented. The posterior edge of the third palp segment is obliquely truncated.

Female ticks of the *D. reticulatus* species lay up to 2700 eggs [130]. Larvae appear on small mammals in May-June, and the peak occurs in June-July [131, 132]. Nymphs are active during July – August. Both larvae and nymphs feed practically on the same hosts. Adult ticks are active during March – April with a peak in April and September – October. In summer, they practically disappear from the vegetation.

Ticks of the *D. reticulatus* species can feed on the blood of more than 60 species of wild and domestic animals and humans [133]. Larvae feed on one host for 2.5-6 days, and nymphs for 4–12 days [134]. In laboratory conditions, females can feed on the host for 7–15 days, and males for 3–5 days [135].

During the spring and autumn of 2017, TNMU students collected ticks in 38 settlements in 33 districts of 9 regions of Ukraine: Transcarpathia, Lviv, Ivano-Frankivsk, Ternopil, Volyn, Rivne, Khmelnytskyi, Vinnytsia and Zhytomyr. 292 specimens of ticks were collected, of which only 17 individuals belonged to the species *I. ricinus*, and the rest belonged to species *D. reticulatus* species. Ticks were collected from humans and 4 species of domestic animals: cats, dogs, cattle and horses. Most ticks were collected from dogs (132 specimens) and cows (116), fewer from cats (10), horses (12), humans (7), and a total of 14 specimens from flags.

After analysing the morphological parameters of the ratio of body length to the width of the abdomen of ticks of the *D. reticulatus* species, the minimum sizes of males not saturated with blood were established (body length – 2.2 mm, width of the abdomen – 1.2 mm) and the maximum sizes of males saturated with blood (5.6 and 3.6, respectively). Thus, at maximum blood saturation, the body length of males increases by 2.5 times, and the width of the abdomen by 3 times.

Knowing the patterns of changes in tick body proportions depending on the time of their feeding will allow making certain predictions regarding the probable infection of the host by pathogens of infectious diseases.

The sizes of female ticks of the *D. reticulatus* species, depending on the degree of saturation of their host's blood, vary in a much larger range. At the same time, some peculiarities of morphological parameters are observed depending on the type of host on which they fed.

Females with minimum body length (3.2 mm) and minimum abdominal width (2.0 mm) were collected from flag. When examining the animals, females with a body length of 3.4 mm and an abdominal width of 2.0 mm were taken. At the same time, the maximally saturated females on dogs had a body length of 13.0 mm and abdomen width of 9.3 mm, on cows – 11.1 and 8.0 mm, respectively, on horses – 8.9 and 5.8 mm. Ticks collected on cats had a maximum body length of 12.5 mm with an abdominal width of 8.0 mm (Figure 20). Thus, when feeding ticks of the *D. reticulatus* species has maximum arthropod sizes on cats and dogs, and somewhat smaller on cows and horses. Based on these parameters, it can be stated that in adult ticks collected on dogs and cats, the maximum body length, compared to the body length of hungry ticks, increases by 4 times, and the width of the abdomen – by 4.7 times. In ticks that feed on cows and horses, these parameters are 3.5 and 4 times and 2.8 and 2.9 times, respectively.

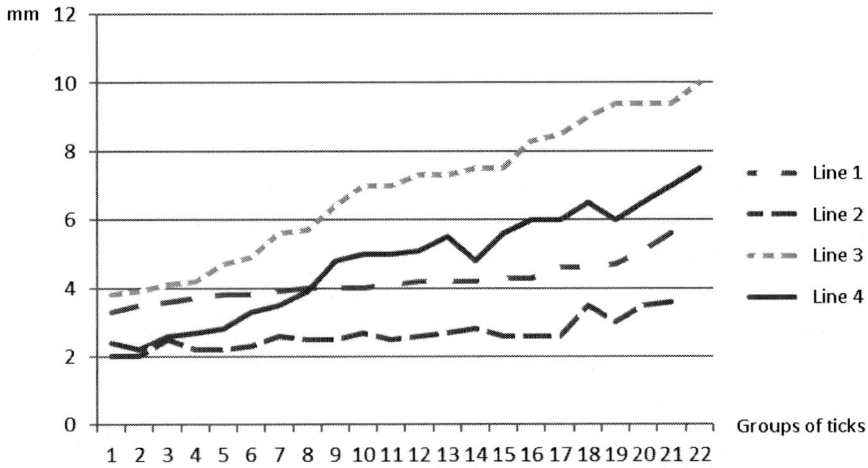

Note. Line 1 – body length of males; line 2 – the width of the abdomen of males; line 3 – body length of females; line 4 – the width of the abdomen of females.

Figure 20. Changes in body length and abdominal width (in mm) of ticks of the *D. reticulatus* species.

Based on the size of ticks of the *D. reticulatus* species that fed on dogs and cows, an analysis of abdominal volume parameters at different degrees of saturation was carried out (Figure 21). It was established that at the minimum saturation of females, when their body length was 4 mm, and the width of the abdomen was 2.7 mm, its volume was more than 15 mm^3. At maximum saturation, when their body length was 13.0 mm and the abdomen width was 9.3 mm, its volume was 558 mm^3. Thus, the volume increased 37 times.

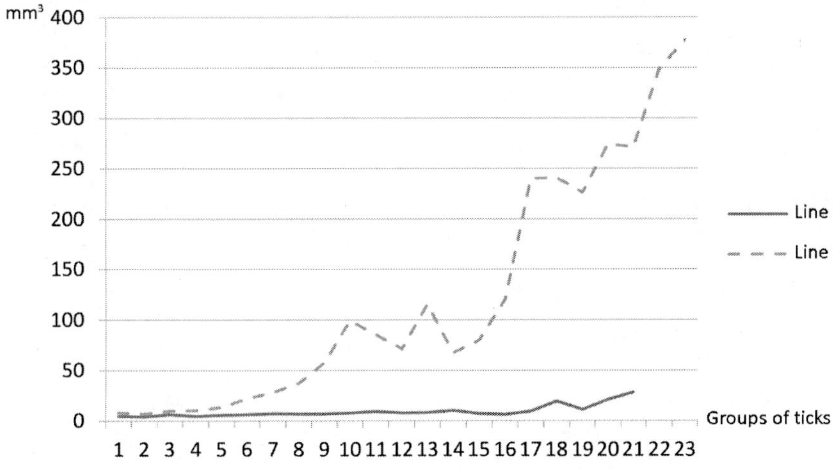

Note. Line 1 – body volume of males; line 2 – body volume of females.

Figure 21. Abdominal volume changes (in mm^3) during feeding of *D. reticulatus* ticks.

A slightly different picture is observed when feeding males. So, at their minimum saturation, when the length of the body was 3.8 mm, and the width of the abdomen was 2.0 mm, the volume of the consumed blood was about 4.5 mm^3. At the maximum saturation of males, when their body length was 5.6 mm, and the width of the abdomen was 3.6 mm, the volume of the blood consumed was 28 mm^3. Thus, the volume of the blood increased only 6.5 times.

The significance of *Dermacentor* ticks in Ukraine and other countries for medicine and veterinary science was reported by Ye. M. Yemchuk [88]. According to her data, ticks at all stages of their development can transmit the pathogens of piroplasmosis and nuttalliosis in horses. Z. M. Nekhoroshykh, O. O. Yehorova, and others [136] indicate the important role of these ticks in transmitting the agent of tularemia. In the conditions of Ukraine, these ticks have also been identified as carriers of the pathogens causing listeriosis, erysipeloid, and brucellosis.

Ticks of the genus *Dermacentor* primarily have veterinary significance. The main pathogen they can transmit to animals is Babesia canis. Babesiosis in animals mostly manifests in a mild form, but it can also have a severe course accompanied by renal and hepatic failure, acute pancreatitis, and so on.

Another common pathogen transmitted by these ticks is *B. caballi*, which causes piroplasmosis in horses. This disease is characterized by fever, loss of appetite, increased heart and respiratory rates, tachycardia, diarrhoea, splenomegaly, anaemia, and others.

Very often, ticks of this genus are carriers of rickettsiae of the *Anaplasma* genus, in particular *A. marginale*, which cause anaplasmosis in cattle. Czech scientists cultivated 38 strains of different microorganisms that have no practical veterinary or medical significance, but were present in ticks of the *D. reticulatus* species collected in the field [137]. Pathogens that can cause serious diseases in humans are *Babesia microti, B. burgdorferi s. s., B. afzelii, B. valaisiana, B. garinii, A. phagocytophilum, Francisella tularensis ssp., Toxoplasma gondii* [138] and others.

In the laboratory of TNMU Centre for Lyme Borreliosis and Other Tick-Borne Diseases Research, ticks were examined for the presence of infectious disease pathogens. Using the PCR method, 10 ticks of the *D. reticulatus* species, which were removed from humans, were studied. It was established that 3 ticks were carriers of *B. burgdorferi s. l.* and *A. phagocytophilum*. Separately, ticks removed from animals were also studied by the PCR method (Table 4). Thus, in 2018, 9 ticks collected in 2017 were analysed. Of them, 8 were carriers of infectious disease agents, of which 7 were found to be *B. burgdorferi s. l.*, in 3 – *A. phagocytophilum*, and in 2 – both pathogens at the same time.

Table 4. Infectious disease agents detected by polymerase chain reaction in *D. reticulatus* ticks collected from humans and animals in 2017–2019

Causative agent	Ticks							
	collected from humans				collected from animals			
	2017	2018	2019	total	2017	2018	2019	total
B. burgdorferi s. l.	0	0	2	2	5	2	0	7
B. miyamotoi	0	0	0	0	0	0	0	0
A. phagocytophilum	0	0	1	1	3	4	0	7
Babesia sp.	0	0	0	0	0	0	5	5
Tick-borne encephalitis virus	0	0	0	0	0	0	2	2
Total	0	0	3	3	8	6	7	21

Of the 14 ticks studied in 2018, 2 were vectors of *B. burgdorferi s. l.*, 4 – *A. phagocytofilum*, including 1 contained both pathogens at the same time. Out of 10 ticks of the *D. reticulatus* species collected in 2019, 5 were carriers of *Babesia sp.*, 2 of tick-borne encephalitis virus, 1 of these ticks contained both pathogens.

Based on the research results, it is possible to generalize that ticks of the species *D. reticulatus*, removed from animals, are more often found to cause infectious diseases. Studies conducted over a period of 3 years show that ticks of the *D. reticulatus* and *I. ricinus* species are capable of carrying all pathogens listed in Table 4. Moreover, ticks are often carriers of two, and sometimes three pathogens at the same time.

5. The Results of In-Depth Acarological Research in Ternopil Region

Mykhaylo Andreychyn
Volodymyr Panychev
Mykola Kashuba
and Andrii Sverstyuk

In many fields of science and practice, there is a need for collecting ticks. This is essential for studying their species diversity, distribution range, characteristics of their biocenosis, the impact of ecological factors, and assessing the state of populations, among other reasons.

From a public health perspective, ticks are of interest as vectors and sources of various zoonotic diseases [139, 140], some of which are common to both humans and animals. Therefore, they are of particular interest in the context of the One Health concept, which emphasizes the interconnectedness of human, animal, and environmental health.

The collection of ticks is carried out to assess epidemiological risks in specific territories, to find out their number, infection, and features of territorial distribution. it is important for many types of human activity: forestry, agriculture, when deploying troops in the field, location of summer recreation camps, tourism, work on homesteads and summer cottages. A component of zooentomological monitoring is the collection of data on the number of ticks and dominant species. For this reason, the areas to be surveyed are selected with the most characteristic landscape of the given area, after that ticks are collected and examined [141, 142].

As of today, Ukraine does not have any active regulatory documents or methodological recommendations regarding the collection of ticks and appropriate tools for this purpose. In practice, traditional methods are used, such as flagging with fabric on a wooden handle, combing collected small mammals, and so on [143, 144]. Therefore, improvement of methods and means of tick collection, their unification, standardization and efficiency remain relevant.

The purpose of the study was to compare the effectiveness of tick collection tools depending on the design of the flag (the number of tick specimens collected using the flag per 1 km of the route).

In accordance with the goal, we compared the effectiveness of traditional and our own patented means:

- traditional flag (waffle fabric measuring 100 × 100 cm on wooden holder);

- flag on an L-shaped device (fluffy flannel size 100 × 100 cm on a metal L-shaped telescopic holder with a spring clip);
- flags on 2 parallel metal rods (fluffy flannel size 100 × 100 cm).

The distinctive feature of comparative assessment is the precise measurement of distance using pedometers. The comparison conditions include using collection tools simultaneously at the same location, ensuring identical weather conditions, terrain, vegetation, one-hour duration, and consistent distance and time duration. The effectiveness of the collection tools was compared across five locations in Ternopil region (Table 5).

On the traditional flag, the average number of ticks collected per flag-kilometre was 3.9 specimens, on the flag with a "L"-shaped handle it was 12.7 specimens, and on the flag with two parallel metal rods it was 13.4 specimens.

Under conditions where all requirements were met, the flag measuring 100×100 cm with two parallel metal rods proved to be more effective. This increased effectiveness is attributed to the fabric covering more tightly and uniformly against the surface, effectively increasing the flag's area used. This is supported by the fact that ticks were found attached across the entire fabric area, whereas on the flag with a wooden handle, they were primarily found in the lower 1/3 to 1/2 of the fabric.

Table 5. The number of ticks collected by various means in 2017 in forestry farms of Ternopil region

Site of collection	Number of ticks per 1 flag-kilometre		
	flag of flannel on 2 metal poles	flag of flannel on L-shaped device	flag of waffle fabric
Buchach Forestry, Dorohychiv Forest Farm, Khmeleva Tract (Dniester Canyon)	20,0	18,0	8,0
Kremenets Forestry, Kremenets Forest Farm, Velyki Berezhtsi Tract	10,0	8,0	1,0
Buchach Forestry, Yazlovets Forest Farm, Beremiany Tract	14,0	11,3	2,4
Ternopil Forestry, Mshanets Hunting Forest Farm, Vertelka Tract	4,0	12,9	2,5
Chortkiv Forestry, Skala-Podilskyi Forest Farm, Mushkativka Tract	19,0	13,1	5,7
The average number of ticks per means of collection	13,4	12,7	3,9

Statistical calculations comparing the effectiveness of different tick collection methods were conducted using Statistica 10.0. To determine the possibility of applying parametric or non-parametric statistical criteria, the input data (Figure 22, a) were checked for compliance with the normal law of distribution of the research results (Figure 22, b–d).

Figure 22 shows that the input data does not follow a normal distribution. This was further confirmed by the values of skewness coefficients, kurtosis, Shapiro-Wilk test, and the small number of collection sites.

Since the experimental data does not follow a normal distribution, parametric tests (such as ANOVA) cannot be used. In this case, it is appropriate to use the non-parametric Kruskal-Wallis test, which allows answering whether a nominal multi-level factor influences a quantitative response, and whether a quantitative factor influences a nominal multi-level response. Mathematically, the Kruskal-Wallis test checks for equality of median values across multiple groups on a quantitative scale.

The requirements for the input data are as follows: the nominal scale should have 3 or more levels, and the data within the compared subgroups should be distributed according to a distribution law different from normal. For graphical distribution, diagrams are used (Figure 23).

The number of ticks collected by various means per 1 flag-kilometre is taken as basic data. Figure 23 graphically shows the number of ticks collected by different means.

The number of tick specimens is the dependent variable, and the means of collection are the independent variables. Figure 23 shows that the diagrams are asymmetric, the medians are not in the centre, so the distribution of the number of ticks collected by different means is an additional confirmation of the non-normal law of distribution of experimental data.

	1 Flag of flannel on 2 metal rods	2 Flag of flannel on L-like device	3 Flag of waffle fabric
1	20	18	8
2	10	8	1
3	14	11,3	2,4
4	4	12,9	2,5
5	19	13,1	5,7

(a)

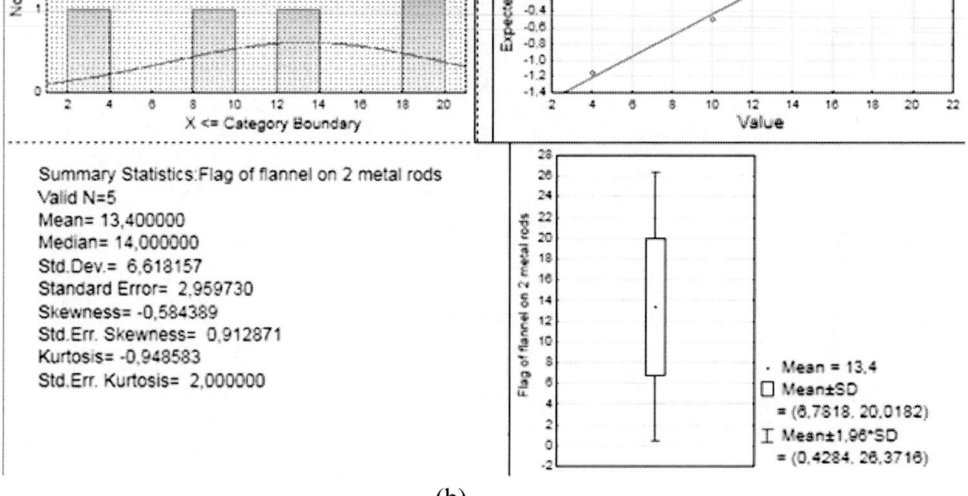

(b)

Figure 22. Continued on next page.

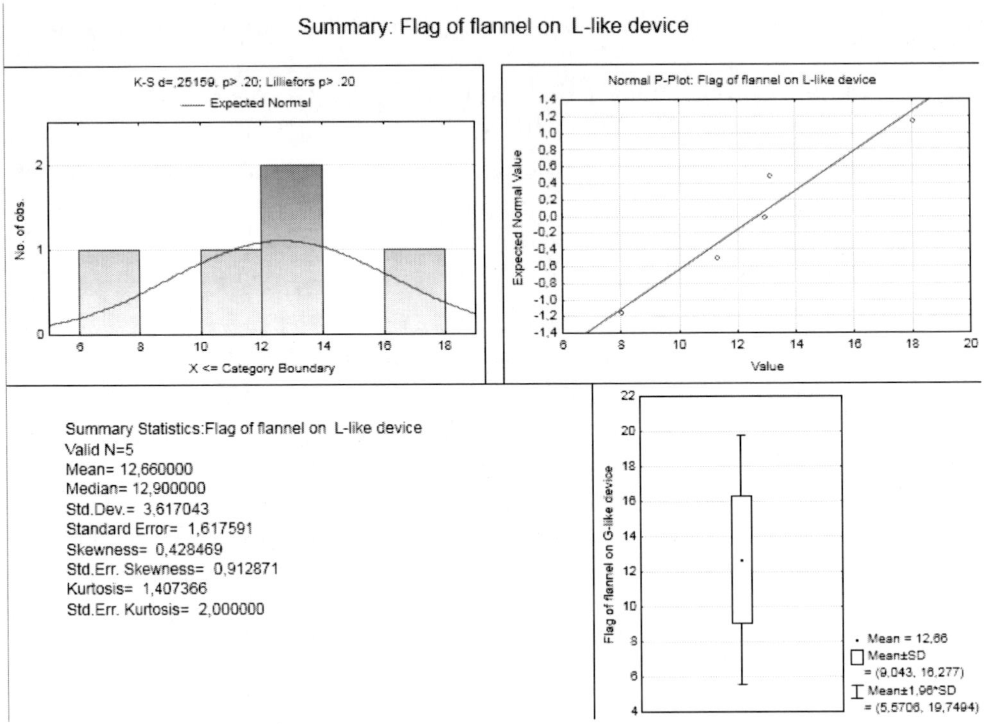

(c)

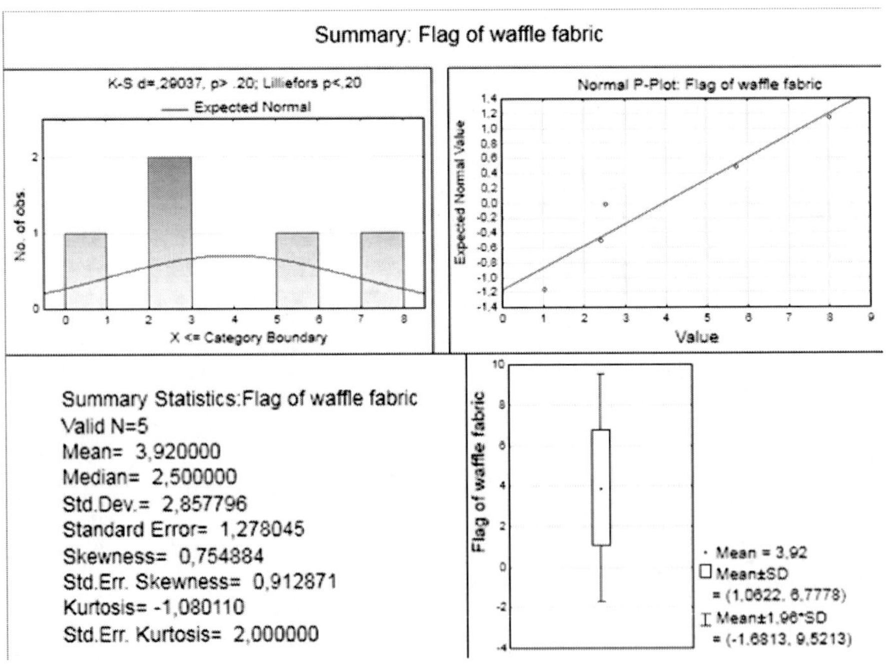

(d)

Figure 22. The results of checking for compliance with the normal law of the distribution of research results: a– input data; b – flag of flannel on 2 metal rods; c – a flag of flannel on L-shaped device; d – a flag of waffle fabric.

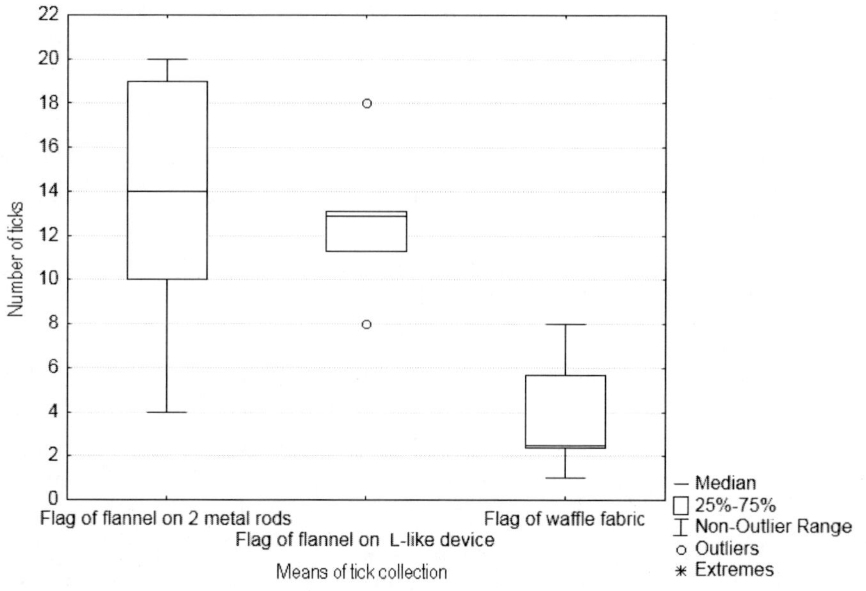

Figure 23. Graphical presentation of the number of ticks collected on 3 devices: a flag of flannel on 2 metal rods, a flag of flannel on an L-shaped device, and a flag of waffle fabric.

When comparing the effectiveness of 3 means of collection, the significance criterion is $p = 0.0216$, which is less than 0.05 (Figure 24, a). This means significant differences in the number of ticks collected on different means. Similar differences were observed when comparing the efficiency of pairs of means of collection: a flag on 2 parallel metal rods and a traditional flag, $p = 0.0283$ (Figure 24, b); a flag on the L-shaped holder and the traditional flag, $p = 0.0119$ (Figure 24, c). When comparing the flag on 2 parallel metal rods and the flag on the L-shaped holder, $p = 0.6015$ (Figure 24, d), which is more than 0.05. This indicates the absence of significant differences in the effectiveness of the application of these means of collection.

Summarizing the obtained results, supported by an appropriate automated mathematical program for intelligent database processing, it can be argued that the flag with two parallel metal rods and the flag with a "L"-shaped handle have significant advantages over the traditional flag for collecting ticks in natural habitats.

5.1. Standardization of Tick Population Indicators

Research and practical activities related to the study and evaluation of specific phenomena and processes require the use of objective criteria. If these criteria are expressed in numerical values and are related to objects, phenomena, or processes, it is preferable to present them in International System (SI) units.

The obtained data should be reproducible and convergent, meaning they should not depend on subjective or other influencing circumstances. The scientific value of research results lies in their reproducibility and comparability. This necessitates the use of standardized methods, and the quantitative indicators obtained should be reflected in a universally accepted system of measurement standards [145].

In practical and scientific epidemiology, there is a need for collecting ticks, particularly for studying their species composition, distribution range, biocenosis characteristics, ecological influences, population status, and infection with pathogens. Such information is essential for assessing epidemic threats, predicting the activity of natural foci of tick-borne infections, and evaluating the stability of the parasitic system, which depends on the stability of its components, specifically in the case of tick populations, where one of the characteristics is population size [146].

Traditionally, to assess the abundance of Ixodidae ticks, so-called zoo-parasitological indices are used, namely: abundance, dominance, detection, and others [146, 147]. These approaches and evaluations do not involve determining the level or density of ticks in specific territories, i.e., they are not oriented towards determining the number of individuals per unit area. The main objective indicator of tick abundance in territories, in our opinion, could be the settlement index or colonization index, which refers to the number of ticks per unit area.

An important component of epidemiological surveillance is predicting the epidemiological situation, which includes assessing the epidemic potential of natural foci of tick-borne infections. Most of these infections are zoonotic, thus they are of interest from the perspective of the One Health concept (human and animal health). However, currently, there are no unified standardized methods for assessing tick habitat infestation in medical and veterinary fields.

This issue needs special attention because it stems from the absence of standardized methods for tick collection, techniques, methodologies, and standardized units of assessment. The collection of ticks for the purpose of assessing their population density significantly differs from collecting ticks to assess their infection, infestation, or species composition.

Methods used in practice involve quantitative assessment expressed as the number of individuals per unit area or unit time, such as the number of ticks collected per flag-kilometre or flag-hour. Based on these, a density index is calculated [139, 146]. While these units of measurement are widely accepted, they are not enforced by current regulatory acts. Results obtained are difficult to compare across different years or regions because in some cases, they are derived from the length of the route in kilometres, and in others, from the time spent in hours, depending on the skills and techniques of the collectors. Each collector's collection technique varies based on their movement speed, intensity and range of flag movements, length of the flag, the part of the fabric in contact with vegetation, direction, and speed of movement. Consequently, the length of the route in an hour is always different. Thus, the indicators obtained in this way do not take into account the surveyed area, and therefore do not accurately characterize the density of tick habitats. The size of the flag and the type of fabric are also not regulated. Some researchers consider the use of indicators such as the number of ticks per averaged accounting hour [148] impractical and incorrect. Others argue that the periodicity of inspection methods should also be regulated [149].

Recognizing the practical value of the traditional flagging method and its use in assessing tick species composition, infection rates, and infestation with pathogenic microorganisms, particularly in average terrain and dense vegetation conditions, we consider it appropriate to propose a patented tool for quantitative assessment of habitat occupancy [150, 151]. This tool consists of a square fabric with sides measuring 1 meter. The front and back sides have metal rods inserted into special loops, ensuring proper stretching and continuous contact of the entire fabric with the ground surface. The weight of the rods facilitates the fabric's adherence to the vegetation cover. The density of contact can be adjusted by varying the weight of the rods. The consistently working fixed area of 1 m^2 allows for calculating the total surveyed area.

	Kruskal-Wallis ANOVA by Ranks; Number of ticks (Spreadsheet_30_10_18) Independent (grouping) variable: Means of tick collection Kruskal-Wallis test: H (2, N=15) =7,668694 p =,0216			
Depend.: Number of ticks	Code	Valid N	Sum of Ranks	Mean Rank
Flag of flannel on 2 metal rods	113	5	53,00000	10,60000
Flag of flannel on L-like device	110	5	49,50000	9,90000
Flag of waffle fabric	107	5	17,50000	3,50000

(a)

	Kruskal-Wallis ANOVA by Ranks; Number of ticks (Spreadsheet_30_10_18) Independent (grouping) variable: Means of tick collection Kruskal-Wallis test: H (1, N=10) =4,810909 p =,0283			
Depend.: Number of ticks	Code	Valid N	Sum of Ranks	Mean Rank
Flag of flannel on 2 metal rods	113	5	38,00000	7,600000
Flag of waffle fabric	107	5	17,00000	3,400000

(b)

	Kruskal-Wallis ANOVA by Ranks; Number of ticks (Spreadsheet_30_10_18) Independent (grouping) variable: Means of tick collection Kruskal-Wallis test: H (1, N=10) =6,321951 p =,0119			
Depend.: Number of ticks	Code	Valid N	Sum of Ranks	Mean Rank
Flag of flannel on L-like device	110	5	39,50000	7,900000
Flag of waffle fabric	107	5	15,50000	3,100000

(c)

	Kruskal-Wallis ANOVA by Ranks; Number of ticks (Spreadsheet_30_10_18) Independent (grouping) variable: Means of tick collection Kruskal-Wallis test: H (1, N=10) =,2727273 p =,6015			
Depend.: Number of ticks	Code	Valid N	Sum of Ranks	Mean Rank
Flag of flannel on 2 metal rods	113	5	30,00000	6,000000
Flag of flannel on L-like device	110	5	25,00000	5,000000

(d)

Figure 24. The results of the application of the non-parametric Kruskel-Wallis test: a – all 3 means of collection; b – 1–3 means; c – 2–3 means; d – 1–2 means.

This approach significantly differs from methods based on route length and duration. Assessing population density by counting individuals relative to area truly reflects habitat density, which we believe holds promise for standardizing metrics. A fixed collection time (1 hour) and average travel speed (approximately 2 km/h), along with clear regulation of inspection frequency, enable comparison of the number of collected ticks with the surveyed area and calculation of a corresponding index that objectively characterizes density, i.e., the number of individuals per unit area.

As of today, various indicators are employed to assess phenomena, demanding standardization of measurement units. Ideally, these units should align with the metric system to ensure universal accessibility of information. The application of such indicators will bring practical epidemiology closer to achieving one of the goals of evidence-based medicine – standardization of activities [152].

An objective assessment of tick population on a territory, combined with other indicators such as infection rates and degree of infestation with pathogenic microorganisms, forms the basis for developing criteria to assess epidemic risks, a task of modern epidemiological surveillance systems. Risk assessment is a scientifically grounded process involving the identification and characterization of hazards, impact assessment, and risk characterization. Epidemiological surveillance of infectious diseases requires quantitative characteristics of the components (driving forces) of the epidemic process, enabling the identification of cause-and-effect relationships. Developing quantitative characteristics of individual components of the epidemic process is important for developing comprehensive risk assessment methodologies.

Ticks and their parasites (pathogens) constitute an important component (parasitic system) of the ecological level of the epidemic process in many natural foci diseases.

Measurement units based on tradition must yield to mathematical and natural data [153, 154]. Counting many living biological objects is performed in accepted practice by calculating their quantity per unit of surveyed area [155].

Over a period of 3 years, acarological surveys were conducted in forest biotopes across different climatic-geographic zones of Ternopil region and park territories in Ternopil city. Based on survey results, a population density index was calculated. The obtained results were compared with the density index determined by traditional methods applied concurrently. To compare specific indicators, a visibility index was calculated [156]. Distances were recorded in meters. The collection duration was 1 hour, with an average speed of movement of 2 km/h.

The research was conducted in 8 biotopes across 5 forestry districts in 3 climatic-geographic zones (Small Polissia, Cold and Warm Podilia (Dniester Canyon)) in Ternopil region, and 5 parks in Ternopil city from 2017 to 2019.

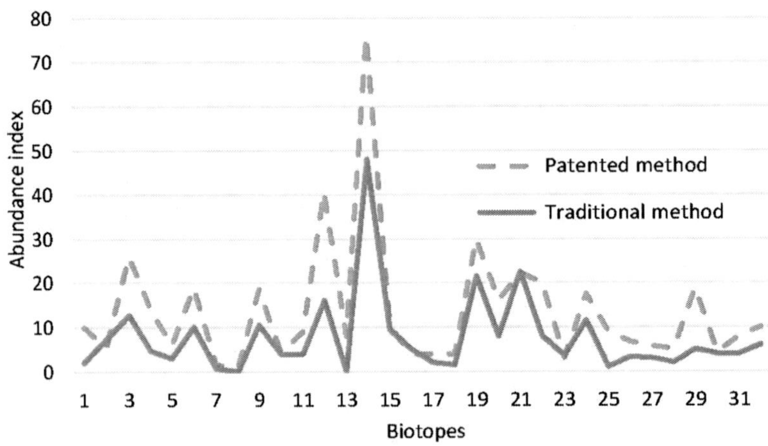

Figure 25. Results of tick collection by patented and traditional methods.

In order to obtain objective data to compare the qualitative and quantitative characteristics of the traditional means of collecting ticks (the flag) and the means we proposed with a permanently working standard surface [157], ticks were collected simultaneously by both methods on the same territories. Routes were planned in advance and their length was determined in advance. The average speed of movement was calculated. The means of collection were inspected at the same time. The work was carried out in the same time interval (10^{00}–12^{00}), temperature, air velocity, and atmospheric pressure were measured. When planning field work, possible changes in the weather, weather phenomena, and the presence of dew were taken into account.

Statistical processing of the obtained results showed that there is a significant difference in the number of ticks collected by traditional and patented methods ($p = 0.027$), which confirms the higher efficiency of the patented method. Figure 25 shows the value of the tick abundance index in the studied 32 biotopes. The abundance index was calculated based on the results of the tick collection by patented and traditional methods.

The obtained results were analysed using the oscillation coefficient. The results of the statistical analysis are shown in Figures 26 and 27.

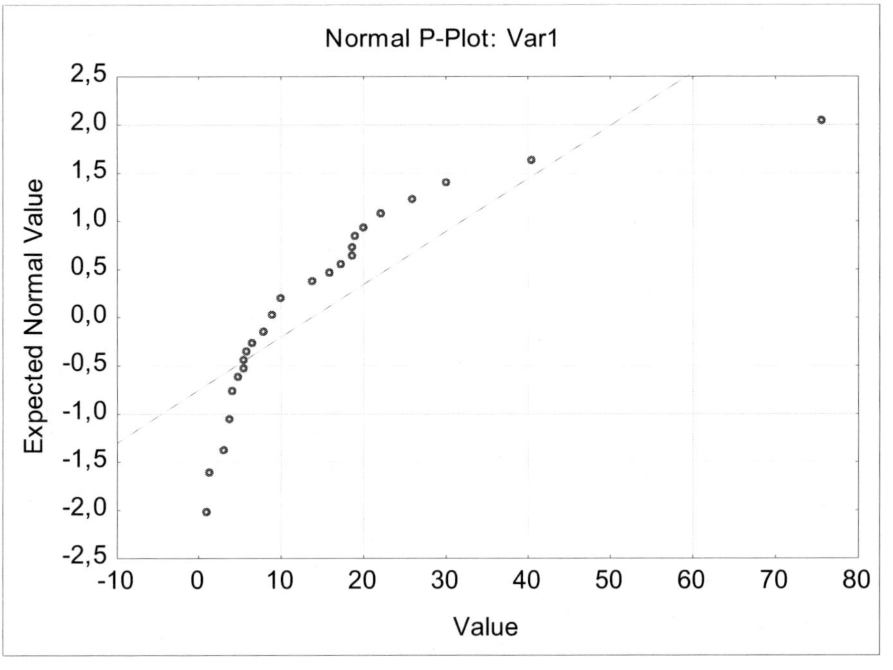

Figure 26. The coefficient of oscillation when using the patented method.

The studied variables are independent, but each of them is closely related to the same general population – the total number of ticks in the surveyed territory. Therefore, the nature of the distribution of ticks in the studied territories, established by the methods we suggest and generally accepted methods, has the same normal distribution. However, the coefficient of oscillation, which reflects the share of the range of variation of a random variable in the average value and which is a relative measure of the absolute dispersion of values in the statistical population in the results of research conducted by our method, is smaller (5.479452) than in the data obtained by the generally accepted method (6.282209).

Therefore, the amount of deviation of the research results from the actual number of ticks in our case is smaller than in the study by the generally accepted method. This allows for a more accurate calculation and assessment of tick population parameters of biotopes or surveyed territories. Such indicators are important for assessing the level of tick danger. Unlike the existing method, the method we proposed allows you to present the results of work in the International System of Units (SI) and conduct quantitative comparisons of your own results with the results of other studies.

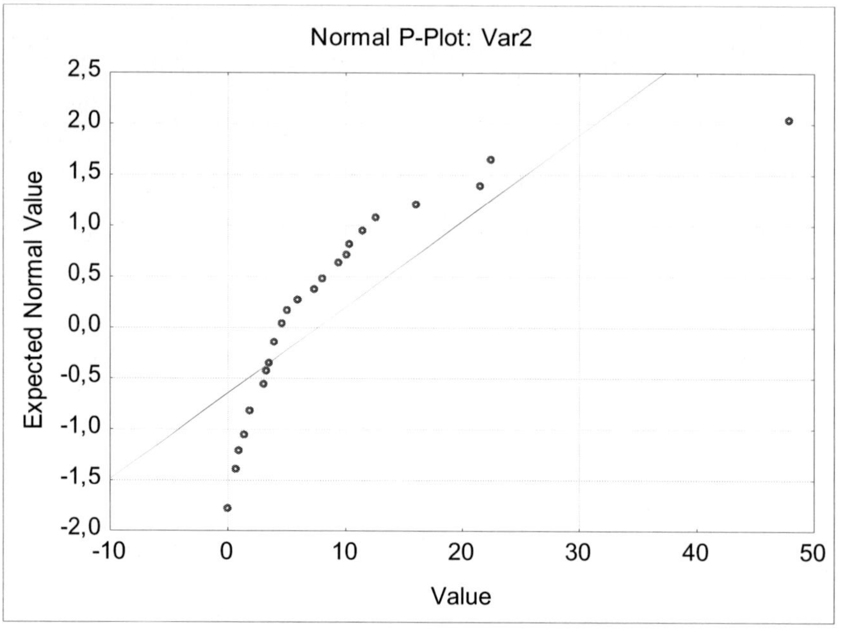

Figure 27. The coefficient of oscillation when using the traditional method.

Using a device with a working surface area of 1 m^2 with sides of 1×1 m and recording the distance in meters travelled in 1 hour (3600 s) through the GPS system in a mobile smartphone application or using a pedometer with a constant average speed of movement of 2 km/h allows to determine (calculate) the surveyed area (S) (1):

$$S = S_1 \times L, \quad (1)$$

where S_1 is the area of the working surface; L is the length of the route.

Population density (index) (M) is calculated according to the formula (2):

$$M = M_1/S, \quad (2)$$

where M_1 is the total number of ticks; S is the surveyed area.

It is possible to calculate indicators per square meter, acre, or hectare.

The practice of collecting ticks indicates that a single contact of the fabric of a flag or the continuously working surface of a tick collection tool with the surveyed area does not capture all existing individuals. Repeat contacts are also effective. The ratio of ticks collected during initial and subsequent contacts can vary, typically ranging from 70% to 30% up to 90% to 10%, averaging around 80% to 20%. This requires the application of an appropriate correction coefficient, which should be 1/5 of the total number of ticks collected. Therefore, the formula (3), supplemented with the coefficient, is as follows:

$$M = M_1 \times 1.2/S, \quad (3)$$

where 1.2 is the correction factor.

The method of assessing the density of tick populations (infestations) in biotopes by counting the number of individuals per unit area or population index is based on the use of the International System of Units (SI), making it universal and allowing for standardized results. The population index is suitable for evaluation and comparison in acarological research across various fields of science and practice, accurately characterizing the degree of tick infestation in an area. It can be used to assess the epidemic risk of relevant zoonotic infectious diseases. The effectiveness of the patented tool and method is statistically higher.

The infection of ticks with pathogenic microorganisms affects the epidemiological well-being of territories, as these arachnids serve as reservoirs and vectors for transmitting pathogens of many zoonotic diseases. Ticks facilitate the circulation of various bacteria in natural foci as an important component of parasitic systems.

5.2. Natural Foci of Tick-Borne Infections and Tick Infestation

In many areas, stable natural foci of diseases transmitted by ticks exist, but their epidemiological potential is insufficiently understood [146]. One reason for this situation could be the lack of information regarding the presence of natural foci of zoonotic infectious diseases, the spectrum of pathogens, and the circulation maintained within parasitic systems and their subsystems, which have emerged and function particularly in urbanized areas. These systems, supported by hosts such as migratory birds and the introduction of mammals, are linked to parasitic systems not only in adjacent territories but also across other countries and continents. It is believed that birds play a significant role in the migration of ticks from one biotope to another.

Thanks to long-term research conducted in the Lviv region, stable natural foci of tick infections with polyhostal and polyvector parasitic systems were discovered. The main vectors are performed by *I. ricinus* and *D. reticulatus* with a significant advantage of the first species [146].

In Ternopil region, for the purpose of assessing natural infection, ticks collected from humans were studied [120]. At the same time, the territorial origin of arthropods was not taken into account. During earlier studies using dark field microscopy, we confirmed infection of ticks with bacteria from the Spirochaetaceae family, and also established the degree of infection [158].

The lack of specific information about pathogens circulating in a certain area is one of the reasons for low or no registration of a number of zoonotic diseases [48, 146, 159]. At the same time, information on the infection of ticks with Borrelia, in particular in the USA, is the basis for establishing the degree of epidemic risk, which determines the tactics of urgent antibacterial prophylaxis of Lyme disease after a tick attack without its laboratory examination.

Ternopil region is located in the forest-steppe zone. The area covered by forests is approximately 199.3 thousand hectares, predominantly consisting of mixed broadleaf forests. Due to specific weather and geographic conditions, three main zones can be identified: Small Polissia in the northern part, Cold Podilia including Opillia in the central part, and Warm Podilia including the Dniester Canyon in the southwest and south of the region. These zones differ in altitude, average annual temperatures, precipitation levels, duration of warm and cold periods, number of sunny and cloudy days, soil types and composition, and belong to different water basins. In Small Polissia, coniferous forests predominate, covering a sandy plain with pine forests adjacent to the Ikva River valley. In the Dniester Canyon, which has a climate similar to the Mediterranean, the biotope is located in the meander of the Dniester River, partially constrained by sculptural-erosion relief features. The biotopes of Podilia are formed by deciduous forests and shrubs.

A total of 8 forest biotopes were identified that best reflect the characteristics specific to each zone. The distance between the northernmost biotope (Velyki Berezhtsi village) and the southernmost (Mushkativka village) is approximately 200 km.

In recent years, like in the entire Ternopil region, there has been a significant increase in LB incidence and the number of populated areas affected. The territory of Ternopil region is recognized as endemic for LB [160].

The aim of the study was to determine the infection rates of ticks with specific pathogens in different weather and geographic zones of Ternopil region (Small Polissia, Cold and Warm Podilia), compare the degrees of tick infection and the spectrum of their pathogens, and investigate the structure of rodent communities as a component of parasitic systems.

During the field seasons of 2017–2019, ticks were collected in 8 forest biotopes, including near Velyki Berezhtsi (Small Polissia zone), Naraiiv, Rai, Vertelka (Cold Podilia zone), Beremiany, Khmeleva, Bila, Mushkativka (Warm Podilia zone). Villages Beremiany and Khmeleva are located in the Dniester Canyon, while villages Rai and Naraiiv are in Opillia. In addition to collecting ticks from vegetation using traditional flags and an improved method, ticks were combed from captured rodents in the same biotopes. The total route length covered was 81.7 km.

A total of 1089 ticks were collected, of which 864 were from vegetation, 225 were combed from caught rodents; 503 ticks were examined by the PCR method for the detection of DNA fragments of pathogenic bacteria, 386 – by the method of dark field microscopy for the presence of Borrelia, 200 ticks were transferred for research to the Lublin Institute of Rural Medicine (Republic of Poland) within the framework of a cooperation agreement with I. Horbachevsky Ternopil National Medical University.

For the PCR investigation, ticks were divided into 62 pools based on the following criteria: collection site, collection method (flagging, combing), species, sex, and developmental stage. Of these pools, 3 were D. reticulatus and 59 were I. ricinus. Samples of biomaterial suspension in a special solution from test kits were prepared from individuals pooled together. For each biotope and climatic-geographical zone, a density index was calculated to characterize the tick population density on the territory.

Ticks were collected from rodents and their numbers were counted using the trap-line method. Traps were checked 24 hours after installation. In total, 4500 trap-days were completed, capturing 390 rodents of 8 species. Generalized data from PCR analysis of ticks collected in forest biotopes from different climatic-geographical zones of Ternopil region are presented in Table 6.

Over the entire period of observation, the lowest average level of the tick abundance index was established in the area of Small Polissia (7.3). In the zone of Cold Podilia, it was 11.1 with variations in biotopes from 3.7 (Vertelka) to 19.1 (Naraiiv). In Warm Podilia zone, the index was 11.2, with fluctuations in biotopes from 8.0 (Khmeleva) to 13.1 (Beremiany). That is, an increase in the index was observed from north to south, from the zone of coniferous forests (Small Polissia) to mixed (forest-steppe) and in the direction of increasing average annual air temperatures (Figure 28).

Table 6. The results of the collection and PCR study of ticks from forest biotopes of different climatic and geographical zones of Ternopil region

Parameter	Zone, biotope											
		Small Polissia		Cold Podilia				Warm Podilia				
	Total	Velyki Berezhtsi	Total	Naraiiv	Rai	Vertelka	Total	Beremiany	Khmeleva	Bila	Mushkativka	Total
Abundance Index	10,5	7,3	7,3	19,1	8,5	3,7	11,1	13,1	8,0	11,1	12,3	11,2
Number of ticks	503	40	40	96	8	46	150	113	89	43	68	313
Number of pools	62	8	8	14	2	5	21	11	8	6	8	33
Number of pools with pathogens	40	4	4	12	2	5	19	7	2	4	4	17
Number of pathogens	56	6	6	15	2	6	23	9	2	7	9	27
% of total number	100,0	10,7	10,7	26,7	3,6	10,7	41,1	10,7	3,6	12,5	16,1	48,2
Including: *B. burgdorferi s. l.*	30	4	4	10	1	3	14	4	1	4	3	12
B. miyamotoi	3	–	–	1	–	1	2	–	–	–	1	1
Babesia sp.	8	–	–	1	1	1	3	–	1	2	2	5
A. phagocytophilum	15	2	2	3	-	1	4	5	-	1	3	9
E. muris	–	–	–	–	–	–	–	–	–	–	–	
E. chaffeensis	–	–	–	–	–	–	–	–	–	–	–	

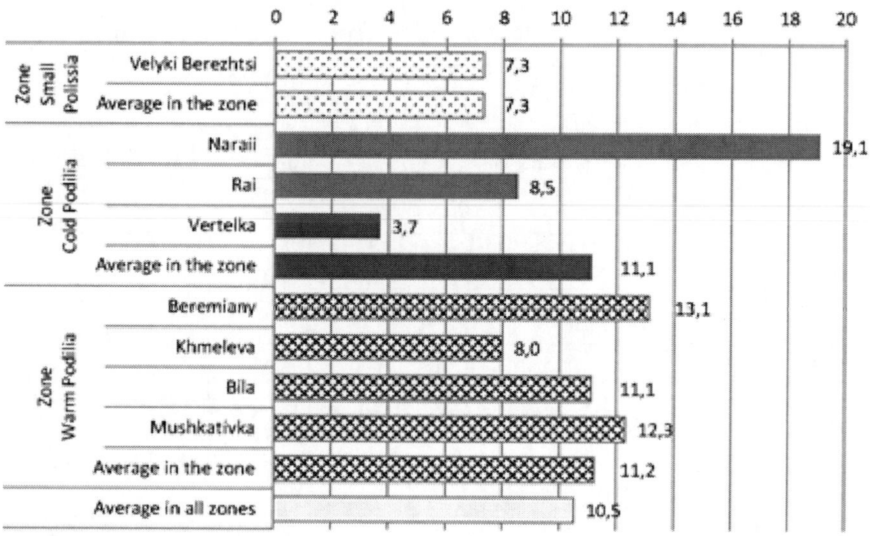

Figure 28. Tick abundance index in forest biotopes in 2017–2019.

Among the ticks collected, 96.2% were individuals of the species I. ricinus, of which 33.2% were females, 30.4% were males, and 36.4% were nymphs. The share of *D. reticulatus* was 3.7% of all collected ticks, 65.6% of them were females, 34.4% were males. Ticks of the *D. reticulatus* species were collected only in 2 biotopes (Velyki Berezhtsi and Naraiiv). Their geographical coordinates: north latitude – 50°5' and 49°31,' east longitude – 25°36' and 24°46,' respectively.

The percentage of rodents caught in traps also increased towards the south and in the zone of Warm Podilia exceeded the average for the zones (Table 7). In this zone, 8 species of mixed rodents were captured, 5 in Small Polissia, and 4 in Cold Podilia. Other researchers also note the relatively low abundance and lower diversity of mixed rodents in coniferous biotopes in the Kremenets Mountains National Park [161]. They highlight the dominance of bank voles in coniferous biotopes. In Velyki Berezhtsi biotope, its relative abundance reached 35.5%, similar to the yellow-necked mouse, likely due to its immediate proximity to the floodplain of the Ikva River.

A high percentage (18.5%) of rodents caught in traps was observed in Warm Podilia zone in the Mushkativka biotope, located within an oak-hornbeam forest and bordering a water body and meadows.

Table 7. Percentage of murine rodents caught in traps in different climatic-geographical zones of Ternopil region

Weather and geographical zone	Number of trap-days	Number of rodents falling into traps	Percentage of falling into traps
Small Polissia	700	31	4,4
Cold Podilia	1350	70	5,2
Warm Podilia	2450	289	11,8
Total	4500	390	8,7

Table 8. Number of the main species of rodents caught in different climatic-geographic zones of Ternopil region

Rodent species	Total number of the caught rodents	Zone					
		Small Polissia		Cold Podilia		Warm Podilia	
		Absolute number	%	Absolute number	%	Absolute number	%
Yellow-necked mouse – Sylvaemus flavicollis	102	11	10,8	29	28,4	62	60,8
Wood mouse – Sylvaemus sylvaticus	149	3	2,0	20	13,4	126	84,6
Striped field mouse – Apodemus agrarius	34	5	13,4	7	20,6	22	64,7
Harvest mouse – Micromys minutus	2	1	50,0	–	–	1	50,0
Common vole – Microtus arvalis sensu stricto	58	–	–	11	19,0	47	81,0
Bank vole – Myodes glareolus	41	11	26,8	10	24,4	20	48,8
Dormouse – Muscardinus avellanarius	1	–	–	–	–	1	100,0
Common shrew – Sorex araneus	3	–	–	–	–	3	100,0

The species composition of caught murine rodents in different weather and geographical zones of Ternopil region is shown in Table 8 and Figure 29.

The results of the study on communities of murine rodents indicate that habitats and climatic-geographic zones differ in the abundance and species composition of these rodents. The most widespread species are the wood mouse and the yellow-necked mouse, which are present in all zones. Their abundance increases from north to south. The bank vole is most abundant in Small Polissia zone. Warm Podilia zone, particularly the southernmost habitat with oak-hornbeam forests and undergrowth dominated by hazel, has the highest rodent abundance and species diversity. Only in this zone were the dormouse and common shrew captured.

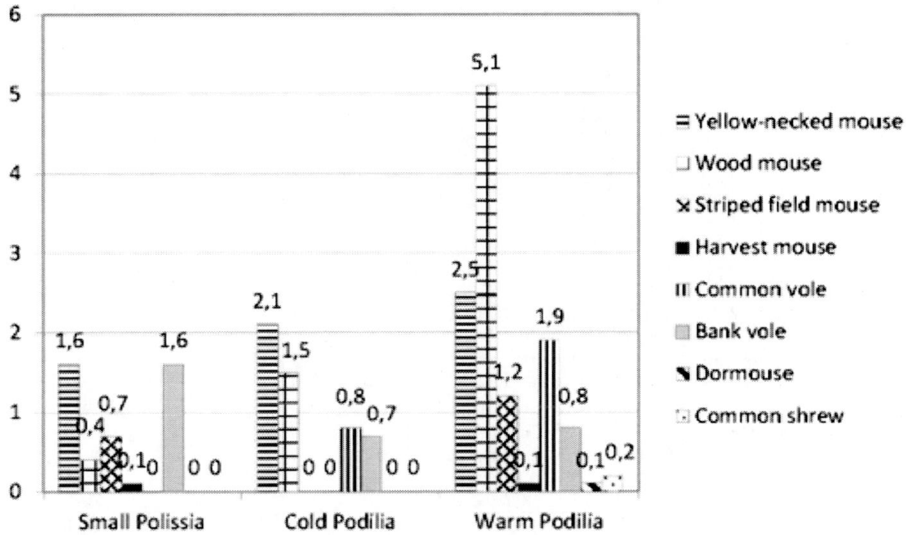

Figure 29. The frequency of entrapment of certain species of rodents in weather and geographical zones of Ternopil region, %.

Table 9. The frequency of detection of pathogens in ticks from certain climatic and geographical zones, %

Pathogen	Zone		
	Small Polissia	Cold Podilia	Warm Podilia
B. burgdorferi s. l.	66,7	60,9	44,5
B. miyamotoi	0	8,7	3,7
Babesia sp.	0	13,0	18,5
A. phagocytophilum	33,3	17,4	33,3
Total	100,0	100,0	100,0

According to tick research conducted by the PCR method, DNA of B. burgdorferi s. l., B. miyamotoi, A. phagocytophilum, *Babesia sp.* was detected in the forest biotopes of Ternopil region (Table 9). At the same time, the causative agents of monocytic ehrlichiosis, i.e., *E. muris* and *E. chaffeensis*, were not found.

The proportion of B. burgdorferi s. l. accounted for 53.6% of all pathogen findings (Figure 30). At the same time, their percentage was 66.7 in the area of Small Polissia, 60.9 in Cold Podilia, and 44.5 in Warm Podilia. That is, the share of these borrelia in the sum of positive findings decreased in the direction from north to south.

At the same time, the percentage of positive results in general and the findings of *Babesia sp.*, *B. miyamotoi* had the opposite trend.

Similar tendencies in Warm Podilia zone are mainly formed by 2 typical forest biotopes, namely: Bila and Mushkativka. On the other hand, 2 biotopes from this zone belonging to the

Dniester Canyon (Beremiany and Khmeleva) are inferior to the first in terms of the percentage of positive results and the spectrum of pathogens. Perhaps this is a manifestation of the autonomy of these biotopes and is due to their less accessibility for wild animals, the predominance among feeders of small rodents, whose migration is sharply limited due to the geological and geographical features of the canyon biotopes. Outside the canyon, these biotopes are surrounded by fields with intensive agriculture, settlements are located nearby, and there is a significant anthropogenic impact.

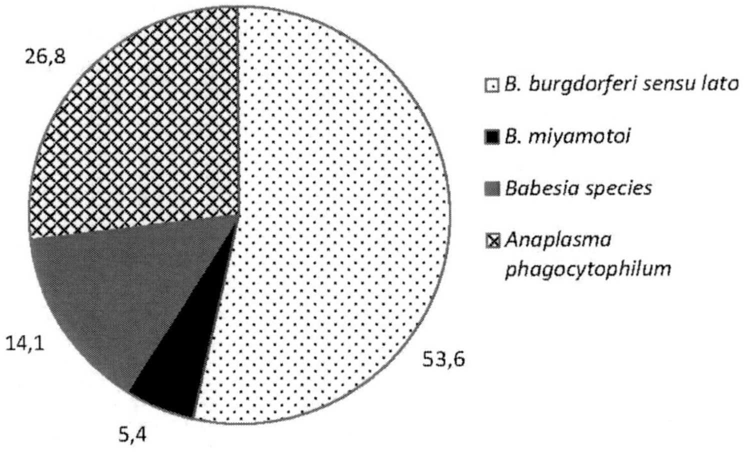

Figure 30. The composition of pathogens detected in tick pools from forest biotopes, %.

The characteristic feature of Small Polissia zone is its predominantly pine forests, with sandy soils influencing the herbaceous cover and resulting in the absence of undergrowth, significant insolation, and lower relative humidity. The findings of ticks in this zone are similar to those near the floodplain of the Ikva River, characterized by the presence of deciduous trees and herbaceous cover similar to meadows. In Small Polissia zone, 56.3% of individuals of the species D. reticulatus were collected, from which 3 pools were formed (one of them positive for *B. burgdorferi s. l.*), and 5 pools from *I. ricinus* (3 of them positive for both *B. burgdorferi s. l.* and *A. phagocytophilum*, with one pool showing these pathogens in combination).

Obviously, the peculiarities of the flora and fauna, geographical remoteness, and weather conditions contributed to the formation of various natural foci of tick-borne infections on the territory of Ternopil region, which differ in the number and composition of transmission vectors, the species composition and number of murine rodents, and the spectrum of pathogens that reside in parasitic systems. Other researchers also point to such differences in different territories of the country [162, 163]. It is worth noting that with a relatively close tick abundance index, the Podilia biotopes differed from Small Polissia biotopes in a larger spectrum of species and percentages of detected pathogens (Figure 31).

The structure of positive results of studies of tick pools attests to the highest prevalence of *B. burgdorferi s. l.* (Figure 32, 33). It prevails both with a combination of pathogens and without their combinations. *B. burgdorferi s. l.* is present in all established variants of the combination of pathogens. The share of *A. phagocytophilum* is 1.4 times smaller, and *Babesia sp.* – 2.5 times. The least common pathogen is *B. miyamotoi*, it was detected in only 3 pools out of 40 positive ones.

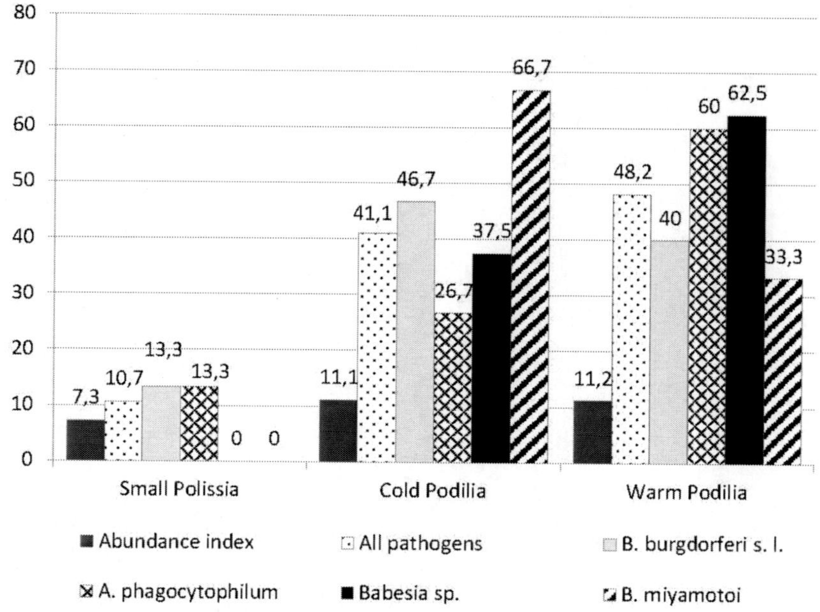

Figure 31. Comparison of the tick abundance index and the percentage of pathogens among those detected in different climatic and geographical zones of Ternopil region.

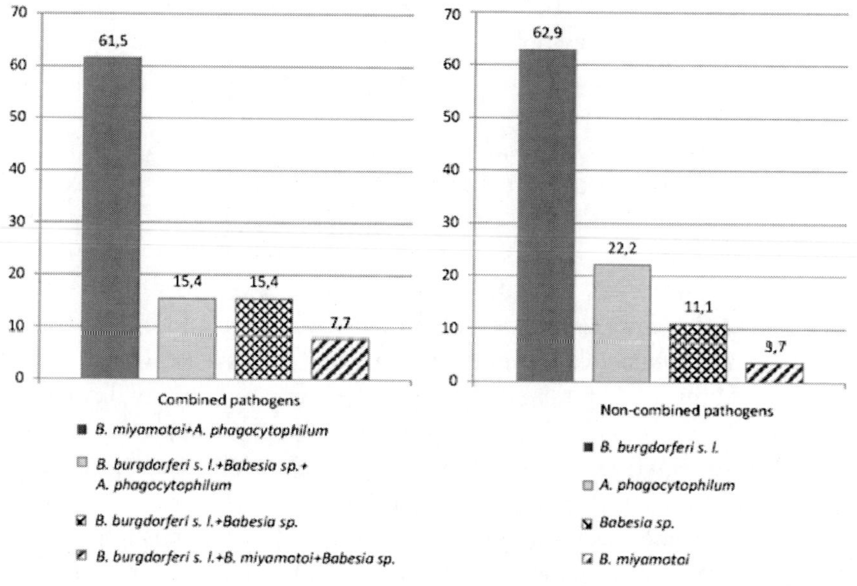

Figure 32. Percentages of infection rate of ticks with pathogens and their combinations in pools.

The ratio of the number of pathogens and pools with a positive result in Small Polissia zone is 1.5 (6/4), in Cold Podilia zone – 1.2 (23/19), in Warm Podilia zone – 1.6 (27/17). That is, the combination of pathogens in one pool is somewhat more often observed in the south of the region in Warm Podilia zone. Here, the coefficient is higher in typical forest biotopes – 2.0 (16/8) and lower in the Dniester Canyon biotopes – 1.2 (11/9).

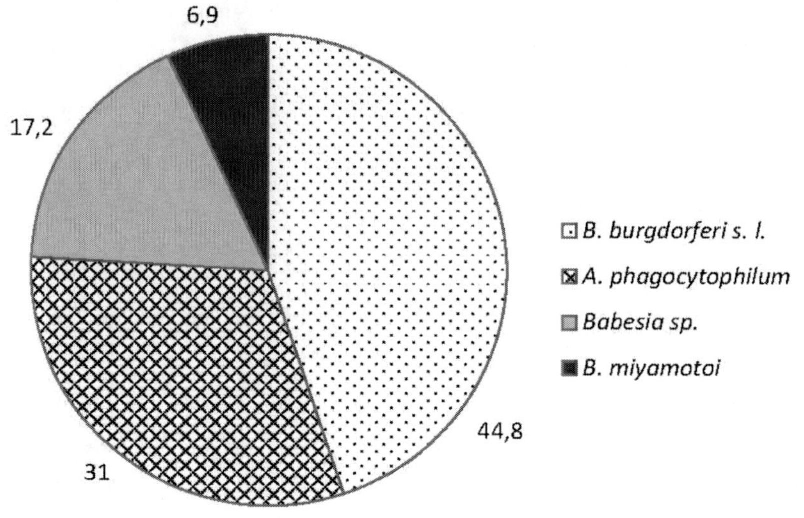

Figure 33. Percentages of pathogens in pools of ticks with combined contamination.

Among ticks, males and females accounted for 72.5% of all detected pathogens, in particular, 80% of *A. phagocytophilum*, 70% of *B. burgdorferi s. l.*, 66.6% of *B. miyamotoi. Babesia sp.* were more often found in pools of larvae and nymphs (62.5%). The higher infection rate of adults with pathogenic bacteria is obviously caused by changes in the number of hosts, because *I. ricinus* and *D. reticulatus* belong to ticks with a three-year development cycle. In the literature, it was also reported that nymphs are less often infected, in particular with anaplasmas, compared to adult ticks [164]. Presumably, this is due to the inability of transphase transmission of individual pathogens.

Thus, there are conditions in the forest biotopes of 3 climatic and geographical zones of Ternopil region and components for sustainable functioning of parasitic systems of natural foci of tick infections. The stability of the systems is ensured by the presence of Borrelia and other pathogens, a sufficient number of ticks, 8 types of rodents and favourable environmental factors.

In forest biotopes, I. ricinus dominates. *D. reticulatus* occurs only in 2 biotopes. The tick abundance index in the Podilia area is higher than in Small Polissia area.

It was established for the first time that ticks in the forest biotopes of Ternopil region are infected with *B. burgdorferi s. l.*, *B. miyamotoi*, *Babesia sp.*, *A. phagocytophilum*. Predominated by *B. burgdorferi s. l.* and *A. phagocytophilum*. *B. miyamotoi* and *Babesia sp.* were found only in Podilia, more often in Warm Podilia.

The number of ticks, the spectrum of pathogens, the species composition, and the number of murine rodents increase from the north (Small Polissia) to the south (Warm Podilia). The dependence between the tick abundance index, the number of hosts and the spectrum of pathogens circulating in rodent populations is observed. Infection of imago with the investigated pathogens is higher than that of larvae and nymphs of ticks.

The results of the collection of ticks, their research by the PCR method, and the detection of DNA fragments of individual bacteria, which are shown in Tables 6, 9 and Figures 28, 30–32, testify to the existence of a direct connection between them. In particular, the correlation coefficient between the tick abundance index and the number of pools with detected bacteria is 0.76; with the number of detected bacteria – 0.80; with the number of detected *B. burgdorferi s. l.* – 0.76. The correlation coefficient between the number of detected *B. burgdorferi s. l.* and the number of pools in which pathogenic bacteria were detected is 0.95; with the number of detected pathogens – 0.92 and with the percentage of the total number of pathogenic bacteria – 0.93. The given correlation coefficients range in the intervals of strong (0.70–0.89) and very strong (0.90–0.99) direct relationship.

However, the situation with the diagnosis of other diseases, in which ticks are also carriers and reservoirs, repeats the recent history of LD. This primarily concerns HGA, babesiosis, granulocytic and monocytic ehrlichiosis. They began to be studied in the USA from the end of the 80s of the last century. A single mechanism of transmission, common reservoirs and vectors contribute to the formation of classic natural foci of transmissible infectious diseases combined with borreliosis.

In urbanized areas, human activities such as neglecting animal keeping requirements, sanitary conditions in settlements, disorder in green zones and residential areas, irregular rodent control measures, establishment of animal shelters, introduction of wild animals, and the overwintering of migratory birds due to warming contribute to an increase in the number of hosts, some of which are infected with pathogens, leading to higher tick density in populated areas.

Table 10. The results of the collection and research of ticks from the parks of Ternopil by the polymerase chain reaction method in 2018–2019

Ticks, pools, pathogens	Park																				Total			
	Taras Shevchenko Park				"Topilche"				"Zahrebellia"				"Zdorovia"				Natsionalnoho vidrodzhennia							
	males	females	nymphs/larvae	total	males	females	nymphs/larvae	total	males	females	nymphs/larvae	total	males	females	nymphs/larvae	total	males	females	nymphs/larvae	total	males	females	nymphs/larvae	total
Number of collected ticks	–	1*	1*	2*	10	18	6	34	51	45	66	162	11	14	12	37	58	34	31	123	130	112	116	358
Pools	–	1	1	2	2	7	3	12	7	6	7	20	2	2	3	7	10	7	5	22	21	23	19	63
Pools with positive results	–	–	1	1	1	4	2	7	6	4	5	15	1	–	2	3	9	6	4	19	17	14	14	45
Number of detected pathogens, including:	–	–	1	1	1	6	3	10	7	7	8	22	2	–	3	5	12	12	4	28	22	25	19	66
B. burgdorferi s. l.	–	–	1	1	–	2		2	4	3	2	9	1	–	2	3	5	6	3	14	10	11	8	29
B. miyamotoi	–	–	–	–	–	2		2		1	1	2	–	–	–	–	2	1	–	3	2	4	1	7
A. phagocyto-philum	–	–	–	–	–	1	1	2	2	2	1	5	1	–		1	3	3	1	7	6	6	3	15
Babesia sp.	–	–	–	–	1	1	2	4	1	1	4	6	–	–	1	1	2	2	–	4	4	4	7	15
E. muris	–	–	–	–	–	–	–	–	–	–	–	–	–	–	–	–	–	–	–	–	–	–	–	–
E. chaffeensis	–	–	–	–	–	–	–	–	–	–	–	–	–	–	–	–	–	–	–	–	–	–	–	–

Note. * – ticks of the *D. reticulatus* species.

During 2018–2019, entomological research was conducted in 5 parks of the city of Ternopil. 358 ticks were collected. They were divided into 63 pools according to such characteristics as: place, time of collection, species, sex, stages of development. Two pools consisted of *D. reticulatus*: female and nymph. The rest of the pools (61) consisted of *I. ricinus*: 111 females, 130 males, 115 larvae and nymphs.

Out of the pool of individuals, a combined sample of biomaterial was prepared, which was a suspension of ticks, using a special solution included in the test system sets.

The material obtained in this way was studied by the PCR method in real time using test systems produced by "Vektor-Best" in order to detect DNA fragments of *B. burgdorferi s. l.*, *B. miyamotoi*, *Babesia sp.*, *A. phagocytophilum*, *E. muris* and *E. chaffeensis*.

The number of ticks, their distribution by genera, sex, stages of development, formation of pools, and the results of molecular genetic studies are shown in Table 10.

The simultaneous circulation of several *Borrelia* genospecies and other pathogenic microorganisms in the tick population results in mixed infections. A number of works are devoted to this problem [165–170]. Modern studies confirm the significant prevalence of ticks in urbanized areas and landscapes and the dominance of *I. ricinus* [171–175].

In the available literature, we have not found information about the causative agents of tick-borne infections in the territory of Ternopil. In the past, episodic entomological surveys of Ternopil were conducted, but they were not systematic. The result of such studies were calculations of the number of ticks using the abundance index.

According to our data, the vector and reservoir of the identified pathogens in the parasitic systems of the park landscapes of Ternopil is *I. ricinus*, which dominates in all 5 parks and accounts for 99.4% of ticks collected during 2 years. Only in one pool DNA fragments of *B. burgdorferi s. l.* were found in *D. reticulatus*.

Table 11. Detection of pathogenic microorganisms in pools with *I. ricinus*

Pathogen	Total	Including	
		in combinations	separately
B. burgdorferi s. l.	28	12	16
B. miyamotoi	7	4	3
Babesia sp.	15	5	10
A. phagocytophilum	15	11	4
E. muris	–	–	–
E. chaffeensis	–	–	–

DNA fragments of pathogenic bacteria were found in 44 pools of *I. ricinus*. In particular, *B. burgdorferi s. l.* – in 28 pools, *B. miyamotoi* – in 7, *Babesia sp.* – in 15, *A. phagocytophilum* – in 15 pools. DNA of *E. muris* and *E. chaffeensis* was not detected (Table 11). No pathogenic bacteria or protozoa were identified in 18 pools, i.e., in 29.3% of the pools with *I. ricinus*.

DNA fragments of several pathogens were found simultaneously in 11 pools. Moreover, DNA fragments of *B. burgdorferi s. l.*, *B. miyamotoi*, *A. phagocytophilum* were detected simultaneously in 4 pools. Also, 4 pools simultaneously contained DNA fragments of *B. burgdorferi s. l.* and *A. phagocytophilum*, 2 pools – *B. miyamotoi* and *A. phagocytophilum*, one pool – *Babesia sp.* and *A. phagocytophilum*. In total, DNA fragments of only one pathogen were detected in 33 pools.

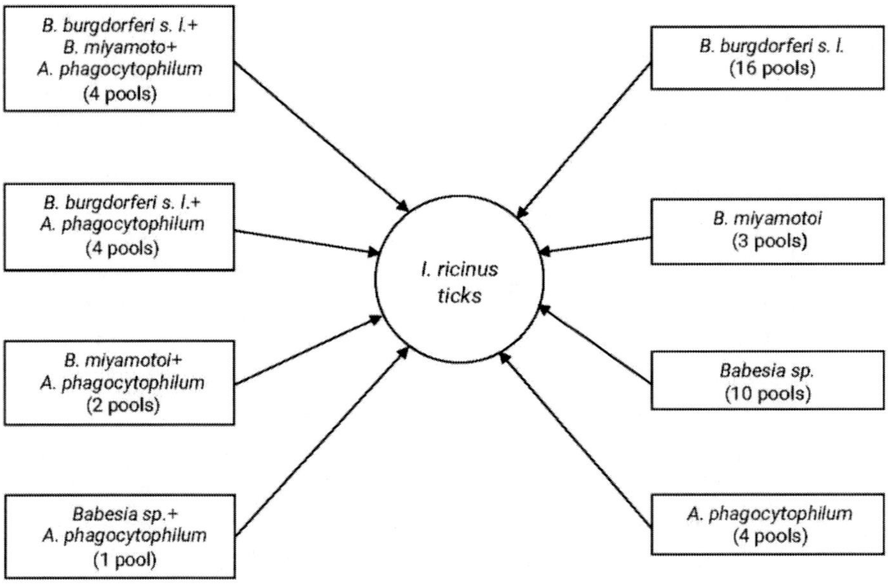

Figure 34. Variants of infection rates of *I. ricinus* tick pools with pathogenic microorganisms in the parks of Ternopil city.

The proportion of *I. ricinus* pools with *B. burgdorferi s. l.* was 45.2; with *B. miyamotoi* – 11.3; with *Babesia sp.* and *A. phagocytophilum* – 24.2 each. No pathogen was found in 29.0% of the pools.

B. burgdorferi s. l. and *Babesia sp.* were detected independently more often than in combinations with other pathogens. *B. miyamotoi* and *A. phagocytophilum* were more often combined with others. Combinations of *B. burgdorferi s. l.* from *Babesia sp.* never occurred (Figure 34).

The obtained results indicate that the most prevalent pathogen in the tick populations of parks in Ternopil city is *B. burgdorferi s. l.* (detected in 46.8% of pools), followed less frequently by *A. phagocytophilum*, and even less frequently by *Babesia sp.* The proportion of pools positive for various pathogens among males, females, and pre-imaginal stages ranges from 57.1% to 14.3%. Overall, the infection rate among adult ticks is higher than that among pre-imaginal developmental stages, except for *B. miyamotoi*. There was no significant difference in infection rates between pools from males and females, except for *B. miyamotoi*. In pools where DNA fragments of multiple pathogens were simultaneously detected, *B. burgdorferi s. l.* (72.7%) and *A. phagocytophilum* (66.6%) were most commonly present.

Thus, urban parks in Ternopil city harbor anthropogenic foci of transmissive infections where circulation of *B. burgdorferi s. l.*, *B. miyamotoi*, *A. phagocytophilum*, and *Babesia sp.* is maintained, with *I. ricinus* being their dominant vector. The recreational function of parks increases the risk of infection for humans. The findings of this study should be utilized for the development and implementation of comprehensive epidemiological measures and in clinical practice.

5.3. Infection of Ixodes Ticks Collected from Humans with Lyme Borreliosis and Other Tick-Borne Infections

Data on the infection of ticks taken from humans with *B. burgdorferi*, *A. phagocytophilum*, *B. miyamotoi*, *Babesia sp.* are extremely scarce [176, 177], and such studies were conducted only abroad.

In the laboratory of TNMU Centre for Lyme Borreliosis and Other Tick-Borne Diseases Research, during 2017–2019, 1,226 ticks collected from humans were examined, of which 1,179 were received from residents of Ternopil and the region, 47 from residents of other regions of Ukraine. It is worth noting that 80.0% of arthropods removed from residents of Ternopil region were extracted by physicians at the emergency department of the Ternopil Municipal Hospital of Emergency Medical Aid, while the rest were removed by patients themselves [120].

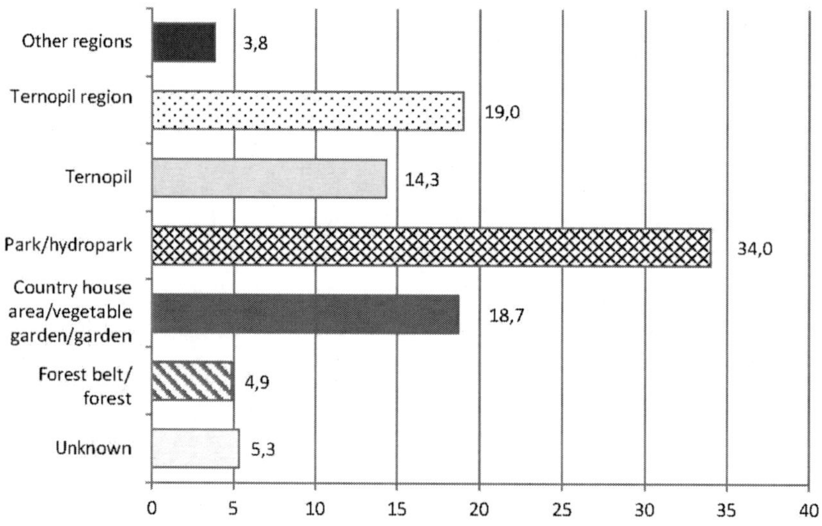

Figure 35. The area where ticks attacked people, %.

According to patients' reports, in 233 cases (19.0%), tick attacks occurred in populated areas of Ternopil region, excluding Ternopil city, and in 47 cases (3.8%), in other regions of Ukraine. In Ternopil city and adjacent villages, 946 episodes (77.2%) of tick attacks on humans were registered. Specifically, residents of the city experienced attacks outside parks in 175 cases (14.3%), in park areas in 417 cases (34.0%), in dacha and gardening plots within the city and nearby villages in 229 cases (18.7%), and within forest belts/forests in 60 cases (4.9%). It should be noted that 65 individuals (5.3%) either could not remember or were unable to specify clearly where the tick attacks occurred (Figure 35).

Tick attacks on people within Ternopil region during 2017–2019 were recorded from February to November. In 2018, one peak was noted – in May, in 2019 – in June (Figure 36), and the first victims began to seek help in February and March, respectively.

In contrast, in 2017, the largest number of victims of tick attacks was registered in September, since the official registration of tick attacks on people in the TNMU laboratory in 2017 began only in July.

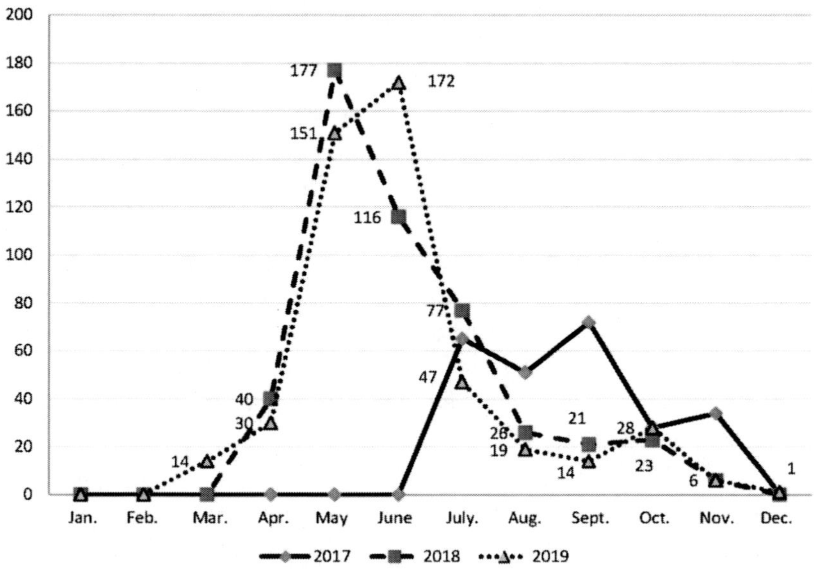

Figure 36. Dynamics of tick attacks on people in Ternopil region in different months during 2017–2019, Absolute number.

Of the 1226 identified ticks, 1212 (98.9%) were assigned to the *I. ricinus* species, 12 (0.9%) to *D. reticulatus*, and 2 (0.2%) to *Rhipiciphalus sanguineus* [105]. The data we received coincide with the results of scientists from Belgium, in whose studies 99.0% of ticks collected from humans belonged to the I. ricinus species [177]. At the same time, in similar studies conducted in Italy, ticks of the specified species were only 59.5% [178]. The results of researchers from Italy also differ significantly regarding the detected share of ticks of the *R. sanguineus species*. In contrast to our results, according to Italian researchers, ticks of this species accounted for 84.0% of the total number of samples [179]. As for ticks of the *D. reticulatus* species, the data we received (0.9%) are consistent with the results of research by scientists from Belgium – 0.3% [177] and are close to reports from Poland, where these ticks were identified in 1.9% of patients who experienced attacks [176].

When identifying 1,212 ticks of the *I. ricinus* species by sex and stage of development, it was noted that there were 391 (32.3%) females, 12 (0.9%) males, most of them 649 (53.5%) were nymphs, 32 (2.6%) were larvae. In 128 (10.6%) ticks, it was not possible to establish the stage of development and sex (Figure 37). According to the literature sources, nymphs accounted for 41.0% [178] of all I. ricinus ticks collected from humans in Italy, 70.0% of all *I. ricinus* ticks collected in Sweden [180], and 81.0% in Belgium and in the UK [181]. The predominance of nymphs over other developmental stages of *I. ricinus* ticks was also reported by scientists from Serbia [182].

Study of nucleic acids of *B. burgdorferi s. l.* (*B. burgdorferi s. s.*, *B. afzelii* and *B. garinii*), *B. miyamotoi*, *A. phagocytophilum* and *Babesia sp.* in ticks was carried out in the laboratory of TNMU Centre for Lyme Borreliosis and Other Tick-Borne Diseases Research. The DNA of the specified bacteria was determined in 441 (36.0%) ticks out of 1226 examined. At the same time, in 394 (89.3%) ticks, the DNA of one pathogen was recognized, in 47 (10.7%) – of several pathogens.

The analysis of 441 infected ticks made it possible to establish that 438 (99.3%) individuals belonged to the *I. ricinus* species and only 3 (0.7%) to the *D. reticulatus* species.

It should be noted that among 438 infected ticks of the *I. ricinus* species, nymphs and adults dominated – 212 (48.4%) and 198 (45.2%), respectively. At the same time, 23 (5.3%) of the examined ticks were delivered in the form of fragments of representatives of the *I. ricinus* species, which could not be identified by stage of development and sex, and 5 (1.1%) were larvae (Figure 38).

According to the detection of bacterial DNA in PCR, infected with borrelia of *B. burgdorferi s. l.* genocomplex, there were 236 (19.2%) ticks out of 1226 examined, which coincides with the literature data, according to which the proportion of ticks infected with these borrelia, in Europe ranges from 0.5 to 85.0% [182–185], in the USA – from 1.0 to 100.0%. The results we obtained are close to the data of scientists from Poland, who found *B. burgdorferi s. l.* in ticks collected from humans in 15.3% of cases [186].

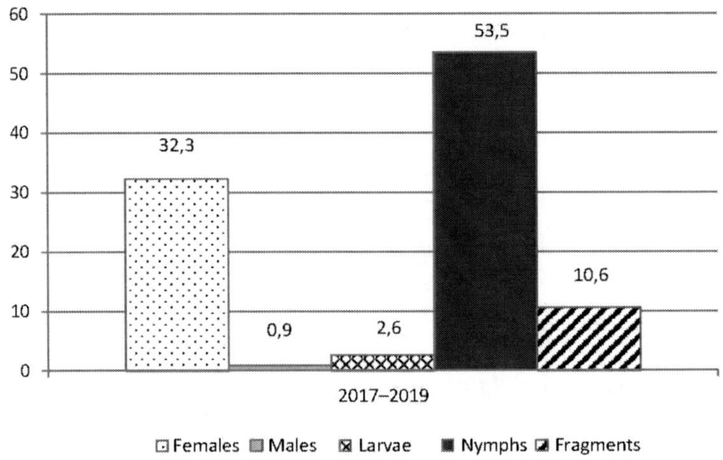

Figure 37. The results of the identification of ticks of the *I. ricinus* species (n = 1226) collected from humans in 2017–2019, by sex and stages of development.

In addition, we detected *B. miyamotoi* DNA in 21 (1.7%) of 1226 ticks collected from humans (Figure 39). The *B. miyamotoi* species genetically belongs to the *Borrelia* group that are the causative agents of tick-borne relapsing fever. Data from the literature sources inform about the presence of these borrelia in many European countries, in particular in the Czech Republic, Denmark, Estonia, France, Germany, the Netherlands, Norway, Poland, Romania, Sweden, and Switzerland [187–190]. The study of the distribution of this species of spirochetes in the territory of Ukraine has only just begun. According to scientific publications, in European countries the natural *B. miyamotoi* infestation of ticks taken from the environment is quite different: in Estonia – 0.4% [191], in Belgium – 1.1% and in the Netherlands – 4.8% [192], in France – 3.0% [193]. In Germany, the above parameter ranges from 1.8 to 2.8% [194].

A. phagocytophilum DNA was detected in 180 (14.7%) ticks out of 1226 examined. The results we obtained are consistent with the data of Italian scientists, according to which the percentage of ticks infected with this pathogen, taken from the environment, ranged from 1.6 to 19.9 [195]. At the same time, the infection rate of ticks with *A. phagocytophilum* was 10.5% [178]. *Babesia sp.* was found only in 4 (0.3%) ticks collected from humans (Figure 39).

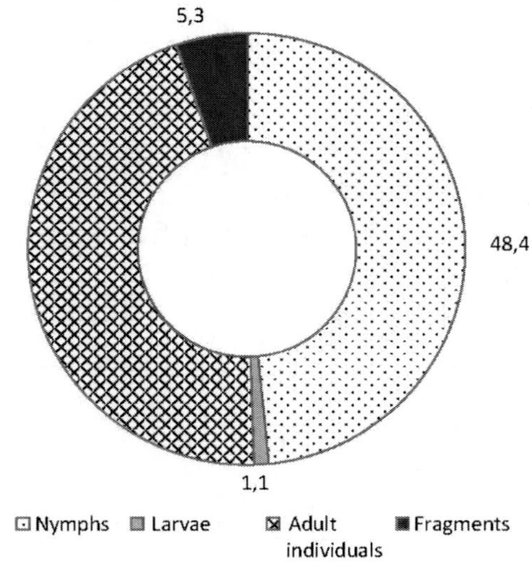

Figure 38. Distribution of infected ticks of the *I. ricinus* species (n = 438) by stages of development, %.

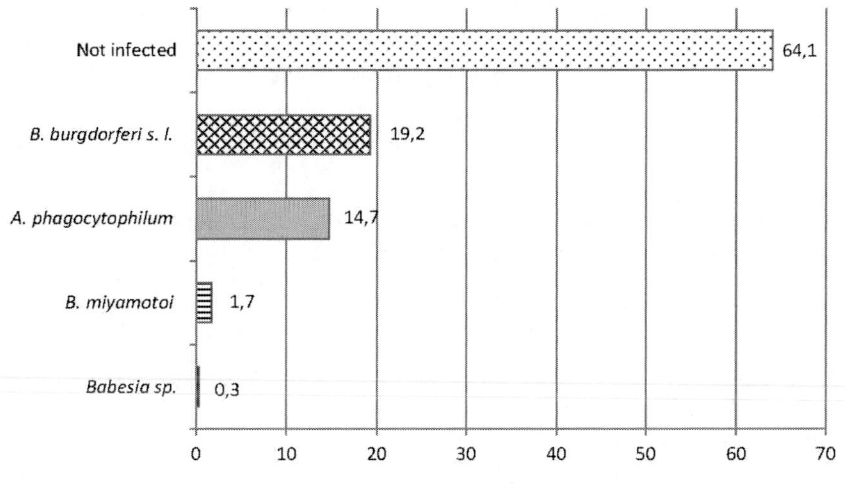

Figure 39. Percentages of ticks infected with pathogens of blood-borne infections (n = 1226) collected from humans in 2017–2019.

Ticks can have several causative agents of transmissible infections at the same time. In our studies, DNA of only one of these pathogens (*B. burgdorferi s. l.*, *B. miyamotoi*, *A. phagocytophilum* or *Babesia sp.*) was detected in 394 (32.0%) ticks out of 1226 examined, while in 47 (3.8%) ticks, multiple pathogens were detected concurrently (Figure 40).

Six types of different combinations have been singled out. Two pathogens of different species were detected in 45 ticks, three in 2, respectively. It is interesting to note that *B. burgdorferi s. l.* is present in all 6 combinations. The second most frequent was *A. phagocytophilum* – 84.4% of all mixed infections. Similar results regarding the infection of ticks with several pathogens were simultaneously published by researchers from Romania and Belgium, in whose papers, the number of such ticks was 3.7 and 3.9%, respectively. At the same time, Italian scientists cite a slightly higher rate of infection of ticks with several pathogens at the same time – 5.7% [177].

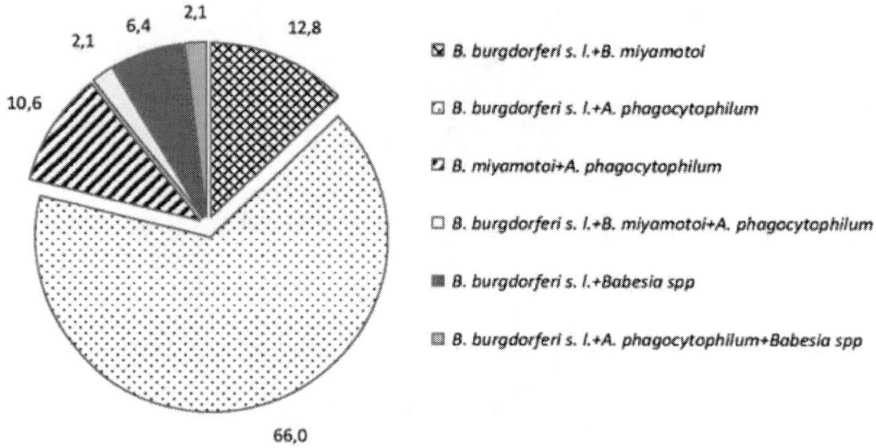

Figure 40. Simultaneous detection of DNA of pathogens of various infections in ticks (n = 47) collected from humans, %.

Thus, the possibility of occurrence of Lyme borreliosis in the form of mono- and mixed infections on the territory of Ukraine has been confirmed in connection with the proven infestation of 36.0% of ticks taken from humans with the causative agents of tick-borne infections: *B. burgdorferi s. l.* – 19.2% of individuals, *A. phagocytophilum* – 14.7%, *B. miyamotoi* – 1.7%, *Babesia sp.* – 0.3%, including 3.8% – with several pathogens.

6. Analysis of Awareness of Different Categories of the Population about Lyme Borreliosis

Mariia Ivanivna Shkilna
Mykhaylo Mykhaylovych Korda
Stepan Yosypovych Zaporozhan
Oleh Liubomyrovych Ivakhiv
Svitlana Oleksiivna Nykytiuk
and Alina Mykolaiivna Petruk

Foresters belong to professional population groups with a high risk of Borrelia infection [196–198]. Awareness of different groups of population regarding LB, in particular students [199–201] and forestry workers [202, 203], and their infestation with B. burgdorferi has been studied in a number of European countries [204, 205]. In Ukraine, similar studies were conducted only among a small number of forestry workers in the Lviv region [206], and the issue of awareness of LB needs further study both in Ternopil region and in other regions.

For the first time, we conducted a survey of 1,070 forestry workers in Volyn, Zhytomyr, Transcarpathian, Ternopil, Khmelnytskyi, Chernivtsi, and Chernihiv regions to find out their knowledge about Lyme borreliosis and to establish the risks of foresters becoming infected with Borrelia during the performance of their professional duties.

723 students of Ternopil national universities (two non-medical and one medical university) were interviewed. Of them, 252 people studied in non-medical higher education institutions (HEIs): 119 Volodymyr Hnatiuk Ternopil National Pedagogical University

(TNPU) and 133 – at Ivan Puluj Ternopil National Technical University (TNTU). Academic buildings and dormitories of TNPU are located near the park and forest zones, and those of TNTU are located in the city centre, far from these zones. The age of students of non-medical higher education institutions is from 18 to 23. The research included 140 males and 112 females.

Also, 471 TNMU students took part in the survey (questionnaire): 164 – 2nd year students, 165 – 4th year students, 142 – 6th year students. The age of students was from 18 to 23; there were 174 males and 297 females. The survey was conducted within the framework of research projects of the European Union. To achieve the aim of the research, a unified questionnaire was used, which was developed by TNMU scientists together with their colleagues from the Pope John Paul II State Higher School (Biała Podlaska, Poland).

All examinees (foresters, students) gave answers to the questions of the unified international questionnaire, which provided the information about the number and places of tick bites, the methods of their removal, the use of repellents before entering the forest area and the inspection of their skin after returning home. In addition, forest workers and patients indicated complaints that bothered them after tick attacks. Subsequently, based on the results of the questionnaire, an analysis of the awareness of forestry workers in a number of regions of Ukraine, students and patients of hospitals in Ternopil regarding LB was carried out, and ways to improve their knowledge regarding the specified problem were also proposed.

Among 1,070 forestry workers in the specified seven regions of Ukraine, there were 972 males and 98 females. The age of the interviewees ranged from 18 to 69 years (Table 12).

Table 12. Age and gender distribution of surveyed forestry workers in seven regions of Ukraine (n = 1070)

Criterion	Total	Region						
		Volyn	Zhytomyr	Transcarpathian	Ternopil	Khmelnytskyi	Chernivtsi	Chernihiv
The number of foresters	1070	147	100	141	339	150	73	120
Males, absolute number (%)	972	120 (81,6)	81 (81,0)	126 (89,4)	332 (97,9)	135 (90,0)	66 (90,4)	112 (93,3)
Females, absolute number (%)	98	27 (18,4)	19 (19,00)	15 (10,6)	7 (2,1)	15 (10,0)	7 (9,6)	8 (6,7)
Average age, years (range)	–	39,14 ± 11,52 (20–62)	39,97 ± 10,64 (20–65)	40,96 ± 12,33 (18–69)	42,37 ± 11,26 (18–62)	42,87 ± 11,44 (20–61)	37,96 ± 10,79 (18–60)	45,26 ± 11,10 (20–63)

The group of the examined foresters included: foresters, forester assistants, forest masters, loggers, tree fellers, machine operators, sorters, tractor operators, workers, administration, gamekeepers and others – mechanics, auto electricians. Among the surveyed foresters, there were more foresters (326; 30.5%), forest masters (254; 23.7%) and administrative workers (185; 17.3%) (Table 13).

The age distribution of interviewed forestry workers was analysed. It was established that foresters of Chernihiv region were significantly older compared to foresters of Volyn, Zhytomyr, Transcarpathian, and Chernivtsi regions ($p < 0.001–0.05$). At the same time, respondents from Ternopil region and Khmelnytskyi region were older only than employees from Chernivtsi region ($p < 0.05$). So, the youngest were the foresters of Chernivtsi region ($p < 0.05$).

Table 13. Distribution of foresters in seven regions of Ukraine according to their professions (n = 1070)

Position		Total	Region						
			Volyn	Zhytomyr	Transcarpathian	Ternopil	Khmelnytskyi	Chernivtsi	Chernihiv
Forester	Absolute number	254	15	22	42	143	14	10	8
	%	23,7	10,2	22,0	29,8	42,3	9,3	13,7	6,7
Forester assistant	Absolute number	60	8	2	4	24	14	4	4
	%	5,6	5,4	2,0	2,8	7,1	9,3	5,4	3,3
Forest master	Absolute number	327	47	24	37	100	10	30	79
	%	30,5	32,0	24,0	26,3	29,4	6,7	41,1	65,9
Logger	Absolute number	38	6	3	4	24	0	0	1
	%	3,6	4,1	3,0	2,8	7,1	0	0	0,8
Tree feller	Absolute number	27	9	3	1	4	10	0	0
	%	2,5	6,1	3,0	0,7	1,2	6,7	0	0
Gamekeeper	Absolute number	18	1	1	4	6	1	1	4
	%	1,7	0,7	1,0	2,8	1,8	0,7	1,4	3,3
Administration	Absolute number	185	45	12	29	13	43	28	15
	%	17,3	30,6	12,0	20,6	3,8	28,6	38,4	12,5
Machine operator	Absolute number	21	0	14	0	0	7	0	0
	%	2,0	0	14,0	0	0	4,7	0	0
Sorter	Absolute number	15	0	9	0	0	6	0	0
	%	1,4	0	9,0	0	0	4,0	0	0
Tractor operator	Absolute number	29	5	0	0	15	9	0	0
	%	2,7	3,4	0	0	4,4	6,0	0	0
Other	Absolute number	96	11	10	20	10	36	0	9
	%	9,0	7,5	10,0	14,2	2,9	24,0	0	7,5

Important data were obtained regarding the work experience of foresters (Table 14). Respondents from Chernihiv region worked the longest – 17 years on average, Khmelnytskyi and Chernivtsi regions – 15 years each ($p < 0.001$-0.05). The length of service of foresters in Volyn, Zhytomyr, and Transcarpathian regions was shorter and did not differ significantly. Foresters from Chernivtsi region spent the least amount of time in the forest, with their working hours significantly lower compared to foresters from the Volyn and Chernihiv regions ($p < 0.05$). It was established that the respondents from the last two regions, as well as from Zhytomyr and Khmelnytskyi, spent the longest time in the forest, performing their professional duties.

The next question of the survey concerned the number of tick attacks on foresters while performing their professional duties. 170 individuals (15.9%) reported one tick attack, 115 (10.7%) reported two attacks, and 385 (35.9%) reported three or more attacks. Workers in forest enterprises in Transcarpathian and Chernivtsi regions experienced the fewest tick attacks. Foresters from Chernihiv region most frequently reported numerous tick attacks, followed somewhat less frequently by workers from Zhytomyr and Khmelnytskyi regions (Table 15). For comparison, survey results from foresters in Lublin Voivodeship, Poland, indicated that 22.7% reported one tick attack, and 8.7% reported two attacks [203], with a higher percentage (58.9%) experiencing three or more attacks. According to other Polish researchers, in surveys of foresters in Podkarpackie Voivodeship, 35.0% reported one tick attack, and an even larger percentage, specifically 60.0-62.0%, reported numerous attacks [202].

More than a third of the people (400; 37.4%) we interviewed did not remember tick bites during their lifetime, despite the fact that the average duration of their stay in the forest during the day while performing their professional duties was from 6 up to 8 hours (Table 15). It is worth noting that the largest number of people who did not remember tick attacks were among the foresters of Transcarpathian and Chernivtsi regions (68.8 and 67.1%, respectively), who spent the least number of hours in the forest during the day (6–7). In contrast to our data, only 10.7% of the interviewees among foresters in Poland did not remember tick attacks [203].

Table 14. Length of service of surveyed foresters of different regions and the time they spend in the forest (n = 731; Me (Lq; Uq))

Region	Group	Length of service, years	Time spent in the forest, hours
Volyn	1	9,0 (4,0; 21,0)	8,0 (4,0; 8,0)
Zhytomyr	2	10,0 (4,0; 15,0)	8,0 (1,5; 8,0)
Transcarpathian	3	10,0 (2,0; 19,0)	7,0 (4,0; 8,0)
Ternopil	4	–	–
Khmelnytsky	5	15,0 (7,0; 23,0)	8,0 (2,0; 8,0)
Chernivtsi	6	15,0 (10,0; 24,0)	6,0 (3,0; 8,0)
Chernihiv	7	17,0 (11,0; 24,0)	8,0 (5,0; 8,0)

Notes: 1. Length of service: the Kruskel-Wallis coefficient H = 44.70; $p < 0.001$; reliability coefficients for the Mann-Whitney test $p_{1,5} < 0.05$; $p_{1,6} < 0.05$; $p_{1,7} < 0.001$; $p_{2,5} < 0.05$; $p_{2,6} < 0.05$; $p_{2,7} < 0.001$; $p_{3,5} < 0.001$; $p_{3,6} < 0.05$; $p_{3,7} < 0.001$. 2. Number of hours in the forest: Kruskel-Wallis coefficient H = 11.16; $p < 0.05$; reliability coefficients for the Mann-Whitney test $p_{1,3} < 0.05$; $p_{1,6} < 0.05$; $p_{6,7} < 0.05$.

The localization of tick bites on the body surface was also determined (Table 16). When analysing the answers received from all foresters, as well as in each region, the following was established: the most frequent site of tick bite was the stomach – in 304 (28.4%) of 1,070 respondents, and in forestry workers of the Chernihiv and Ternopil regions, this localization of attacks was reported significantly more often than in Transcarpathian and Chernivtsi regions. According to the data of Polish scientists, among the mentioned foresters of the Lublin Voivodeship, the stomach was also the most frequent place for tick bites, but much more often – in 56.0% of the respondents [203]. The next most frequent types of bites were multiple areas of tick bite – in 294 (27.5%) of all respondents, they were most often indicated by foresters in Chernihiv region, 4 times less often in Transcarpathia. Every fourth interviewed forester (270; 25.2%) from all regions had ticks attached to their lower limbs. The largest number of such was found among forestry workers in the Chernihiv and Ternopil regions, the smallest – in Transcarpathian and Chernivtsi regions. Among foresters in neighbouring Poland, tick attacks on the lower limbs were significantly more frequent – 53.7% [203]. Tick bites on the hands, neck, and back of the body were mentioned much less often. It should be noted that the smallest number of interviewed foresters named the head area as the site of tick bites. Thus, in Chernivtsi region there was no such affected person, in Ternopil region – only 1, at the same time in Volyn region, 7.5% of respondents pointed to this area affected by ticks.

Table 15. The number of tick attacks examined by foresters of different regions (n = 1070; Me (Lq; Uq))

Region	Group	Number of attacks							
		1		2		3 and more		do not remember	
		Absolute number	%	Absolute number	%	Absolute number	%	Absolute number	%
Volyn	1	23	15,65 (9,78; 21,52)	16	10,88 (5,85; 15,91)	50	34,01 (26,35; 41,67)	58	39,46 (31,56; 47,36)
Zhytomyr	2	14	14,00 (7,20; 20,80)	15	15,00 (8,00; 22,00)	43	43,00 (33,30; 52,70)	28	28,00 (19,20; 36,80)
Transcarpathian	3	14	9,93 (4,99; 14,87)	7	4,96 (1,38; 8,54)	23	16,31 (10,21; 22,41)	97	68,79 (61,14; 76,44)
Ternopil	4	66	19,47 (15,25; 23,69)	44	12,98 (9,40; 16,56)	130	38,35 (33,17; 43,53)	99	29,20 (24,36; 34,04)
Khmelnytskyi	5	27	18,00 (11,85; 24,15)	17	11,33 (6,26; 16,40)	65	43,33 (35,40; 51,26)	41	27,33 (20,20; 34,46)
Chernivtsi	6	7	9,59 (2,84; 16,34)	6	8,22 (1,92; 14,52)	11	15,07 (6,86; 23,28)	49	67,12 (56,34; 77,90)
Chernihiv	7	19	15,83 (9,30; 22,36)	10	8,33 (3,39; 13,27)	63	52,50 (43,57; 61,43)	28	23,33 (15,76; 30,90)

Notes: 1. $p < 0.001$ for Pearson's χ^2-test in groups in general. 2. $p < 0.001$ for Pearson's χ^2 test when comparing groups 1, 3; 2, 3; 2, 6; 3, 4; 3, 5; 3, 7; 4, 6; 5, 6; 6, 7. 3. $p < 0.05$ for Pearson's χ^2 test when comparing groups 1, 6; 1, 7.

Table 16. Localization of tick bites in examined foresters of different regions (n = 1070; Me (Lq; Uq))

Location of tick bites	Region, groups					
	Volyn		Zhytomyr		Transcarpathian	
	1		2		3	
	Absolute number	%	Absolute number	%	Absolute number	%
Upper extremities	18	12,24 (6,94; 17,54)	20	20,00 (12,16; 27,84)	8	5,67 (1,85; 9,49)
Lower extremities	34	23,13 (16,31; 29,95)	32	32,00 (22,86; 41,14)	17	12,06 (6,68; 17,44)
Neck	15	10,20 (5,31; 15,09)	7	7,00 (2,00; 12,00)	5	3,55 (0,50; 6,60)
Front part of the trunk	31	21,09 (14,50; 27,68)	21	21,00 (13,02; 28,98)	6	4,26 (0,93; 7,59)
Back part of the trunk	12	8,16 (3,73; 12,59)	14	14,00 (7,20; 20,80)	8	5,67 (1,85; 9,49)
Head	11	7,48 (3,23; 11,73)	3	3,00 (0; 6,34)	2	1,42 (0; 3,37)
Abdomen	39	26,53 (19,39; 33,67)	28	28,00 (19,20; 36,80)	20	14,18 (8,42; 19,94)
Several locations	47	31,975 (24,43; 39,51)	29	29,00 (20,11; 37,89)	14	9,93 (4,99; 14,87)

Table 16. Continued

Location of tick bites	Region, group							
	Ternopil		Khmelnytskyi		Chernivtsi		Chernihiv	
	4		5		6		7	
	Absolute number	%	Absolute number	%	Absolute number	%	Absolute number	%
Upper extremities	50	14,75 (10,98; 18,52)	18	12,00 (6,80; 17,20)	9	12,33 (4,79; 19,87)	14	11,67 (5,93; 17,41)
Lower extremities	92	27,14 (22,41; 31,87)	52	34,67 (27,05; 42,29)	11	15,07 (6,86; 23,28)	32	26,67 (18,76; 34,58)
Neck	15	4,42 (2,23; 6,61)	13	8,67 (4,17; 13,17)	4	5,48 (0,26; 10,70)	13	10,83 (5,27; 16,39)
Front part of the trunk	76	22,42 (17,98; 26,86)	43	28,67 (21,43; 35,91)	9	12,33 (4,79; 19,87)	45	37,50 (28,84; 46,16)
Back part of the trunk	24	7,08 (4,35; 9,81)	25	16,67 (10,71; 22,63)	5	6,85 (1,06; 12,64)	25	20,83 (13,56; 28,10)
Head	1	0,29 (0; 0,86)	6	4,00 (0,86; 7,14)	0	0	6	5,00 (1,10; 8,90)
Abdomen	123	36,28 (31,16; 41,40)	39	26,00 (18,98; 33,02)	8	10,96 (3,79; 18,13)	47	39,17 (30,44; 47,90)
Several locations	97	28,61 (23,80; 33,42)	46	30,67 (23,29; 38,05)	10	13,70 (5,81; 21,59)	51	42,50 (33,60; 51,34)

Notes: 1. $p = 0.002$ for Pearson's χ^2-test in groups in general. 2. Pearson's χ^2-criterion in case of tick bites in different areas: upper extremities ($p = 0.05$); lower extremities ($p < 0.001$); neck ($p = 0.06$); front part of the trunk ($p < 0.001$); back part of the trunk ($p < 0.001$); head ($p < 0.001$); abdomen ($p < 0.001$); several locations ($p < 0.001$).

Forestry workers were also asked what methods they used to remove ticks. Most often, respondents of all regions used several methods of removing ticks – 318 (29.7%). Foresters of Chernihiv region used several methods the largest number of times both compared to forest workers from other regions and compared to other methods of tick removal. The least number of respondents who removed ticks in several ways were those from Transcarpathia and Chernivtsi region. Another common way among foresters to remove ticks was to pull them out with the fingers. 300 (28.0%) of all respondents used this method. However, among foresters in the Lublin Voivodeship, there were slightly more of them – 36.6% [203].

It is noteworthy that workers of forestry in the Zhytomyr, Ternopil and Chernihiv regions more frequently removed ticks by hand, while this practice was significantly less common in Transcarpathia and Chernivtsi. Furthermore, only 4.6% of the surveyed foresters sought medical help for tick removal, nearly three times lower than the rate among foresters in the Lublin Voivodeship of Poland, where it was 14.2%."

One in five forestry workers across all regions disinfected the site of a tick bite (216; 20.2%). This practice was most common among foresters in the Ternopil and Khmelnytskyi regions, and least common in Transcarpathia (Table 17).

During the survey, foresters were asked about their complaints. The most common were pain in the joints, head, and/or muscles. These symptoms were least frequently reported by foresters in the Ternopil, Transcarpathian, Zhytomyr, and Chernivtsi regions. Respondents from all regions less frequently mentioned facial nerve damage, swollen lymph nodes, difficulty concentrating, and fever. It was found out that the largest number of respondents – 152 (14.2%) – complained of joint pain ($p < 0.001$). In a separate analysis of the frequency of detection of this complaint by region, it was established that the number of people who associated pain in the joints with the fact of being bitten by ticks was different: from 4 (2.8%)

cases in Transcarpathian to 46 (38.3%) in Chernihiv region ($p < 0.001$). The largest number of foresters who associated headache with tick bite were from Khmelnytskyi region, the least number – in Transcarpathian, Ternopil, and Chernivtsi regions ($p < 0.001$). Respondents from Khmelnytskyi region most often complained of muscle pain that occurred after being bitten by ticks. At the same time, none of the foresters of Chernivtsi and Transcarpathian regions expressed such a complaint.

It is worth noting that only 2.7 and 3.3% of respondents from Chernihiv and Khmelnytskyi regions and 1 (0.29%) respondent from Ternopil region indicated inflammation of the joints, which they noted after a tick attack ($p < 0.001$).

The frequency of the use of repellents by interviewed forestry workers was also determined (Table 18). It was established that the majority of respondents – 607 (56.7%) – did not use protective equipment at all. In particular, the highest percentage of those who did not use repellents was among foresters in Chernivtsi region (90.4%), the lowest – among respondents from Ternopil region (16.8%) ($p < 0.05$). Occasionally, repellents were used by forestry workers in Chernihiv, Volyn, and Khmelnytskyi regions – 29.17, 25.17, and 24.00%, respectively, and only 3.24% in Ternopil region.

Table 17. Methods of removing ticks by foresters of different regions (n = 1070; Me (Lq; Uq))

Method of tick removal	Region							
	Volyn		Zhytomyr		Transcarpathian		Ternopil	
	Absolute number	%	Absolute number	%	Absolute number	%	Absolute number	%
Removed by a doctor	4	2,72 (0,09; 5,35)	4	4,00 (0,16; 7,84)	3	2,13 (0; 4,51)	21	6,19 (3,62; 8,76)
Removed by another person	14	9,53 (4,78; 14,28)	12	12,00 (5,63; 18,37)	7	4,96 (1,38; 8,54)	22	6,49 (3,87; 9,11)
Pulled out with fingers	43	29,25 (21,90; 36,60)	37	37,00 (27,54; 46,46)	14	9,93 (4,99; 14,87)	127	37,46 (32,31; 42,61)
Removed with simple movements	2	1,36 (0; 3,23)	5	5,00 (0,73; 9,27)	3	2,13 (0; 4,51)	22	6,49 (3,62; 8,76)
Unscrewed with tweezers	19	12,93 (7,51; 18,35)	22	22,00 (13,88; 30,12)	6	4,26 (0,93; 7,59)	19	5,60 (3,15; 8,05)
Scratched with a fingernail	10	6,80 (2,73; 10,87)	8	8,00 (2,68; 13,32)	0	0	16	4,72 (2,46; 6,98)
Rinsed with a disinfectant solution	1	0,68 (0; 2,01)	1	1 (0; 2,95)	2	1,42 (0; 3,37)	13	3,83 (1,79; 5,87)
Covered with oil	20	13,61 (8,07; 19,15)	14	14,00 (7,20; 20,80)	12	8,51 (3,90; 13,12)	67	19,76 (15,52; 24,00)
The place of tick bite was disinfected after its removal	21	14,29 (8,63; 19,95)	13	13,00 (6,41; 19,59)	7	4,96 (1,38; 8,54)	97	28,61 (23,80; 33,42)
Other removal methods	0	0	3	3,00 (0; 6,34)	8	5,67 (1,85; 9,49)	11	3,24 (1,36; 5,12)
Several methods of removal	37	25,17 (18,15; 32,19)	27	27,00 (18,30; 35,70)	16	11,35 (6,11; 16,59)	125	36,87 (31,73; 42,01)

Table 17. Continued

Method of tick removal	Region					
	Khmelnytskyi		Chernivtsi		Chernihiv	
	Absolute number	%	Absolute number	%	Absolute number	%
Removed by a doctor	5	3,33 (0,46; 6,20)	2	2,74 (0; 6,48)	10	8,33 (3,39; 13,27)
Removed by another person	18	12,00 (6,80; 17,20)	2	2,74 (0; 6,48)	25	20,83 (13,56; 28,10)
Pulled out with fingers	30	20,00 (13,60; 26,40)	10	13,70 (5,81; 21,59)	39	32,50 (24,12; 40,88)
Removed with simple movements	15	10,00 (5,20; 14,80)	2	2,74 (0; 6,48)	13	10,83 (5,27; 16,39)
Unscrewed with tweezers	39	26,00 (18,98; 33,02)	4	5,48 (0,26; 10,70)	41	34,17 (25,68; 42,66)
Scratched with a fingernail	5	3,33 (0,46; 6,20)	3	4,11 (0; 8,66)	11	9,17 (4,01; 14,33)
Rinsed with a disinfectant solution	10	6,67 (2,68; 10,66)	1	1,37 (0; 4,04)	3	2,50 (0; 5,29)
Covered with oil	24	16,00 (10,13; 21,87)	4	5,48 (0,26; 10,70)	18	15,00 (8,61; 21,39)
The place of tick bite was disinfected after its removal	43	28,67 (21,43; 35,91)	7	9,59 (2,84; 16,34)	28	23,33 (15,76; 30,90)
Other removal methods	4	2,67 (0,09; 5,25)	1	1,37 (0; 4,04)	0	0
Several methods of removal	56	37,33 (29,59; 45,07)	6	8,22 (1,92; 14,52)	51	42,50 (33,66; 51,34)

Notes: 1. $p < 0.001$ for Pearson's χ^2-test in groups in general. 2. Pearson's χ^2 test for different methods of removing ticks: removed by a doctor ($p = 0.12$); removed by another person ($p < 0.001$); pulled out with fingers ($p < 0.001$); removed with simple movements ($p < 0.01$); unscrewed with tweezers ($p < 0.001$); scratched with a fingernail ($p = 0.01$); rinsed with a disinfectant solution ($p= 0.03$); covered with oil ($p= 0.01$); the place of tick bite was disinfected after its removal ($p < 0.001$); other methods of removal ($p= 0.03$); several methods of removal ($p < 0.001$).

Table 18. Frequency of repellents use by foresters of different regions when staying in forest/park zones (n = 1070; Me (Lq; Uq))

Region	Group	Repellents application					
		never		rarely		often	
		Absolute number	%	Absolute number	%	Absolute number	%
Volyn	1	104	70,75 (63,40; 78,10)	37	25,17 (18,15; 32,19)	6	4,08 (0,88; 7,28)
Zhytomyr	2	79	79,00 (71,02; 86,98)	20	20,00 (12,16; 27,84)	1	1,00 (0; 2,95)
Transcarpathian	3	118	83,69 (77,59; 89,79)	22	15,60 (9,61; 21,59)	1	0,71 (0; 2,10)
Ternopil	4	57	16,81 (12,83; 20,79)	11	3,24 (1,36; 5,12)	2	0,59 (0; 1,41)
Khmelnytskyi	5	104	69,33 (61,95; 76,71)	36	24,00 (17,17; 30,83)	9	6,00 (2,20; 9,80)
Chernivtsi	6	66	90,41 (83,66; 97,16)	6	8,22 (1,92; 14,52)	1	1,37 (0; 4,04)
Chernihiv	7	79	65,83 (57,34; 74,32)	35	29,17 (21,04; 37,30)	6	5,00 (1,10; 8,90)

Note. $p < 0.01$ for Pearson's χ^2 test in general; $p < 0.05$ for Pearson's χ^2 test when comparing groups 1, 3; 1, 6; 3, 7; 5, 6; 6, 7.

It is good to note that there are at least 1-2 foresters in Zhytomyr, Transcarpathian, Chernivtsi, and Ternopil regions, and 6 in Volyn and Chernihiv region and 9 – in Khmelnytskyi region, repellents are still used often ($p< 0.05$). At the same time, it is known that only 22.8% of foresters in Poland do not use repellents, while the rest use them [203].

The next question in the questionnaire was whether forestry workers inspect their own skin after returning from forest/park areas (Figure 41).

It is worth noting that 40.1% of all surveyed foresters in 7 regions often examined their skin after returning from forest/park zones. This procedure was most often carried out by forestry workers in the Zhytomyr and Khmelnytskyi regions (48.0 and 44.7%, respectively), somewhat less often – in Ternopil region (35.4%) ($p > 0.05$). 41.9% of all respondents rarely examined their own skin after returning from forest/park areas.

The largest number of such persons was in Volyn (53.1%), the smallest – in Transcarpathia (29.1%). The fact that 193 (18.0%) of the surveyed forestry workers of Ukraine, upon returning from the forest zone (the area where they perform their professional duties), do not conduct a self-examination of the skin at all, is of considerable concern. The largest number of these are in Transcarpathia (29.1%), the least number in Volyn (8.8%) ($p < 0.05$), while only 3.0–4.0% of foresters in neighbouring Poland do not examine their skin after returning from forest [203].

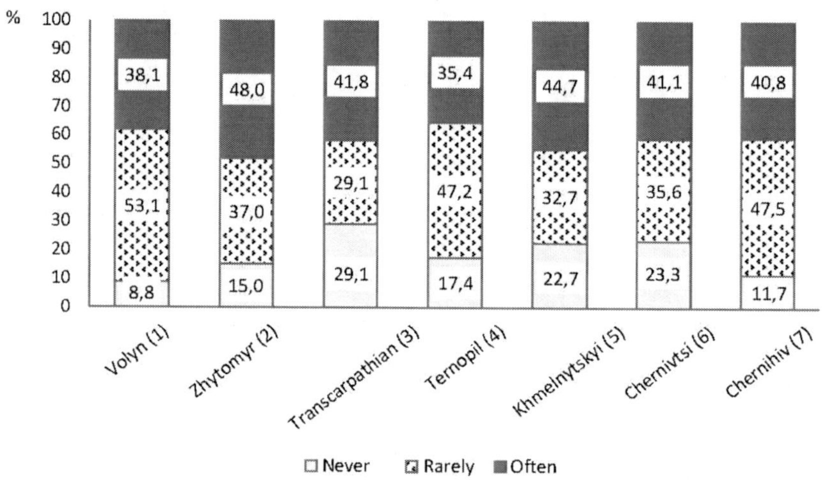

Note. $p < 0.001$ for Pearson's χ^2 test in general; $p < 0.05$ for Pearson's χ^2 test when comparing regions: 1, 3; 1, 6; 3, 7; 5, 6; 6, 7.

Figure 41. Frequency of inspection of the skin by foresters of different regions after returning from forest/park zones (n = 1070), %.

Next, we studied the level of awareness of forestry workers in the specified regions regarding LB and other tick-borne infections (Table 19). Half of the interviewed foresters assessed their knowledge of the above-mentioned issues as insufficient – 537 (50.2%) people, every fourth (267; 24.9%) claimed that they were minimal, and only 90 (8.4%) forestry workers considered their knowledge sufficient. Foresters from Volyn and Chernivtsi region were the least informed, and those from Ternopil region and Transcarpathia were the most informed.

The next question in the questionnaire was how sufficient, in the opinion of foresters, was the data on LB and other tick-borne infections in mass media (Table 20). About half (512; 47.8%) of the interviewed forestry workers believed that the above-mentioned issue is not sufficiently covered in mass media, and only 90 (8.4%) people answered that there is enough information. Foresters of Transcarpathia said more often that the mass media pay sufficient attention to the coverage of issues related to Lyme disease and other tick-borne infections ($p < 0.05$).

Table 19. Awareness of forestry workers in some regions of Ukraine regarding Lyme borreliosis and other tick-borne infections (n = 1070; Me (Lq; Uq))

Region	Group	Level of awareness							
		insufficient		minimal		medium		sufficient	
		Absolute number	%	Absolute number	%	Absolute number	%	Absolute number	%
Volyn	1	96	65,31 (57,62; 73,00)	33	22,45 (15,70; 29,20)	15	10,20 (5,31; 15,09)	3	2,04 (0; 4,33)
Zhytomyr	2	45	45,00 (35,25; 54,75)	24	24,00 (15,63; 32,37)	22	22,00 (13,88; 30,12)	9	9,00 (3,39; 14,61)
Transcarpathia	3	51	36,17 (28,24; 44,10)	50	35,46 (27,56; 43,36)	24	17,02 (10,82; 23,22)	16	11,35 (6,11; 16,59)
Ternopil	4	155	45,72 (40,42; 51,02)	70	20,65 (16,34; 24,96)	66	19,47 (15,25; 23,69)	48	14,16 (10,45; 17,87)
Khmelnytskyi	5	76	50,67 (42,67; 58,67)	39	26,00 (18,98; 33,02)	24	16,00 (10,13; 21,87)	11	7,33 (3,16; 11,50)
Chernivtsi	6	45	61,64 (50,49; 72,79)	18	24,66 (14,77; 34,55)	9	12,33 (4,79; 19,87)	1	1,37 (0; 4,04)

Note. $p < 0.001$ for Pearson's χ^2 test in general; $p < 0.05$ for Pearson's χ^2 test when comparing groups 1, 2; 13; 1, 4; 1, 5; 2, 6, 2, 7; 3, 4; 3, 6; 3, 7; 4, 6; 4, 7.

Table 20. The opinion of foresters of some regions of Ukraine regarding the sufficiency of data on Lyme borreliosis and other tick-borne infections in mass media (n = 1070; Me (Lq; Uq))

Region	Group	Information							
		insufficient		minimal		medium		sufficient	
		Absolute number	% (95% CI)	Absolute number	% (95% CI)	Absolute number	% (95% CI)	Absolute number	% (95% CI)
Volyn	1	74	50,34 (42,26; 58,42)	47	31,97 (24,43; 39,51)	18	12,24 (6,94; 17,54)	8	5,44 (1,77; 9,11)
Zhytomyr	2	55	55,00 (45,25; 64,75)	23	23,00 (14,75; 31,25)	16	16,00 (8,81; 23,19)	6	6,00 (1,35; 10,65)
Transcarpathia	3	52	36,88 (28,92; 44,84)	48	34,04 (26,22; 41,86)	23	16,31 (10,21; 22,41)	18	12,77 (7,26; 18,28)
Ternopil	4	149	43,95 (38,67; 49,23)	64	18,88 (14,71; 23,05)	82	24,19 (19,63; 28,75)	43	12,68 (9,14; 16,22)
Khmelnytskyi	5	79	52,67 (44,68; 60,66)	42	28,00 (20,81; 35,19)	20	13,33 (7,89; 18,77)	9	6,00 (2,20; 9,80)
Chernivtsi	6	39	53,42 (41,98; 64,86)	20	27,40 (17,17; 37,63)	13	17,81 (9,03; 26,59)	1	1,37 (0; 4,04)
Chernihiv	7	64	53,33 (44,40; 62,26)	36	30,00 (21,80; 38,20)	15	12,50 (6,58; 18,42)	5	4,17 (0,59; 7,75)

Note. $p < 0.001$ for Pearson's χ^2 test in general; $p < 0.05$ for Pearson's χ^2 test when comparing groups 1, 3; 1, 4; 2, 3; 2, 4; 3, 4; 3, 5; 3, 6; 3, 7; 4, 5; 4, 6; 4, 7.

Finally, it was found out whether the surveyed forestry workers want to improve their knowledge about LB and other ticks of infections (Figure 42).

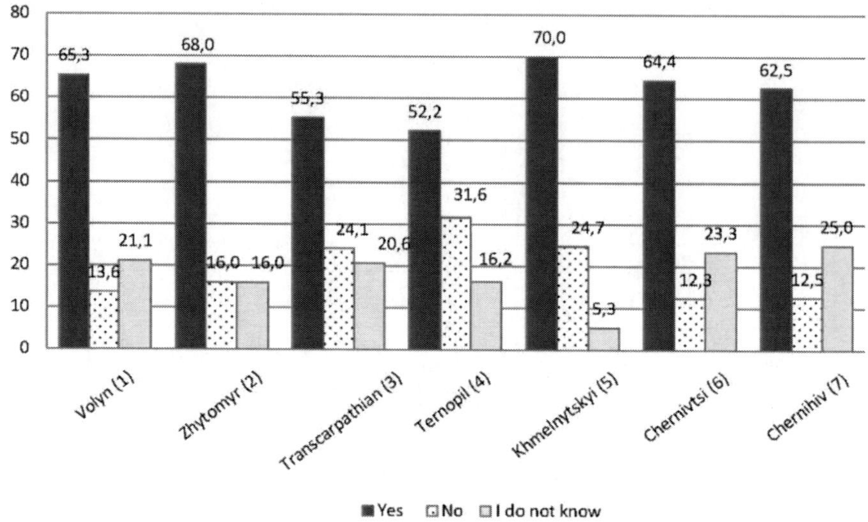

Note. $p < 0.001$ for Pearson's χ^2 test in general; $p < 0.05$ for Pearson's χ^2 test when comparing groups 1, 4; 1, 5; 2, 4; 2, 5; 3, 5; 4, 5; 4, 6; 4, 7; 5, 6; 5, 7.

Figure 42. Desire of interviewed foresters to expand their knowledge about Lyme borreliosis (n = 1070), %.

It is good to note that 646 (60.4%) respondents had a desire to expand their knowledge about Lyme disease and other tick-borne infections. Most of them are in the Khmelnytskyi and Zhytomyr regions. However, it is of great concern that every fifth (238; 22.2%) respondent categorically believes that there is no need to expand their knowledge about these infectious diseases, almost half of them (107; 44.9%) were identified among foresters of Ternopil region, at the same time in the region, 16.2% of respondents are not sure of the need to expand their knowledge about these diseases [207–210].

Therefore, in Ternopil and Transcarpathian regions, the fewest foresters expressed a desire to expand their knowledge about Lyme disease, with the highest number indicating no interest in doing so. Based on the data provided, it can be concluded that for the prevention of Lyme disease and other tick-borne infections, it is necessary to provide foresters with appropriate protective gear (clothing and footwear), repellents, and special individual devices (tick removers) for tick removal, and mandate their use. Additionally, there is a need to increase the level of sanitary education through occupational safety engineers, family doctors, infectious disease departments of universities, and regional and national mass media.

It is necessary to classify forestry workers of Ukraine as a high-risk group for Lyme borreliosis, and this infectious disease must be classified as a professional disease of foresters.

In 2017–2018, academic staff of TNMU Department of Infectious Diseases, Epidemiology, Skin and Venereal Diseases studied the level of knowledge of the 2nd, 4th and 6th year students regarding LB (Table 21) [211].

Table 21. Gender composition of the surveyed students of I. Horbachevsky Ternopil National Medical University (n = 471; Me (Lq; Uq))

Year of study	Males		Females	
	Absolute number	%	Absolute number	%
2	59	35,98 (28,63; 43,33)	105	64,02 (56,67; 71,37)
4	65	39,39 (31,93; 46,85)	99	60,00 (52,53; 67,47)
6	50	35,21 (26,96; 42,33)	93	65,49 (57,67; 73,31)

136 (28.9%) respondents indicated the fact of tick attacks during their life, while it should be noted that the smallest number of such persons appeared among the 4th-year students ($p < 0.05$) (Table 22). At the same time, among the respondents of the 2nd year, those who were attacked by ticks were twice as many as among the 4th-year students. The number of 6th-year students who were attacked by ticks once was almost the same as that of the 2nd-year students.

The next step was to reveal the number of tick attacks experienced by students (Table 23).

Table 22. Data on tick attacks on students of I. Horbachevsky Ternopil National Medical University (n = 471; Me (Lq; Uq))

Tick attacks	Students					
	2-nd year		4-th year		6-th year	
	Absolute number	%	Absolute number	%	Absolute number	%
There were attacks	56	34,15 (26,89; 41,41)	28	16,97 (11,24; 22,70)	52	36,62 (28,70; 44,54)
No attacks or cannot recollect	108	65,85 (58,59; 73,11)	137	83,03 (77,30; 88,76)	90	63,38 (55,46; 71,30)

Note. $p < 0.05$ for Pearson's χ^2-test when comparing 2nd- and 4th-, 4th- and 6th-year students.

Table 23. The number of tick attacks on students of I. Horbachevsky Ternopil National Medical University (n = 136; Me (Lq; Uq))

Number of tick attacks	Students					
	2-nd year		4-th year		6-th year	
	Absolute number	%	Absolute number	%	Absolute number	%
1–2	47	28,66 (21,74; 35,58)	26	15,76 (10,20; 21,32)	34	23,94 (16,92; 30,96)
3 and more	9	5,49 (2,00; 8,98)	2	1,21 (0; 2,88)	18	12,68 (7,21; 18,15)

Note. $p < 0.05$ for Pearson's χ^2-test when comparing 2nd- and 4th- year students, 4th- and 6th-year students.

It was found that only one instance of tick attachment was reported by 107 (22.8%) out of 471 respondents, with the fewest affected individuals being on the 4th year ($p < 0.05$), while the highest, nearly twice as many, were noted on the 2nd year. However, respondents who experienced tick attachment more than 3 times were most prevalent on the 6th year: twice as many compared to the 2nd year and nine times more than the 4th year. The data we obtained are significantly lower than the results from international studies, where 51.3% of medical students from Pope John Paul II State School of Higher Education, Poland, and Presov University in Slovakia reported a single episode of tick attachment [201].

Table 24. Localization of tick bites among students of I. Horbachevsky Ternopil National Medical University (n = 471; Me (Lq; Uq))

Localization of tick bites	Students					
	2-nd year		4-th year		6-th year	
	Absolute number	%	Absolute number	%	Absolute number	%
1. Arms	14	8,54 (4,26; 12,82)	7	4,24 (1,17; 7,31)	7	4,93 (1,37; 8,49)
2. Legs	16	9,76 (5,22; 14,30)	6	3,64 (0,78; 6,50)	29	20,42 (13,79; 27,05)
3. Neck	10	6,10 (2,44; 9,76)	2	1,21 (0; 2,88)	4	2,82 (0,10; 5,54)
4. Front part of the trunk	5	3,05 (0,42; 5,68)	5	3,03 (0,41; 5,65)	7	4,93 (1,37; 8,49)
5. Back part of the trunk	1	0,61 (0; 1,80)	1	0,61 (0; 1,80)	1	0,70 (0; 2,07)
6. Head	5	3,05 (0,42; 5,68)	2	1,21 (0; 2,88)	3	2,11 (0; 4,47)
7. Abdomen	7	4,27 (1,18; 7,36)	6	3,64 (0,78; 6,50)	16	11,27 (6,07; 16,47)
8. Other	4	2,44 (0,08; 4,80)	0	0	5	3,52 (0,49; 6,55)

Note. Answers 1, 4–6, 8: p> 0.05 for Pearson's χ^2 test; Answer 2: $p < 0.05$ for Pearson's χ^2 test when comparing the 2nd and 4th, 2nd and 6th, 4th and 6th years; Answer 3: $p < 0.05$ for Pearson's χ^2 test when comparing the 2nd and 4th years; Answer 7: $p < 0.05$ for Pearson's χ^2 test when comparing the 2nd and 6th, 4th and 6th years.

The next survey question concerned the localization of tick bites among students (Table 24). The most common areas for tick bites reported by students of all years were legs (10.8%), abdomen (6.2%), and hands (5.9%). Meanwhile, ticks were least likely to attach to the legs of 4th-year students ($p < 0.05$). Second-year students reported the above-mentioned localization almost three times more often than fourth-year students, while sixth-year students reported it almost five times more often. Tick attachment to the abdomen of sixth-year students was more frequent compared to second- and fourth-year students, almost twice and three times more often, respectively. Attachments to the head, neck, and torso were noted less frequently. Only one student from each year reported tick attachment to the back of the torso [212]. The data we obtained align with the survey results from medical students in Poland and Slovakia, where legs, abdomen, and hands were also the most common areas for tick bites [201].

Interesting responses were obtained regarding the methods of tick removal. Most commonly, students removed ticks themselves with tweezers – 59 (12.5%). Sixth-year students performed this procedure more frequently than fourth-year students, and slightly more often compared to second-year students (p> 0.05). In contrast, the majority of surveyed students from Poland (36.7%) and Slovakia (62.9%) sought help from others for tick removal [201]. Only 45 (9.6%) of the surveyed medical students used a doctor or nurse for tick removal, with second-year students seeking medical help slightly more often than fourth-year students. Forty (8.5%) of the respondents used oil to suffocate ticks, with second-year students performing this procedure significantly more often than fourth-year students ($p < 0.05$). Thirty-two (6.9%)

students disinfected the attachment site after tick removal, with no significant difference observed among the students of the same year (Table 25).

Table 25. Methods of tick removal by students of I. Horbachevsky Ternopil National Medical University (n = 471; Me (Lq; Uq))

Method of tick removal	Students					
	2nd year		4th year		6th year	
	Absolute number	%	Absolute number	%	Absolute number	%
1. Removed by a doctor/nurse	21	12,80 (7,69; 17,91)	10	6,0 (2,42; 9,70)	14	9,86 (4,96; 14,76)
2. Removed by another person	–	–	–	–	–	–
3. Pulled out with fingers	6	3,66 (0,79; 6,53)	2	1,21 (0; 2,88)	4	2,82 (0,10; 5,54)
4. Removed with simple movements	8	4,88 (1,58; 8,18)	2	1,21 (0; 2,88)	2	1,41 (0; 3,35)
5. Twisted out with tweezers	20	12,20 (7,19; 17,21)	12	7,27 (3,31; 11,23)	27	19,01 (12,56; 25,46)
6. Scraped off with a fingernail	1	0,61 (0; 1,80)	0	0	2	1,41
7. Poured with disinfectant solution	9	5,49 (2,00; 8,98)	4	2,42 (0,08; 4,76)	8	5,63 (1,84; 9,42)
8. Smeared with oil	19	11,59 (6,69; 16,49)	7	4,24 (1,17; 7,31)	14	9,86 (4,96; 14,76)
9. The site of the tick bite was disinfected after removal	15	9,15 (4,74; 13,56)	10	6,06 (2,42; 9,70)	17	11,97 (6,63; 17,31)
10. Other methods	1	0,61 (0; 1,80)	1	0,61 (0; 1,80)	1	0,70 (0; 2,07)

Note. Answers 1, 3, 4, 6, 7, 9, 10: $p > 0.05$ for Pearson's χ^2 test; answer 5: $p < 0.05$ for Pearson's χ^2 test when comparing 4th and 6th courses; answer 8: $p < 0.05$ for Pearson's χ^2 test when comparing 2nd and 4th years.

Significant concern was raised regarding the information about medical students' inspection of their skin after returning from the forest. It was found that 43 (9.1%) students never inspected their skin, while inspection was rare – ranging from 31.5% of fourth-year students to 46.5% of sixth-year students (Figure 43). Among medical students from Poland and Slovakia, the corresponding figure was 49.4% [201]. Notably, the highest percentage (60.6%) of students who always performed this procedure belonged to the 4th year of our university ($p < 0.05$). Only 44.4% of sixth-year students always inspected their skin, while second-year students did so slightly more often at 51.8%, and fourth-year students most frequently at 60.6%, significantly more compared to sixth-year students.

The situation regarding the use of repellents by future doctors before entering forest and park areas is alarming (Table 26). It is concerning that 275 (58.4%) of all students do not use repellents at all, with the highest proportion among sixth-year students – 54.23%. A significantly smaller and nearly equal percentage of second- and fourth-year students – 35.98% and 36.36%, respectively – do not use repellents. Only 13.8% of all TNMU students and 16.4% of future doctors from Poland and Slovakia [201] always use repellents before entering forested areas. Rare use of protective factors is reported by 41.6% of respondents from Ukraine and 48.9% from Poland and Slovakia.

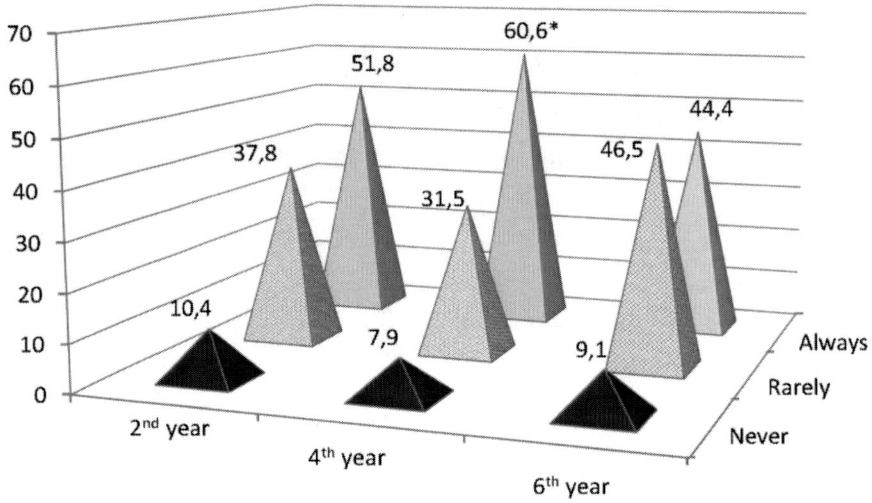

Note. * – $p < 0.05$ for Pearson's χ^2 test when comparing 4th and 6th years.

Figure 43. Examination of the skin by students of I. Horbachevsky Ternopil National Medical University after returning from the forest, %.

During the spring of 2017, the staff of the Department of Infectious Diseases, Epidemiology, Dermatology, and Venereal Diseases at Ternopil National Medical University studied the level of knowledge among students of non-medical higher education institutions in Ternopil regarding LB (Table 27) [213].

Table 26. Use of repellents by students of I. Horbachevsky Ternopil National Medical University (n = 471; Me (Lq; Uq))

Answer options	Students					
	2-nd year		4-th year		6-th year	
	Absolute number	%	Absolute number	%	Absolute number	%
1. I do not use repellents	59	35,98 (28,63; 43,33)	60	36,36 (29,02; 43,70)	77	54,23 (46,04; 62,42)
2. I rarely use repellents	80	48,78 (41,13; 56,43)	78	47,27 (39,65; 54,89)	52	36,62 (28,70; 44,54)
3. I always use repellents	25	15,24 (9,74; 20,74)	27	16,36 (10,72; 22,00)	13	9,15 (4,41; 13,89)

Note. $p < 0.05$ for Pearson's χ^2 test when comparing 2nd and 6th, 4–6 courses; answers 2 and 3: $p > 0.05$ for Pearson's χ^2 test.

Table 27. Gender composition of surveyed students of non-medical universities in Ternopil (n = 252; Me (Lq; Uq))

University	Males		Females	
	Absolute number	%	Absolute number	%
TNPU	19	15,97 (9,39; 22,55)	100	84,03 (77,45; 90,61)
TNTU	121	90,98 (86,11; 95,85)	12	9,02 (4,15; 13,89)

Note. $p < 0.001$ for Pearson's χ^2 test.

Over a third of respondents (38.1% of individuals) from both higher education institutions in Ternopil experienced tick attacks (Table 28).

Table 28. Number of tick attacks on students of non-medical universities in Ternopil (n = 252; Me (Lq; Uq))

Tick attacks	Students			
	TNPU		TNTU	
	Absolute number	% (95% CI)	Absolute number	% (95% CI)
There were attacks	54	45,76 (36,81; 54,71)	42	31,58 (23,68; 39,48)
1–2	31	57,41(48,53; 66,29)	30	71,43 (63,75; 79,11)
3 and more	23	42,59 (33,71; 51,47)	12	28,57 (20,89; 36,25)
There were none or they do not remember	65	54,24 (45,29; 63,19)	91	68,42* (60,52; 76,32)

Note. * – between the characteristics of attacks on students within one higher education institution, $p < 0.05$ for Pearson's χ^2 test.

Tick attacks were more frequently reported by students of TNPU ($p < 0.05$). This can be partly explained by the fact that the university's educational buildings and dormitories are located near park and forest zones in Ternopil, whereas TNTU is situated in the city centre, far from these areas. One hundred fifty-six (61.9%) respondents from both universities did not recall ever experiencing tick attacks in their lifetime; however, significantly more respondents from TNTU fell into this category ($p < 0.05$).

Regarding the number of tick attacks experienced by students, it was found that among all surveyed non-medical higher education students, 35 (13.9%) individuals reported more than 3 attacks in their lifetime, with nearly twice as many at TNPU compared to TNTU. Nearly twice as many students from both universities (61 or 24.6%) reported experiencing one attack. The number of affected individuals in each university was approximately the same (see Table 28).

Students from both TNPU and TNTU reported nearly the same number of attacks per person – 31 and 30 respectively. However, students from TNPU reported more than 3 attacks nearly twice as often – 23 compared to 12 at TNTU ($p < 0.05$).

Interesting data was obtained regarding the localization of tick attacks among students of Ternopil universities (see Table 29). The most common locations for tick bites were noted as legs (19 at TNPU and 13 at TNTU), abdomen (22 and 9 respectively), hands (14 and 7), and neck (11 and 8). These findings align with the results of surveys conducted among non-medical higher education students in Latvia and Poland [200], where legs were also the most common location for tick bites (7% of respondents from Poland and 38.2% from Latvia), and the torso was least affected [200].

It should be noted that ticks attached to the abdomen area significantly more frequently in students of TNPU compared to TNTU – 22 and 9 times respectively ($p < 0.05$). Incidences of attacks on the front and back torso were mentioned less frequently by students of both universities – 10 and 11 cases respectively. Only 5 individuals from both universities reported ticks attaching to the head.

The next question in the survey concerned the use of repellents by non-medical university students before entering forested areas (Figure 44). It was found that a small percentage of respondents use repellents before entering forested areas – only 1.6% and 12.0% of TNPU and TNTU students, respectively. In Poland, these products are also used by 12.1% of non-medical university students, while in Latvia they are used slightly more frequently – 16.1% [200]. A significant portion of students never used repellents – 47.1% and 39.9% respectively, while nearly half of the respondents used them rarely – 48.1% and 51.3% respectively.

Table 29. Localization of tick bites in students of non-medical universities in Ternopil (n=252; Me (Lq; Uq))

Localization of tick bites	Students					
	TNPU			TNTU		
	Absolute number	%	Number of attacks	Absolute number	%	Number of attacks
1. Arms	14	11,76 (5,97; 17,55)	2,5 (1,0; 3,0)	7	5,26 (1,47; 9,05)	1,0 (1,0; 2,0)
2. Legs	19	15,97 (9,39; 22,55)	2,0 (1,0; 2,0)	13	9,77 (4,72; 14,82)	1,0 (1,0; 1,0)
3. Neck	11	9,24 (4,04; 14,44)	1,0 (1,0; 1,0)	8	6,02 (1,98; 10,06)	1,0 (1,0; 1,0)
4. Front part of the trunk	7	5,88 (1,65; 10,11)	1,0 (1,0; 2,0)	3	2,26 (0; 4,79)	1,0 (1,0; 1,0)
5. Back part of the trunk	7	5,88 (1,65; 10,11)	1,0 (1,0; 2,0)	4	3,01 (0,11; 5,91)	1,5 (1,0; 2,5)
6. Head	2	1,68 (0; 3, 99)	1,5 (1,0; 2,0)	3	2,26 (0; 4,79)	1,0 (1,0; 1,0)
7. Abdomen	22	18,49 (11,51; 25,47)	1,0 (1,0; 2,0)	9	6,77 (2,50; 11,04)	1,0 (1,0; 1,0)
8. Other	3	2,52 (0; 5,34)	1,0 (1,0; 2,0)	6	4,51 (0,98; 8,04)	1,0 (1,0; 1,0)

Note. Answers from 1 to 4: $p > 0.05$ for Pearson's χ^2 test; answer 7: $p < 0.05$ for Pearson's χ^2 test.

Table 30. Methods of tick removal by students of non-medical universities in Ternopil (n = 252; Me (Lq; Uq))

Method of tick removal	Students			
	TNPU		TNTU	
	Absolute number	%	Absolute number	%
1. Removed by a doctor/nurse	12	10,08 (4,67; 15,49)	17	12,78 (7,11; 18,45)
2. Removed by another person	0	0	0	0
3. Pulled out with fingers	4	3,36 (0,12; 6,60)	4	3,01 (0,11; 5,91)
4. Removed with simple movements	8	6,72 (2,22; 11,22)	3	2,26 (0; 4,79)
5. Twisted out with tweezers	15	12,61 (6,65; 18,57)	10	7,52 (3,04; 12,00)
6. Scraped off with a fingernail	4	3,36 (0,12; 6,60)	1	0,75 (0; 2,22)
7. Poured with disinfectant solution	6	5,04 (1,11; 8,97)	5	3,76 (0,53; 6,99)
8. Smeared with oil	20	16,81 (10,09; 3,53)	10	7,52 (3,04; 12,00)
9. The site of the tick bite was disinfected after removal	15	12,61 (6,65; 18,57)	8	6,02 (1,98; 10,06)

Note. Answers from 1 to 7, 9: $p > 0.05$ for Pearson's χ^2 test; answer 8: $p < 0.05$ for Pearson's χ^2 test.

The survey regarding tick removal methods (Table 30) revealed that the majority of respondents from both TNPU and TNTU applied oil to the tick before removal (30 students). It is noteworthy that twice as many TNPU respondents used this method compared to TNTU ($p < 0.05$). In contrast, none of the students from Poland used oil to remove ticks, and only 1% of respondents from Latvia did so [214]. Medical assistance from a doctor or nurse was used by only 10.3% of surveyed students, while 9.9% of respondents from both universities removed ticks themselves with tweezers. In Poland and Latvia, this method was used by 27.4% of non-medical university students [200].

The information that 3.4% of students from TNPU did not inspect their skin after returning from the forest at all is alarming, compared to 12.8% among respondents from TNTU ($p < 0.05$) (Figure 45).

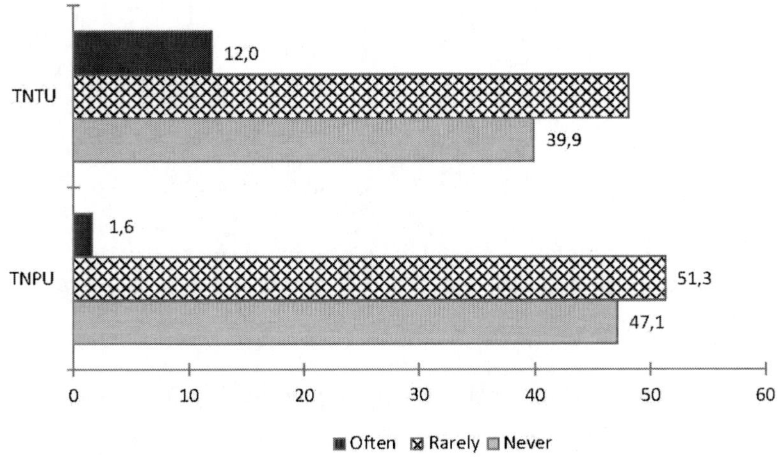

Figure 44. Frequency of repellents use by students of non-medical universities in Ternopil before entering the forest zone, %.

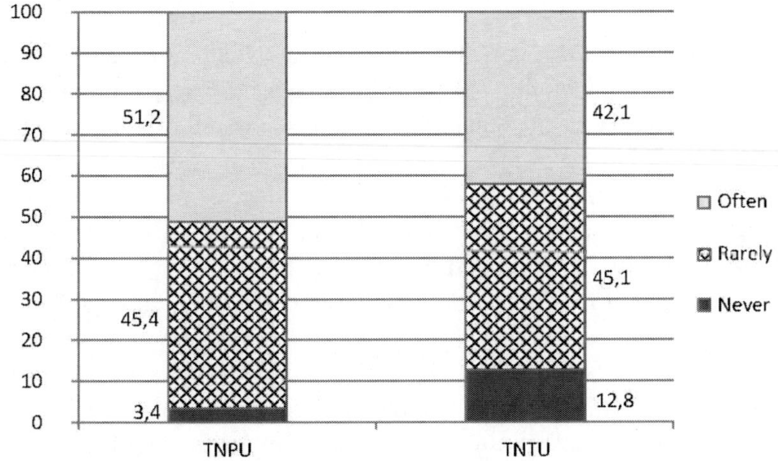

Figure 45. The frequency of examination of the skin by students of non-medical universities in Ternopil after returning from the forest, %.

Skin inspections after returning from the forest were conducted rarely at about the same frequency among students of both TNPU (45.4%) and TNTU (45.1%). However, this inspection was slightly more frequent among TNPU students (51.2% vs. 42.1%), possibly due to a higher proportion of female students who tend to be more attentive to their skin. These findings are similar to the results of surveys among non-medical university students in Latvia and Poland [200]: 54% of respondents from Latvia and 43.7% from Poland often inspect their skin after returning from the forest, while 14.9% and 5.5%, respectively, never do. In Czechia, 11.0% of students do not inspect their skin after returning from the forest [199].

Thus, the survey conducted among 1070 employees of forestry enterprises across 7 regions (Volyn, Zhytomyr, Transcarpathian, Ternopil, Khmelnytskyi, Chernivtsi, and Chernihiv) allowed establishing that the least number of tick attacks were reported by foresters in Transcarpathian and Chernivtsi regions, while their colleagues from Chernihiv region most frequently reported multiple tick attacks. Over a third of respondents did not recall tick attachments despite spending 6-8 hours in the forest during workdays. The abdomen was the most common attachment site (28.4% of respondents), followed closely by multiple attachment sites (27.5%), with every fourth forester reporting lower limb attachments. Most respondents (29.7%) employed multiple methods to remove ticks, while only 4.6% sought medical assistance. Approximately one in five forestry workers disinfect the attachment site, most commonly in Ternopil and Khmelnytskyi regions, and least commonly in Transcarpathian region.

Forestry workers most commonly complained of joint, head, and muscle pain; respondents mentioned fever, swollen lymph nodes, and facial nerve involvement less frequently. Changes were noted more often by forest workers from Volyn, Khmelnytskyi, Chernivtsi, and Chernihiv regions.

A majority (56.7%) of respondents did not use any protective measures at all, with forestry workers from Chernivtsi region (90.4%) least likely to use them. Skin inspections after leaving forest/park areas were conducted frequently by 40.1% of all surveyed forestry workers, led by respondents from Zhytomyr and Khmelnytskyi regions – 48.0% and 44.7% respectively. Rarely performed by 41.9% of all respondents, this was most common in Volyn (53.1%) and least in Transcarpathia (29.1%). Nearly one-fifth (18.0%) of forest workers never conducted self-examinations of their skin.

Half of the surveyed forestry workers rated their knowledge of LB and other tick-borne infections as insufficient, with another quarter (24.9%) considering it minimal. Approximately half (47.8%) of the respondents stated that there is insufficient information about Lyme disease and other tick-borne borreliosis in mass media. The majority (60.4%) expressed a desire to expand their knowledge about these illnesses.

Based on the analysis of survey results among 2nd, 4th, and 6th-year students of Ternopil National Medical University, it was found that 28.9% of respondents experienced at least one tick bite episode during their lifetime, with the fewest occurrences among 4th-year students ($p < 0.05$). Second-year students experienced twice as many tick attacks compared to fourth-year students. Among students of all years, ticks most commonly attached to the legs (10.8%), abdomen (6.2%), and hands (5.9%). Attachments to the legs were least common among fourth-year students ($p < 0.05$), occurring almost three times more frequently among second-year students and almost five times more frequently among sixth-year students. Attachments to the abdomen were most common among sixth-year students compared to second- and fourth-year students, occurring almost twice and three times more frequently, respectively. Respondents mentioned tick attacks on the head, neck, and torso less frequently.

Most students removed ticks themselves with tweezers (12.5%), and sixth-year students did this more frequently than fourth-year students ($p < 0.05$). Only 9.6% of medical students sought help from a doctor or nurse to remove ticks, with second-year students doing so slightly more often than fourth-year students. 8.5% of respondents applied oil to ticks, with second-year students doing this significantly more often than fourth-year students ($p < 0.05$). Only

6.9% of students disinfected the site of tick attachment after removal, with a similar number across all years. It was found that 9.1% of students never inspected their skin after leaving the forest. Only 44.4% of sixth-year students, 51.8% of second-year students, and 60.6% of fourth-year students always performed this inspection, which was more frequent compared to sixth-year students ($p < 0.05$). A total of 58.4% of all students never applied repellents, with sixth-year students using them the least. Only 11.7% of respondents always used repellents.

The survey included 252 students: 119 from Volodymyr Hnatiuk Ternopil National Pedagogical University and 133 from Ivan Puluj Ternopil National Technical University. More than a third of respondents (96 individuals) from both universities experienced tick attacks, with ticks attacking students of TNPU more frequently ($p < 0.05$) and almost twice as frequently noting more than 3 attacks of these arthropods.

The most common attachment sites for ticks noted by students from both universities were legs, abdomen, hands, and neck. Significantly more ticks attached to the abdomen of students from TNPU compared to students from TNTU ($p < 0.05$). Respondents from both universities mentioned tick attacks on the front and back of the torso and head much less frequently. Most respondents from both universities applied oil to ticks before removal, but twice as many respondents from TNPU used this method ($p < 0.05$). Students from both universities often removed ticks themselves with tweezers. Only 10.3% of all respondents sought help from a doctor or nurse to remove ticks.

In general, 3.4% of students from TNPU and 12.8% from TNTU did not inspect their skin after leaving the forest, and about 45% of respondents from both universities did this rarely, with students from TNPU inspecting slightly more often. A significant portion of respondents from both universities never applied repellents, and almost half of the respondents used them infrequently. Only a small percentage (1.6% and 12.0%) of respondents used repellents before entering the forest area.

7. Epidemiological Features of Lyme Borreliosis in Patients with Erythematous and Non-Erythematous Forms of the Disease

Mariia Shkilna
Mykhaylo Andreychyn
and Oleh Ivakhiv

Two groups of patients were examined in the study. The first group consisted of 146 patients with EM of LB, who received outpatient and inpatient treatment at Ternopil Regional Clinical Dermatovenereologic Dispensary and the infectious diseases department of the Ternopil Municipal Emergency Hospital from 2015 to 2020. There were 63 males (43.2%) and 83 females (56.8%) in this group, with ages ranging from 19 to 79 years and a mean age of 43.09 ± 14.29 years. The majority of the examined patients (124; 84.9%) were of working age (up to 60 years) [215].

The second group included 90 patients with non-erythema migrans (NEM) form of LB, who were treated as outpatients and inpatients at various medical institutions in Ternopil during 2015-2020: Ternopil Regional Clinical Dermatovenerologic Dispensary, infectious diseases department of Ternopil Municipal Hospital of Emergency Medical Aid, Ternopil Regional

Phthisiopulmonological Medical Centre, and Ternopil University Hospital. There were 33 men (36.7%) and 57 women (63.3%) in the group ($p < 0.05$). City residents predominated among those surveyed – 56 (62.2%) compared to 34 (37.8%) ($p < 0.05$). Their average age was (43.1 ± 14.3) years. The majority of patients (78; 86.7%) were of working age (up to 60 years) [216].

Through the survey, patients were questioned about the number of tick attacks, methods, and timing of tick removal (Table 31).

It was found that patients with NEM form of LB reported occurrences of more than 3 tick attacks almost twice as often as those with EM form – 41.8% versus 21.1%, while the percentage of individuals who experienced 1 and 2 tick attacks was almost similar between the groups – 26.0% and 9.6%, respectively, compared to 28.9% and 11.1%. It is worth noting that those who had no ticks or could not remember any tick attacks but associated the onset of clinical symptoms with visiting forests, gardens, or city parks were more common among patients with NEM LB than those with EM form – 38.9% versus 22.6% ($p < 0.05$). Perhaps this is because the signs of NEM LB appear much later than EM, causing patients to forget about tick bites.

Regarding the method of tick removal, the majority of respondents from both groups equally often pulled out ticks with their fingers – 21.9% and 21.1%, respectively. They also removed ticks with simple movements – 11.0% and 8.9%, and treated the bite site with a disinfectant solution – 13.7% and 20.0% of individuals. However, patients with EM LB twisted the tick out twice as often as those with NEM LB – 12.3% versus 5.5%, while seeking medical help was less frequent among them – 8.2% versus 17.8%. Almost every tenth respondent removed the tick with simple movements (11.0% and 8.9%, respectively) or applied oil to the bite site (9.6% and 10.0%). Only patients with EM LB sought help from others (11; 7.5%).

Table 31. Characteristics of tick attacks, methods, and timing of their removal in patients with erythema migrans and non-erythema migrans forms of Lyme borreliosis

Criterion		Patients with LB			
		EM (n = 146)		NEM (n = 90)	
		Absolute number	%	Absolute number	%
Number of bites	0	38	26,0	26	28,9
	2	14	9,6	10	11,1
	Many (more than 3)	61	41,8	19	21,1
	There were none or they do not remember	33	22,6	35	38,9
Method of tick removal	Removed by a doctor/nurse	12	8,2	16	17,8
	Removed by another person	11	7,5	–	–
	Pulled out with fingers	32	21,9	19	21,1
	Removed with simple movements	16	11,0	8	8,9
	Twisted out with tweezers	18	12,3	5	5,5
	Scraped off with a fingernail	4	2,7	3	3,3
	Poured with disinfectant solution	2	1,4	3	3,3
	Smeared with oil	14	9,6	9	10,0
	The site of the tick bite was disinfected after removal	20	13,7	18	20,0
	Other	13	8,9	5	5,5
Timing of tick removal, hour	Up to 12	27	18,5	19	21,1
	13–24	24	16,5	15	16,7
	25–48	11	7,5	6	6,7
	After a few days	13	8,9	5	5,5
	Unknown	71	48,6	36	40,0

When analysing the survey results, it was found that most often patients from both groups removed ticks within 12 hours after the attack – 18.5% and 21.1%, respectively. Between 13 to 24 hours after the attack, it was 16.5% and 16.7%, between 25 to 48 hours – 7.5% and 6.7%, and later than that – 8.9% and 5.5% of individuals. Nearly half of the respondents from both groups (48.6% and 40.0%, respectively) could not recall or did not remember the time of tick removal. Further, the survey explored the location where the affected individuals experienced tick attacks (Figure 46).

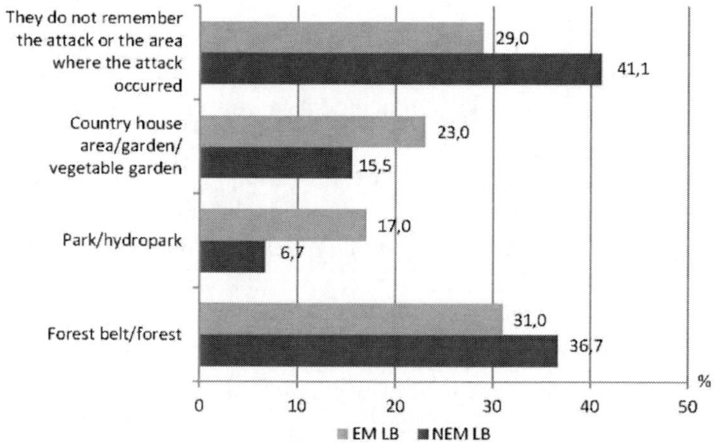

Figure 46. The locality where tick attacks occurred on people who later developed erythematous (n = 146) and non-erythematous forms of Lyme borreliosis (n = 90), %.

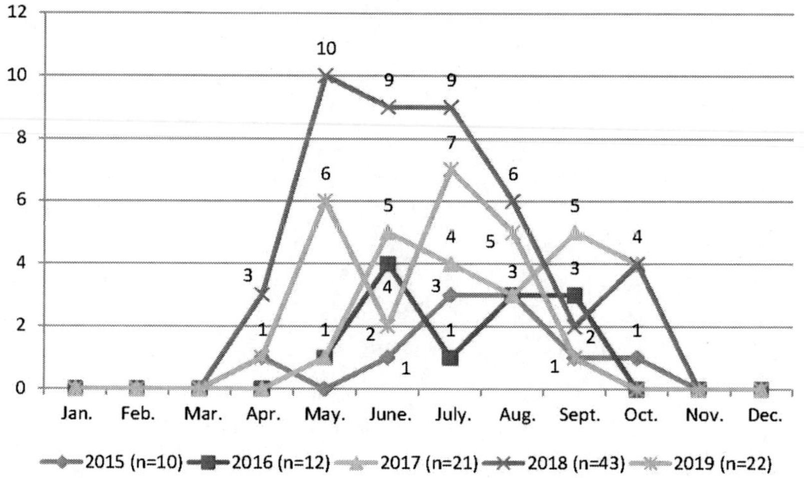

Figure 47. Seasonality of tick attacks on patients with erythema migrans form of Lyme borreliosis in 2015-2019 (n = 108), Absolute number.

Most commonly, these incidents occurred during leisure time in forest clearings and forests (in 31.0% of EM LB patients and 36.7% of NEM LB patients) or while working in backyard plots (in 23.0% and 15.5%, respectively), less frequently during leisure time in park areas (17.0% and 6.7%, respectively). Patients with NEM LB were slightly more likely to not remember the location of tick attacks compared to EM LB patients – 41.1% versus 29.0% of respondents.

An analysis of the seasonality of tick attacks was conducted on 108 EM LB patients who were under observation during 2015-2019 (Figure 47). This analysis excluded 36 patients who did not specify the month of tick attacks and 2 respondents who were under observation in 2020.

It was established that patients registered tick attacks from March to November. In 2016 and 2017, two peaks were noted in June and September, while in 2018 and 2019, peaks occurred in May and July.

Regarding the localization of tick bites in individuals with erythema migrans Lyme disease (EM LD), it was found that the majority of patients indicated ticks attaching to the lower extremities ($p < 0.05$) (Figure 48). Tick attachments were reported approximately equally on the hands, anterior trunk, and abdomen – 14.3%, 13.2%, and 12.3% respectively. Less frequently, patients reported attacks on the posterior trunk, neck, and head – 6.2%, 2.1%, and 1.2% respectively. It is worth noting that 28 individuals out of 146 (19.2%) with EM LD associated their symptoms with tick bites, but they could not specify the exact attachment site.

For patients with non-erythema migrans Lyme disease (NEM LD), the possibility of combined organ involvement was considered. Therefore, the percentage of individuals predominantly affected in various organs or systems was initially determined. Specifically, 46 out of 90 examined individuals (51.1%) were found to have musculoskeletal system involvement (1st group), 23 (25.6%) predominantly had cardiovascular system involvement (2nd group), and 21 (23.3%) had morphoea (3rd group) (Table 32).

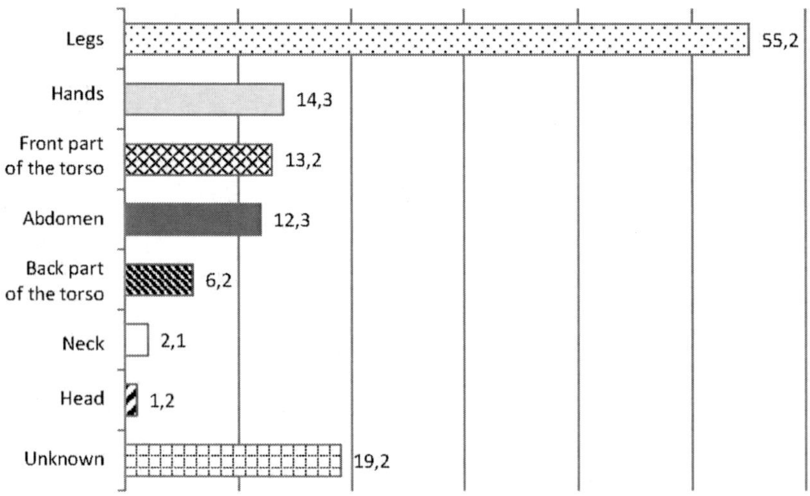

Figure 48. Localization of tick bites in patients with the erythematous form of Lyme borreliosis (n = 146), %.

When surveying patients, the localization of tick attachments was also investigated (Figure 49). The most frequent sites of tick bites among patients with predominantly cardiovascular system involvement were the legs – in 9 out of 23 respondents (39.1%), among those with morphoea – in 8 out of 21 (38.1%), and among those with predominantly musculoskeletal system involvement – in 12 out of 46 (26.1%). It is noteworthy that patients with cardiovascular system involvement most commonly reported tick attacks on the anterior trunk, posterior trunk, and abdomen – 30.4%, 17.4%, and 21.7% respectively. Only 1 out of 23 individuals (4.3%) with predominantly cardiovascular system involvement reported tick bites on the head ($p < 0.05$).

Therefore, among patients with EM LD, more than 3 tick attacks were noted in 41.8% of individuals, with nearly a quarter unable to recall the tick attachment but associating their symptoms with visits to forested park areas or dachas. Most commonly after attachment, patients removed ticks by pulling them out (21.9%), twisting them (12.3%), or using simple movements or oil application (each around 10%). Only 8.2% sought medical assistance. More than a third of patients removed ticks within the first day after attachment, while almost half could not specify the removal time. Tick attacks were most frequently registered during stays in forested areas (31.0%) or on suburban plots (23.0%), less often in park zones (17.0%), with 29.0% unable to recall.

Table 32. Patients with the erythematous form of Lyme borreliosis with predominant damage to certain organs and systems (n = 90)

Predominant damage to	Number of patients	
	Absolute number	%
Locomotor apparatus	46	51,1
Cardiovascular system	23	25,6
Skin (morphea)	21	23,3

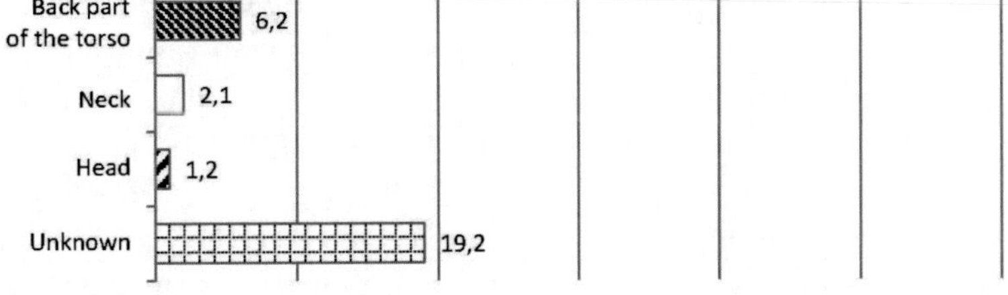

Note. * – the difference is significant with respect to patients of other groups within the same localization ($p < 0.05$).

Figure 49. Places of tick bites in patients who later developed non-erythematous Lyme borreliosis: 1st group – predominantly with musculoskeletal system involvement (n = 27); 2nd group – predominantly with cardiovascular system involvement (n = 23); 3rd group – with morphoea (n = 21), %.

Tick attacks were documented from March to November with peaks in May-July and September in different years. A significant majority of patients pointed to tick attachments on their lower extremities ($p < 0.05$), while every fifth individual could not clearly identify the attachment site.

Among patients with NEM LD, every fifth reported more than 3 tick attacks, and 38.9% could not recall such attacks. Of the 90 patients examined, 46 predominantly had musculoskeletal system involvement, 23 had cardiovascular system involvement, and 21 had skin involvement. The legs were most commonly reported as the site of tick attachment: in individuals with predominantly cardiovascular system involvement – in 39.1%, with morphoea – in 38.1%, and with musculoskeletal system involvement – in 26.1%. Patients with predominantly cardiovascular system involvement reported the highest number of tick attacks on the anterior trunk, posterior trunk, and abdomen.

8. Interactive Medical Map (Based on Geographic Information System)

Stepan Podobivskyi
and Mykhaylo Korda

The medical geographic information system (GIS) for tick-borne infections is a specialized medical cartographic and analytical resource designed for the collection, storage, accumulation, analysis, and visualization of information regarding the distribution of tick-borne infections in specific regions. This interactive map provides analytical information covering a wide range of infections to achieve a comprehensive understanding of the current situation related to diseases and their impact on human and animal health. Through this map, users can access a full set of functionalities including map navigation, manipulation of vector layers, spatial analysis, address and simple parameter-based searching, real-time database updates and editing, a wide array of analytical capabilities such as graph displays, spatial and statistical analysis, data security protection from distortion and unauthorized access, multi-user access, and group database editing.

The interactive map created within the medical GIS framework includes 10 layers, with 9 dedicated to different species of ticks. Each tick specimen on the map is identified by its Latin name, life stage (imago, larva, nymph), precise geographic localization of tick attacks on humans, the location where the tick was removed from an animal or caught in nature, morphological characteristics of the tick (body length, gnathosoma, idiosoma width), method of acquisition, presence of infectious disease agents, temporary host, and the researcher's name and surname. One layer (the 10th) displays patients who have experienced tick attacks. The map also displays information such as the patient's identification code, address, occupation, diagnosis upon seeking medical attention and after examination, date of detection of LD agents, and obtained results.

The real-time online medical GIS displays research results on ticks, infections caused by them, and patient examination data for those who have experienced tick bites in specific regions of Ukraine and Ternopil city. It contains concise information on cases of Ixodes tick attacks on humans and domestic animals, their distribution in various biotopes of Ternopil and 38 settlements across 13 Ukrainian regions. Special attention is given to employees of certain forestry enterprises in Ternopil, Zhytomyr, Chernihiv, Khmelnytskyi, Volyn, Rivne, and Transcarpathian regions.

The map shows 615 cases of *Ixodes ricinus* tick attacks and 95 cases of *Dermacentor reticulatus* tick attacks (Figure 50).

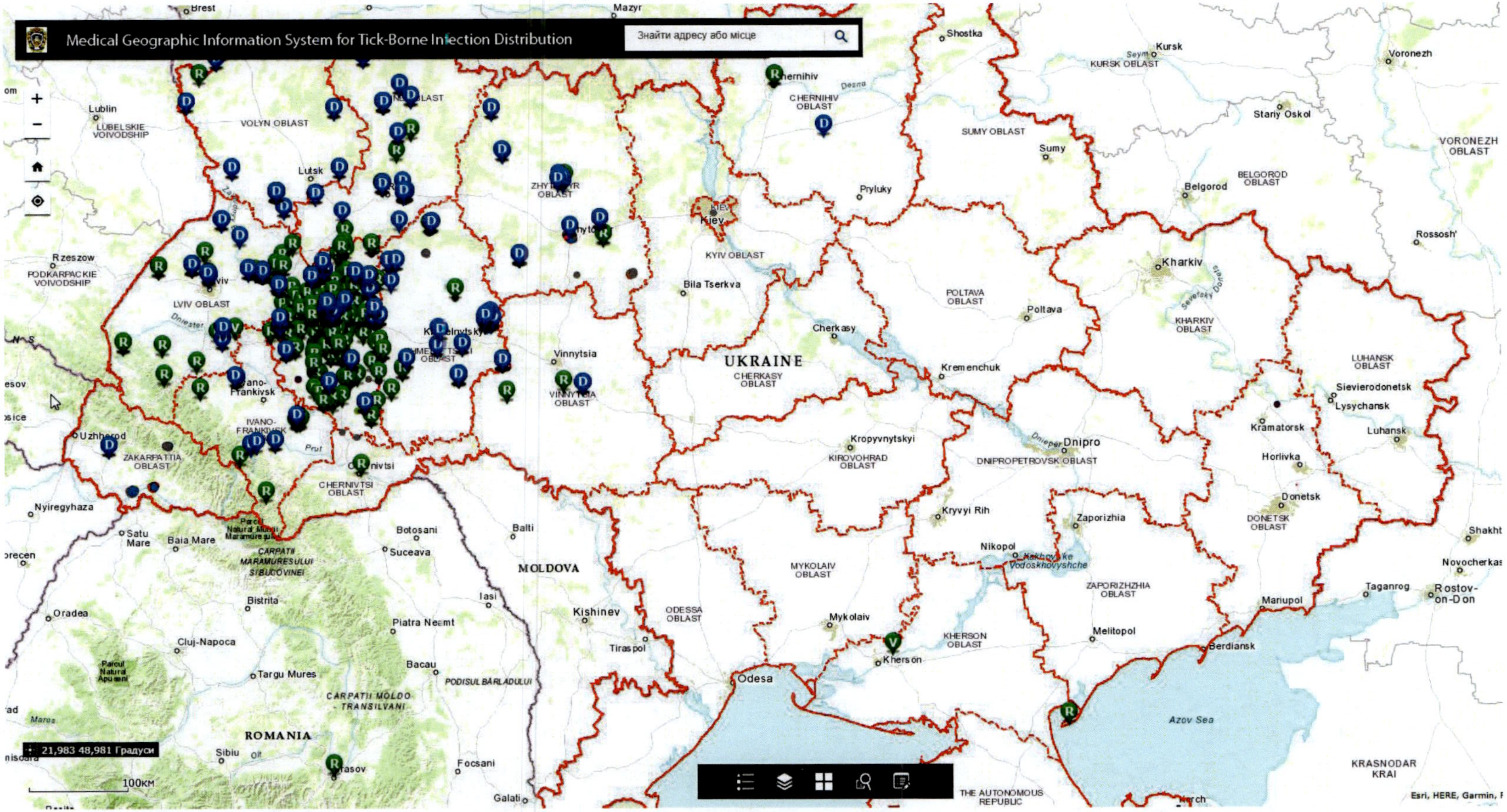

Note. The stages of tick development are highlighted by colours: green – nymphs; blue – females; red – larvae; R – *I. ricinus*; D – *D. reticularis*.

Figure 50. Map of places where ticks attack people.

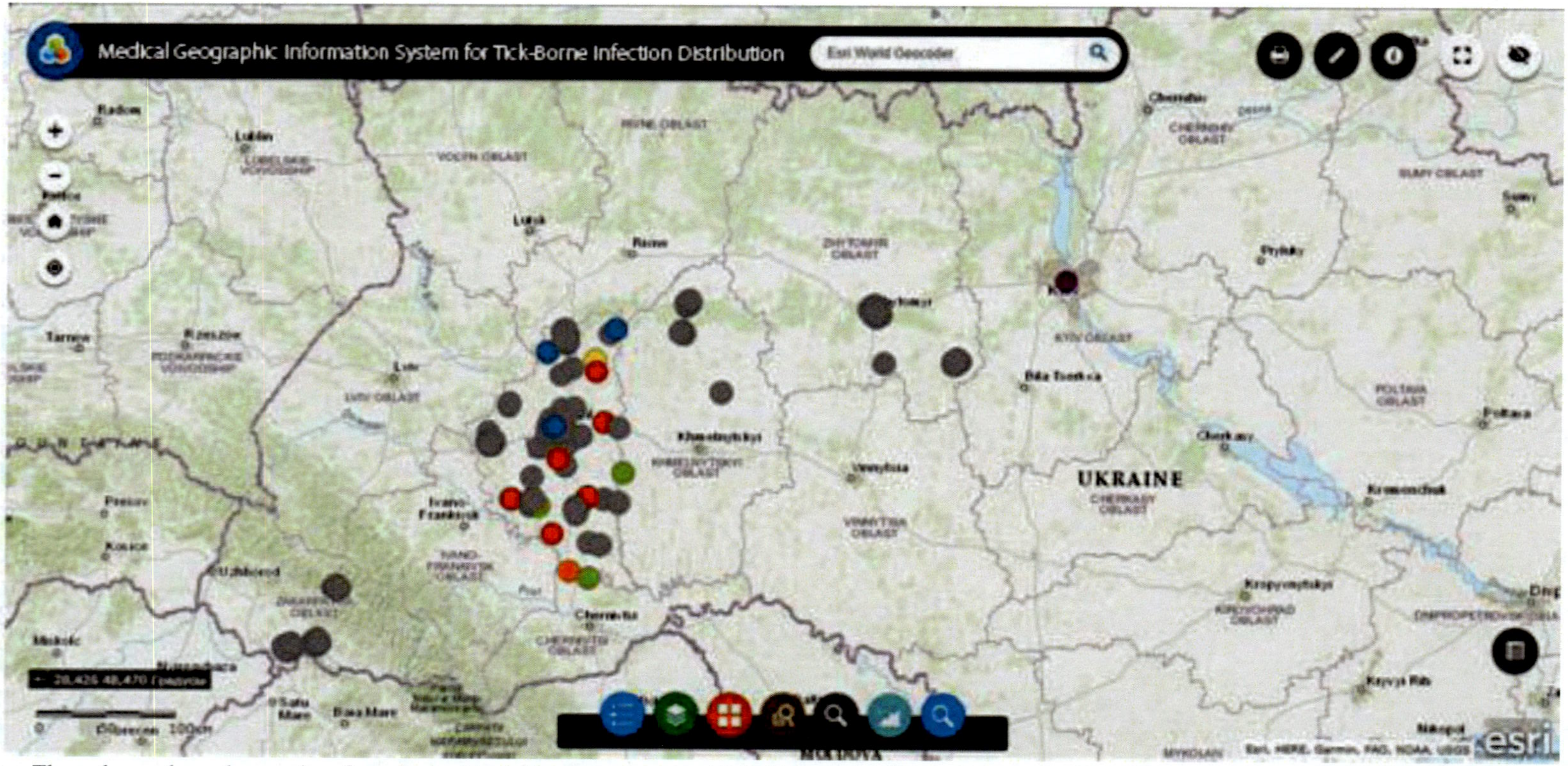

Note. The colours show the results of serological tests for the presence of IgM/IgG antibodies to *B. burgdorferi s. l.*: grey – positive; blue – intermediate; red is negative.

Figure 51. Data on foresters affected by ticks in Ukraine.

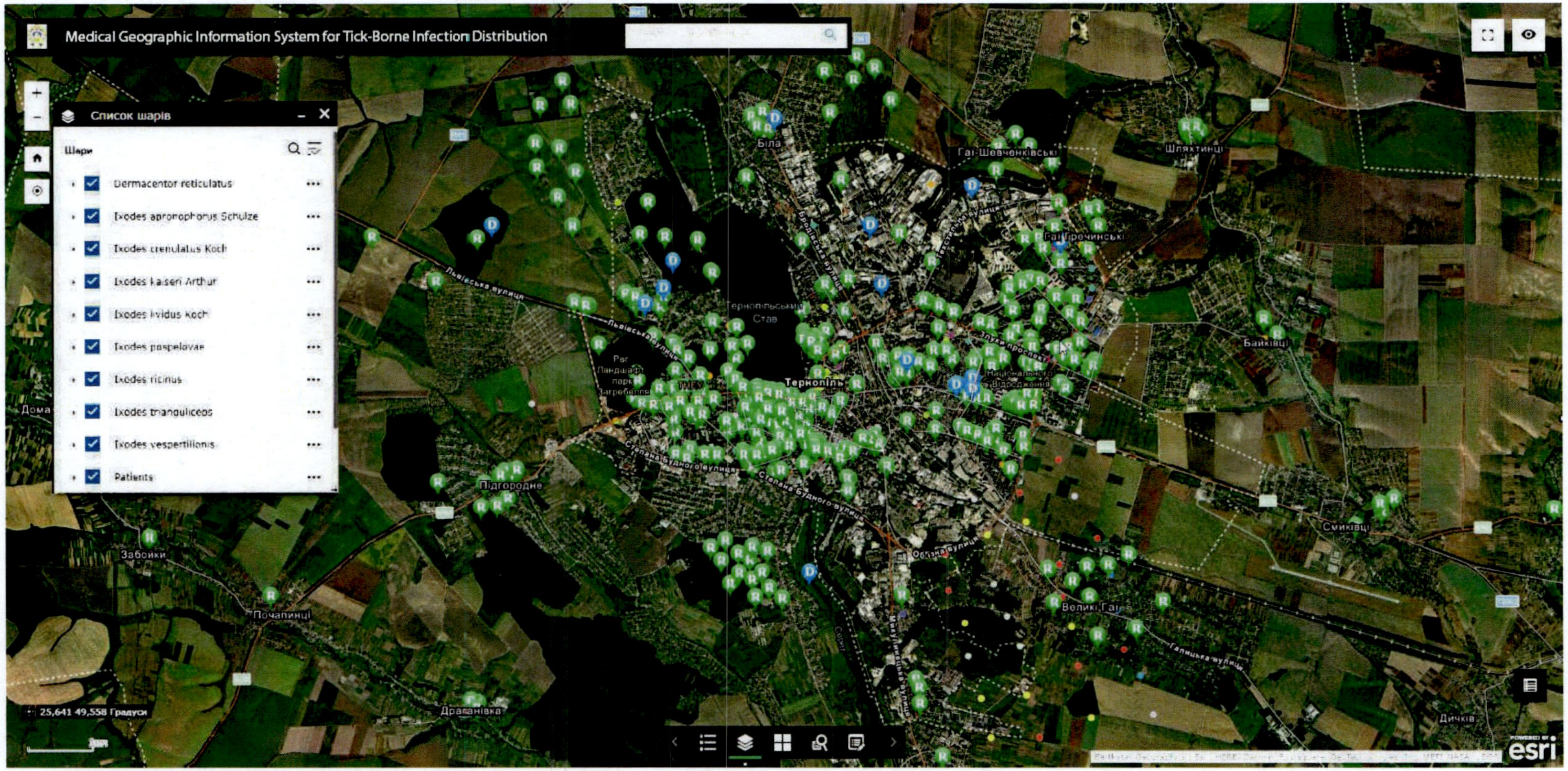

Note. The stages of development of ticks of the species *I. ricinus* (R) are highlighted by colours: green – nymphs; blue – females; red – larvae.

Figure 52. Biotopes of the distribution of ticks in the city of Ternopil.

In addition to the locations and other information about ticks, the GIS we have created also contains data about patients from whom these ticks were removed from the body surface. Currently, the map includes data on 1070 forestry workers from Ternopil, Zhytomyr, Chernihiv, Khmelnytskyi, Volyn, Rivne, and Transcarpathian regions of Ukraine (Figure 51), as well as 355 patients with erythematous and non-erythematous forms of Lyme borreliosis who were treated on an outpatient and inpatient basis during 2015-2020 at Ternopil Regional Clinical Dermatovenereological Dispensary, the infectious diseases department of Ternopil City Municipal Hospital Emergency Aid, Ternopil Regional Phthisiopulmonology Medical Centre, and Ternopil University Hospital.

The map integrates responses from a Unified International Questionnaire, detailing the frequency and specific locations of tick attacks, information about repellent use before entering forest zones, and self-examination of skin upon returning. Additionally, it records complaints reported after tick bites.

Furthermore, the map indicates dates of antibody detection to *B. burgdorferi s. l.* antigens (*B. burgdorferi s. s.*, *B. afzelii*, and *B. garinii*) in patients' blood serum using the ELISA and immunoblot, along with laboratory-confirmed LD results among foresters in the specified Ukrainian regions and hospital patients in Ternopil.

Subsequently, we briefed the administration of the State Forest Resources Agency of Ukraine and regional forest management administrations, including those in Ternopil, Zhytomyr, Chernihiv, Khmelnytskyi, Volyn, Rivne, and Transcarpathian regions, about the results of examinations conducted on forestry workers registered in the medical GIS. Infectious disease specialists in these regions received relevant information for further treatment of infected foresters.

An essential component of the medical GIS is the creation of topographic maps that include street names in populated areas, building numbering, and other details useful for pinpointing tick distribution within cities and villages. However, for delineating tick distribution zones over larger areas, physical maps or satellite images of the respective areas are more practical. This approach provides a visual representation of the biotopes where these ticks are prevalent (Figure 52).

The above information was shared with the staff of Ternopil Regional Public Health Centre and Ternopil Regional Laboratory Centre of the Ministry of Health of Ukraine for monitoring the sanitary and epidemiological situation of the environment, recreational and leisure zones, forests, forest belts, and other natural or artificial plantations in Ternopil city and the region.

The information on tick infestations in Ternopil city and the region, as well as the areas of their distribution, provided by us and the employees of Ternopil Regional Laboratory Centre of the Ministry of Health of Ukraine, allowed the staff of the "Preventive Disinfection" municipal enterprise to timely carry out disinsection of 5 areas of the city: Taras Shevchenko Park, "Vidrodzhennia," "Topilche," "Staryi Park," and "Zdorovia," significantly reducing the number of ticks in these areas and thus the incidence of these arthropods on humans and the likelihood of their infection with researched pathogens.

Therefore, we proposed modern approaches to monitoring the infestation of Ixodes ticks in nature and preventing the population from being affected by the pathogens of infectious diseases they transmit.

A geographic information system has been created, which provides spatial-geographical visualization of the spread of tick-borne infections and displays the localization of the detected pathogens of these diseases. This allows for statistical-visual analysis and comparative analysis of tick distribution, including those infected with Borrelia and other pathogens, according to the natural-geographical conditions of the region.

The geographic information system improves the visual-spatial perception of the correlation between natural conditions and the spread of tick-borne infections. This enables the assessment of threats to public health and the control of the spread of tick-borne infections, as well as the overall coverage of the sanitary-epidemiological situation of the region. It helps integrate into a unified visual-statistical geography the detection of tick vectors of infections, their quantity, types, morphology, infection rates with various transmissible pathogens, and the prevalence of diseases associated with them.

Conclusion

More than 50 species of the Borrelia genus are currently known, of which 7 species have been identified in Ukraine. These are predominantly transmitted by Ixodes ricinus and Dermacentor reticulatus ticks and are capable of causing various forms of Lyme borreliosis. The spontaneous infection rate of ticks collected from the environment with B. Burgdorferi s. l. complex spirochetes ranges from 7.0% to 25.0%, with an average of 17.0%. In-depth surveys across different population categories revealed that forestry workers, who operate directly in natural biotopes, are most frequently affected by ticks. Based on the study findings, interactive maps have been developed using a medical geographic information system. These maps reflect the dynamics of tick distribution, seasonal stage variation, and infection rates during specific time periods.

References

[1] Galdwin, M., Trattler, B. *Spirochetes: Clinical Microbiology Made Ridiculously Simple.* MedMaster, Inc; 2009. 393 p.

[2] Wang, G., Schwartz, I., Genus, I. I. Borrelia Swellengrebel 1907, 582AL. In: *Bergey's Manual of Systematic Bacteriology.* New York: Springer; 2011. Vol. 3; p. 484-498.

[3] Winn, W., Allen, S., Janda, W., Koneman, E., Procop, G., Schreckenberger, P., Woods, G. *Koneman's Colour Atlas and Textbook of Diagnostic Microbiology,* 6th ed. Baltimore: Lippincot Williams and Wilkins; 2006. 1535 p.

[4] LeClair, R. J. *LibreTexts.* Medicine [Internet]. Bacterial Infections of the Circulatory and Lymphatic Systems; 2024 [cited 2025 Feb 3]. Available from: https://med.libretexts.org/Courses/Virginia_Tech_Carilion_School_of_Medicine/Block_V_Preparation_Materials/17:_Systemic_Infections/17.04:_Circulatory_and_Lymphatic_System_Infections/17.4.02:_Bacterial_Infections_of_the_Circulatory_and_Lymphatic_Systems.

[5] Preac-Mursic, V., Wilske, B., Schierz, G. European Borrelia burgdorferi isolated from humans and ticks culture conditions and antibiotic susceptibility. *Zentralbl Bakteriol Mikrobiol Hyg A.* 1986;263(1-2):112-8. doi: 10.1016/s0176-6724(86)80110-9.

[6] Woitzik, P., Linder, S. Molecular Mechanisms of Borrelia burgdorferi Phagocytosis and Intracellular Processing by Human Macrophages. *Biology* (Basel). 2021;10(7):567. doi: 10.3390/biology10070567.

[7] Garrity, G., Bell, J., Lilburn, T. *Taxonomic Outline of the Prokaryotes. Bergey's Manual of Systematic Bacteriology.* 2nd ed. New York: Springer-Verlag; 2004. 399 p. doi: 10.1007/bergeysoutline200405.

[8] Miklossy, J., Kasas, S., Zurn, A. D., McCall, S., Yu, S., McGeer, P. L. Persisting atypical and cystic forms of Borrelia burgdorferi and local inflammation in Lyme neuroborreliosis. *J Neuroinflammation.* 2008;5:40. doi: 10.1186/1742-2094-5-40.

[9] Shapiro, E. D. Clinical practice. Lyme disease. *N Engl J Med.* 2014;370(18):1724-31. doi: 10.1056/NEJMcp1314325.

[10] Cameron, D. J., Johnson, L. B., Maloney, E. L. Evidence assessments and guideline recommendations in Lyme disease: the clinical management of known tick bites, erythema migrans rashes and persistent disease. *Expert Rev Anti Infect Ther.* 2014;12(9):1103-35. doi: 10.1586/14787210.2014.940900.

[11] Popovych, O. Lyme borreliosis: current problem of infectiology (Clinical Lecture). *Actual Infectology.* 2022;(3.12):114-22. doi: 10.22141/2312-413x.3.12.2016.81725. [in Ukrainian].

[12] Stupica, D., Lusa, L., Ruzić-Sabljić, E., Cerar, T., Strle, F. Treatment of erythema migrans with doxycycline for 10 days versus 15 days. *Clin Infect Dis.* 2012;55(3):343-50. doi: 10.1093/cid/cis402.

[13] Barthold, S. W,. Hodzic, E., Imai, D. M., Feng, S., Yang, X., Luft, B. J. Ineffectiveness of tigecycline against persistent Borrelia burgdorferi. *Antimicrob Agents Chemother.* 2010;54(2):643-51. doi: 10.1128/AAC.00788-09.

[14] Hunfeld, K. P., Kraiczy, P., Norris, D. E., Lohr, B. The *In Vitro* Antimicrobial Susceptibility of Borrelia burgdorferi sensu lato: Shedding Light on the Known Unknowns. *Pathogens.* 2023;12(10):1204. doi: 10.3390/pathogens12101204.

[15] Johnson, R. C., Schmid, G. P., Hyde, F. W., Steigerwalt, A. G., Brenner, D. J. Borrelia burgdorferi sp. nov.: etiologic agent of Lyme disease. *Int J Syst Bacteriol.* 1984;34: 496-497. doi: 10.1099/00207713-34-4-496.

[16] Nunes, M., Parreira, R., Maia, C., Lopes, N., Fingerle, V., Vieira, M. L. Molecular identification of Borrelia genus in questing hard ticks from Portugal: Phylogenetic characterization of two novel Relapsing Fever-like Borrelia sp. *Infect Genet Evol.* 2016;40:266-274. doi: 10.1016/j.meegid.2016.03.008.

[17] Colunga-Salas, P., Sánchez-Montes, S., Volkow, P., Ruíz-Remigio, A., Becker, I. Lyme disease and relapsing fever in Mexico: An overview of human and wildlife infections. *PLoS One.* 2020;15(9):e0238496. doi: 10.1371/journal.pone.0238496.

[18] Talagrand-Reboul, E., Boyer, P. H., Bergström, S., Vial, L., Boulanger, N. Relapsing Fevers: Neglected Tick-Borne Diseases. *Front Cell Infect Microbiol.* 2018;8:98. doi: 10.3389/fcimb.2018.00098.

[19] Clark, K. L., Leydet, B. F., Threlkeld, C. Geographical and genospecies distribution of Borrelia burgdorferi sensu lato DNA detected in humans in the USA. *J Med Microbiol.* 2014;63(Pt 5):674-684. doi: 10.1099/jmm.0.073122-0.

[20] Michelet, L., Delannoy, S., Devillers, E., Umhang, G., Aspan, A., Juremalm, M., Chirico, J., van der Wal, F. J., Sprong, H., Boye Pihl, T. P., Klitgaard, K., Bødker, R., Fach, P., Moutailler, S. High-throughput screening of tick-borne pathogens in Europe. *Front Cell Infect Microbiol.* 2014;4:103. doi: 10.3389/fcimb.2014.00103.

[21] Trevisan, G., Bonin, S., Ruscio, M. A Practical Approach to the Diagnosis of Lyme Borreliosis: From Clinical Heterogeneity to Laboratory Methods. *Front Med (Lausanne).* 2020;7:265. doi: 10.3389/fmed.2020.00265.

[22] Turianytsia, S. M., Andrashko, Y. V., Petrov, V. O., Sakal, M. M. Dynamics of the situation regarding Lyme disease in Zakarpattia [Internet]. Clinical Immunology. Allergology. *Infectology.* 2012 [cited 4 Feb 2025]; (1–2):61-64. Available from: https://kiai.com.ua/ua/archive/2012/1-2%2850-51%29/pages-34-39/dinamika-situaciyi-shchodo-hvorobi-layma-na-zakarpatti [in Ukrainian].

[23] Nebogatkin, I., Shulhan, A. Epidemiological and epizootic features of Lyme disease in 2019 in Ukraine. *Actual Infectology.* 2020;8(5-6):44-8. doi: 10.22141/2312-413x.8.5-6.2020.217959. [in Ukrainian].

[24] Talaska, T. Focus on Lyme-Borreliosis [Internet]. Milano: divisione di Springer-Verlag Italia Srl; 2013. *Epidemiological, biological, and ecological aspects of Lyme borreliosis;* [cited 5 Feb 2025]; pp. 5-25. Available at: https://novodx.net/borrelia/Borrelia%20(English).pdf.

[25] Rudenko, N., Golovchenko, M., Grubhoffer, L., Oliver, J. H. Jr. Updates on Borrelia burgdorferi sensu lato complex with respect to public health. *Ticks Tick Borne Dis.* 2011 Sep;2(3):123-8. doi: 10.1016/j.ttbdis.2011.04.002.

[26] Margos, G., Gofton, A., Wibberg, D., Dangel, A., Marosevic, D., Loh, S. M., Oskam, C., Fingerle, V. The genus Borrelia reloaded. *PLoS One.* 2018;13(12):e0208432. doi: 10.1371/journal.pone.0208432.

[27] Szekeres, S., Coipan, E. C,. Rigó, K., Majoros, G., Jahfari, S., Sprong, H., Földvári, G. Eco-epidemiology of Borrelia miyamotoi and Lyme borreliosis spirochetes in a popular hunting and recreational forest area in Hungary. *Parasit Vectors.* 2015;8:309. doi: 10.1186/s13071-015-0922-2.

[28] Kubiak, K., Szczotko, M., Dmitryjuk, M. Borrelia miyamotoi-An Emerging Human Tick-Borne Pathogen in Europe. *Microorganisms.* 2021;9(1):154. doi: 10.3390/microorganisms9010154.

[29] Kiewra, D., Stańczak, J., Richter, M. Ixodes ricinus ticks (Acari, Ixodidae) as a vector of Borrelia burgdorferi sensu lato and Borrelia miyamotoi in Lower Silesia, Poland - preliminary study. *Ticks Tick Borne Dis.* 2014;5(6):892-7. doi: 10.1016/j.ttbdis.2014.07.004.

[30] Komarenko, N. S., Vynohrad, N. O. Species varietion of borrelia and theirimportance for regional pathology. *Annals of Mechnikov Institute* [Internet]. 2011 [cited 1 Feb 2025];(3):20-22. Available at: https://www.imiamn.org.ua/journal/3_2011/PDF/6.pdf. [in Ukrainian].

[31] Krause, P. J., Narasimhan, S., Wormser, G. P., Rollend, L., Fikrig, E., Lepore, T., Barbour, A., Fish, D. Human Borrelia miyamotoi infection in the United States. *N Engl J Med.* 2013;368(3):291-3. doi: 10.1056/NEJMc1215469.

[32] Hovius, J. W., de Wever, B., Sohne, M., Brouwer, M. C., Coumou, J., Wagemakers, A., Oei, A., Knol, H., Narasimhan, S., Hodiamont, C. J., Jahfari, S., Pals, S. T., Horlings, H. M., Fikrig, E., Sprong, H., van Oers, M. H. A case of meningoencephalitis by the relapsing fever spirochaete Borrelia miyamotoi in Europe. *Lancet.* 2013;382(9892):658. doi: 10.1016/S0140-6736(13)61644-X.

[33] *American Society for Microbiology [Internet].* [cited 5 Feb 2025]. Available at: http://www.textbookofbacteriology.net/Lyme.html.

[34] Barer, M. R., Irving, V., Swonn, E., Perera, N. Medical Microbiology. A Guide to Microbial Infections: Pathogenesis, Immunity, Laboratory Diagnosis, and Control. In 2 vols. Vol 1. *Kyiv: Medicine;* 2020. 433 c. [in Ukrainian].

[35] Shyrobokov, V. P., (ed.). Medical Microbiology. Virology. Immunology. *Vinnytsia: Nova Knyha*; 2011. 952 p. [in Ukrainian].

[36] Ružić-Sabljić, E., Maraspin, V., Cimperman, J., Strle, F., Lotrič-Furlan, S., Stupica, D., Cerar, T. Comparison of isolation rate of Borrelia burgdorferi sensu lato in two different culture media, MKP and BSK-H. *Clin Microbiol Infect.* 2014;20(7):636-41. doi: 10.1111/1469-0691.12457.

[37] Walter, K. S., Carpi, G., Caccone, A., Diuk-Wasser, M. A. Genomic insights into the ancient spread of Lyme disease across North America. *Nat Ecol Evol.* 2017;1(10):1569-1576. doi: 10.1038/s41559-017-0282-8.

[38] Carroll, J. A., El-Hage, N., Miller, J. C., Babb, K., Stevenson, B. Borrelia burgdorferi RevA antigen is a surface-exposed outer membrane protein whose expression is regulated in response to environmental temperature and pH. *Infect Immun.* 2001;69(9):5286-93. doi: 10.1128/IAI.69.9.5286-5293.2001.

[39] Byram, R., Gaultney, R. A., Floden, A. M., Hellekson, C., Stone, B. L., Bowman, A., Stevenson, B., Johnson, B. J., Brissette, C. A. Borrelia burgdorferi RevA Significantly Affects Pathogenicity and Host Response in the Mouse Model of Lyme Disease. *Infect Immun.* 2015;83(9):3675-83. doi: 10.1128/IAI.00530-15.

[40] Mannelli, A., Bertolotti, L., Gern, L., Gray, J. Ecology of Borrelia burgdorferi sensu lato in Europe: transmission dynamics in multi-host systems, influence of molecular processes and effects of climate change. *FEMS Microbiol Rev.* 2012;36(4):837-61. doi: 10.1111/j.1574-6976.2011.00312.x.

[41] Zadorozhna, V. I., Rudenko, A. O., Klius, V. Yu. Lyme-borreliosis is a particularly dangerous infection. Threats and risks. *Veterynarna medytsyna* [Internet]. 2017 [cited 1 Feb 2025];103:30-2. Available at: https://www.jvm.kharkov.ua/sbornik/103/1_5.pdf. [in Ukrainian].

[42] Jaenson, T. G., Värv, K., Fröjdman, I., Jääskeläinen, A., Rundgren, K., Versteirt, V., ... & Golovljova, I. *First evidence of established populations of the taiga tick Ixodes persulcatus* (Acari: Ixodidae) in Sweden. Parasites & Vectors. 2016. 9, 1-8. https://doi.org/10.1186/s13071-016-1658-3

[43] Lewis, L. A., Radulović, Ž. M., Kim, T. K., Porter, L. M., Mulenga, A. Identification of 24h Ixodes scapularis immunogenic tick saliva proteins. *Ticks Tick Borne Dis.* 2015;6(3):424-34. doi: 10.1016/j.ttbdis.2015.03.012.

[44] Yevstafiev, I. L., Evstarev, E. Laimas disease: epizootical aspect. *The Journal of V. N. Karazin Kharkiv National University, series "Medicine"* [Internet]. 2002 [cited 2025 Feb 5];(4):42-6. Available from: https://periodicals.karazin.ua/medicine/article/view/7349. [in Ukrainian].

[45] Hauck, D., Jordan, D., Springer, A., Schunack, B., Pachnicke, S., Fingerle, V., Strube, C. Transovarial transmission of Borrelia spp., Rickettsia spp. and Anaplasma phagocytophilum in Ixodes ricinus under field conditions extrapolated from DNA detection in questing larvae. *Parasit Vectors.* 2020;13(1):176. doi: 10.1186/s13071-020-04049-7.

[46] Chitimia-Dobler L. TBEV-transmission and natural cycles. У: Dobler G, Erber W, Bröker M, Chitimia-Dobler L., Schmit H. J., редактори. *The TBE Book* [Internet]. 7th ed. Chapter 5. Global Health Press Pte Ltd; 2024 [cited 8 Feb 2025]. p. 71-89. Available at: https://tbenews.com/tbe/chapter-5-tbev-transmission-and-natural-cycles. doi: 10.33442/26613980_TBE-7.

[47] Estrada-Peña, A., Fernández-Ruiz, N. Is composition of vertebrates an indicator of the prevalence of tick-borne pathogens? *Infect Ecol Epidemiol.* 2022;12(1):2025647. doi: 10.1080/20008686.2022.2025647.

[48] Boulanger, N., Boyer, P., Talagrand-Reboul, E., Hansmann, Y. Ticks and tick-borne diseases. *Med Mal Infect.* 2019;49(2):87-97. doi: 10.1016/j.medmal.2019.01.007.

[49] Teodorowicz, P., Weiner, M. Current methods used to identify and genotype spirochaetes Borrelia burgdorferi. *Health Problems of Civilization.* 2020;14(2):71-82. doi: 10.5114/hpc.2020.93808.

[50] Kulias, S. M. Current opinion on peculiarities of specific diagnostics, treatment and prevention of Lyme borreliosis [Internet]. *Biomedical and biosocial anthropology.* 2013 [cited 2025 Feb 3];(20):245-51. Available from: http://nbuv.gov.ua/UJRN/bba_2013_20_62. [in Ukrainian].

[51] Lischer, C. J., Leutenegger, C. M., Braun, U., Lutz, H. Diagnosis of Lyme disease in two cows by the detection of Borrelia burgdorferi DNA. *Vet Rec.* 2000;146(17):497-9. doi: 10.1136/vr.146.17.497.

[52] Bouchard, C., Dibernardo, A., Koffi, J., Wood, H., Leighton, P. A., Lindsay, L. R. N Increased risk of tick-borne diseases with climate and environmental changes. *Can Commun Dis Rep.* 2019;45(4):83-89. doi: 10.14745/ccdr.v45i04a02.

[53] Bouchard, C., Beauchamp, G., Leighton, P. A., Lindsay, R., Bélanger, D., Ogden, N. H. Does high biodiversity reduce the risk of Lyme disease invasion? *Parasit Vectors.* 2013;6:195. doi: 10.1186/1756-3305-6-195.

[54] Bouchard, C., Leighton, P. A., Beauchamp, G., Nguon, S., Trudel, L., Milord, F., Lindsay, L. R., Bélanger, D., Ogden, N. H. Harvested white-tailed deer as sentinel hosts for early establishing Ixodes scapularis populations and risk from vector-borne zoonoses in southeastern Canada. *J Med Entomol.* 2013;50(2):384-93. doi: 10.1603/me12093.

[55] Levi, T., Kilpatrick, A. M., Mangel, M., Wilmers, C. C. Deer, predators, and the emergence of Lyme disease. *Proc Natl Acad Sci U S A.* 2012;109(27):10942-7. doi: 10.1073/pnas.1204536109.

[56] Nebogatkin, I., Shulhan, A. Epidemiological and epizootic features of Lyme disease in 2019 in Ukraine. *Actual Infectology.* 2020;8(5-6):44-8. doi: 10.22141/2312-413x.8.5-6.2020.217959. [in Ukrainian].

[57] Karbowiak, G., Biernat, B. The role of particular tick developmental stages in the circulation of tick-borne pathogens affecting humans in Central Europe. 2. Tick-borne encephalitis virus. *Ann Parasitol.* 2016;62(1):3-9. doi: 10.17420/ap6201.25.

[58] Steinbrink, A., Brugger, K., Margos, G., Kraiczy, P., Klimpel, S. The evolving story of Borrelia burgdorferi sensu lato transmission in Europe. *Parasitol Res.* 2022;121(3):781-803. doi: 10.1007/s00436-022-07445-3.

[59] Černý, J., Lynn, G., Hrnková, J., Golovchenko, M., Rudenko, N., Grubhoffer, L. Management Options for Ixodes ricinus-Associated Pathogens: A Review of Prevention Strategies. *Int J Environ Res Public Health.* 2020;17(6):1830. doi: 10.3390/ijerph17061830.

[60] Tokarz, R., Lipkin, W. I. Discovery and Surveillance of Tick-Borne Pathogens. *J Med Entomol.* 2021;58(4):1525-1535. doi: 10.1093/jme/tjaa269.

[61] Tsioka, K., Saratsis, A., Pappa, S., Papa, A. Pathogens Detected in Questing Ixodes ricinus Ticks in a Mountainous Area in Greece. *Pathogens.* 2024;13(6):449. doi: 10.3390/pathogens13060449.

[62] Dantas-Torres, F., Chomel, B. B., Otranto, D. Ticks and tick-borne diseases: a One Health perspective. *Trends Parasitol.* 2012;28(10):437-46. doi: 10.1016/j.pt.2012.07.003.

[63] Cutler, S. J., Vayssier-Taussat, M., Estrada-Peña, A., Potkonjak, A., Mihalca, A. D., Zeller, H. Tick-borne diseases and co-infection: Current considerations. *Ticks Tick Borne Dis.* 2021;12(1):101607. doi: 10.1016/j.ttbdis.2020.101607.

[64] Sprong, H., Azagi, T., Hoornstra, D., Nijhof, A. M., Knorr, S., Baarsma, M. E., Hovius, J. W. Control of Lyme borreliosis and other Ixodes ricinus-borne diseases. *Parasit Vectors*. 2018 Mar 6;11(1):145. doi: 10.1186/s13071-018-2744-5.

[65] Nebbak, A., Dahmana, H., Almeras, L., Raoult, D., Boulanger, N., Jaulhac, B., Mediannikov, O., Parola, P. Co-infection of bacteria and protozoan parasites in Ixodes ricinus nymphs collected in the Alsace region, France. *Ticks Tick Borne Dis*. 2019;10(6):101241. doi: 10.1016/j.ttbdis.2019.06.001.

[66] Kalmár, Z., Dumitrache, M. O., D'Amico, G., Matei, I. A., Ionică, A. M., Gherman, C. M., Lupşe, M., Mihalca, A. D. Multiple Tick-Borne Pathogens in Ixodes ricinus Ticks Collected from Humans in Romania. *Pathogens*. 2020;9(5):390. doi: 10.3390/pathogens9050390.

[67] Cook, M. J. Lyme borreliosis: a review of data on transmission time after tick attachment. *Int J Gen Med*. 2014;8:1-8. doi: 10.2147/IJGM.S73791.

[68] Cotté, V., Sabatier, L., Schnell, G., Carmi-Leroy, A., Rousselle, J. C., Arsène-Ploetze, F., Malandrin, L., Sertour, N., Namane, A., Ferquel, E., Choumet, V. Differential expression of Ixodes ricinus salivary gland proteins in the presence of the Borrelia burgdorferi sensu lato complex. *J Proteomics*. 2014;96:29-43. doi: 10.1016/j.jprot.2013.10.033.

[69] Pospisilova, T., Urbanova, V., Hes, O., Kopacek, P., Hajdusek, O., Sima, R. Tracking of Borrelia afzelii Transmission from Infected Ixodes ricinus Nymphs to Mice. *Infect Immun*. 2019 May 21;87(6):e00896-18. doi: 10.1128/IAI.00896-18.

[70] National Institute for Health and Care Excellence [Internet]. *Lyme disease. NICE guideline* [NG95]; April 11 2018 [cited 5 Feb 2025]. Available at: https://www.nice.org.uk/guidance/NG95.

[71] Chemych, M., Lutai, I. Lyme disease. Modern issue condition. *East Ukr Med J*. 2020;8(2):230-41. doi: 10.21272/eumj.2020;8(2):230-41. [in Ukrainian].

[72] Ben Said, M., Belkahia, H., Alberti, A., Abdi, K., Zhioua, M., Daaloul-Jedidi, M., Messadi, L. First molecular evidence of [i]Borrelia burgdorferi[/i] sensu lato in goats, sheep, cattle and camels in Tunisia. *Ann Agric Environ Med*. 2016;23(3):442-7. doi: 10.5604/12321966.1219184.

[73] Lakos, A., Solymosi, N. Maternal Lyme borreliosis and pregnancy outcome. *Int J Infect Dis*. 2010;14(6):e494-8. doi: 10.1016/j.ijid.2009.07.019.

[74] Waddell, L. A., Greig, J., Lindsay, L. R., Hinckley, A. F., Ogden, N. H. A systematic review on the impact of gestational Lyme disease in humans on the fetus and newborn. *PloS One*. 2018;13(11):e0207067. doi: 10.1371/journal.pone.0207067.

[75] Tylewska-Wierzbanowska, S., Chmielewski, T. Tick-borne bacterial diseases in Poland. *Health Problems of Civilization*. 2017; 11(2): 56-65. doi: 10.5114/hpc.2017.69017.

[76] Shostakovych-Koretska, L., Budayeva, I., Cherginets, A., Mavrutenkov, V., Marchenko, N. Lyme Borreliosis: Diagnosis and Treatment Issues. *Actual Infectology*. 2014;(2.03):34-8. doi: 10.22141/2312-413x.2.03.2014.82346. [in Ukrainian].

[77] Mysterud, A., Stigum, V. M., Jaarsma, R. I., Sprong, H. Genospecies of Borrelia burgdorferi sensu lato detected in 16 mammal species and questing ticks from northern Europe. *Sci Rep*. 2019;9(1):5088. doi: 10.1038/s41598-019-41686-0.

[78] Scott, J. D., Anderson, J. F., Durden, L. A., Smith, M. L., Manord, J. M., Clark, K. L. Prevalence of the Lyme Disease Spirochete, Borrelia burgdorferi, in Blacklegged Ticks, Ixodes scapularis at Hamilton-Wentworth, Ontario. *Int J Med Sci*. 2016;13(5):316-24. doi: 10.7150/ijms.14552.

[79] Strzelczyk, J. K., Gaździcka, J., Cuber, P., Asman, M., Trapp, G., Gołąbek, K., Zalewska-Ziob, M., Nowak-Chmura, M., Siuda, K., Wiczkowski, A., Solarz, K. Prevalence of Borrelia burgdorferi sensu lato in Ixodes ricinus ticks collected from southern Poland. *Acta Parasitol*. 2015;60(4):666-74. doi: 10.1515/ap-2015-0095.

[80] Potkonjak, A., Kleinerman, G., Gutiérrez, R., Savić, S., Vračar, V., Nachum-Biala, Y., Jurišić, A., Rojas, A., Petrović, A., Ivanović, I., Harrus, S., Baneth, G. Occurrence of Borrelia burgdorferi Sensu Lato in Ixodes ricinus Ticks with First Identification of Borrelia miyamotoi in Vojvodina, Serbia. *Vector Borne Zoonotic Dis*. 2016;16(10):631-5. doi: 10.1089/vbz.2016.2008.

[81] Jahfari, S., Hofhuis, A., Fonville, M., van der Giessen, J., van Pelt, W., Sprong, H. Molecular Detection of Tick-Borne Pathogens in Humans with Tick Bites and Erythema Migrans, in the Netherlands. *PloS Negl Trop Dis*. 2016;10(10):e0005042. doi: 10.1371/journal.pntd.0005042.

[82] Ragagli, C., Mannelli, A., Ambrogi, C., Bisanzio, D., Ceballos, L. A., Grego, E., Martello, E., Selmi, M., Tomassone, L. Presence of host-seeking Ixodes ricinus and their infection with Borrelia burgdorferi sensu lato in the Northern Apennines, Italy. *Exp Appl Acarol.* 2016;69(2):167-78. doi: 10.1007/s10493-016-0030-9.

[83] Estrada-Peña, A., Cutler, S., Potkonjak, A., Vassier-Tussaut, M., Van Bortel, W., Zeller, H., Fernández-Ruiz, N., Mihalca, A. D. An updated meta-analysis of the distribution and prevalence of Borrelia burgdorferi s.l. in ticks in Europe. *Int J Health Geogr.* 2018;17(1):41. doi: 10.1186/s12942-018-0163-7.

[84] Walter, K. S., Carpi, G., Evans, B. R., Caccone, A., Diuk-Wasser, M. A. Vectors as Epidemiological Sentinels: Patterns of Within-Tick Borrelia burgdorferi Diversity. *PloS Pathog.* 2016;12(7):e1005759. doi: 10.1371/journal.ppat.1005759.

[85] Chiappa, G., Perini, M., Cafiso, A., Nodari, R., Wilhelmsson, P., Lindgren, P. E., Omazic, A., Ullman, K., Moutailler, S., Kjellander, P., Bazzocchi, C., Grandi, G. A Novel High Discriminatory Protocol for the Detection of Borrelia afzelii, Borrelia burgdorferi Sensu Stricto and Borrelia garinii in Ticks. *Pathogens.* 2022;11(11):1234. doi: 10.3390/pathogens11111234.

[86] Stanek, G., Wormser, G. P., Gray, J., Strle, F. Lyme borreliosis. *Lancet.* 2012;379(9814):461-73. doi: 10.1016/S0140-6736(11)60103-7.

[87] Coipan, E. C., Jahfari, S., Fonville, M., Oei, G. A., Spanjaard, L., Takumi, K., Hovius, J. W., Sprong, H. Imbalanced presence of Borrelia burgdorferi s.l. multilocus sequence types in clinical manifestations of Lyme borreliosis. *Infect Genet Evol.* 2016;42:66-76. doi: 10.1016/j.meegid.2016.04.019.

[88] Sprong, H., Azagi, T., Hoornstra, D., Nijhof, A. M., Knorr, S., Baarsma, M. E., Hovius, J. W. Control of Lyme borreliosis and other Ixodes ricinus-borne diseases. *Parasit Vectors.* 2018;11(1):145. doi: 10.1186/s13071-018-2744-5.

[89] Strnad, M., Hönig, V., Růžek, D., Grubhoffer, L., Rego, R. O. M. Europe-Wide Meta-Analysis of Borrelia burgdorferi Sensu Lato Prevalence in Questing Ixodes ricinus Ticks. *Appl Environ Microbiol.* 2017;83(15):e00609-17. doi: 10.1128/AEM.00609-17.

[90] Karbowiak, G., Biernat, B., Szewczyk, T., Sytykiewicz, H. The role of particular tick developmental stages in the circulation of tick-borne pathogens affecting humans in Central Europe. 1. The general pattern. *Ann Parasitol.* 2015;61(4):221-8. doi: 10.17420/ap6104.11.

[91] Nosek, J., Sixl, W.. Central-European Ticks (Ixodoidea). Key for determination. *Mitteilungen Abt Fur Zool Am Landesmus Joanneum Graz* [Internet]. 1972 [cited 6 Feb 2025];1:61-92. Available at: https://www.zobodat.at/pdf/MittZoolJoan_01_1972_0061-0092.pdf.

[92] Estrada-Peña, A., Mihalca, A. D., Petney, T. N. Ticks of Europe and North Africa. *A Guide to Species Identification.* Springer Cham; 2017. 404 p. doi: 10.1007/978-3-319-63760-0.

[93] Balashov, Yu. S. Bloodsucking ticks (Ixodoidea) – vectors of disease in man and animals. *Miscellaneous Publications of the Entomological Society of America.* 1972;8(5):376 p. doi: 10.4182/HKTD2318.

[94] Barbour, A. G., Burgdorfer, W., Hayes, S. F., Péter, O., Aeschlimann, A. Isolation of a cultivable spirochete from Ixodes ricinus ticks of Switzerland. *Curr Microbiol.* 1983;(8):123-126. doi: 10.1007/BF01566969.

[95] de la Fuente, J., Estrada-Pena, A., Venzal, J. M., Kocan, K. M., Sonenshine, D. E. Overview: Ticks as vectors of pathogens that cause disease in humans and animals. *Front Biosci.* 2008;13:6938-46. doi: 10.2741/3200.

[96] Keirans, J. Systematics of the Ixodida (Argasidae, Ixodidae, Nuttalliellidae): an overview and some problems. In: Fivaz B, Petney T, Horak I, eds. *Tick Vector Biology. Medical and Veterinary Aspects.* Berlin: Springer-Verlag; 1992. P. 1-21.

[97] Guglielmone, A. A., Robbins, R. G., Apanaskevich, D. A., Petney, T. N., Estrada-Pea, A., Horak, I. G., Shao, R. Barker S. C. The Argasidae, Ixodidae and Nuttalliellidae (Acari: Ixodida) of the world: a list of valid species names [Internet]. *Zootaxa.* 2010 [cited 6 Feb 2025]; 2528: 1–28. Available at: http://hdl.handle.net/2263/17278.

[98] Yemchuk, E. M. Fauna of Ukraine: in forty vol. Vol. 25, *Ixodes Ticks*. Kyiv: Publishing House of the Academy of Sciences of the Ukrainian SSR; 1960. 163 p. [in Ukrainian].

[99] Podobivskyi, S. S., Fedoniuk, L. Ya. On the species composition, biology, and significance of Ixodes ticks of Western Ukraine [Internet]. *Scientific Issues of Ternopil Volodymyr Hnatiuk National Pedagogical University*. Series: Biology. 2017 [cited 6 Feb 2025];(2):123-29. Available at: http://dspace.tnpu.edu.ua/bitstream/123456789/8069/1/Podobivskij%2c%20Fedonyuk.pdf [in Ukrainian].

[100] Fedoniuk, L. Ya., Podobivskyi, S. S. Morphological 99eculiarities of ixodidae populations in Ternopil region and neighbouring regions of Western Ukraine [Internet]. *Bulletin of Biological and Medical Problems.* 2017[cited 6 Feb 2025]; 2(4):152-155. Available at: https://repository.pdmu.edu.ua/server/api/core/bitstreams/763f57d3-ecb1-4066-a535-e0be6b31b4f1/content [in Ukrainian].

[101] Bowman, A. S., Nuttall, P. A., Eds. *Ticks: Biology, Disease and Control.* Cambridge University Press; 2008. 506 p.

[102] Mihalca, A. D., Dumitrache, M. O., Sándor, A. D., Magdaş, C., Oltean, M., Györke, A., Matei, I. A., Ionică, A., D'Amico, G., Cozma, V., Gherman, C. M. Tick parasites of rodents in Romania: host preferences, community structure and geographical distribution. *Parasit Vectors*. 2012;5:266. doi: 10.1186/1756-3305-5-266.

[103] Keve, G., Sándor, A. D., Hornok, S. Hard ticks (Acari: Ixodidae) associated with birds in Europe: Review of literature data. *Front Vet Sci*. 2022;9:928756. doi: 10.3389/fvets.2022.928756.

[104] Kocianová, E. Ticks (Ixodidae) from passerine birds in the Carpathian region. *Wiener klinische Wochenschrift*. 2006;118(23-24):759-64. doi: 10.1007/s00508-006-0729-4.

[105] Fedoniuk, L. Ya., Podobivskyi, S. S., Korda, M. M., Klishch, I. M., Andreychyn, M. A., Shkilna, M. I. Morpho-physiological features and medical significance of ixodic mites of ixodes latr. And dermacentor fabr. Generations – humans and animals ectoparasites in Western Ukraine. *World of Medicine and Biology*. 2018;(1):173-177. doi: 10.26724/2079-8334-2017-4-62-173-177 [in Ukrainian].

[106] Stanko, M. Ecology of Ixodes ricinus immatures on Apodemus agrarius (Muridae) in the lowland ecosystems conditions. *Wiad Parazytol.* 1995;41(3):329-36.

[107] Kahl, O., Gray, J. S. The biology of Ixodes ricinus with emphasis on its ecology. *Ticks Tick Borne Dis.* 2023;14(2):102114. doi: 10.1016/j.ttbdis.2022.102114.

[108] Radolf, J. D., Strle, K., Lemieux, J. E., Strle, F. Lyme Disease in Humans. *Curr Issues Mol Biol.* 2021;42:333-84. doi: 10.21775/cimb.042.333.

[109] Venclíková, K., Betášová, L., Sikutová, S., Jedličková, P., Hubálek, Z., Rudolf, I. Human pathogenic borreliae in Ixodes ricinus ticks in natural and urban ecosystem (Czech Republic). *Acta Parasitol.* 2014;59(4):717-20. doi: 10.2478/s11686-014-0296-1.

[110] Woldehiwet, Z. The natural history of Anaplasma phagocytophilum. *Vet Parasitol.* 2010;167(2-4):108-22. doi: 10.1016/j.vetpar.2009.09.013.

[111] Strle, F. Human granulocytic ehrlichiosis in Europe. *Int J Med Microbiol.* 2004;293 (37):27-35. doi: 10.1016/s1433-1128(04)80006-8.

[112] Di Domenico, M., Pascucci, I., Curini, V., Cocco, A., Dall'Acqua, F., Pompilii, C., Cammà, C. Detection of Anaplasma phagocytophilum genotypes that are potentially virulent for human in wild ruminants and Ixodes ricinus in Central Italy. *Ticks Tick Borne Dis*. 2016;7(5):782-787. doi: 10.1016/j.ttbdis.2016.03.012.

[113] Boletska, T. O., Chemych, M. D. Lyme disease, anaplasmosis, and ehrlichiosis in Sumy region. Current Issues in Theoretical and Practical Medicine: *Proceedings of the 2nd International Scientific-Practical Conference for Students and Young Scientists;* April 16–18, 2014; Sumy. Sumy; 2014. P. 119. [in Ukrainian].

[114] Malyi, V. P., Shepileva, N. V., Tkachenko, L. V. Tick-borne infections in Kharkiv region. *International Medical Journal.* 2010;16(3):99-102. [in Russian].

[115] Beletskaya, H. V., Lozinsky, I. N., Morochkovsky, R. S. Current state of tick-borne infections in the border regions of Ukraine and the Republic of Belarus. In: *Current Issues in Infectious Pathology: Proceedings of the 6th Congress of Infectiologists of the Republic of Belarus*; May 29–30, 2014; Vitebsk. Vitebsk; 2014. P. 41–43. [in Russian].

[116] Ben, I. I., Biletska, G. V., Korolyuk, O. V., Morochkovsky, R. S., Shulgan, A. M. Granulocytic anaplasmosis in humans in Western Ukraine: epidemiological and laboratory studies [Internet*].*

Collected Scientific Works of P. L. Shupyk NMA of Ukraine. 2013 [cited 6 Feb 2025];22(2):320-323. Available at: http://nbuv.gov.ua/UJRN/Znpsnmapo_2013_22%282%29__51 [in Ukrainian].

[117] Zelenukhina, O. V., Kovryha, N. Ya., Chebotok, Ye. M. Monitoring of natural focal infections transmitted by Ixodes ticks in Zaporizhzhia region. *Problems of Military Health Protection.* 2015;44(2):135-138. [in Ukrainian].

[118] Fedoniuk, L. Ya., Podobivskyi, S. S. Results of the study of the biology and epidemiology of Ixodes ticks in 2018 in Ternopil region [Internet]. Medical-Biological Aspects and Multidisciplinary Integration in the Concept of Human Health: *Proceedings of the All-Ukrainian Conference with International Participation;* April 9–11, 2020; Ternopil. Ternopil; 2020 [cited 6 Feb 2025]. Vol. 1. P. 201-202. Available at: https://repository.tdmu.edu.ua/handle/123456789/16964 [in Ukrainian].

[119] Podobivskyi, S. S. Study of the biology and epidemiology of Ixodes ticks in Ternopil region in 2019. Medical-Biological Aspects and Multidisciplinary Integration in the Concept of Human Health: *Proceedings of the All-Ukrainian Conference with International Participation;* April 9–11, 2020; Ternopil. Ternopil; 2020 [cited 6 Feb 2025]. Vol. 1. P. 158-160. Available at: https://repository.tdmu.edu.ua/handle/123456789/16964 [in Ukrainian].

[120] Shkilna, M. I., Andreychyn, M. A., Podobivsky, S. S., Fedoniuk, L. Ya., Panychev, V. A., Ivakhiv, O. L., Vyshnevska, N. Yu., Marchuk, O. M., Korda, M. M., Klishch, I. M. Tick infestation collected from humans in Ukraine with bacterial pathogens of some diseases. *Bukovyna Medical Bulletin.* 2020;24(1):195-201. doi: 10.24061/2413-0737.XXIV.1.93.2020.26 [in Ukrainian].

[121] Akimov, I. A., Nebogatkin, I. V. *Ixodid ticks of urban landscapes of Kyiv.* Kyiv; 2016. 156 p. [in Russian].

[122] Akimov, I. A., Nebogatkin, I. V. Ixodid ticks of Kyiv – urbozoological and epizootological aspects. *Zoology Bulletin.* 2002;36 (1): 91-5. [in Russian].

[123] Rizzoli, A., Silaghi, C., Obiegala, A., Rudolf, I., Hubálek, Z., Földvári, G., Plantard, O., Vayssier-Taussat, M., Bonnet, S., Spitalská, E., Kazimírová, M. Ixodes ricinus and Its Transmitted Pathogens in Urban and Peri-Urban Areas in Europe: New Hazards and Relevance for Public Health. *Front Public Health.* 2014;2:251. doi: 10.3389/fpubh.2014.00251.

[124] Krause, P. J., Fish, D., Narasimhan, S., Barbour, A. G. Borrelia miyamotoi infection in nature and in humans. *Clin Microbiol Infect.* 2015 Jul;21(7):631-9. doi: 10.1016/j.cmi.2015.02.006. Epub 2015 Feb 18. PMID: 25700888; PMCID: PMC4470780.

[125] Turianin, I. I. On the parasitic fauna of some terrestrial vertebrates in the Transcarpathian region. Reports and Communications of Uzhhorod University. *Series: Biology.* 1958;(2):76-9. [in Russian].

[126] Turianin, I. I. Problems of Parasitology. Kyiv; 1963. Composition of vertebrate hosts of ticks of the genus Ixodoidea Latr. *In the Soviet Carpathians;* p. 36-8. [in Russian].

[127] Turianin, I. I. Ecology of Insects and Other Terrestrial Invertebrates of the Soviet Carpathians. Uzhhorod; 1964. *On the peculiar foci of Ixodes ticks in some points of the Ukrainian Carpathians;* p. 85-7. [in Russian].

[128] Nebogatkin, I. V. Ixodes ricinus and Dermacentor reticulatus (Acari: Ixodida: Ixodidae) in southern Ukraine. *Ukrainian Entomofaunistica* [Internet]. 2018 [cited 4 Feb 2025];9(1):43-57. Available at: https://drive.google.com/open?id=1vi9dljvKMU6XPuybwWTIGQJ2vXDuL8YH [in Ukrainian].

[129] Fedoniuk, L. Ya., Podobivskyi, S. S. Spread of Dermacentor reticulatus ticks in Ukraine. Clinical and Experimental *Pathology.* 2020;19(3):128-37. doi: 10.24061/1727-4338.XIX.3.73.2020.18 [in Ukrainian].

[130] Šimo, L., Kocáková, P., Slávíková, M., Kubes, M., Hajnicka, V., Vancova, I., Slovak, M. Dermacentor reticulatus (Acari, Ixodidae) female feeding in laboratory. *Biologia Bratislava.* 2004;59:655-60.

[131] Nowak, M. Discovery of Dermacentor reticulatus (Acari: Amblyommidae) populations in the Lubuskie Province (Western Poland). *Exp Appl Acarol.* 2011 Jun;54(2):191-7. doi: 10.1007/s10493-010-9422-4.

[132] Pfäffle, M., Littwin, N., Petney, T. Host preferences of immature Dermacentor reticulatus (Acari: Ixodidae) in a forest habitat in Germany. *Ticks Tick Borne Dis.* 2015;6(4):508-15. doi: 10.1016/j.ttbdis.2015.04.003.

[133] Földvári, G., Široký, P., Szekeres, S., Majoros, G., Sprong, H. Dermacentor reticulatus: a vector on the rise. *Parasit Vectors.* 2016;9(1):314. doi: 10.1186/s13071-016-1599-x.

[134] Paziewska, A., Zwolińska, L., Harris, P. D., Bajer, A., Siński, E. Utilisation of rodent species by larvae and nymphs of hard ticks (Ixodidae) in two habitats in NE Poland. *Exp Appl Acarol.* 2010;50(1):79-91. doi: 10.1007/s10493-009-9269-8.

[135] Slovák, M., Labuda, M., Marley, S. E. Mass laboratory rearing of Dermacentor reticulatus ticks (Acarina, Ixodidae) *Biologia, Bratislava.* 2002;57(2):261-6.

[136] Nehoroshikh, Z. M., Yegorova, O. O., Gaydash, O. M., Dzhurtubaeva, G. M., Pylypenko, N. V., Protsishyna, N. M., Kovbasyuk, O. V. Monitoring of natural foci of tularemia in the Southern region of Ukraine. *Current Infectology.* 2018; 6(5):275-7. doi: 10.22141/2312-413x.6.5.2018.146774 [in Ukrainian].

[137] Rudolf, I., Mendel, J., Sikutová, S., Svec, P., Masaríková, J., Nováková, D., Bunková, L., Sedlácek, I., Hubálek, Z. 16S rRNA gene-based identification of cultured bacterial flora from host-seeking Ixodes ricinus, Dermacentor reticulatus and Haemaphysalis concinna ticks, vectors of vertebrate pathogens. *Folia Microbiol (Praha).* 2009 Sep;54(5):419-28. doi: 10.1007/s12223-009-0059-9.

[138] Dwużnik, D., Mierzejewska, E. J., Drabik, P., Kloch, A., Alsarraf, M., Behnke, J. M., Bajer, A. The role of juvenile Dermacentor reticulatus ticks as vectors of microorganisms and the problem of 'meal contamination.' *Exp Appl Acarol.* 2019;78(2):181-202. doi: 10.1007/s10493-019-00380-6.

[139] On approval of the guidelines Non-specific prevention of transmissible natural focal infections transmitted by Ixodes ticks, Order of the Ministry of Health of Ukraine № 369, May 13, 2013, *Zakon Online* [Internet], [cited 4 Feb 2025] (Ukraine). Available at: https://zakononline.com.ua/documents/show/6557365573. [in Ukrainian].

[140] On improving the measures for the prevention of tick-borne encephalitis in Ukraine, Order of the Ministry of Health of Ukraine № 431, Aug 30, 2005, *Zakon Online* [Internet], [cited 4 Feb 2025] (Ukraine). Available at: https://zakononline.com.ua/documents/show/53697___53697. [in Ukrainian].

[141] On enhancing the diagnostic and preventive measures for Ixodes tick-borne borreliosis in Ukraine, Order of the Ministry of Health of Ukraine from №. 218, May 16, 2005, *Zakon Online* [Internet], [cited 4 Feb 2025] (Ukraine). Available at: https://zakononline.com.ua/documents/show/8393783937. [in Ukrainian].

[142] Kooyman, F. N. J., Zweerus, H., Nijsse, E. R., Jongejan, F., Wagenaar, J. A., Broens, E. M. Monitoring of ticks and their pathogens from companion animals obtained by the "tekenscanner" application in The Netherlands. *Parasitol Res.* 2022;121(7):1887-1893. doi: 10.1007/s00436-022-07518-3.

[143] Newman, B. C., Sutton, W. B., Wang, Y., Schweitzer, C. J., Moncayo, A. C., Miller, B. T. A standardized method for the construction of a tick drag/flag sampling approach and evaluation of sampling efficacy. *Exp Appl Acarol.* 2019;79(3-4):433-446. doi: 10.1007/s10493-019-00429-6.

[144] Harrison, A., Bennett, N. C. The importance of the aggregation of ticks on small mammal hosts for the establishment and persistence of tick-borne pathogens: an investigation using the R(0) model. *Parasitology.* 2012;139(12):1605-13. doi: 10.1017/S0031182012000893.

[145] On Standardization, Law of Ukraine № 1315-VII, Jun 5, 2014, *Verkhovna Rada of Ukraine* [Internet], [cited 4 Feb 2025] (Ukraine). Available at: https://zakon.rada.gov.ua/laws/show/en/1315-18?lang=uk#Text [in Ukrainian].

[146] Biletska, H. V., Semenyshyn, O. V., Ben, I. I. Modern parasitic systems of tick-borne infections in Lviv region. In: *Strategy and Tactics of Combating Infectious Diseases.* October 17–18, 2012; Kharkiv. Kharkiv; 2012. P. 126–32. [in Ukrainian].

[147] Boehnke, D., Brugger, K., Pfäffle, M., Sebastian, P., Norra, S., Petney, T., Oehme, R., Littwin, N., Lebl, K., Raith, J., Walter, M., Gebhardt, R., Rubel, F. Estimating Ixodes ricinus densities on the landscape scale. *Int J Health Geogr.* 2015;14:23. doi: 10.1186/s12942-015-0015-7.

[148] Ehrmann, S., Liira, J., Gärtner, S., Hansen, K., Brunet, J., Cousins, S. A. O., Deconchat, M., Decocq, G., De Frenne, P., De Smedt, P., Diekmann, M., Gallet-Moron, E., Kolb, A., Lenoir, J., Lindgren, J., Naaf, T., Paal, T., Valdés, A., Verheyen, K., Wulf, M., Scherer-Lorenzen, M. Environmental drivers of Ixodes ricinus abundance in forest fragments of rural European landscapes. *BMC Ecol.* 2017;17(1):31. doi: 10.1186/s12898-017-0141-0.

[149] Jung Kjær, L., Soleng, A., Edgar, K. S., Lindstedt, H. E. H., Paulsen, K. M., Andreassen, Å. K., Korslund, L., Kjelland, V., Slettan, A., Stuen, S., Kjellander, P., Christensson, M., Teräväinen, M., Baum, A., Klitgaard, K., Bødker, R. Predicting the spatial abundance of Ixodes ricinus ticks in southern

Scandinavia using environmental and climatic data. *Sci Rep.* 2019;9(1):18144. doi: 10.1038/s41598-019-54496-1.

[150] Panychev, V. O., Pavlyshyn, A. V., Andreychyn, M. A. Device for tick catching. *Patent* 123825. March 12, 2018. [in Ukrainian].

[151] Panychev, V. O., Pavlyshyn, A. V., Andreychyn, M. A. Method of tick catching in natural environment. *Patent* 123848. March 12, 2018. [in Ukrainian].

[152] Kyseliov, S. M. Basic principles of evidence-based medicine: educational guide. *Zaporizhzhia;* 2018. P. 118 p. [in Ukrainian]

[153] Milton, M. [Internet]. Using the laws of nature to establish the laws of measurement. *Message on the occasion of World Metrology Day–2018;* 2018 [cited 4 Feb 2025]. Available at: https://www.ukrcsm.kiev.ua/images/news/2018-05-20/Directors_Message_WMD_2018_Milton_Uk.docx [in Ukrainian].

[154] YouTube.ua [Internet]. [Video], *Why is the metric system so important TED Ed*?; Nov. 12 2023 [cited 4 Feb 2025]; [5 min., 45 s]. Available at: https: https://youtu.be/A1VPAXLHxSk?feature=shared. [in Ukrainian].

[155] Randolph, S. E. Tick ecology: processes and patterns behind the epidemiological risk posed by ixodid ticks as vectors. *Parasitology*. 2004;129:S37-65. doi: 10.1017/s0031182004004925.

[156] Holiachenko, O. M. *Social medicine and healthcare organization: textbook*. Kyiv: Medicine; 2011. 208 p. [in Ukrainian].

[157] Panychev, V. O., Sverstiuk, A. S., Avsiukevych, O. Y., Velychko, S. V., Savchuk, I. M. Comparison of the effectiveness of tick-catching devices depending on the design of the flag. *Infectious Diseases*. 2018;(4):20-5. doi: 10.11603/1681-2727.2018.4.9772 [in Ukrainian].

[158] Panychev, V., Dautov, A., Pavelieva, M., Hodovana, N. Some results of assessing the number and Borrelia infection in mites from various natural sites of Ternopil. Epidemiological risk assessment. In: *Third Annual BTRP Ukraine Regional One Health Research Symposium*. April 16-20, 2018; Kyiv. Kyiv; 2018. P. 72.

[159] Klymnyuk, S. I., Romanyuk, L. B., Shkilna, M. I. Modern concepts of granulocytic anaplasmosis in humans. *Infectious Diseases*. 2017;(3):4-9. doi: 10.11603/1681-2727.2017.3.8220. [in Ukrainian].

[160] Vasilyeva, N. A., Ivakhiv, O. L., Kachor, V. O., Avsyukevich, O. E., Voloshyn, S. B., Prodan, A. M., Gerasymenko, O. A., Velychko, S. V., Biletska, H. V., Semenyshyn, O. B. Lyme Disease in the Ternopil Region. *Infectious Diseases.* 2011;(20):50–53. doi: 10.11603/1681-2727.2011.2.577. [in Ukrainian].

[161] Krasovska, A. Rodent (Muridae) assemblages of the Kremenets Mountains National Nature Park. *Proceedings of the Teriological School.* 2017;15:28-34. doi: http://doi.org/10.15407/ptt2017.15.028. [in Ukrainian].

[162] Mangombi-Pambou, J. B., Granjon, L., Flirden, F., Kane, M., Niang, Y., Davoust, B., Fenollar, F., Mediannikov, O. *Molecular Survey of Rodent-Borne Infectious Agents in the Ferlo Region, Senegal.* Genes (Basel). 2023;14(5):1107. doi: 10.3390/genes14051107.

[163] Biletska, H. V., Lozynskyi, I. M., Ben, I. I., Semenyshyn, O. B., Shulgan, A. M., Legeza, K. M. Methodical recommendations on epidemiology, clinical course, laboratory diagnostics, and prevention of granulocytic anaplasmosis in humans. Clinical Immunology. *Allergology. Infectology* [Internet]. 2012 [cited 2025 Feb 4];(10):5-15. Available from: https://kiai.com.ua/ua/archive/2012/10%2859%29/pages-5-15/metodichni-rekomendaciyi-z-epidemiologiyi-kliniki-laboratornoyi-diagnostiki-ta-profilaktiki-granulocitarnogo-anaplazmozu-lyudini [in Ukrainian].

[164] Klitgaard, K., Kjær, L. J., Isbrand, A., Hansen, M. F., Bødker, R. Multiple infections in questing nymphs and adult female Ixodes ricinus ticks collected in a recreational forest in Denmark. *Ticks Tick Borne Dis.* 2019;10(5):1060-1065. doi: 10.1016/j.ttbdis.2019.05.016.

[165] Malyi, V. P., Shepileva, N. V. Tick-borne Infections (Lyme Disease, Granulocytic Anaplasmosis, and Monocytic Ehrlichiosis) in the Kharkiv Region. Clinical Immunology. Allergy. *Infectology.* 2013;(2):49-52. [in Ukrainian].

[166] Wójcik-Fatla, A., Zając, V., Sawczyn, A., Sroka, J., Cisa,k E., Dutkiewicz, J. Infections and mixed infections with the selected species of Borrelia burgdorferi sensu lato complex in Ixodes ricinus ticks collected in eastern Poland: a significant increase in the course of 5 years. *Exp Appl Acarol.* 2016;68(2):197-212. doi: 10.1007/s10493-015-9990-4.

[167] Pawełczyk, A., Bednarska, M., Hamera, A., Religa, E., Poryszewska, M., Mierzejewska, E. J., Welc-Falęciak, R. Long-term study of Borrelia and Babesia prevalence and co-infection in Ixodes ricinus and Dermacentor recticulatus ticks removed from humans in Poland, 2016-2019. *Parasit Vectors.* 2021;14(1):348. doi: 10.1186/s13071-021-04849-5.

[168] Knoll, S., Springer, A., Hauck, D., Schunack, B., Pachnicke, S., Fingerle, V., Strube, C. Distribution of Borrelia burgdorferi s.l. and Borrelia miyamotoi in Ixodes tick populations in Northern Germany, co-infections with Rickettsiales and assessment of potential influencing factors. *Med Vet Entomol.* 2021;35(4):595-606. doi: 10.1111/mve.12537.

[169] Zubriková, D., Wittmann, M., Hönig, V., Švec, P, Víchová, B., Essbauer, S., Dobler, G., Grubhoffer, L., Pfister, K. Prevalence of tick-borne encephalitis virus and Borrelia burgdorferi sensu lato in Ixodes ricinus ticks in Lower Bavaria and Upper Palatinate, Germany. *Ticks Tick Borne Dis.* 2020;11(3):101375. doi: 10.1016/j.ttbdis.2020.101375.

[170] Raileanu, C., Moutailler, S., Pavel, I., Porea, D., Mihalca, A. D., Savuta, G., Vayssier-Taussat, M. Borrelia Diversity and Co-infection with Other Tick Borne Pathogens in Ticks. *Front Cell Infect Microbiol.* 2017 Feb 14;7:36. doi: 10.3389/fcimb.2017.00036.

[171] Reye, A. L., Stegniy, V., Mishaeva, N. P., Velhin, S., Hübschen, J. M., Ignatyev, G., Muller, C. P. Prevalence of tick-borne pathogens in Ixodes ricinus and Dermacentor reticulatus ticks from different geographical locations in Belarus. *PLoS One.* 2013;8(1):e54476. doi: 10.1371/journal.pone.0054476.

[172] Grochowska, A., Milewski, R., Pancewicz, S., Dunaj, J., Czupryna, P., Milewska, A. J., Róg-Makal, M., Grygorczuk, S., Moniuszko-Malinowska, A. Comparison of tick-borne pathogen prevalence in Ixodes ricinus ticks collected in urban areas of Europe. *Sci Rep.* 2020;10(1):6975. doi: 10.1038/s41598-020-63883-y.

[173] Bezrukyi, Ye. S., Koziar, B. Ye., Ischuk, I. S. On the epidemiological situation of Lyme disease in the city of Ternopil. In: *Environment and Health*; April 25-26, 2013; Ternopil. Ternopil; TSMU, 2013. p. 10-1. [in Ukrainian].

[174] Akimov, I. A., Nebogatkin, I. V. Dynamics of the number and ecological features of ticks (Acari, Ixodidae) in the urbanized landscapes of Kyiv since the beginning of the 21st century. *Scientific Journal of M. P. Drahomanov NPU.* Series 20: Biology [Internet]. 2011 [cited 2025 Feb 4];3:98-109. Available from: http://nbuv.gov.ua/UJRN/Nchb_020_2011_3_19. [in Ukrainian].

[175] Zintl, A., Zaid, T., McKiernan, F., Naranjo-Lucena, A., Gray, J., Brosnan, S., Browne, J., O'Connor, J., Mee, J. F., Good, B., Gillingham, E. L., Vaux, A. G. C., Medlock, J. Update on the presence of Ixodes ricinus at the western limit of its range and the prevalence of Borrelia burgdorferi sensu lato. *Ticks Tick Borne Dis.* 2020;11(6):101518. doi: 10.1016/j.ttbdis.2020.101518.

[176] Didyk, Y. M., Blaňárová, L., Pogrebnyak, S., Akimov, I., Petko, B., Víchová, B. Emergence of tick-borne pathogens (Borrelia burgdorferi sensu lato, Anaplasma phagocytophilum, Ricketsia raoultii and Babesia microti) in the Kyiv urban parks, Ukraine. *Ticks Tick Borne Dis.* 2017;8(2):219-225. doi: 10. 1016/j.ttbdis.2016.10.002.

[177] Lernout, T., De Regge, N., Tersago, K., Fonville, M., Suin, V., Sprong, H. Prevalence of pathogens in ticks collected from humans through citizen science in Belgium. *Parasit Vectors.* 2019;12(1):550. doi: 10.1186/s13071-019-3806-z.

[178] Otranto, D., Dantas-Torres, F., Giannelli, A., Latrofa, M. S., Cascio, A., Cazzin, S., Ravagnan, S., Montarsi, F., Zanzani, S. A., Manfredi, M. T., Capelli, G. Ticks infesting humans in Italy and associated pathogens. *Parasit Vectors.* 2014;7:328. doi: 10.1186/1756-3305-7-328.

[179] Mancini, F., Vescio, M. F., Toma, L., Di Luca, M., Severini, F., Cacciò, S. M., Mariano, C., Nicolai, G., Laghezza Masci, V., Fausto, A. M., Pezzotti, P., Ciervo, A. Detection of tick-borne pathogens in ticks collected in the suburban area of Monte Romano, Lazio Region, Central Italy. *Ann Ist Super Sanita.* 2019;55(2):143-50. doi: 10.4415/ANN_19_02_06.

[180] Lindblom, P., Wilhelmsson, P., Fryland, L., Sjöwall, J., Haglund, M., Matussek, A., Ernerudh, J., Vene, S., Nyman, D., Andreassen, A., Forsberg, P., Lindgren, P. E. Tick-borne encephalitis virus in ticks detached from humans and follow-up of serological and clinical response. *Ticks Tick Borne Dis.* 2014;5(1):21-8. doi: 10.1016/j.ttbdis.2013.07.009.

[181] Cull, B., Pietzsch, M. E., Hansford, K. M., Gillingham, E. L., Medlock, J. M. Surveillance of British ticks: An overview of species records, host associations, and new records of Ixodes ricinus distribution. *Ticks Tick Borne Dis.* 2018;9(3):605-614. doi: 10.1016/j.ttbdis.2018.01.011.

[182] Simin, V., Lalošević, D., Mijatović, D., Tomanović, S., Miljević, M., Čabrilo, B., Bogdan, I., Banović, P. Borellia burgdorferi infection in removed ticks and anti-Borrelia antibodies in infested patients admitted to the Pasteur institute, *Novi Sad. Veterinarski glasnik.* 2020;74(2):164-77. doi: 10.2298/ VETGL200527008S.

[183] Rollend, L., Fish, D., Childs, J. E. Transovarial transmission of Borrelia spirochetes by Ixodes scapularis: a summary of the literature and recent observations. *Ticks Tick Borne Dis.* 2013;4(1-2):46-51. doi: 10.1016/j.ttbdis.2012.06.008.

[184] Ogden, N. H., Margos, G., Aanensen, D. M., Drebot, M. A., Feil, E. J., Hanincová, K., Schwartz, I., Tyler, S., Lindsay, L. R. Investigation of genotypes of Borrelia burgdorferi in Ixodes scapularis ticks collected during surveillance in Canada. *Appl Environ Microbiol.* 2011;77(10):3244-54. doi: 10.1128/ AEM.02636-10.

[185] Nelder, M. P., Russell, C. B., Sheehan, N. J., Sander, B., Moore, S., Li, Y., Johnson, S., Patel, S. N., Sider, D. Human pathogens associated with the blacklegged tick Ixodes scapularis: a systematic review. *Parasit Vectors.* 2016;9:265. doi: 10.1186/s13071-016-1529-y.

[186] Gałęziowska, E., Rzymowska, J., Najda, N., Kołodziej, P., Domżał-Drzewicka, R., Rząca, M., Muraczyńska, B., Charzyńska-Gula, M., Szadowska-Szlachetka, Z., Ślusarska, B., Guty, E. Prevalence of Borrelia burgdorferi in ticks removed from skin of people and circumstances of being bitten - research from the area of Poland, 2012-2014. *Ann Agric Environ Med.* 2018;25(1):31-5. doi: 10.5604/12321966.1233906.

[187] Crowder, C. D., Carolan, H. E., Rounds, M. A., Honig, V., Mothes, B., Haag, H., Nolte, O., Luft, B. J., Grubhoffer, L., Ecker, D. J., Schutzer, S. E., Eshoo, M. W. Prevalence of Borrelia miyamotoi in Ixodes ticks in Europe and the United States. *Emerg Infect Dis.* 2014 Oct;20(10):1678-82. doi: 10.3201/eid2010.131583.

[188] Dibernardo, A., Cote, T., Ogden, N. H., Lindsay, L. R. The prevalence of Borrelia miyamotoi infection, and co-infections with other Borrelia spp. in Ixodes scapularis ticks collected in Canada. *Parasit Vectors.* 2014;7:183. doi: 10.1186/1756-3305-7-183.

[189] Iwabu-Itoh, Y., Bazartseren, B., Naranbaatar, O., Yondonjamts, E., Furuno, K., Lee, K., Sato, K., Kawabata, H., Takada, N., Andoh, M., Kajita, H., Oikawa, Y., Nakao, M., Ohnishi, M., Watarai, M., Shimoda, H., Maeda, K., Takano, A. Tick surveillance for Borrelia miyamotoi and phylogenetic analysis of isolates in Mongolia and Japan. *Ticks Tick Borne Dis.* 2017;8(6):850-857. doi: 10.1016/j. ttbdis.2017.06.011.

[190] Wagemakers, A., Jahfari, S., de Wever, B., Spanjaard, L., Starink, M. V., de Vries, H. J. C., Sprong, H., Hovius, J. W. Borrelia miyamotoi in vectors and hosts in The Netherlands. *Ticks Tick Borne Dis.* 2017;8(3):370-374. doi: 10.1016/j.ttbdis.2016.12.012.

[191] Geller, J., Nazarova, L., Katargina, O., Järvekülg, L., Fomenko, N., Golovljova, I. Detection and genetic characterization of relapsing fever spirochete Borrelia miyamotoi in Estonian ticks. *PLoS One.* 2012;7(12):e51914. doi: 10.1371/journal.pone.0051914.

[192] Cochez, C., Heyman, P., Heylen, D., Fonville, M., Hengeveld, P., Takken, W., Simons, L., Sprong, H. The Presence of Borrelia miyamotoi, A Relapsing Fever Spirochaete, in Questing Ixodes ricinus in Belgium and in The Netherlands. *Zoonoses Public Health.* 2015 Aug;62(5):331-3. doi: 10.1111/zph. 12154.

[193] Cosson, J. F., Michelet, L., Chotte, J., Le Naour, E., Cote, M., Devillers, E., Poulle, M. L., Huet, D., Galan, M., Geller, J., Moutailler, S., Vayssier-Taussat, M. Genetic characterization of the human relapsing fever spirochete Borrelia miyamotoi in vectors and animal reservoirs of Lyme disease spirochetes in France. *Parasit Vectors.* 2014;7:233. doi: 10.1186/1756-3305-7-233.

[194] Venczel, R., Knoke, L., Pavlovic, M., Dzaferovic, E., Vaculova, T., Silaghi, C., Overzier, E., Konrad, R., Kolenčík, S., Derdakova, M., Sing, A., Schaub, G. A., Margos, G., Fingerle, V. A novel duplex real-time PCR permits simultaneous detection and differentiation of Borrelia miyamotoi and Borrelia burgdorferi sensu lato. *Infection.* 2016;44(1):47-55. doi: 10.1007/s15010-015-0820-8.

[195] Corrain, R., Drigo, M., Fenati, M., Menandro, M. L., Mondin, A., Pasotto, D., Martini, M. Study on ticks and tick-borne zoonoses in public parks in Italy. *Zoonoses Public Health.* 2012;59(7):468-76. doi: 10.1111/j.1863-2378.2012.01490.x.

[196] Grillon, A., Sauleau, E., Boulanger, N. Risk of Ixodes ricinus Bites in a Population of Forestry Workers in an Endemic Region in France. *Pathogens.* 2024;13(8):696. doi: 10.3390/pathogens13080696.

[197] Jahfari, S., Herremans, T., Platonov, A. E., Kuiper, H., Karan, L. S., Vasilieva, O., Koopmans, M. P., Hovius, J. W., Sprong, H. High seroprevalence of Borrelia miyamotoi antibodies in forestry workers and individuals suspected of human granulocytic anaplasmosis in the Netherlands. *New Microbes New Infect.* 2014;2(5):144-9. doi: 10.1002/nmi2.59.

[198] Jovanovic, D., Atanasievska, S., Protic-Djokic, V., Rakic, U., Lukac-Radoncic, E., Ristanovic, E. Seroprevalence of Borrelia burgdorferi in occupationally exposed persons in the Belgrade area, Serbia. *Braz J Microbiol.* 2015;46(3):807-14. doi: 10.1590/S1517-838246320140698.

[199] Nejezchlebova, H., Kiewra, D., Žákovská, A., Ovesná, P. Students' attitudes to tick risks. *Ann Agric Environ Med.* 2016;23(3):437-41. doi: 10.5604/12321966.1219183.

[200] Pańczuk, A., Tokarska-Rodak, M., Tarelkina, I., Voita, D. Prevention of Lyme borreliosis among students from Poland and Latvia. Hygeia. *Public Health.* [Internet]. 2018 [cited 1 Feb 2025];53(3):307-12. Available at: http://www.h-ph.pl/hyg.php?opc=AR&lng=pl&art=719.

[201] St Pierre, S. E., Gould, O. N., Lloyd, V. Knowledge and Knowledge Needs about Lyme Disease among Occupational and Recreational Users of the Outdoors. *Int J Environ Res Public Health.* 20205; 17(1):355. doi: 10.3390/ijerph17010355.

[202] Lewandowska, A., Kruba, Z., Filip, R. Epidemiology of Lyme disease among workers of forest inspectorates in Poland. *Ann Agric Environ Med* [Internet]. 2013 [cited 2025 Feb 4];20(2):329-31. Available from: https://www.aaem.pl/pdf-71937-9164?filename=9164.pdf.

[203] Pańczuk, A., Tokarska-Rodak, M., Plewik, D., Paszkiewicz, J. Tick exposure and prevalence of Borrelia burgdorferi antibodies among hunters and other individuals exposed to vector ticks in eastern Poland. *Rocz Panstw Zakl Hig.* 2019;70(2):161-168. doi: 10.32394/rpzh.2019.0066.

[204] Chmielewska-Badora, J., Moniuszko, A., Żukiewicz-Sobczak, W., Zwoliński, J., Piątek, J., Pancewicz, S. Serological survey in persons occupationally exposed to tick-borne pathogens in cases of co-infections with Borrelia burgdorferi, Anaplasma phagocytophilum, Bartonella spp. and Babesia microti. *Ann Agric Environ Med* [Internet]. 2012 [cited 2025 Feb 4];19(2):271-4. Available from: https://www.aaem.pl/pdf-71773-8999?filename=8999.pdf.

[205] Tokarska-Rodak, M., Plewik, D., Kozioł-Montewka, M., Szepeluk, A., Paszkiewicz, J. Risk of occupational infections caused by Borrelia burgdorferi among forestry workers and farmers. *Med Pr Work Health Saf.* 2014;65(1):109-17. doi: 10.13075/mp.5893.2014.017. [in Polish].

[206] Zinchuk, O. M. *Lyme Borreliosis: Clinical-Immunopathogenetic Features and Emergency Preventive Treatment* [Author's Abstract]. Kyiv; 2010. 41 c. [in Ukrainian].

[207] Tokarska-Rodak, M., Shkilna, M., Krajewska, M., Pańczuk, A., Weiner, M., Pawłowicz, E., Korda, M., Klishch, I., Andreychyn, M. The evaluation of hunters and foresters' knowledge of the possible ways of preventing Borrelia burgdorferi infections. *Med Pr.* 2020;71(1):59-68. doi: 10.13075/mp.5893.00841. [in Polish]

[208] Shkilna, M. I., Vasylieva, N. A., Ivakhiv, O. L. Epidemiological situation of Lyme borreliosis among workers of forestry enterprises in Ternopil region. In: *Actual problems of epidemiology of infectious, parasitic and non-infectious diseases;* May 12-13, 2016; Lviv. Lviv; 2016. p. 241-312. [in Ukrainian].

[209] Shkilna, M. I., Korda, M. M., Klishch, I. M., Andreychyn, M. A. Lyme borreliosis – an actual problem for forestry workers in Ternopil region. In: *Modern infectious diseases. Biological safety and biosecurity;* Oct 12-13, 2016; Kyiv. Kyiv; 2016. p. 162-63. [in Ukrainian].

[210] Shkilna, M. I. Awareness of foresters in Ternopil and Zhytomyr regions regarding Lyme borreliosis. In: *Epidemiological and clinical complications of infectious and parasitic diseases in modern conditions;* Oct 5-6, 2017; Zhytomyr. Zhytomyr; 2017. p. 164-65. [in Ukrainian].

[211] Nykytyuk, S., Pańczuk, A., Shkilna, M., Tokarska-Rodak, M., Szepeluk, A., Melnyk, L., Korda, M. Awareness of tick-borne bacterial infection in the students of non-medical universities in Ternopil region (Western Ukraine). *Health Problems of Civilization.* 2017;11(2):99-102. doi: 10.5114/hpc.2017.69026.

[212] Shkilna MI, Nykytiuk SO, Tkachuk NI. Awareness about Lyme borreliosis among students of some higher educational institutions of Ternopil. In: *Achievements in Clinical and Experimental Medicine* [Internet]; June 14, 2017; Ternopil. Ternopil: TNMU, Ukrmedkniga; 2017 [cited 4 Feb 2025]. p. 113-5. Available at: https://repository.tdmu.edu.ua/bitstream/handle/1/8519/ЗБІРНИК.pdf?sequence=1&isAllowed=y. [in Ukrainian].

[213] Shkilna, M. I. Awareness of students of non-medical universities in Ternopil regarding Lyme borreliosis. In: *Modern infectious diseases. Etiology, epidemiology, diagnostics, treatment, prevention, biological safety*; Oct 12-13, 2017; Kyiv. Kyiv; 2017. P. 218-19. [in Ukrainian].

[214] Pańczuk, A., Tokarska-Rodak, M., Mikuľáková, W., Kendrová, L., Magurová, D. Exposure to ticks and undertaking Lyme borreliosis prevention activities among students from Poland and Slovakia. *Ann Agric Environ Med.* 2019;26(2):217-21. doi: 10.26444/aaem/99089.

[215] Shkilna, M. I. Clinical-epidemiological features of erythema migrans in residents of Ternopil region. *Dermatology and Venereology.* [Internet]. 2019;(1):37–41. Available from: http://idvamnu.com.ua/wp-content/uploads/2019/04/2019_01-Shkilna.pdf. [in Ukrainian].

[216] Shkilna, M., Korda, M., Gumenna, R., Andreychyn, M., Miller, L., Klishch, I., Shtokailo, S., Zaporozhan, S. O., Hook, M. Analysis of patients' awareness in Ternopil hospitals regarding Lyme disease. In: *Public health in the social and educational space – current challenges and development prospects* [Internet]; September 25-26, 2019; Ternopil. Ternopil: TNMU, Ukrmedkniga; 2019 [cited 4 Feb 2025]. p. 64-5. Available at: https: https://repository.tdmu.edu.ua/bitstream/handle/123456789/12506/Матеріали%20симпозіуму.pdf?sequence=1&isAllowed=y. [in Ukrainian].

[217] Podobivskyi, S. S., Fedonyuk L. Y., Korda, M. M., Klishch, I. M., Andreychyn, M. A., Shkilna, M. I., Podobivskyi, V. S., Nikityuk, S. O. Implementation of the medical geoinformation system in research of ixodes ricinus and mite's infections in Ukraine. *Infectious Diseases.* 2019;(3):38-45. doi: 10.11603/1681-2727.2019.3.10634 [in Ukrainian].

[218] Podobivskyi, S. S., Fedonyuk, L. Y., Korda, M. M., Klishch, I. M., Andreychyn, M. A., Shkilna, M. I., Podobivskyi, V. S., Nikityuk, S. O. Implementation of the medical geoinformation system in research of ixodes ricinus and mite's infections in Ukraine. In: *Achievements in Clinical and Experimental Medicine* [Internet]; 13 Jun. 2019; Ternopil. Ternopil: TNMU, Ukrmedkniga; 2019 [cited 4 Feb 2025]. pp. 21-3. Available at: https://repository.tdmu.edu.ua/bitstream/handle/123456789/11017/МАТЕРИАЛИ%20КОНФЕРЕНЦИІІ.pdf?sequence=9&isAllowed=y. [in Ukrainian].

Chapter 3

The Clinical Manifestations of Lyme Borreliosis with Elements of Pathogenesis

Mykhaylo Andreychyn[1]
Mariia Shkilna[2]
Oleh Ivakhiv[3]
Serhii Andreychyn[4]
Nataliia Bilkevych[5]
Vitaliy Hlushok[6]
Mariana Huk[7]
Inna Ishchuk[8]
Nataliia Kavetska[9]
Vasyl Kopcha[10]
Larysa Melnyk[11]
Ruslan Semenyna[12]
Svitlana Shkrobot[13]
Svitlana Smiyan[14]
and Valentyna Yuskevych[15]

[1]Academician of the National Academy of Medical Sciences of Ukraine,
Honoured Master of Sciences and Technologies of Ukraine, DSc in Medicine, Professor,
Head of the Department of Infectious Diseases with Epidemiology, Dermatology and Venerology,
I. Horbachevsky Ternopil National Medical University, Ternopil, Ukraine
[2]DSc in Medicine, Professor, Department of Infectious Diseases with Epidemiology,
Dermatology and Venerology, I. Horbachevsky Ternopil National Medical University, Ternopil, Ukraine
[3]Honoured Doctor of Ukraine, PhD in Medicine, Associate Professor,
Department of Infectious Diseases with Epidemiology, Dermatology and Venerology,
I. Horbachevsky Ternopil National Medical University, Ternopil, Ukraine
[4]DSc in Medicine, Professor, Head of the Department of Internal Medicine Propaedeutics and Phthisiology,
I. Horbachevsky Ternopil National Medical University, Ternopil, Ukraine
[5]PhD in Medicine, Associate Professor, Department of Internal Medicine Propaedeutics and Phthisiology,
I. Horbachevsky Ternopil National Medical University, Ternopil, Ukraine

In: Lyme Borreliosis
Editors: Mykhaylo Andreychyn, Mykhaylo Korda, Maria Shkilna and Oleh Ivakhiv
ISBN: 979-8-89530-657-4

[6]PhD in Medicine, Associate Professor, Department of Infectious Diseases with Epidemiology, Dermatology and Venerology, I. Horbachevsky Ternopil National Medical University, Ternopil, Ukraine
[7]PhD in Medicine, Assistant Professor, Department of Infectious Diseases with Epidemiology, Dermatology and Venerology, I. Horbachevsky Ternopil National Medical University, Ternopil, Ukraine
[8]PhD in Medicine, Associate Professor, Department of Infectious Diseases with Epidemiology, Dermatology and Venerology, I. Horbachevsky Ternopil National Medical University, Ternopil, Ukraine
[9]PhD in Medicine, Associate Professor, Department of Internal Medicine Propaedeutics and Phthisiology, I. Horbachevsky Ternopil National Medical University, Ternopil, Ukraine
[10]DSc in Medicine, Professor, Department of Infectious Diseases with Epidemiology, Dermatology and Venerology, I. Horbachevsky Ternopil National Medical University, Ternopil, Ukraine
[11]PhD in Medicine, Assistant Professor, Department of Infectious Diseases with Epidemiology, Dermatology and Venerology, I. Horbachevsky Ternopil National Medical University, Ternopil, Ukraine
[12]General Director of the Ternopil Regional Clinical Dermatology and Venereology Dispensary, Ternopil Regional Council, Ternopil, Ukraine
[13]Honoured Master of Sciences and Technologies of Ukraine, DSc in Medicine, Professor, Head of the Department, Department of Neurology, I. Horbachevsky Ternopil National Medical University, Ternopil, Ukraine
[14]Honoured Master of Sciences and Technologies of Ukraine, DSc in Medicine, Professor, Head of the Department of Internal Medicine No.2, I. Horbachevsky Ternopil National Medical University, Ternopil, Ukraine
[15]PhD in Medicine,
Municipal Non-Profit Enterprise "Ternopil Regional Clinical Hospital" of the Ternopil Regional Council, Emergency Physician, Ternopil, Ukraine

Abstract

The chapter presents current perspectives on the pathogenesis and clinical manifestations of Lyme borreliosis. Following a tick bite, Borrelia spirochetes penetrate the skin and begin to multiply locally. Within several weeks, the pathogen disseminates via the bloodstream or lymphatic system to other tissues and organs (joints, heart, nervous system). In response to the infection, pro-inflammatory cytokines are produced, contributing to the development of clinical symptoms. In some cases, autoimmune reactions may occur, promoting the progression of chronic lesions.

Lyme disease follows a staged course, including: an early localized stage (characterized by intoxication symptoms and the appearance of erythema migrans); a disseminated stage (with widespread erythema and involvement of the nervous system – meningitis, radiculitis, peripheral paresis; cardiac manifestations – heart block, myocarditis; and joint involvement – arthralgia or arthritis); and a late stage (marked by chronic arthritis, chronic encephalopathy, encephalitis, encephalomyelitis, cerebrovascular neuroborreliosis, meningoradiculoneuritis, atrophic acrodermatitis, and localized scleroderma).

Keywords: Lyme borreliosis, pathogenesis, clinical presentation, disease stages, skin manifestations, neuroborreliosis, cardiovascular involvement, joint form

1. Introduction

The clinical presentation of Lyme borreliosis reflects the stages of pathogen dissemination within the host and the corresponding immune response. Initial replication of Borrelia in the skin, followed by hematogenous and lymphatic dissemination, along with the pathogen's ability to persist in tissues over extended periods, underlie the sequential development of clinical manifestations. Depending on the disease stage, symptoms may range from localized cutaneous lesions to systemic neurological, cardiac, and articular disorders. Given the broad spectrum of symptoms – from facial paralysis to cognitive dysfunction – Lyme borreliosis is often referred to as the "great imitator." Understanding the pathogenic mechanisms is crucial for accurate diagnosis, assessing the risk of chronic progression, and timely treatment. Of particular interest is the potential impact of Lyme borreliosis on the course of concomitant chronic infections, a subject that remains insufficiently addressed in the literature.

2. Clinical Classification

Oleh Ivakhiv
and Inna Ishchuk

E. Asbrink proposed the initial clinical classification of this disease in 1982, which was significantly expanded by A. Steere in 1989 and 1991. The classification distinguishes the period of early infection, which includes Stage 1 – localized infection (1-3 weeks from the onset of illness) and Stage 2 – disseminated infection (within 1 month), as well as the period of late infection (2-6 months from the onset of illness) [1, 2].

As of today, the clinical classification of LB looks as follows [3]:

- By form: latent; manifest.
- By stage: localized (primary effect stage); disseminated (generalized); persistent (chronic); residual (post-Lyme syndrome).
- By predominant site of involvement: skin; nervous system; joints; heart; mixed.
- By course: acute (up to 3 months); subacute (3 to 6 months); chronic (over 6 months), continuous; recurrent.
- By severity: mild; moderate; severe.
- By infectivity status: seropositive, seronegative.
- By presence of complications [4].

The division into stages is quite arbitrary and largely relies on clinical manifestations and temporal characteristics from the moment of infection. It is important to note that the disease can progress gradually from one stage to another or may initially manifest in any stage without a preceding stage being evident.

According to European authors, LB manifests as skin disease in 80-90% of patients, whereas involvement of other organs and systems is noted in approximately 10-20% of individuals [5-7].

3. Skin Lesions

Mariia Shkilna
Ruslan Semenyna
and Vitaliy Hlushok

During the bite of an infected tick or when it is crushed, Borrelia penetrate the human body, where they trigger an inflammatory allergic reaction and form a primary lesion clinically manifested by the development of erythema. The expansion of the zone of hyperaemia at the site of entry is due to centrifugal spread of the pathogen [8]. Through the lymphatic vessels, bacteria enter regional lymph nodes, causing lymphadenitis. These changes correspond to Stage 1 of the disease. Due to hematogenous dissemination, Borrelia penetrate various organs and tissues, including the skin, heart, central nervous system, joints, and others, forming metastatic foci of infection [9]. Bacterial destruction is accompanied by the release of endotoxin, which initiates a cascade of immunopathological reactions [8, 10].

The ability of B. burgdorferi to intracellularly parasitize ensures the possibility of a chronic course of the disease with late relapses and prolonged persistence of the pathogen in the body (over 10 years) [11, 12]. Chronic (late-stage) infection, irreversibly affecting certain target organs such as skin (chronic atrophic acrodermatitis, anetodermia), joints (chronic arthritis or late-stage arthritis), nervous system (progressive encephalomielitis, encephalopathy), and eyes (progressive keratitis), develops as a result of prolonged pathogenic influence of the pathogen on organs and systems with pronounced autoimmune pathological process [13]. Circulating immune complexes (CIC), autoantibodies, interleukins exhibit damaging effects [8, 14]. Immunity in LB is non-sterile, similar to other spirochaetoses. There is a suggestion that reinfection may occur in individuals who have already had the disease, after 2-7 years [4].

In 1997, the nucleotide sequence of the linear chromosome of *B. burgdorferi s. s.* (strain B31) was determined, consisting of 910,725 base pairs. 853 genes were identified. In addition to the chromosomal structure, nucleotide sequences of 9 circular and 11 linear plasmids were discovered [15-17]. Changes (drift) in the plasmid genome are associated with Borrelia's evasion phenomenon from the host's immune defences. It has been shown that the Borrelia genome lacks tox+ genes encoding toxin synthesis – virulence factors [18]. Borrelia pathogenicity is determined by surface proteins of the pathogen, as well as immunopathological reactions. Moreover, phage DNA of lysogenic strains of Borrelia may carry markers of antibiotic resistance [16].

It has been established that the major surface antigenic proteins OspA, OspB, and OspC, which distinguish individual strains [19], can vary significantly, thereby allowing for prolonged (over many years) persistence of the pathogen in the human body [20]. Many antigenic determinants of the outer membrane of Borrelia species are similar to each other and even to certain bacteria of other genera, which explains the possibility of cross-immune reactions [21–23].

The study of certain indicators of cellular and humoral immunity in patients with Lyme borreliosis confirms changes in reactivity of the immune system. Results from international studies of immune reactions in patients with borreliosis unequivocally demonstrate the prevalence of cellular immunity, where T-lymphocytes and macrophages activated by Th1 play a key role [24]. This is supported by the presence of macrophage and T-cell infiltrates in erythema migrans and target organs. This mechanism, driven by phagocytic activity and cytotoxic T-lymphocytes, is aimed at localizing and eliminating Borrelia [15].

The pathogenesis of Borrelia infection is influenced by both the pathogenic action of the pathogen and the characteristics of the host's immune response [25]. Virulence factors of B. burgdorferi, such as surface Osp proteins (lipoproteins of the outer membrane) [26], activate macrophages, dendritic cells, T- and B-lymphocytes, which secrete specific proteinaceous communicative substances – cytokines [27, 28]. These cytokines are highly specific regulatory peptides produced by cells of the immune system and organs involved in the inflammatory process.

Currently, three mechanisms of Borrelia long-term persistence in the host's body are known: suppression of the immunogenicity of surface proteins (antigenic drift), inactivation of effector organisms, antigenic mimicry, and residence in the extracellular matrix [23].

To protect against the host's immune response, Borrelia are capable of suppressing the opsonizing function of complement using their surface proteins (e.g., Fhbp protein, OspE and OspF lipoproteins), which bind to the complement regulatory protein H-factor; stimulate synthesis of anti-inflammatory cytokines (IL-10); attach plasminogen to their surface via OspA; and interact with components of the extracellular matrix [23, 25].

It has been found that *B. burgdorferi s. s.* is associated with joint damage, while *B. garinii* and *B. bavariensis* are linked to the development of meningoradiculitis, and *B. afzelii* with skin lesions [29, 30–35]. In Germany, Hungary, and Slovenia, *B. spielmanii* is often the etiological agent [29].

The incubation period of the disease ranges from 1 to 53 days (typically 7–14 days on average) [4, 21, 22, 36]. A short incubation period (1–6 days) is characteristic of the erythema stage of localized infection. For non-erythematous forms of Lyme borreliosis, a longer incubation period (8–45 days) is typical, which can be explained by prolonged dissemination of Borrelia from the tick bite site (primary focus) and subsequent spirochaetaemia [37].

The onset of Lyme borreliosis is usually gradual. Patients often complain of rapid fatigue, general malaise, moderate headache, dizziness, nausea, sleep disturbances, and increased irritability. Body temperature may remain within the physiological norm or rise to 37.5–38°C, sometimes accompanied by chills. Hyperthermia typically lasts 2–7 days. Lyme borreliosis may also manifest with myalgias, arthralgias, lymphadenopathy, catarrhal symptoms, and vegetative symptoms such as scleritis, conjunctivitis, hyperhidrosis, facial and neck skin erythema [1, 36].

At the site of the pathogen's entry, the development of primary affection characterized by EM is typical, presenting as a round red spot that gradually expands centripetally, reaching 15–20, and sometimes up to 70 cm in diameter [38, 39]. As the erythema expands, its central part undergoes regression, with a distinct mark from the tick bite visible as a reddish dot. The periphery of the lesion exhibits the most intense redness, and the edges of the erythema may be raised, forming a ridge. The frequency of EM occurrence ranges from 27% to 90% [44, 96, 162, 163].

Currently, typical and atypical variants of EM are distinguished [7, 40]. Clinical signs of typical EM include a ring-shaped erythema with clear borders, located around the site of tick attachment.

Signs of typical EM include:

- The time interval between the tick bite and the appearance of erythema typically ranges from 3 days to several weeks.
- Centripetal spread of erythema.
- Well-defined erythema that does not rise above the surface of the surrounding skin, with a diameter of at least 5 cm.
- A tick bite mark is present in the centre of the erythema.
- Several clinical variants of typical EM are identified:
- Round or "elongated oval" shape.
- Urticarial.
- Linear.
- Incomplete ring.

It can be difficult to diagnose primary skin lesions based on clinical signs alone. In such cases, it is referred to as atypical EM [40, 41].

Several variants of atypical EM are distinguished:

- Monochromatic (total), uniformly coloured.
- With pronounced central necrosis.
- Small-sized (<5 cm).
- With vesicular elements in the centre.
- With haemorrhagic elements in the centre.
- Infiltrated, not macular.
- Visualized only when exposed to heat.
- No visible tick bite site.

Sometimes, in addition to one erythema, secondary (daughter) erythemas of smaller size may appear at the site of the tick bite [41, 42]. Sometimes, secondary ring-shaped elements appear around the primary spot, benign lymphocytoma (painful reddish thickening of swollen skin). Regional lymphadenitis may occur (in 41% of cases), less frequently – generalized lymphadenopathy [4, 7]. Moderate or absent itching and discomfort are typical in the area of Mum.

As a rule, stage 1 lasts from 3 to 30 days and ends with complete recovery, the likelihood of which is significantly increased with adequate antibacterial therapy [4].

If EM persists for 4 weeks or longer, it is called chronic EM [7]. Serological testing results can detect anti-Borrelia IgG antibodies in the majority of cases (approximately 80%), and sometimes IgM antibodies as well [43]. Erythema may disappear spontaneously without antibiotic treatment, but Borrelia can persist even without visible inflammatory reactions and after a latent period, leading to further pathological manifestations in internal organs. Otherwise, even after body temperature normalizes and EM disappears, the disease progresses to the stage of disseminated infection [36].

The second stage of the disease (early disseminated) begins 4 weeks after the end of the early localized infection stage and is characterized by dissemination of the pathogen and involvement of various organs and systems – skin, musculoskeletal system, nervous and cardiovascular systems [1].

During this period, patients may experience numerous erythematous rashes on the skin, called multiple erythema migrans (MEM), usually smaller than the first. Occasionally, short-term polymorphic rash (roseolar, macular, urticarial) and lymphocytomas appear. MEM may be associated with systemic manifestations and acute neurological symptoms [1, 7, 44].

The main signs of MEM are as follows: disseminated, round or oval redness on the skin; ring-shaped or homogeneous erythema; in children, symmetric erythema on the face; persisting for several days or weeks; possible recurrence of erythema in the same places; possible combination with acute neurological symptoms [45–47].

Inflammation phenomena in the area of erythema usually persist for several weeks without treatment. After its disappearance, approximately half of the patients experience skin peeling lasting from several days to 3 weeks, and sometimes skin hyperpigmentation, which usually disappears within several months.

We examined 146 patients with EM LB who were treated on an outpatient and inpatient basis at Ternopil Regional Dermatovenerological Dispensary and the infectious diseases department of the Ternopil City Municipal Emergency Hospital from 2015 to 2020. There were 63 men (43.2%) and 83 women (56.8%) aged 19 to 79 years, with a mean age of (43.09 ± 14.29) years. Most of those examined (124; 84.9%) were of active working age (up to 60 years).

It was found that the largest number of patients (59; 40.4%) could not indicate when the erythema appeared after the tick bite ($p < 0.05$) (Figure 1). Among those who indicated the time of onset of EM after tick attachment, 24 (16.4%) mentioned 3 days and 22 (15.1%) mentioned 30 days. Somewhat less often, 7 and 14 days: 16 (11.0%) and 13 (8.9%) patients, respectively, 3 weeks and 3 months – only 7 (4.8%) and 5 (3.4%).

A ring-shaped reddening with clearly demarcated contours, which is located around the site of tick suction and was at least 5 cm in diameter (typical EM), was found in most of the examined patients – 94 (64.38%) ($p < 0.05$). (Table 1). The rest were diagnosed with an atypical form of EM.

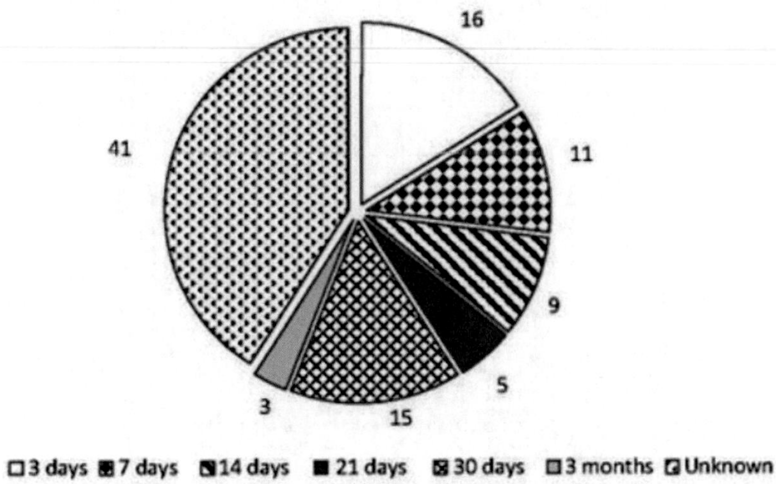

Figure 1. The onset times of erythema migrans after tick attachment in patients with erythematous Lyme borreliosis (n = 146), %.

Figures 2–7 show typical EM variants observed in examined patients.

Table 1. Types of erythema migrans in examined patients with Lyme borreliosis (n = 146)

Erythema migrans	Absolute number	Percentage
Typical	94	64,4*
Atypical	52	35,6

Note. * – the difference is significant, $p < 0.05$.

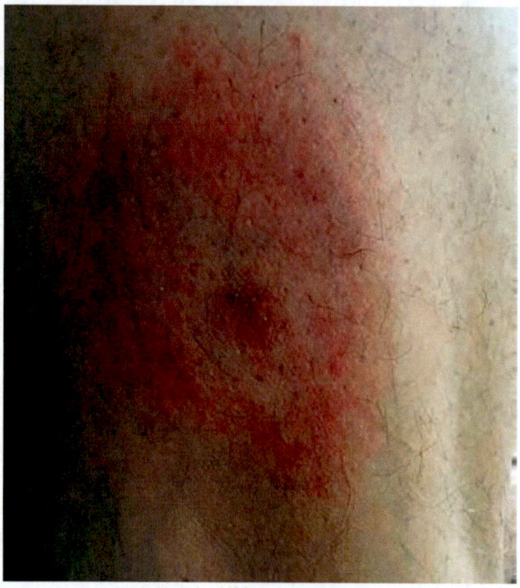

Figure 2. Erythema migrans on the outer surface of the left thigh, typical, in the form of a stretched oval. Patient K., 44 years old. Diagnosis: Lyme borreliosis, erythema form. Acute course.

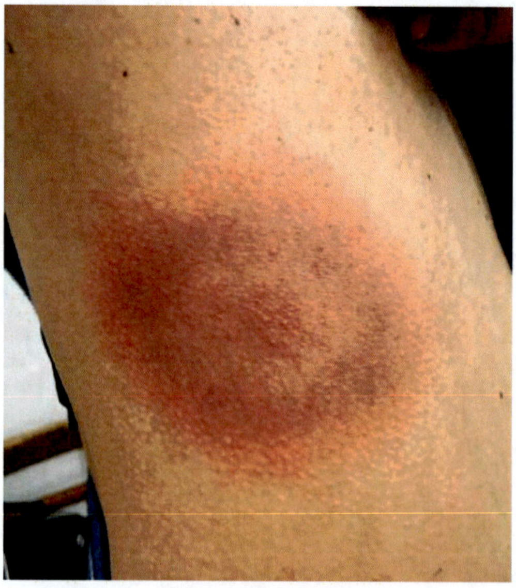

Figure 3. Erythema migrans on the inner surface of the right thigh, typical, in the form of a stretched oval. Patient S., 56 years old. Diagnosis: Lyme borreliosis, erythema form. Acute course.

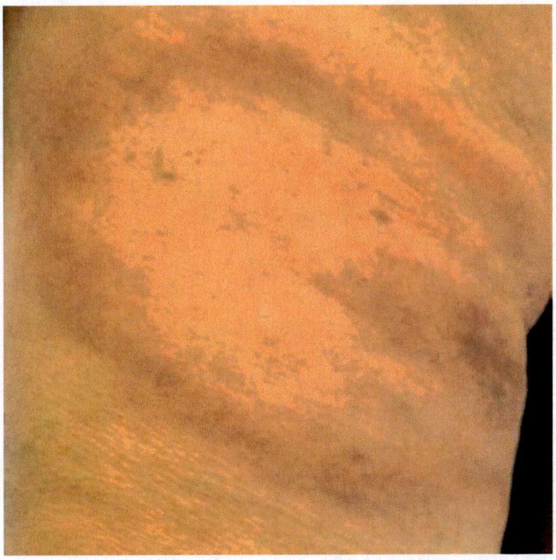

Figure 4. Erythema migrans on the inner surface of the right thigh, typical, urticarial. Patient G., 62 years old. Diagnosis: Lyme borreliosis, erythema form. Subacute course.

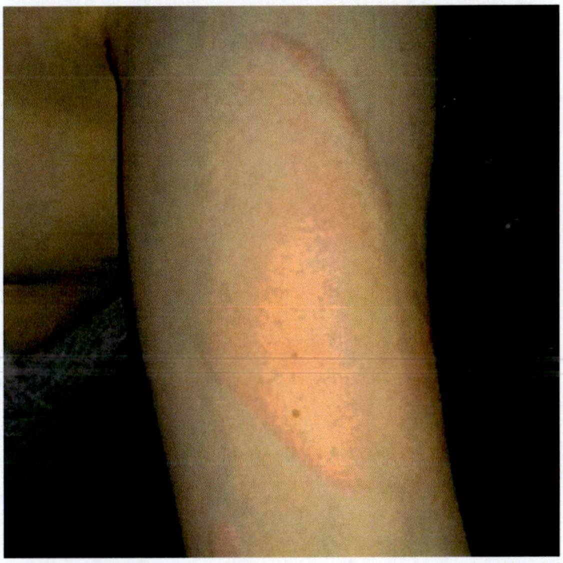

Figure 5. Erythema migrans on the inner surface of the left shoulder, typical, urticarial. Patient U., 41 years old. Diagnosis: Lyme borreliosis, erythema form. Subacute course.

In the examined patients, in addition to typical EM, a number of atypical forms of erythema were observed (Table 2).

Figures 8-12 show subtypes of atypical EM, which were noted in the examined patients.

It was found that in 138 patients (94.5%), there was one erythema, while in only 8 patients (5.5%), multiple erythemas were present on different parts of the body. Only in 1 person, 3 consecutive erythemas were observed on the outer surface of the left shin.

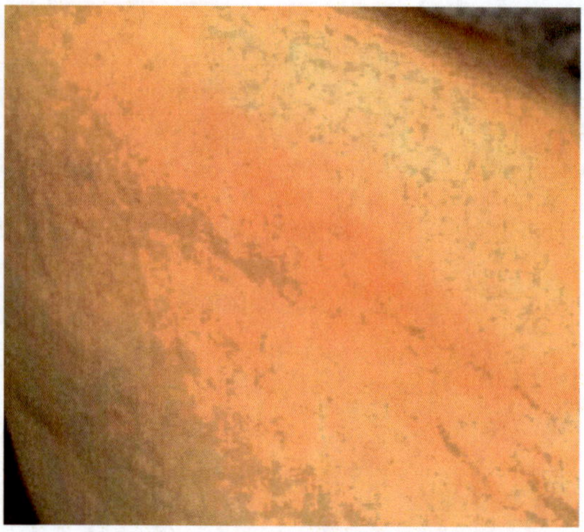

Figure 6. Erythema migrans on the inner surface of the right thigh, typical, linear. Patient K., 53 years old. Diagnosis: Lyme borreliosis, erythema form. Acute course.

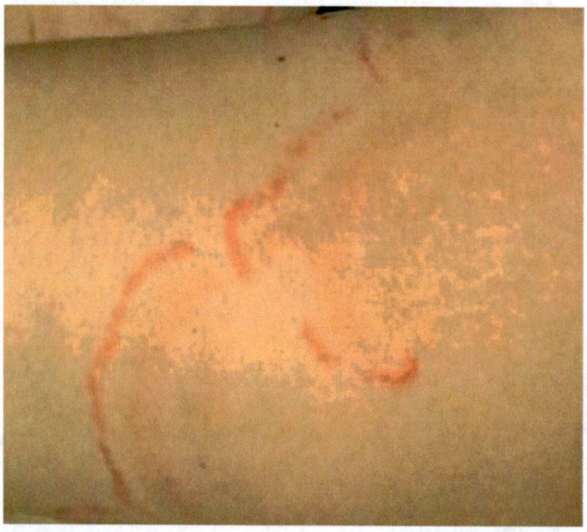

Figure 7. Erythema migrans on the outer surface of the left thigh, typical, with partial border (contour). Patient D., 19 years old. Diagnosis: Lyme borreliosis, erythema form. Acute course.

Table 2. Types and subtypes of erythema migrans in the examined patients (n = 146)

Type of erythema migrans	Absolute number	Percentage
Typical (subtypes):	94	64,4
Stretched oval	72	76,6*
Urticarial	10	10,6
Linear	1	1,1
Incomplete circle	11	11,7
Atypical (subtypes):	52	35,6
Monochrome, evenly coloured	45	86,5*
With pronounced necrosis in the centre	1	1,9
Small-sized erythema (<5 cm)	1	1,9
With vesicular elements in the centre	2	3,9
With haemorrhagic elements in the centre	3	5,8

Note. * – the difference is significant between the types of EM within the subgroup, $p < 0.05$.

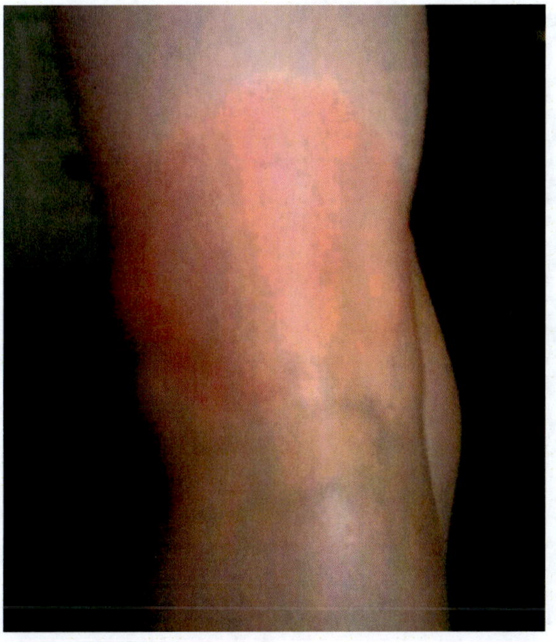

Figure 8. Erythema migrans on the outer surface of the left thigh, solid, atypical erythema. Patient S., 35 years old. Diagnosis: Lyme borreliosis, erythema form. Acute course.

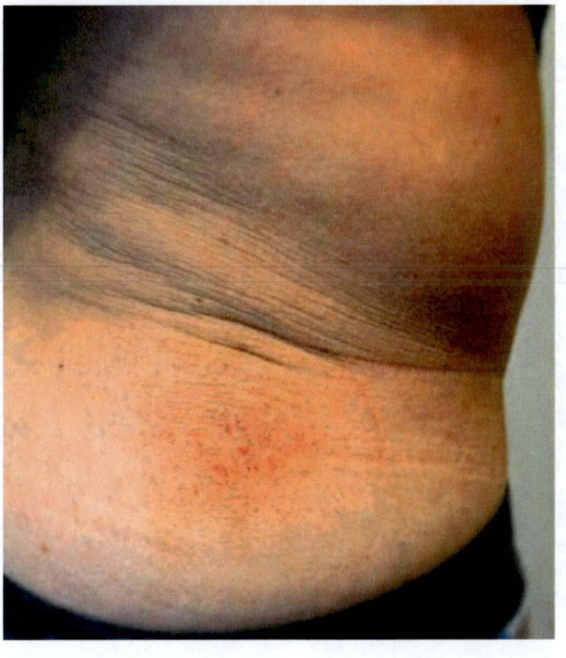

Figure 9. Erythema migrans on the back of the torso, atypical, erythema with vesicular rash. Patient H., 36 years old. Diagnosis: Lyme borreliosis, erythema form. Subacute course.

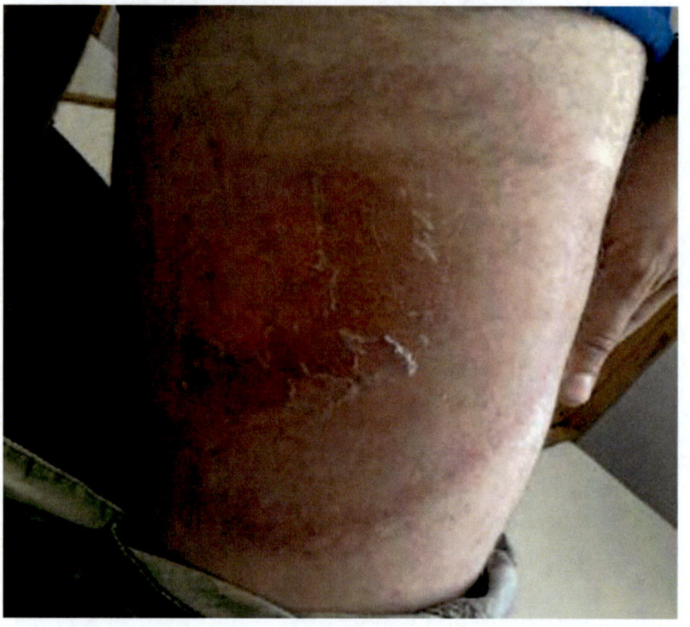

Figure 10. Erythema migrans on the front surface of the thigh, atypical, erythema with vesicular rash. Patient M., 46 years old. Diagnosis: Lyme borreliosis, erythema form. Subacute course.

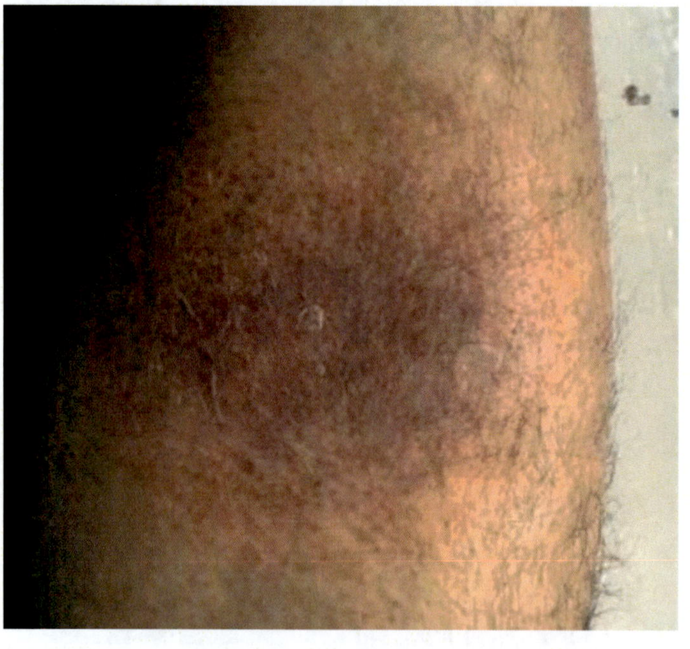

Figure 11. Erythema migrans on the outer surface of the left shin, atypical, without clear borders, with haemorrhagic elements in the centre. Patient M., 34 years old. Diagnosis: Lyme borreliosis, erythema form. Acute course.

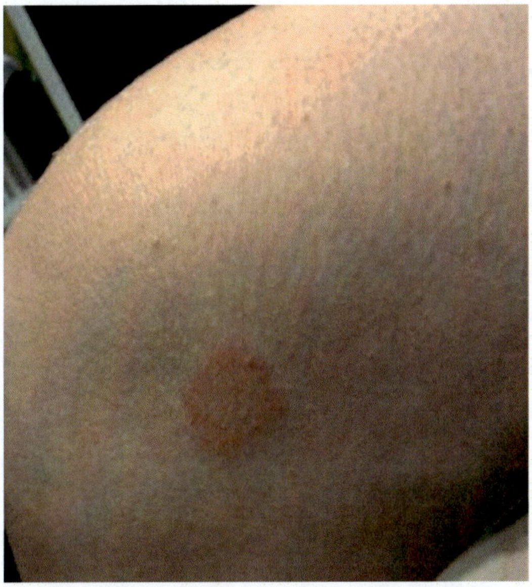

Figure 12. Erythema migrans on the front of the torso, atypical, small-sized rash (<5 cm). Patient Ch., 34 years old. Diagnosis: Lyme borreliosis, erythema form. Acute course.

An example of clinical case.

Patient P. (Figure 13), 18 years old, presented with complaints of multiple rashes on the arms, legs, and torso. The illness has been ongoing for 3 months. She was observed in the outpatient department of Ternopil Regional Clinical Dermatovenerological Dispensary due to idiopathic urticaria.

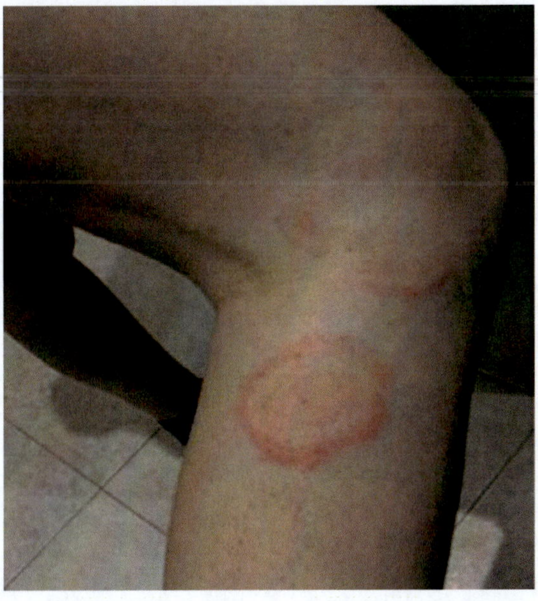

Figure 13. Multiple erythema migrans on the left shin, typical, urticarial. Patient P., 18 years old. Diagnosis: Lyme borreliosis, erythema form. Chronic course.

During the initial examination, the patient complained of swelling of the left forearm area with mild itching. From her medical history, it is known that the patient and her family members did not suffer from allergic diseases. The patient denies any harmful habits. She considers herself ill for about 30-35 days. The disease started gradually with the appearance of isolated rashes on the left forearm area, which disappeared on their own. Within a week, the number of elements increased, prompting her to seek dermatological consultation. A diagnosis of acute urticaria, unspecified, was made. Loratadine (Claritin), a second-generation antihistamine, was prescribed at 10 mg per day. Detoxification therapy was carried out with the enterosorbent Polysorb, 1-2 g three times a day for 7-10 days. During treatment, the condition slightly improved. However, after 3 days, the rashes reappeared, but they were larger, clustered, and spread to other parts of the body. The patient was referred to a clinical immunologist, who confirmed urticaria and supplemented the treatment prescribed by the dermatologist with topical glucocorticoid ointment Prednisolone for 14 days, with gradual discontinuation. After completing the treatment, the rashes reappeared. None of the doctors considered the possibility of a tick bite in the patient's history.

Objective examination: The general condition of the patient is satisfactory, body temperature is 36.8°C. On the skin areas of the outer surface of the left forearm, shin, and back, there are urticarial-like elements measuring 7–10 cm in diameter, with clearly defined raised edges. Upon detailed history taking, it was determined that 3 months ago, after returning from the forest, on the second day, a small unidentified "insect" was found on the front surface of the chest near the nipple, which the patient removed herself (by applying oil) and disposed of.

Complete blood count: Red blood cells – 4.4×10^{12} cells/L, haemoglobin – 135 g/L, haematocrit – 0.9, leukocytes – 7.6×10^{9} cells/L, eosinophils – 4%, band neutrophils – 4%, segmented neutrophils – 63%, lymphocytes – 24%, monocytes – 5%, ESR (erythrocyte sedimentation rate) – 5 mm/hour.

Blood analysis for IgM antibodies to B. burgdorferi complex was conducted. The result obtained was 95 AU/mL (results were evaluated quantitatively. ≥ 22 AU/mL was considered positive, 16–22 AU/mL was considered intermediate, ≤ 16 AU/mL was considered negative).

Therefore, detailed history regarding the tick bite incident and the lack of response to basic therapy for presumed urticaria allowed the diagnosis of atypical erythema migrans, presenting as multiple urticarial-like elements.

Subsequently, among the examined patients, it was investigated whether EM occurred at the site of tick attachment or in distant locations. This question was answered by 87 out of 146 patients (excluding 33 patients who did not remember the tick bite incident and 26 individuals who could not clearly indicate the location of tick attachment on their body surface).

EM was significantly more often registered at the site of tick attachment – in 72 cases (82.76% (95% CI 75.11; 90.89)) compared to 15 cases (17.24% (95% CI 9.11; 24.89)) with distant localization from the site of tick attachment ($p < 0.001$). These data are consistent with reports from researchers in Slovenia and Austria, who noted EM appearance at the tick bite site in 58.0% and 73.0% respectively [48].

We studied the influence of the season and the locality where the tick bite occurred on the localization of erythema. The results of statistical analysis did not reveal a significant effect of these factors on erythema localization (the significance of both two-sided exact Fisher's test and Pearson's chi-squared test exceeded the statistically significant threshold, $p < 0.05$, in all cases). However, odds ratio analysis revealed that in the case of tick bites occurring in autumn, the risk of EM occurrence at the bite site is lower compared to bites occurring in spring and summer, as indicated by a statistically significant odds ratio (OR) of 0.31 (95% CI 0.10–0.98, p = 0.046) (Table 3).

Table 3. Dependence of the localization of erythema migrans on the body in patients with Lyme borreliosis, taking into account the season and the locality where tick bites occurred (n = 87)

Parameter		Localization of EM		P-value of Fisher's exact test	OR	95% CI
		at the site of tick attack	in a remote area			
Season	spring	14	2	p1 = 0,73	1,60	0,32–7,90
	summer	43	6	p2 = 0,25	2,17	0,70–6,77
	autumn	15	7	p3 = 0,05*	0,31*	0,10–0,98
Locality	forest belt/forest	33	8	p4 = 0,56 p5 = 0,99	0,63	0,20–2,02
	park/hydropark	14	2	p6 = 0,76	1,45	0,29–7,22
	country house area/vegetable garden/garden	25	4		1,33	0,38–4,67

Notes:
1. * – significance level, $p < 0.05$.
2. p_1 – significance of the criterion in pairwise comparison of spring/summer+autumn groups.
3. p_2 – significance of the criterion in pairwise comparison of summer/spring+autumn groups.
4. p_3 – significance of the criterion in pairwise comparison of autumn/spring+summer groups.
5. p_4 – significance of the criterion in pairwise comparison of forest belt-forest/park-hydropark+ country house area-vegetable garden-garden groups.
6. p_5 – significance of the criterion in pairwise comparison of park-hydropark/forest belt-forest+ country house area -vegetable garden-garden groups.
7. p_6 – significance of the criterion in pairwise comparison of country house area -vegetable garden-garden/forest strip-forest+park-hydropark groups.

However, the number of tick bite sites had a statistically significant impact on the location of EM occurrence (p < 0.05) (Table 4). The results of the odds ratio analysis showed that the risk of EM occurrence at the bite site was statistically significantly lower when ticks attached to multiple areas of the body compared to attachment in a single body part (OR = 0.28, 95% CI 0.09–0.89, p = 0.031). It was found that the presence of tick attachment to a specific body part increases the likelihood of EM occurrence at the bite site (OR = 3.63, 95% CI 1.12–11.68, p = 0.031).

The duration of EM in patients with localized LB was analysed. It was found that on average it was observed for 30 (19; 59) days.

Dependencies between the duration of EM considering the time of tick removal from the patient's body after its attack (Kruskal-Wallis test significance coefficient, p = 0.95) and the time of its occurrence after attachment were not established (Kruskal-Wallis test significance coefficient, p = 0.31).

The results of the statistical analysis of EM duration based on patients' gender, age, and the number of tick attacks also did not show a significant influence of these factors (significance of two-sided exact Fisher's test and Pearson's chi-square test exceeded the statistical threshold, p < 0.05).

It was found that the duration of EM in patients with LB who experienced tick attacks in autumn was statistically shorter compared to those attacked in summer (Table 5, Figure 14).

Table 4. Frequency of occurrence of erythema migrans in patients with Lyme borreliosis taking into account the number of tick bite sites and their localization (n = 87)

Parameter		EM localization		P-value of Fisher's exact test	OR	95% CI
		at the site of the bite, n (%)	in a remote area, n (%)			
Number of bite sites	one	58 (80,56)	8 (53,33)	p = 0,04*	3,63*	1,12–11,68
	several	14 (19,44)	7 (46,67)		0,28*	0,09–0,89
Localization of tick bite sites	upper limbs	7 (12,07)	0	p = 0,58	2,48	0,12–47,46
	lower limbs	39 (67,24)	6 (75,00)	p = 0,99	0,68	0,13–3,71
	front part of torso	6 (10,34)	0	p = 0,99	2,10	0,11–40,88
	back part of the torso	3 (5,17)	0	p = 0,99	1,07	0,05–22,64

Note. * – significance level, $p < 0.05$; OR – odds ratio for EM at the bite site.

During the survey of 87 patients with erythema migrans form of LB who clearly indicated the location of tick attacks, the localization of these arachnids' attachment on the body surface was also investigated (Table 3.6). It was found that the most frequent site of tick attachment was the lower limbs, in 45 (51.7%) individuals. The next most frequent areas of attachment were multiple regions of tick bites in 21 (23.9%) patients. It should be noted that none of the respondents experienced tick bites on the head or neck, $p < 0.05$.

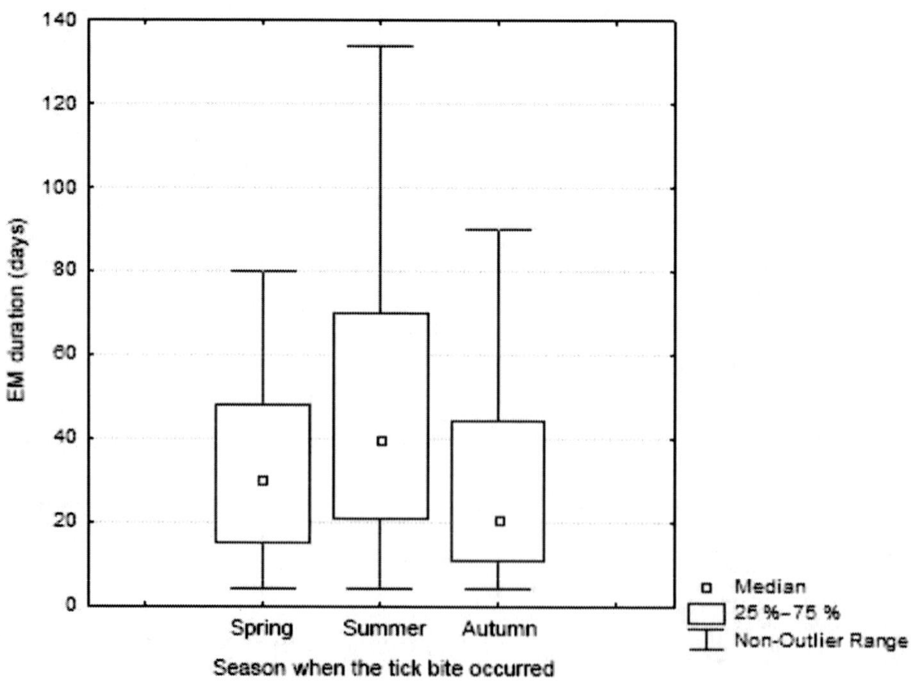

Figure 14. Duration of erythema migrans depending on the season when the tick bite occurred.

Table 5. The duration of erythema migrans in patients with Lyme borreliosis, considering the season when tick bites occurred (Me (Lq; Uq))

Parameter	Season			Kruskal-Wallis test and its significance, p	Mann-Whitney U test significance
	spring	summer	autumn		
Group	1	2	3		
EM duration, days	30,0 (15,0; 48,0)	40,0 (21,0; 70,0)	11,0 (20,5; 44,0)	H = 6,37 p = 0,04*	p1-2 = 0,206 p1-3 = 0,412 p2-3 = 0,015*

Note. The level of statistical significance according to the Bonferroni correction for intergroup comparisons, $p < 0.017$; * – statistically significant difference in indicators; p_{1-2} – significance of the criterion when comparing groups.

It was found that the duration of erythema significantly differed among groups of patients with different tick bite localizations (Kruskal-Wallis test significance coefficient, p = 0.008) (Table 7; Figure 15).

Table 6. Localization options of tick bites in patients with erythema migrans in Lyme borreliosis (n = 87; Me (Lq; Uq))

Tick Bite Localization		Absolute Number	Percentage	95% CI
Upper limbs	Total	17	19,54	11,21; 27,87
	Only this localization	7	8,05	2,33; 13,77
	Combined with other sites	10	11,49	4,79; 18,19
	This localization + lower limbs	2	2,30	0; 5,45
	Upper limbs + neck	1	1,15	0; 3,39
	This localization + lower limbs + torso (front)	4	4,60	0,20; 9,00
	This localization + lower limbs + abdomen	3	3,45	0; 7,29
Lower limbs	Total	61	70,11	60,49; 79,73
	Only this localization	45	51,72*	41,22; 62,22
	Combined with other sites	16	18,39	10,25; 26,53
	This localization + torso (front)	3	3,45	0; 7,29
	This localization + torso (back)	1	1,15	0; 3,39
	This localization + abdomen	3	3,45	0; 7,29
Neck	Total	1	1,15	0; 3,39
	Only this localization	0	0	–
	Combined with other sites	1	1,15	0; 3,39
Front part of the torso	Total	15	17,24	9,30; 25,18
	Only this localization	6	6,90	1,57; 12,23
	Combined with other sites	9	10,34	3,94; 16,74
	This localization + abdomen	2	2,30	0; 5,45
Back part of the torso	Total	6	6,90	1,57; 12,23
	Only this localization	3	3,45	0; 7,29
	Combined with other sites	3	3,45	0; 7,29
	This localization + abdomen	2	2,30	0; 5,45
Head	Total	0	0	–
Abdomen	Total	15	17,24	9,30; 25,18
	Only this localization	5	5,75	0,86; 10,64
	Combined with other sites	10	11,49	4,79; 18,19
Multiple other sites		21	23,86	14,90; 32,82

Table 7. Duration of erythema migrans in patients with Lyme borreliosis, taking into account the localization of tick bites (Me (Lq; Uq))

Group	Site of tick bite					
	upper limbs	lower limbs	front part of the torso	back part of the torso	abdomen	multiple sites
	1	2	3	4	5	6
EM duration	50,5 (20,0; 87,0)	33,5 (19,5; 51,0)	20,0 (13,0; 44,0)	8,0 (5,0; 11,0)	90,0 (75,0; 120,0)	21,0 (14,0; 44,0)
The Kruskal-Wallis criterion (H) and its significance criterion (p) H = 15,776, p = 0,008*						
Mann-Whitney U test significance	p1-2 = 0,412 p1-3 = 0,171 p1-4 = 0,046 p1-5 = 0,144 p1-6 = 0,210	p2-3 = 0,364 p2-4 = 0,027 p2-5 = 0,003* p2-6 = 0,180	p3-4 = 0,245 p3-5 = 0,016 p3-6 = 0,745	p4-5 = 0,053 p4-6 = 0,114	p5-6 = 0,010	–

Note. The level of statistical significance according to Bonferroni corrections for intergroup comparisons, $p < 0.007$; * – statistically significant difference; p_{1-2}, p_{1-3}, p_{1-4}, p_{1-5}, p_{1-6}, p_{2-3}, p_{2-4}, p_{2-5}, p_{2-6}, p_{3-4}, p_{3-5}, p_{3-6}, p_{4-5}, p_{4-6}, p_{5-6} – significance of the criterion in intergroup comparisons.

Upon pairwise comparison of groups, it was found that the duration of EM was longer when ticks bit the abdomen compared to bites on the lower extremities: 90 (75; 120) days versus 33.5 (19.5; 51.0) days (p = 0.003). Differences in the duration of EM between ticks biting the front torso and abdomen (p = 0.016), as well as abdomen in multiple sites (p = 0.010), were close to the level of statistical significance (p = 0.007 according to Bonferroni correction), indicating a tendency towards differences in EM duration depending on the bite location.

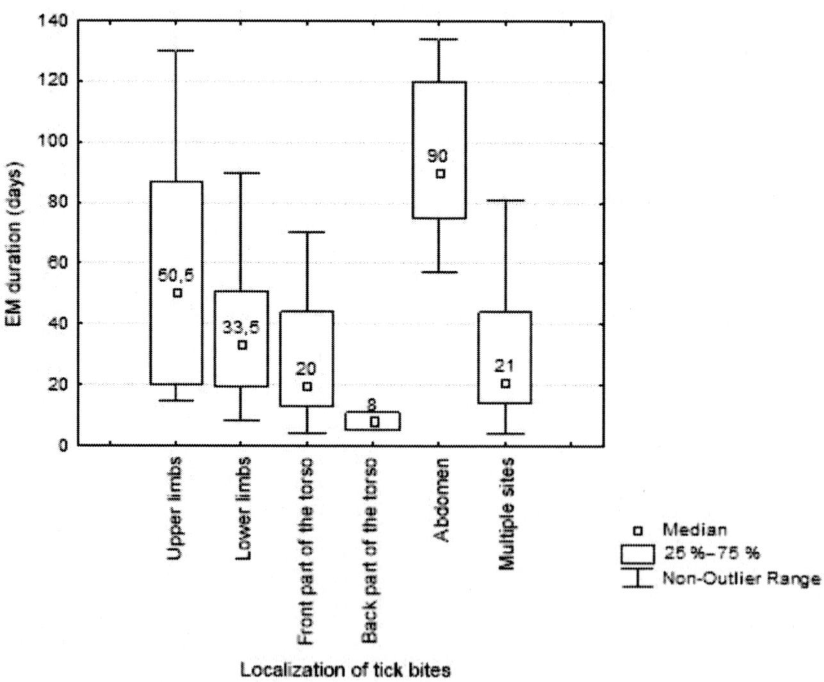

Figure 15. The dependence of the duration of erythema migrans in examined individuals with Lyme borreliosis on the localization of tick bites.

Table 8. The frequency of detection of the main clinical signs of Lyme borreliosis in patients with erythema migrans

Syndrome	Patients with EM (n = 146)	
	Absolute number	%
EM without signs of dissemination	96	65,8
EM with dissemination		
Intoxication	17	11,6
Cardiovascular system involvement	8	5,5
Musculoskeletal system involvement	16	10,9
Nervous system involvement	9	6,2
Total	146	100,0

Table 9. Comparison of clinical symptoms in examined patients with erythema migrans in Lyme borreliosis depending on the location of tick bites (n = 87)

Symptoms		Site of tick bite					
		Upper limbs (n = 7)	Lower limbs (n = 45)	Front part of the torso (n = 6)	Back part of the torso (n = 3)	Abdomen (n = 5)	Multiple sites (n = 21)
Fever	Absolute number	0	7	3	1	0	2
	%	0	15,56	50,00*	33,33	0	9,52
Headache	Absolute number	2	9	2	2	0	5
	%	28,57	20,00	33,33	66,67	0	23,81
Myalgia	Absolute number	0	4	0	0	1	2
	%	0	8,89	0	0	20,00	9,52
Arthralgia	Absolute number	2	11	5	2	1	9
	%	28,57	24,44*	83,33*	66,67	20,00	42,86
Lymphadenopathy	Absolute number	0	0	1	0	0	1
	%	0	0	16,67	0	0	4,76
Increased fatigue	Absolute number	1	4	0	2	0	1
	%	14,29	8,89	0	66,67*	0	4,76
Palpitations	Absolute number	0	1	0	0	0	0
	%	0	2,22	0	0	0	0
Neurological symptoms	Absolute number	1	0	0	0	0	0
	%	14,29	0	0	0	0	0
Drowsiness	Absolute number	0	2	0	0	0	1
	%	0	4,44	0	0	0	4,76
Combination of symptoms	Absolute number	2	11	3	2	0	5
	%	28,57	24,44	50,00	66,67	0	23,81
Absence of symptoms	Absolute number	4	16	1	0	3	10

Note. * – the difference is significant in pairwise comparisons of groups using exact two-sided Fisher's test, $p < 0.05$.

Table 10. Probability of clinical symptoms in patients with erythema migrans form of Lyme borreliosis depending on the site of tick bite (n = 87)

Symptom		Site of tick bite					
		upper limb	lower limb	front part of the torso	back part of the torso	abdomen	Multiple sites
Fever	OR	0,33	1,11	7,10*	3,00	0,47	0,53
	95% CI	0,02–6,19	0,34–3,60	1,26–40,12	0,25–35,72	0,02–8,97	0,11–2,59
Headache	OR	1,38	0,70	1,75	7,33	0,28	1,06
	95% CI	0,25–7,71	0,26–1,92	0,30–10,34	0,63–85,53	0,01–5,23	0,33–3,38
Myalgia	OR	0,65	1,27	0,76	1,48	3,17	1,28
	95% CI	0,03–12,60	0,27–6,03	0,04–14,94	0,07–31,38	0,30–33,00	0,23–7,16
Arthralgia	OR	0,74	0,39*	11,20*	4,00	0,46	1,61
	95% CI	0,14–4,08	0,16–0,97	1,24–100,90	0,35–46,03	0,05–4,28	0,59–4,40
Increased fatigue	OR	1,74	0,93	0,67	26,00*	0,80	0,42
	95% CI	0,18–16,57	0,22–3,97	0,03–12,87	2,05–329,69	0,04–15,70	0,05–3,64
Skin itching	OR	0,92	4,00	1,07	2,12	1,31	0,78
	95% CI	0,05–18,21	0,43–37,34	0,05–21,57	0,10–46,36	0,06–26,96	0,08–7,34
Combination of symptoms	OR	1,12	0,81	3,05	6,00	0,23	0,83
	95% CI	0,20–6,24	0,31–2,10	0,57–16,33	0,52–69,58	0,01–4,33	0,27–2,61

Note. * – statistically significant difference for odds ratio (OR), $p < 0.05$.

Table 11. Probability of the impact of tick removal method on clinical manifestations in patients with erythema migrans Lyme borreliosis (n = 87)

Symptom		Methods of tick removal			
		Pulled out with fingers	Removed with a strong motion, twisted or scratched with a fingernail	Disinfected with a disinfectant solution, applied oil	Several methods
Fever	OR	0,11	0,04*	3,71	1,45
	95% CI	0,01–2,12	0,01–0,27	0,30–46,48	0,33–6,44
Headache	OR	0,27	1,64	1,47	1,56
	95% CI	0,05–1,33	0,46–5,82	0,12–17,36	0,50–4,89
Myalgia	OR	1,71	0,77	1,42	0,92
	95% CI	0,26–11,20	0,08–7,45	0,06–31,12	0,14–5,92
Arthralgia	OR	0,82	1,74	1,14	0,74
	95% CI	0,25–2,77	0,52–5,87	0,10–13,38	0,24–2,23
Increased fatigue	OR	8,6	0,31	1,76	0,44
	95% CI	0,83–89,13	0,02–6,13	0,08–39,70	0,04–4,49
Skin itching	OR	0,19	0,77	6,88	2,22
	95% CI	0,01–3,70	0,08–7,45	0,51–93,15	0,34–14,33
Combination of symptoms	OR	0,43	0,95	5,87	1,33
	95% CI	0,11–1,73	0,26–3,53	0,50–69,43	0,43–4,10

Note. * – the difference is significant for odds ratio (OR), $p < 0.05$.

During the analysis of patient complaints, it was determined that out of 146 examined individuals with EM form of Lyme borreliosis, 96 (65.8%) reported only one complaint – skin colour change resembling EM. The remaining 50 (34.2%) individuals also reported other manifestations of the illness (Table 8).

Among them were patients predominantly affected in various organs and systems, as well as those with combined organ involvement. It was noted that signs of intoxication and musculoskeletal system involvement were mostly observed, $p < 0.05$.

The frequency of fever occurrence in patients with EM varied depending on the localization of tick bites. In particular, it was found that fever was significantly more common in individuals with ticks attached to the front torso compared to patients with ticks attached elsewhere (statistical significance by two-sided Fisher's exact test, $p = 0.04$) (Table 9). Fever due to ticks attached to the front torso was recorded in 23.08% (95% CI 0.18; 45.98) of all EM cases.

It was found that the frequency of arthralgia occurrence in EM cases was significantly higher when ticks were attached to the lower limbs and front torso compared to other body areas – statistical significance by two-sided Fisher's exact test was $p = 0.046$ and $p = 0.017$, respectively (Table 9). Among all individuals with arthralgia, 36.67% (95% CI 19.43; 53.91) reported tick bites on the lower limbs in their medical history, and 16.67% (95% CI 69.99; 96.67) reported tick bites on the front torso.

Patients with EM LB who had ticks attached to the back torso more frequently reported increased fatigue compared to individuals with ticks attached in other locations – the significance of the two-sided exact Fisher's test was $p = 0.02$. Among individuals with complaints of increased fatigue and a history of ticks attaching to the back torso, 25.0% (95% CI 0; 55.01) were recorded.

It was found that tick bites on the lower limbs in individuals with EM LB reduce the risk of developing arthralgia. Conversely, attachment of these arachnids to the front torso increases the risk of arthralgia by 11 times (Table 10).

The attachment of ticks to the front of the torso increases the likelihood of fever by 7 times in patients with EM (OR = 7.10; 95% CI 1.26–40.12; $p < 0.05$), while attachment to the back increases the likelihood of developing increased fatigue in patients with EM by 26 times ($p < 0.05$) (Table 10).

Next, we investigated whether the method of tick removal affects the occurrence of clinical manifestations in patients with EM. It was found that removal by energetic movement, twisting, or scraping with nails reduces the likelihood of developing fever (OR = 0.04; 95% CI 0.01–0.27; $p < 0.05$) (Table 11).

Significant differences were found in the frequency of clinical manifestations in patients with EM depending on the time of their occurrence after tick attachment. Specifically, headaches occurred in 66.7% of cases when EM developed several months after the tick bite, which significantly exceeded the frequency observed with earlier onset of erythema (odds ratio from Fisher's exact test, $p = 0.02$) (Table 12).

Combination of symptoms in EM was statistically less frequently registered when EM occurred after the 30th day following tick bite, constituting 5.56%, whereas when EM appeared within the first 7 days – 31.58%; from the 8th to the 14th day – 38.46%; from the 15th to the 21st day – 18.18%; from the 22nd to the 30th day – 37.50%; and after several months – 50.00% ($p = 0.03$) (Table 12).

Table 12. Clinical symptoms in patients with Lyme borreliosis taking into account the time of its appearance after tick bites (n = 87)

Symptoms		Time after tick bite, day					
		up to 7	8–14	15–21	22–30	30–60	in a few months
Fever	Absolute number	4	3	2	2	0	1
	%	21,05	23,08	18,18	25,00	0	16,67
Headache	Absolute number	2	3	2	2	4	4
	%	10,53	23,08	18,18	25,00	22,22	66,67*
Myalgia	Absolute number	2	0	2	1	0	1
	%	10,53	0	18,18	12,50	0	16,67
Arthralgia	Absolute number	5	5	1	5	5	4
	%	26,32	38,46	9,09	62,50	27,78	66,67
Lymphadenopathy	Absolute number	1	0	0	1	0	0
	%	5,26	0	0	12,50	0	0
Increased fatigue	Absolute number	1	3	1	1	0	0
	%	5,26	23,08	9,09	12,50	0	0
Palpitations	Absolute number	0	0	1	0	0	0
	%	0	0	9,09	0	0	0
Neurological symptoms	Absolute number	0	1	0	0	0	0
	%	0	7,69	0	0	0	0
Drowsiness	Absolute number	0	0	0	1	0	0
	%	0	0	9,09	12,50	0	0
Skin itching	Absolute number	1	1	1	0	0	0
	%	5,26	7,69	9,09	0	0	0
Combination of symptoms	Absolute number	6	5	2	3	1	3
	%	31,58	38,46	18,18	37,50	5,56*	50,00
Absence of symptoms	Absolute number	12	5	2	1	11	0
	%	63,16*	38,46	18,18	12,50	61,11	0

Note. * – the difference is significant when comparing groups in pairs using Fisher's exact two-sided test, $p < 0.05$.

It was noted that in 63.2% of patients in whom EM occurred within the first 7 days after tick attachment, there were no other clinical symptoms, significantly more often than in cases where EM occurred between 8 and 30 days and after several months ($p = 0.03$). Close to the level of statistical significance ($p = 0.06$) was the absence of clinical symptoms when EM developed between 30 and 60 days. At the same time, in patients in whom EM appeared two months after tick bite, there were no other symptoms.

The frequency of arthralgia detection when EM occurred between the 15th and 21st days after tick bite was lower (9.09%) compared to other groups; however, if erythema developed after 2 months, the percentage of those who experienced arthralgia was highest – 66.67% (Table 12).

Table 13. The probability of the timing of the appearance of erythema migrans following tick bites influencing the development of other clinical manifestations in patients (n = 87)

Symptom		Time after tick bite, day					
		up to 7	8–14	15–21	22–30	30–60	in a few months
Fever	OR	1,6	1,77	1,20	1,90	0,10	1,05
	95% CI	0,42–6,07	0,41–7,69	0,22–6,40	0,33–10,78	0,01–1,75	0,11–9,92
Headache	OR	0,32	1,03	0,73	1,16	0,97	8,62*
	95% CI	0,07–1,56	0,25–4,26	0,14–3,73	0,21–6,33	0,27–3,45	1,42–52,20
Myalgia	OR	1,53	0,32	3,33	1,77	0,21	2,56
	95% CI	0,26–9,10	0,02–6,07	0,53–20,91	0,18–17,40	0,01–3,99	0,25–26,36
Arthralgia	OR	0,64	1,31	0,19	3,92	0,71	4,57
	95% CI	0,20–2,05	0,38–4,53	0,02–1,59	0,85–17,98	0,22–2,28	0,78–26,92
Lymphadenopathy	OR	3,06	0,90	1,09	9,43	0,60	2,08
	95% CI	0,18–51,39	0,04–19,76	0,05–24,15	0,53–167,84	0,03–13,08	0,09–48,05
Increased fatigue	OR	0,57	5,9*	1,18	1,77	0,26	0,87
	95% CI	0,06–5,18	1,04–33,45	0,12–11,88	0,18–17,40	0,01–4,76	0,04–17,23
Skin itching	OR	1,53	2,54	3,15	1,11	0,43	1,48
	95% CI	0,13–17,86	0,21–30,32	0,26–38,05	0,05–23,20	0,02–8,69	0,07–31,98

Note: * – the difference is significant for odds ratio (OR), $p < 0.05$.

It was found that the risk of developing headache increased in patients when EM developed several months after tick attachment (OR = 8.6; 95% CI 1.42–52.20; p = 0.02) (Table 13).

The impact of the factor such as EM appearance after 30 days on the occurrence of symptom complex was confirmed by odds ratio assessment (OR = 0.12; 95% CI 0.01–0.95; p = 0.04).

Analysing odds ratios, it was noted that when EM appeared between days 15 and 21, the risk of developing arthralgia could practically quadruple (p = 0.07), and when EM appeared after 2 months, it could increase by 4.5 times (p = 0.09). There was also an increased likelihood of developing increased fatigue when EM appeared between 8 and 14 days (OR = 5.9; 95% CI 1.04–33.45; p = 0.04).

The severity of the disease, calculated by the sum of points, corresponded to mild in 110 (75.3%) patients, moderate in 28 (19.2%), and severe in 8 (5.5%).

Thus, a larger proportion of patients with EM indicated tick attachment to the lower limbs ($p < 0.05$), every fifth patient could not clearly specify the site of tick bites. EM after tick bite more often occurred after 3 (16.4%) and 30 (15.1%) days; however, the largest number of patients (40.4%) could not specify the time of erythema appearance ($p < 0.05$). Typical forms of EM were significantly more frequently registered ($p < 0.05$), among which elongated oval-shaped erythemas predominated; among atypical forms were total erythematous rashes. One erythema was diagnosed in 94.5% of patients, several in others. EM significantly more often occurred at the site of tick attachment (82.8%), compared to locations distant from the bite site (17.2%) ($p < 0.001$). The risk of developing EM at the site of tick bite was lower when bitten in autumn than in spring and summer (OR = 0.31; 95% CI 0.10–0.98, p = 0.046), and when attached in multiple places on the body compared to attachment in a single area (OR = 0.28; 95% CI 0.09–0.89, p = 0.031).

In 50 (34.2%) out of 146 patients, other clinical manifestations of LB were diagnosed, besides the pathognomonic sign – EM. Arthralgia and fever occurred significantly more often when ticks attached to the front torso; arthralgia also occurred during attacks on the lower limbs, and increased fatigue occurred in the back part of the torso. Itchiness and drowsiness in patients more frequently occurred when EM was present in remote areas from the attachment site. Headaches were mostly reported when EM appeared 2 months after tick bite; combined clinical symptoms were significantly less troubling when EM developed between 30-60 days, and the risk of arthralgia increased when erythema appeared between 15-21 days. If EM occurred within the first week after tick bite, no other clinical manifestations of LB were present. A mild course of EM was observed in the majority (75.3%) of examined patients, of moderate severity in 19.2%, and severe in only 5.5% of individuals [49, 50].

Skin lesions in LB also manifest as benign lymphocytoma of the skin, chronic atrophic acrodermatitis (CAA), and localized scleroderma (morphea) [41]. Benign lymphocytoma of the skin is more commonly observed in women and children, less frequently in men and elderly individuals [7]. It is primarily located in the region of the earlobe, areola of the breast, face, and groin areas. It manifests with nodular elements, tumour-like formations, or poorly demarcated infiltrates in the dermis. Multiple (or solitary) nodules the size of a pea appear most frequently, with skin colour ranging from bluish-red to brownish-grey. These formations are characterized by their painlessness, with patients mainly concerned about cosmetic defects. Studies have shown that in European residents, this skin condition is most often associated with B. afzelii and B. garinii [36, 39].

CAA is a typical form of chronic LB. It develops slowly over several years (from six months to three or more years). It is predominantly registered in older age, typically in women [7]. CAA usually localizes on the extensor surfaces of the hands and feet, less frequently on the forearms and shins. Skin lesions can be symmetrical or only affect one limb. During its initial development (ooedematous stage), the affected skin area appears swollen. Subsequently, as the processes of skin and subcutaneous tissue atrophy progress, the epidermis becomes thinner and takes on a cigarette paper-like appearance, under which the mesh of blood vessels becomes visible [4, 51].

Today, many researchers believe in a close etiopathogenetic link between localized (focal) scleroderma and localized atrophic skin lesions (morphea) on one hand, and LB on the other [52]. Recent research results have confirmed the borrelial aaetiology of this dermatological syndrome. Borrelia were detected in skin biopsies of patients with localized scleroderma. Positive results of polymerase chain reaction (PCR) and serological tests (elevated levels of anti-Borrelia antibodies) also confirm the etiological significance of Borrelia in every other patient with localized scleroderma [7, 39, 53].

It is presumed that the skin changes in localized scleroderma represent initial manifestations of CAA, which should be considered as pseudoscleroderma [54]. Skin lesions typically form 8-24 months after primary infection. The most commonly observed disseminated superficial plaque-like form of scleroderma appears as plaques or spots ranging in size from 1 to 5 cm, oval or round in shape, with colours ranging from pink, wax-like white, to brown. Sometimes, dermato-sclerosis is observed in the centre of lesions, with a ring of purple colour at the periphery. Skin lesions primarily localize on the torso [51].

In separate studies, it has been noted that in some patients, predominantly residents of Europe, localized scleroderma (LS) is one of the manifestations of late LB [52–56]. Despite immunological and biochemical studies conducted, the nature of localized asymmetric skin inflammation followed by sclerosis remains unclear [55]. For instance, the role of B. burgdorferi as an etiological factor of localized scleroderma has been investigated [57–60].

Arguments supporting the association with B. burgdorferi in localized scleroderma include an erythematous ring similar to erythema migrans in LB, and the effectiveness of treatment with penicillin [58]. The significance of B. burgdorferi as an etiological factor, particularly in Ukraine, requires further research.

According to literature data, in some patients from Austria, Germany, Italy, and Ukraine with these dermatological syndromes, elevated levels of anti-Borrelia antibodies were detected in the blood [52, 53]. Additionally, positive clinical dynamics were observed during antibiotic treatment. All of this allows considering these syndromes as manifestations of borreliosis [53].

We observed 90 patients with LB between 2015-2020 who underwent outpatient and inpatient treatment at Ternopil Regional Clinical Dermatovenereological Dispensary, the infectious diseases department of the Ternopil City Municipal Hospital Emergency Medical Care, Ternopil Regional Tuberculosis and Pulmonology Medical Centre of Ternopil Regional Council, and the Ternopil University Hospital. There were 33 (36.7%) men and 57 (63.3%) women ($p < 0.05$). The majority of those examined were urban residents, compared to rural residents, with 56 (62.2%) versus 34 (37.8%) respectively ($p < 0.05$). Their average age was (43.1±14.3) years.

Skin lesions were noted in 25 (27.8%) out of 90 patients with LB. It is necessary to note that besides morphea, which was diagnosed in 21 (23.3%) patients of this group (Figure 16, 17), one patient each had Weber-Christian panniculitis, erythema annulare, and allergic dermatitis, while two had urticaria and pityriasis rosea. The comparison group consisted of 25 patients with morphea without accompanying LB, matched by age and gender to the distribution of examined patients (Figure 18).

The legs were the most common site of tick bites in patients with morphea – in 8 (38.1%) out of 21, followed less frequently by the front torso (19.0%), hands, and abdomen (each 14.3%). Subsequently, the timing of clinical manifestations of the illness was clarified. It is necessary to note that 9 (42.9%) patients could not clearly indicate the timing of disease symptoms because they did not remember the date of tick attachment to the body surface, although they associated skin lesions with being in an endemic area for LB (forest, backyard, or park). Most respondents who remembered the time of tick attachment had clinical symptoms after 7 months or later – 10 (83.3%), while the rest had symptoms after 3-6 months [61].

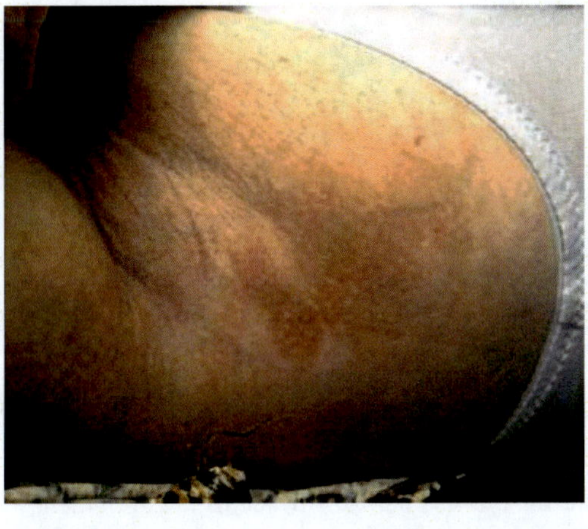

Figure 16. Limited focal skin atrophy in the right inguinal region. Patient K., 52 years old. Diagnosis: Lyme borreliosis. Morphea. Chronic course.

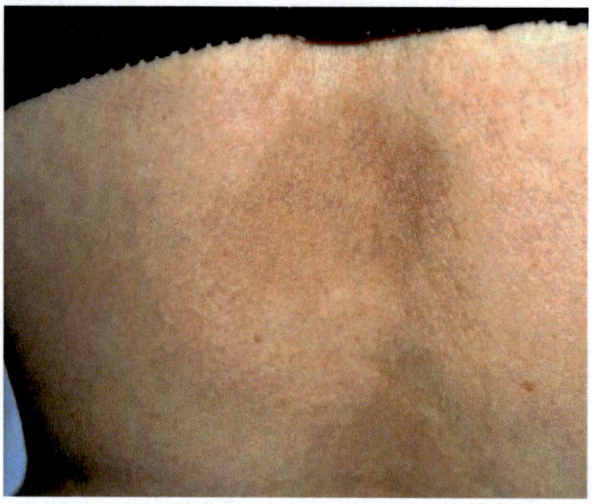

Figure 17. Limited focal skin atrophy on the back. Patient S., 56 years old. Diagnosis: Lyme borreliosis. Morphea. Chronic course.

The analysis of clinical manifestations of morphea allowed the following conclusions: the appearance of lesions of the disease was associated with the site of tick attachment in 7 (33.3%) out of 21 patients. In these patients, foci of superficial scleroderma were more frequently localized on the abdomen and coincided with the site of tick bite (Table 14).

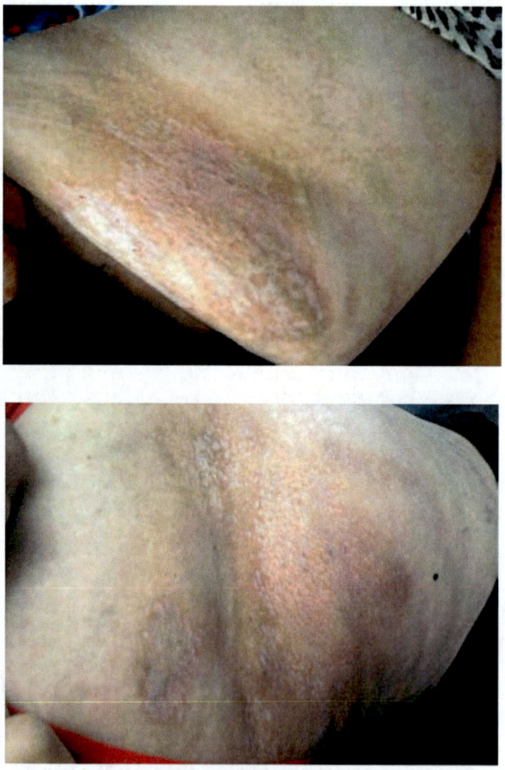

Figure 18. Foci of scleroderma on the anterior surface of the abdomen. Patient S., 58 years old. Diagnosis: Lyme borreliosis. Morphea. Chronic course.

Table 14. Clinical symptoms of skin involvement (morphea) in patients with non-erythematous Lyme borreliosis and without Lyme borreliosis

Characteristics of lesions		Patients with morphea			
		with LB (n = 21)		without LB (n = 25)	
		Absolute number	%	Absolute number	%
Number	One or up to three	11	52,4	20	80,0
	multiple, 4 and more	10	47,6**	5	20,0
Localization	face	–	–	2	8,0
	neck	–	–	1	4,0
	chest	4	19,1	8	32,0
	abdomen	10	47,6*	7	28,0
	back	7	33,3	6	24,0
	upper limbs	4	19,1	2	8,0
	lower limbs	5	23,8	12	48,0*
Modified skin score by G. P. Rodnan		1,14±0,13		2,44±0,18*	

Notes:
1. * – the difference is significant within the group according to the localization of lesions, $p < 0.05$.
2. ** – the difference is significant between groups, $p < 0.05$.

Additionally, comparisons were made between manifestations of morphea in patients with LB and in individuals without tick-borne borreliosis who had similar skin lesions (25 patients). It was found that in individuals with morphea associated with LB, both solitary and multiple lesions were equally frequently recorded (11 and 10 individuals, respectively). However, in contrast to the comparison group, multiple lesions were significantly more common among them – in 10 (47.6%) compared to 5 (20.0%) ($p < 0.05$), while solitary lesions were somewhat less frequent – in 11 (52.4%) compared to 20 (80.0%) (Table 14).

As for the localization of morphea lesions, they predominantly occurred on the abdomen (at the site of tick attachment) in patients with LB – in 10 individuals (47.6%) compared to 7 (28.0%) in the comparison group ($p < 0.05$). In patients without LB, skin involvement primarily affected the legs – in 12 (48.0%) cases, more frequently than in LB patients (5; 23.8%). To assess the degree and severity of skin changes (induration), the modified Rodnan skin score was used. It was found that this coefficient was significantly higher in the comparison group (morphea without LB) compared to patients with morphea and LB – 2.44 ± 0.18 versus 1.14 ± 0.13 ($p < 0.05$) [62].

Thus, skin manifestations were observed in 27.8% of patients with localized scleroderma associated with LB: morphea – 21 cases, urticaria – 2, lichen planus – 2, Weber-Christian panniculitis – 1, erythema annulare – 1 patient. A third of the patients reported the appearance of morphea lesions at the site of tick bite, more frequently on the abdomen. In patients with morphea and LB, as opposed to those with morphea without LB, solitary and multiple lesions were equally frequent, but multiple lesions were significantly more common. In patients without LB, morphea was predominantly located on the legs, more so than in LB patients. The modified Rodnan skin score was significantly higher in patients with morphea without LB compared to those with LB ($p < 0.05$).

Another manifestation of skin involvement in LB is Pansclerotic morphea (Pasini-Pierini atrophy), which develops 6 months (up to 4 years) after Borrelia infection. Lesions present as multiple confluent areas of hyperpigmentation (diameter of individual lesions 5–10 cm) predominantly localized on the trunk. Unlike systemic manifestations of connective tissue diseases, atrophoderma does not involve esophagitis or basal pneumosclerosis [7, 52, 63].

4. Lesions of the Musculoskeletal System

Svitlana Smiyan
and Valentyna Yuskevych

LB, often referred to as a multisystem disease, is frequently called the "new great imitator" due to the variety of clinical manifestations resembling syphilis [64, 65]. It is a complex immune-mediated disease of infectious origin, characterized by inflammatory or "rheumatic" features. From these perspectives, LB serves as a unique model in humans for studying the infectious aaetiology of rheumatic diseases [66].

Increasingly relevant is the study of this pathology in rheumatological practice. Significant attention is given to identifying musculoskeletal lesions among the complex-to-diagnose localized scleroderma associated with LB, many of which may present under the guise of various rheumatic diseases [67]. Tissue damage and symptoms in LB are driven by an inflammatory reaction induced by the bacterium and its antigens. In untreated patients, the disease can exhibit a wide spectrum of clinical manifestations involving joints, skin, and the heart. A small percentage (≈10%) of individuals retain fibromyalgia that does not respond to prolonged antimicrobial therapy. Today, knowledge of the ecological, epidemiological, microbiological, and immunological aspects of LB has been successfully integrated into a concept explaining these mechanisms [68].

Information about the hematogenous spread of spirochetes has been known since the early 1980s [69, 70]. Despite the complexity of detecting spirochaetaemia, a high proportion of constitutional and rheumatological symptoms provides substantial evidence for the systemic nature of LB, even in cases of localized processes [71, 72]. The identification of characteristic metabolic [73] and proteomic [74] changes in the blood of early LB patients further indicates a systemic process regardless of the presence of clinical signs of dissemination. Research results using cultured umbilical vein endothelial cells have demonstrated that Borrelia quickly adhere to vascular endothelium and subsequently attach to subendothelial matrix components through intercellular junctions (transmigration) [75, 76]. Intravital confocal microscopy in real-time mode has confirmed that transmigration through capillaries and post-capillary venules is a multi-step process involving only a small percentage of GFP-expressing spirochetes (GFP – green fluorescent protein – a tool for visualizing spatial and temporal patterns of gene expression *in vivo*) injected intravenously into mice [77, 78]. Besides the skin, the heart, joints, and nervous system become the most significant distant foci of involvement.

4.1. Lyme Arthritis

Lyme arthritis is the most common and serious "rheumatological" manifestation of spirochaetal infection, with an incubation period for joint involvement lasting from 3 to 6 months and longer [79–81]. It is assumed that spirochetes typically enter the joints long before clinical symptoms appear [82]. In some patients, episodes of arthralgia may precede clinical arthritis [83]. The presence of high-titre antibodies to multiple *B. burgdorferi* antigens in the serum of Lyme arthritis patients [84, 85] aligns with the concept of a period of joint quiescence before the onset of clinically evident arthritis [19]. Twenty genotypes of *B. burgdorferi s. l.* have been identified

[86], nine of which infect humans: *B. burgdorferi s. s.*, *B. garinii*, *B. afzelii*, *B. bavariensis*, *B. bissetii*, *B. kurtenbachii*, *B. lusitaniae*, *B. spielmanii*, *B. valaesiana* [87]. *B. burgdorferi s. s.* possesses the highest arthrogenic potential, causing arthritis in 46% of infected patients in the United States [88].

B. burgdorferi employs several mechanisms to evade innate and acquired human immunity. Several *B. burgdorferi* lipoproteins, collectively known as complement regulator-acquiring surface proteins (CRASPs), can bind to factor H, a factor H-like protein in the body that prevents bacterial destruction [89, 90]. Thus, after entering, Borrelia avoids antibodies, which is crucial for its survival. To achieve this, *B. burgdorferi* alters lipoproteins expressed on its outer membrane, replacing OspC with VlsE. Based on structural similarities, these two proteins may perform similar physiological functions. However, unlike OspC, VlsE undergoes extensive antigenic variation to evade the immune response. *B. burgdorferi* mutants secreting non-variable VlsE cannot reinfect an organism previously infected with *B. burgdorferi*, whereas bacteria secreting variable VlsE can [91]. Additionally, *B. burgdorferi* produces a protease that participates in direct tissue damage mechanisms in Lyme arthritis [92].

Lyme arthritis is considered to be monoarticular or oligoarticular arthritis of large joints, characterized by episodes of inflammation with swelling, large effusions, and mild pain [93]. Knee joint involvement is most common, but other joints such as the ankle, shoulder, elbow, or wrist can also be affected; isolated involvement of small joints is atypical [93, 94]. Cases of untreated arthritis lasting from several days to months with spontaneous recovery have also been described [80]. According to a recent CDC report (Centre for Disease Control and Prevention), of approximately 150,000 registered cases of Lyme disease in the United States reported between 1992 and 2006, up to 30% presented with arthritis. In contrast, in Europe, fewer than 10% of *B. burgdorferi*-infected individuals develop arthritis [94, 95].

Joint involvement in LB is caused by hematogenous spread of borreliae and their entry into joint tissues during the early days and weeks of the disease. During this period, specific immune response to borreliae is minimal and characterized by the formation of antibodies against flagellar antigen, surface antigen of the outer membrane – protein C, and heat shock proteins of the bacterium. Over the next few months, a combined cellular and humoral immune response develops against many spirochaetal polypeptides, coinciding with the period of pronounced specific immune response and arthritis development.

B. burgdorferi is a potential inducer of interleukin-1 (IL-1), which is a cytokine with pro-inflammatory effects on synoviocytes and chondrocytes and may contribute to cartilage and bone destruction. Concentrations of IL-1β and its natural antagonist IL-1α vary under conditions of different disease courses: high IL-1α and low IL-1β concentrations are associated with rapid regression of arthritis attacks, whereas patients with the opposite cytokine ratio experience a more sluggish and prolonged arthritis course. Involvement of the synovial membrane is characterized by hyperplasia of synovial cells, vessel proliferation, and pronounced infiltration of mononuclear cells, reflecting a morphological manifestation of delayed hypersensitivity immune response. IL-17 plays a crucial role in the development of Lyme arthritis. Experimental evidence shows that neutralization of endogenous IL-17 leads to reduced local inflammation and production of pro-inflammatory cytokines, suggesting the potential therapeutic efficacy of IL-17 antibodies in treating this condition [96, 97].

Moreover, significant Th17-dependent immune reactions are often observed in patients with Lyme arthritis, which may help control early infection. However, excessive Th17-dependent reactions following disease resolution may become unfavourable due to potentiation of autoimmune mechanisms associated with antibiotic-resistant arthritis, resulting from increased synthesis of matrix metalloproteinase-10 that supports pathological processes in joint structures [98, 99].

In later stages of infection, particularly stage 2 (known in humans as early disseminated infection, presenting with inflammation in multiple locations) and stage 3 (known as late infection, typically associated with arthritis), inflammatory effects may be an important function of Toll-like receptor (TLR) signalling [100]. In Lyme arthritis, polymorphism in TLR1 (leading to decreased TLR1 expression) is associated with increased levels of pro-inflammatory cytokines and development of persistent arthritis after antibiotic therapy [101]. In all tissues infected by *B. burgdorferi*, mononuclear cell infiltrates appear, including CD4+ and CD8+ T-cells, as well as vascular anomalies, indicating spirochetes are located in or around blood vessels. However, inflammatory infiltrates differ at different stages of the disease in various infected areas. For example, macrophages are abundant in heart lesions, while B cells and plasma cells predominate in synovial lesions during stage 3 of the disease in patients with antibiotic-resistant Lyme arthritis. Spirochaetal presence in synovial areas triggers joint inflammation characterized by an exudate rich in neutrophils. Binding of spirochaetal lipoprotein to Toll-like receptor 2 prompts neutrophils to produce pro-inflammatory cytokines: IL-1, TNF-α, IL-8, and IL-15 [103]. Neutrophils also facilitate spirochete elimination through phagocytosis. Additionally, spirochaetal stimulation of macrophages leads to release of pro-inflammatory mediators typical of M1 macrophages, including TNF-α, IL-1β, IL-12, IL-18, and nitric oxide [104]. Th1 lymphocytes also play a role in joint inflammation. *Ex vivo* studies demonstrate that T-lymphocytes activated by *B. burgdorferi* components from patients with Lyme arthritis produce interferon-gamma (IFN-γ) [105].

Associated with Th1 inflammation is not the sole possible immunological pathway in the development of Lyme arthritis. It has been described that *B. burgdorferi* is a strong inducer of IL-10, which suppresses Th1 activity and may promote immune tolerance to the microorganism [106].

In the study by Kuo et al., it was demonstrated that arthritis observed in IFN-γ-deficient mice depended on IL-17 [107]. Significant roles of pro-inflammatory IL-17 in the induction of severe destructive Lyme arthritis were shown in the IFN-γ-deficient mouse model. However, administration of antibodies against IL-17 or IL-17 receptor on the day of infection and daily thereafter for 11 days reduced swelling and eliminated the development of severe destructive Lyme arthritis [108]. Thus, the development of arthritis in this mouse model can be explained by a combined effect involving IL-17 production and correspondingly low presence of CD4+ CD25+ T-lymphocytes. IL-17 and CD4+ CD25+ T-lymphocytes play a significant role in protection against Borrelia-induced arthritis, mediated by IL-17 neutralization [109]. Similar results have been reported in humans [110].

Patients with Lyme arthritis also have high levels of CD56+ natural killer (NK) cells in synovial fluid [111]. It has been hypothesized that CD56+ NK cells may either enhance or attenuate immune reactions. The presence of CD56+ NK cells producing IFN-γ in synovial fluid indicates that these cells contribute to spirochete destruction [112]. FoxP3+ regulatory T-cells in synovial fluid also play a role in Lyme arthritis. Low levels of these cells lead to slowed arthritis development [113]. *In vitro* studies have shown that phagocytic cells, including macrophages, monocytes, neutrophils, microglial dendritic cells, can effectively destroy *B. burgdorferi*. Both T cells and natural killer T cells (NKT cells) are quickly recruited to bacterial sites and participate in enhancing antibody responses to bacteria. Diacylglycerol and glycolipid present in the spirochete's outer membrane can directly activate invariant NKT cells, which play an important role in infection control and enhancing phagocytosis [114].

Studies in animals and humans have shown that neutrophils, which are particularly effective in *B. burgdorferi* destruction, are not present in sufficient quantities during the 24-hour EM period, while T cells, dendritic cells, and monocytes are preserved. Artificially increasing neutrophil levels in animals has shown that *B. burgdorferi* rapidly disappears after penetrating the dermis, indicating an important protective role of neutrophils [115].

Over several weeks or months, innate and acquired immune mechanisms can reduce bacterial numbers such that systemic manifestations of Lyme disease decrease even without antibiotic treatment. However, spirochetes can survive in untreated patients for several years, leading to persistent disease symptoms in some cases [72]. The main pathological features of Lyme arthritis include consequences of immunopathological autoimmune reactions, manifested by synovitis with characteristic morphological changes such as synovial cell hyperplasia, nonspecific villous hypertrophy, lymphoplasmocytic infiltration, follicle formation, and fibrin deposition. Concurrently, due to intravascular persistence of borreliae, microcirculatory damage resembling obliterative endarteritis occurs. In untreated individuals, synovial pannus forms in the perichondral part of the synovial membrane – vascular and fibrous tissue ingrown into cartilage and its destruction. Histopathological examination of joints in infected experimental animals has demonstrated significant structural damage with marked synovial hyperplasia and hypertrophy, where neutrophilic infiltrates cause erosion of joint cartilage and superficial bone destruction. Alongside this, an increase in collagen formation and fibroblasts leads to fibrosis and ankylosis, resulting in overall joint deformity. Moreover, experiments have indicated that B. burgdorferi infection induces bone loss in mice, occurring via trabecular bone and independent of osteoblast inhibition, but rather due to disrupted bone formation (reduced osteoblast survival and/or osteoblast apoptosis induction) [117].

Synovial biopsy of untreated Lyme arthritis reveals synovial hypertrophy with vascular proliferation, a mixed infiltrate containing T-cells, B-cells, and follicular dendritic cells [118, 119]. Joint fluid in patients with Lyme arthritis contains significantly elevated levels of cytokines and chemokines associated with innate and adaptive immune responses, particularly high levels of IFN-γ-induced chemokines CXCL9 and CXCL10, consistent with tissue findings. The levels of these mediators are nominally lower in serum, confirming the hypothesis that these immune responses occur locally in the joints [120, 121]. Besides inflammatory mediators, enzymes that degrade the extracellular matrix, such as matrix metalloproteinases (MMPs), contribute to cartilage and bone erosions [122]. MMPs have been detected in synovial fluid of Lyme arthritis patients [123], and *ex vivo* experiments demonstrate their production by *B. burgdorferi*-stimulated cartilage explants [124], chondrocytes [125], and monocytes [126].

The pathogenesis of Lyme arthritis remains enigmatic from several perspectives. While hematogenous spread of spirochetes to joints or periarticular tissues undoubtedly occurs, attempts to culture live spirochetes from synovial fluid have generally been unsuccessful, with only two documented exceptions [127, 128]. In 1994, Nocton et al., [129] made two pivotal observations: 1) DNA of *B. burgdorferi* can be detected in synovial fluids of the majority (75 out of 88) of Lyme arthritis patients; 2) PCR-positive patients typically respond well to antimicrobial therapy. Cure of arthritis with antibiotics in PCR-positive patients confirms that inflammation triggered by spirochetes is pivotal in the arthritis process. However, it remains unknown where the spirochetes harbouring detectable DNA are located and what precisely initiates the inflammatory process after an anticipated quiescent period. In mouse experiments, spirochetes do not penetrate actual joint spaces but are visualized in collagen-rich periarticular structures [82, 130].

Although Lyme arthritis usually resolves with appropriate antibiotic therapy, some patients (estimated around 10%) develop persistent proliferative synovitis characterized by synovial hyperplasia, vascular damage, intense inflammation, and fibrosis, termed post-infectious antibiotic-resistant Lyme arthritis [131]. Patients diagnosed with this condition are seropositive but typically lack PCR signal for *B. burgdorferi* DNA in joints [85]. The question of how spirochetes initiate a localized, dysregulated inflammatory process that persists after their eradication remains contentious [132, 133]. Increased prevalence of certain HLA alleles, also linked to rheumatoid arthritis [134], has prompted the hypothesis that antibiotic-resistant Lyme arthritis represents an autoimmune process induced by infection, mediated through molecular mimicry [135]. Further research has shown molecular similarity of OspA sequence to hLFA-1 sequence [136], and demonstrated that HLA-DR alleles excessively expressed in patients with antibiotic-resistant arthritis bind to OspA epitopes [137]. The implications of these publications for public health were significant, as OspA was an antigenic component of a Lyme disease vaccine released around the same time [138], and unfounded concerns about autoimmune reactions due to OspA vaccination contributed to the commercial failure and withdrawal of the vaccine from the market [139, 140].

Supporting the concept of spirochete-induced autoimmune reactions, four new autoantigens have been identified: ECGF, ApoB-100, annexin A2, and MMP10, which are targets of T- and B-cell responses in patients with refractory Lyme arthritis [121, 141–143].

Despite the aaetiology remaining unclear, in recent years, much attention has been devoted to dysregulated inflammatory processes underlying post-infectious Lyme arthritis [143]. For instance, patients with a specific single nucleotide polymorphism in TLR1, particularly infected with *B. burgdorferi* RST1 strains, appear prone to excessive Th1-associated inflammation [101]. Compared to the antibiotic-sensitive variant of Lyme arthritis, patients with post-infectious arthritis had lower levels of CD4+ CD25+ regulatory T-cells in their synovial fluids, and their regulatory T-cells were less effective in suppressing Th1 effector responses [113]. High throughput RNA sequencing revealed a sustained IFN-γ response in synovium, inversely correlating with the expression of tissue repair genes, and promoting differentiation of fibroblast-like synoviocytes into immune effector cells believed to enhance and perpetuate these dysregulated Th1 responses [144, 145].

Recently, an alternative or complementary mechanism of persistent inflammation based on innate immunity has been proposed. Jutras et al., [146] reported that *B. burgdorferi* cannot recycle peptidoglycan but disperses its fragments (murapeptides) in its environment. They hypothesized that peptidoglycan fragments disseminated in synovial fluid prior to bacterial eradication trigger chronic activation of NOD2-dependent arthritogenic pathways. Thus, infection with certain Borrelia strains in genetically predisposed individuals appears to lay the groundwork for a dysregulated immune response characterized by high levels of IFN-γ, causing synovial tissue hypertrophy, inhibiting tissue repair, and promoting development of autoimmune T- and B-cell processes in joints. Residual microbes, such as peptidoglycans, which may persist in the absence of active spirochaetal infection, could further sustain these reactions.

A perplexing feature of LB is the gradual onset of musculoskeletal symptoms, which may persist after completion of a full course of treatment, with some patients developing chronic inflammatory arthritis resistant to antibiotic therapy. Experimental findings indicate that *B.*

burgdorferi antigens persist in cartilage for extended periods post-etiotropic therapy and stimulate synthesis of TNF-α from macrophages, contributing to the chronicity of joint processes [147].

Clinical manifestations of LB are typically classified by disease duration (acute and chronic). This division is conventional. Joint involvement variants are divided into:

1. Benign recurrent arthritis – occurs after EM, within a period ranging from several days to a month from onset. Characterized by asymmetric mono- or oligoarthritis syndrome, recurring predominantly in large joints resembling reactive arthritis, lasting up to 5 years with stable symptoms.
2. Chronic arthritis. Every tenth patient with Lyme arthritis (predominantly positive for HLA-DR2 and -DR4) demonstrates chronic arthritis with pannus formation, erosive cartilage processes, bursitis, enthesopathies, and ligamentitis. In advanced stages, signs of inflammatory (osteoporosis, cortical and marginal erosions, cartilage loss) and degenerative (meniscal ossification, osteophytes, cysts, subchondral sclerosis) processes are observed.

EM is a characteristic sign of infection and is found most frequently in 70% of patients. EM is the sole external manifestation of LB detectable during clinical examination of individuals with acute arthralgia. However, in most patients with arthritis, EM either never develops or remains unnoticed. Nearly half of patients exhibit signs of systemic inflammation (malaise, fatigue, headache, arthralgia, myalgia, subfebrile body temperature, and lymphadenopathy). Typically, episodes of Lyme arthritis are short-lived and affect a single large joint, with the knee joint being involved most frequently (90% of cases). Less commonly affected joints include the elbows, ankles, hips, and wrists. Recurrences of arthritis occur over periods ranging from months to years in ≤50% of patients, even with adequate therapy, involving the same or different joints [148]. Arthritis typically starts suddenly with moderate pain (VAS from 20 to 60 mm) and inflammatory syndrome. Typical joint syndrome features include:

- Involvement of large joints hips, knees, shoulders;
- Absence of axial skeleton involvement;
- Mono- or oligoarthritis;
- Moderate synovitis;
- Accompanying tendonitis, tenosynovitis, bursitis, enthesopathies, fibrositis;
- Involvement of muscles – myositis, myalgia;
- Neurological manifestations.

Occasionally, clinical practice encounters atypical Lyme arthritis situations involving hip joints resembling septic coxitis, especially in children, characterized by significant elevation of ESR and absence of fever [149, 150]. Cases of Lyme arthritis developing on prosthetic joints have also been described in the scientific literature [151].

Without adequate treatment, recurrent Lyme arthritis progresses chronically with persistent hypertrophic synovitis and secondary osteoarthritis, erosions, deformities, necessitating treatment similar to autoimmune arthritis (e.g., rheumatoid arthritis).

The disease history, clinical manifestations, and symptoms, especially the appearance of EM, play a crucial role in the diagnosis of Lyme arthritis. However, the main diagnostic methods involve laboratory verification of borrelial infection, which helps in decision-making in more complex disease cases.

During synovial membrane biopsy, deposits of fibrin, hypertrophy of villi, vessel proliferation, and pronounced plasma cell and lymphocytic infiltration are observed. In some cases, spirochetes are detected with silver staining. The leukocyte count in synovial fluid ranges from 5×10^2–11×10^4 cells/mL, predominantly composed of segmented neutrophils. Increased protein content, normal or decreased glucose levels, and typically negative tests for rheumatoid and antinuclear factors are noted. Isolation of spirochete cultures allows for a definitive diagnosis, although this is rarely achieved.

Routine clinical examinations often reveal slightly elevated ESR, while C-reactive protein (CRP) levels remain mostly unchanged; rheumatoid factor is rarely detected. Ultrasound of the joints shows synovial thickening, increased fluid accumulation, combined changes in periarticular tissues, tendonitis, enthesitis, muscle thickening, and ooedema. Ultrasonography may be useful in detecting subclinical synovitis and assessing disease sequelae, but this method is not specific and is not used in differential diagnosis [152].

Radiological examination during the acute stage reveals changes in periarticular tissues; in chronic cases, there is cartilage thinning, subchondral cysts, periarticular osteoporosis, erosions, osteophytes, and Baker's cysts.

Diagnostic criteria for Lyme arthritis [153, 154]:

1. Mono- and oligoarthritis (especially affecting the knee joint with hypertrophic synovitis, Baker's cysts).
2. Endemic area of residence.
3. Optional presence of EM or tick bite history.
4. Presence of antibodies to *B. burgdorferi* in ELISA and specific IgG in immunoblot.
5. Possible positive result for B. burgdorferi DNA in PCR of synovial fluid.

Differential diagnosis of Lyme arthritis is conducted based on the primary arthritic syndrome with diseases such as rheumatoid arthritis, reactive arthritis, and osteoarthritis. In cases of concomitant extra-articular involvement with inflammatory syndrome, patients are examined for systemic lupus erythematosus, scleroderma, and lymphoproliferative disorders. The presence of isolated arthritic syndrome, without inflammatory changes, rheumatoid factor, or antibodies to cyclic citrullinated peptide (aCCP), as well as involvement of large joints, allows exclusion of rheumatoid arthritis due to insufficient criteria according to EULAR 2010 guidelines. Conversely, chronic synovitis, Baker's cysts, varying patient age including young and middle-aged, raise doubts about the diagnosis of primary osteoarthritis in cases with obvious radiological signs combined with erosions and osteoporosis, prompting investigation for chronic infectious arthritis with secondary osteoarthritis. Absence of urinary-genital system involvement (urethritis, vaginitis) and eye manifestations (conjunctivitis) allows exclusion of reactive arthritis.

In some cases, LB may masquerade as systemic connective tissue diseases and lymphoproliferative syndromes. Negative specific tests for these conditions in individuals residing in LB endemic areas help exclude them and necessitate examination for borrelial infection.

Risk stratification for Lyme arthritis occurrence is performed in patients with a history of tick bites, presence of EM, and atypical course of arthritic syndrome in individuals residing in LB endemic areas, regardless of the season.

The prognosis of Lyme arthritis is generally favourable; even without treatment, about 10% of patients recover, while after appropriate antibiotic therapy, 90% of patients achieve recovery.

We examined 67 patients diagnosed with *B. burgdorferi*-associated arthritis treated at the rheumatology department of Ternopil University Hospital [155]. The diagnosis was confirmed by immunoblot results: at least 2 IgM antibodies and 5 IgG antibodies to Borrelia antigens were detected. Among those examined, acute progression was observed in 28 patients and chronic in 39. The study involved determining the type of joint involvement (mono-, oligo-, or polyarthritis), joint count—number of painful and swollen joints according to DAS 28 [156]. Pain syndrome was assessed using VAS in mm, joint ultrasound, and markers of inflammatory processes in blood.

Among those examined were 42 women and 25 men, all of working age, with mean ages for women (34.78 ± 5.92) years and men (46.92 ± 7.39) years. The leading syndrome among those examined was noted as pain syndrome with high VAS values (68.42 ± 4.11) mm.

The number of painful joints was (5.15 ± 2.08), and the average number of swollen joints was (4.15 ± 2.67) cases. Monoarthritis was observed in 41.8%, oligoarthritis in 35.8%, and polyarthritis in 22.4% of patients.

In cases of monoarthritis, hypertrophic synovitis of mostly knee joints with Baker's cysts (according to ultrasound data) was diagnosed in nearly all patients. Classic manifestations of arthritis (Figure 19, 20), characterized by moderate to severe inflammatory processes, were observed in 24 patients and were associated with positive RF and aCCP tests in 13.4%, elevated CRP levels were registered in 38.8% of cases. Signs of spondyloarthralgic syndrome without sacroiliitis were found in 10.4% of patients.

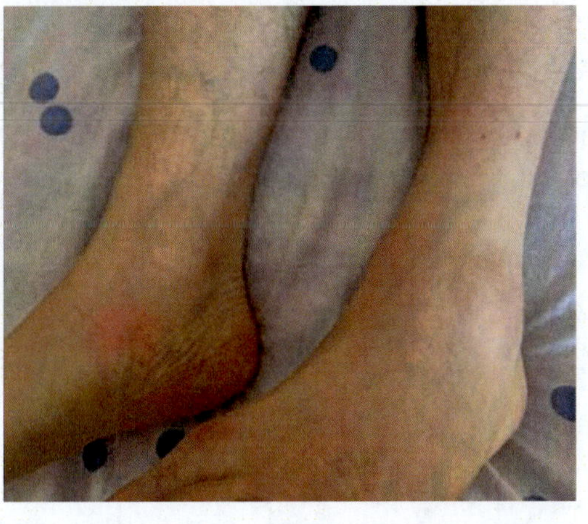

Figure 19. Patient C. (Ternopil University Hospital, Rheumatology Department, Head of Department O. S. Makhovska), initial diagnosis: reactive arthritis of the left ankle joint, subsequently confirmed as Lyme arthritis.

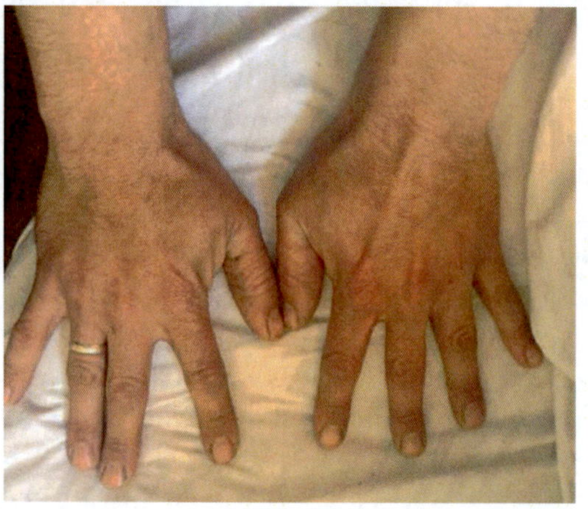

Figure 20. Patient R. (Ternopil University Hospital, Rheumatology Department, Head of Department O. S. Makhovska), initial diagnosis: rheumatoid polyarthritis (symmetrical involvement of the wrists with elevated levels of aCCP and RF), subsequently confirmed as Lyme arthritis.

Treatment of the patients involved in the study consisted of using etiotropic and symptomatic agents – NSAIDs.

The use of etiotropic agents ("Doxycycline" 200 mg per day for 30 days) was most effective in cases of acute arthritis, as evidenced by a decrease in VAS, local inflammatory changes clinically and by ultrasound already by (6.48 ± 1.37) days. At the same time, it was noted that in most patients with chronic disease progression, significant improvement was observed by (12.36 ± 3.72) days of treatment. It is worth noting that therapy was ineffective in 9 (32.1%) patients, who subsequently were prescribed "Methotrexate" at a dose of 15 mg per week for 6 months.

The observations allowed to formulate conclusions that the frequency of Lyme arthritis joint involvement, according to various authors, reaches up to 60%, depending on the geographic region, with arthritis often recorded under conditions of Lyme borreliosis. Difficulties in early diagnosis stem from the lack of information about tick bites, leading to chronicity of the process and delaying treatment and recovery of patients. It remains relevant to determine the indications for Lyme borreliosis examination in individuals with arthralgic syndrome, especially in endemic areas for Lyme borreliosis.

It is necessary to note that acute or chronic manifestations of Lyme arthritis clinically can mimic any inflammatory joint disease, and rheumatic joint diseases in turn can mask the course of infectious involvement. Progressive joint syndrome becomes more intense, indicating a tendency towards chronicity and similarity in progression to rheumatoid arthritis and osteoarthritis with hypertrophic synovitis and Baker's cysts, accompanied by high intensity of pain syndrome (VAS over 65 mm).

The results of etiotropic treatment demonstrated highest efficacy in acute arthritis compared to chronic cases. Further scientific and practical developments are needed to establish clear indications for Lyme borreliosis examination in patients with arthritic syndrome.

4.2. Rheumatoid Arthritis Associated with *B. burgdorferi*

With each passing year, the study of infectious arthritis in rheumatology practice becomes increasingly relevant, as arthritis associated with *B. burgdorferi* is a serious medical-biological and socio-medical issue due to its tendency to chronicity and the development of musculoskeletal impairments, leading to adverse outcomes such as prolonged disability and various degrees of invalidity across different age groups and genders. Common features of Lyme arthritis with inflammatory joint diseases contribute to mutual masking. The necessity for differential diagnosis remains pertinent especially when suspecting rheumatoid arthritis (RA), particularly in atypical courses and ineffectiveness of disease-modifying therapy. Arthritis syndrome in rheumatology is marked by numerous inflammatory joint diseases, but the issue of their combination with infectious agents remains relevant and requires further study. It is known that LB, including its late manifestation, arthritis, can present with an isolated course, while in other cases, it can trigger mechanisms leading to other forms of arthritis and complicate their course. Inflammatory arthritis such as RA, reactive arthritis, or psoriatic arthritis, osteoarthritis, can develop within months after LB, purportedly triggered by spirochaetal infection [157, 158]. Recent research results in this direction by Arvikar et al., indicate that in cases of inflammatory arthritis developing against the background of LB, clinicians need to distinguish between three possibilities: patients with active joint infection, those with post-infectious Lyme arthritis, and those with another form of inflammatory arthritis arising after LB [159]. On the other hand, clinical practice has identified variants of RA progression that poorly respond to standard therapy, and the search for reasons for such situations does not exclude an infectious nature, including *B. burgdorferi*. Today, it is known that joint involvement is a late manifestation of LB. However, while some patients may report tick bites or the presence of EM, arthritis can manifest as a disease without prior LB symptoms or signs [160, 161]. Severe late-stage arthropathy was characterized in studies by synovial hyperplasia, infiltration of mononuclear cells into the synovial membrane, formation of inflammatory exudate over the synovial cell membranes (formation of pannus), cartilage destruction, and erosion of bones and joints [162]. From a clinical perspective, Lyme arthritis typically asymmetrically affects large synovial joints [163]. In over 90% of cases, the knee joint is affected. It has been proven that the ankle joint is the second most frequently involved joint in the pathological process [164].

Considering the commonalities between RA and Lyme arthritis, we conducted an analysis of the clinical course of these conditions at our clinic. Under observation were 63 patients aged 19 to 73 years – 19 (30.15%) males and 44 (69.85%) females who sought treatment at the rheumatology department of Ternopil University Hospital [165]. Patients were divided into 2 groups: 34 (group 1) with RA associated with *B. burgdorferi* and 29 (group 2) with isolated RA. The diagnosis of RA was verified according to classification criteria (ACR/EULAR 2010). Pain intensity was assessed using VAS, and disease activity was characterized using the DAS-28 disease activity score. IgM and IgG antibodies to *B. burgdorferi* antigens were determined using immunoblotting.

The results of the analysis of clinical characteristics of patients (Table 15) showed that the duration of the disease was significantly lower in patients with RA associated with *B. burgdorferi* compared to those with isolated RA ($p < 0.05$). Regarding arthralgic status assessed by VAS, a significant increase in pain sensations ($p < 0.05$) was noted in patients with RA associated with *B. burgdorferi*. The number of painful and swollen joints was significantly higher in individuals with RA associated with *B. burgdorferi* ($p < 0.05$). A similar trend was observed in the analysis of the disease activity index (DAS-28), which demonstrated that patients with isolated RA were in the moderate disease activity stage (3.2-5.1), while those with B. burgdorferi-associated RA had high disease activity (>5.1).

Evaluation of instrumental examination data showed that the number of patients with structural radiographic changes was higher among those with RA associated with *B. burgdorferi*, as was the presence of Baker's cysts. These data indicate that the presence of *B. burgdorferi* adversely affects the clinical course of RA.

Analysis of laboratory indicators in the examined patients (Table 16) revealed that half of the patients with isolated RA did not have anti-CCP antibodies, while the other half did. In contrast, in the cohort examined with RA associated with B. burgdorferi, the number of patients with positive anti-CCP antibodies was 4.5 times higher compared to those without these antibodies. Evaluating ESR levels, it was found that in the majority of patients with RA associated with *B. burgdorferi*, the ESR exceeded 40 mm/h, indicating high inflammatory activity, whereas in the group examined with isolated RA, the same percentage of individuals had ESR levels within 20-40 mm/h. Significantly lower CRP levels were observed in patients with isolated RA compared to those with RA associated with *B. burgdorferi* ($p < 0.05$).

Thus, among patients under our observation, RA associated with *B. burgdorferi* was diagnosed in 53.97% of individuals, and this condition was associated with intense pain syndrome with high VAS values, high inflammatory syndrome activity, presence of hypertrophic synovitis, mainly of the knee joint, with Baker's cysts, which together contribute to the progression of arthritis in patients and lead to a more severe clinical course of the disease. We believe that early detection of *B. burgdorferi* and its elimination may contribute to a less aggressive course of RA.

Table 15. Clinical characteristics of patients with rheumatoid arthritis associated with *B. burgdorferi* and with isolated rheumatoid arthritis

Parameter	Patients	
	with rheumatoid arthritis associated with B. burgdorferi, n = 34 (53,97%)	with isolated rheumatoid arthritis, n = 29 (46,03%)
Age, years	49,6 ± 6,7	57,82 ± 4,6
Gender:		
– men	11 (32,35%)	8 (27,59%)
– women	23 (67,65%)	21 (72,41%)
Duration of disease, years	5,21 ± 3,08	13,68 ± 1,47*
VAS, mm	68,85 ± 3,22	54,21 ± 4,86*
Morning stiffness:		
≤30, min	2 (5,88%)	5 (17,24%)
30–60, min	7 (20,59%)	18 (62,07%)
≥60, min	25 (73,53%)	6 (20,69%)
Number of painful joints	13,12 ± 1,62	5,08 ± 2,96*
Number of swollen joints	15,62 ± 3,1	6,18 ± 2,34*
DAS-28	6,9 ± 1,2	3,5 ± 0,89*
Number of patients with structural changes on X-ray (Ro-gram)	26 (76,47%)	12 (41,38%)
Number of patients with Baker's cysts on ultrasound	14 (41,18%)	2 (6,9%)

Note. * – significant difference between groups, $p < 0.05$.

Table 16. Changes in laboratory indicators of patients with rheumatoid arthritis associated with *B. burgdorferi* and with isolated rheumatoid arthritis

Parameter	Patients	
	with rheumatoid arthritis associated with B. burgdorferi, n = 34 (53,97%)	with isolated rheumatoid arthritis, n = 29 (46,03%)
aCCP		
negative	6 (17,65%)	14 (48,28%)
positive	28 (82,35%)	15 (51,72%)
RF		
negative	9 (26,47%)	19 (65,52%)
positive	25 (73,53%)	10 (34,48%)
ECR, mm/h		
normal	3 (8,82%)	7 (24,14%)
20–40	9 (26,47%)	18 (62,07%)
more than 40	22 (64,71%)	4 (13,79%)
CRP, g/L	14,98 ± 3,92	6,1 ± 1,27*

Note. * – significant difference between groups, $p < 0.05$.

A study was conducted at our clinic on stratifying factors affecting the quality of life of patients with RA associated with *B. burgdorferi* and isolated RA (44 (48.9%) and 46 (51.1%) individuals, respectively) based on surveys using the Health Assessment Questionnaire-Disability Index (HAQ-DI) and the Short Form Medical Outcomes Study (SF-36) questionnaires. Using the SF-36 questionnaire, indicators were assessed on eight scales: Physical Functioning (PF), Role-Physical Functioning (RP), Bodily Pain (BP), General Health (GH), Vitality (VT), Social Functioning (SF), Role Emotional (RE), and Mental Health (MH), as well as calculated two health components: Physical (PCS) and Psychological (MCS). Each scale ranged from 0 to 100; higher scores indicated better quality of life in that parameter. The patient's functional status was assessed using the HAQ-DI health status questionnaire, which includes 20 questions grouped into 8 scales of 2-3 questions each, relating to the patient's daily life activity. Responses to the questions were evaluated on a scoring scale from 0 to 3:

- 0 – without difficulty;
- 1 – with some difficulty;
- 2 – with much difficulty;
- 3 – unable to do.

HAQ has 25 possible values. Values from 0 to 1.0 define minimal life activity impairments, from 1.1 to 2.0 – moderate, from 2.1 to 3.0 – severe life activity impairments [166].

It is known that isolated RA and complications of this severe disease result in very poor quality of life for patients [167]. Prolonged searching for the infectious cause of arthritis, delay in examination for Lyme borreliosis due to atypical course of arthritis syndrome [168], leads to difficulties in early diagnosis of *B. burgdorferi*-associated arthritis and timely initiation of etiotropic treatment [169]. Significant impact of the disease on RA includes changes in the patient's personality occurring during the first year of illness from diagnosis [170].

In such cases, only timely intervention by a multidisciplinary team of specialists in the treatment and rehabilitation of arthritis patients will enable them to avoid changes in self-awareness and contribute to reducing the number of negative consequences of the disease affecting patients' quality of life [171]. Starting from the first stage of adequate treatment and rehabilitation, symptomatic relief can be achieved, remission periods prolonged, work capacity maintained, personality changes prevented, and the patient's daily life improved [170].

Important aspects and consequences of arthritis include increasing disability and loss of work capacity, which play a significant role in the social and emotional functioning of the patient. Since disease progression is unpredictable, patients worry about the future, concerned about increasing mobility limitations and side effects of treatment. They fear losing the ability to self-care, which negatively affects their self-awareness and all spheres of life [172]. Due to the increasing incidence of Lyme borreliosis and the possibility of chronic disease, it is important to continue studying psychosocial factors related to the quality of life of patients that affect perception of the disease and coping abilities [173]. There is an opinion that inflammation is a sign of depression, as elevated levels of pro-inflammatory cytokines are observed even in the absence of autoimmune disease [174]. In addition, results from a systematic review of 32 studies reporting cytokine levels before and after antidepressant treatment showed significant decreases in IL-4, IL-6, and IL-10 in peripheral blood after therapy [175]. The severity of Lyme borreliosis and its complications underline the need for earlier diagnosis and an innovative approach to treatment [176]. Without timely antibiotic therapy for Lyme borreliosis, more than 60% of patients develop Lyme arthritis – a late manifestation of the disease characterized by symptoms of joint swelling and pain similar to RA [177].

The results of the conducted studies demonstrated that all patients had moderate RA activity. Age and gender did not significantly differ between patients with RA and RA associated with *B. burgdorferi.*

A thorough analysis of quality of life and functional status indicators in patients with RA associated with B. burgdorferi and isolated RA showed a decrease in all scales according to the SF-36 and HAQ-DI questionnaires, indicating a deterioration in the quality of life of patients in both groups (Table 17). Patients with RA associated with *B. burgdorferi* had significantly lower scores on the SF-36 scale and all its components: physical functioning, social functioning, role emotional functioning, and mental health. No significant differences were found in the individuals of both groups regarding physical functioning and role physical functioning indicators, but pain and general health status in patients with RA associated with *B. burgdorferi* were significantly different. Therefore, the PCS scale score in patients with RA associated with *B. burgdorferi* was lower, although no significant difference was found in this parameter between patient groups.

Thus, significant reduction in physical activity in patients with RA associated with *B. burgdorferi* compared to patients with isolated RA was observed not only due to significantly higher pain intensity and decreased overall health but also due to the important role played by the psychological state of the patients. The HAQ-DI score according to the specific questionnaire in individuals with isolated RA ranged from 1.1 to 2.0, corresponding to moderate impairment in activities of daily living, whereas in patients with RA associated with *B. burgdorferi*, this index ranged from 2.1 to 3.0 on the scale of values, indicating a greater impact of the disease on the daily activities of patients.

Table 17. Quality of life and functional status indicators in patients with rheumatoid arthritis associated with *B. burgdorferi* and those with isolated rheumatoid arthritis

Parameter	Patients		Significance coefficient p
	with rheumatoid arthritis associated with B. burgdorferi, n = 44 (48,9%)	with isolated rheumatoid arthritis PA, n = 46 (51,1%)	
	1	2	3
HAQ-DI	2,1 ±0,05	1,7 ± 0,09	0,01*
SF-36 scale			
physical functioning (PF)	31,79 ± 2,14	35,75 ± 4,01	0,27
role physical functioning (RF)	44,11 ± 2,89	46,20 ± 3,97	0,74
pain (BP)	28,86 ± 2,75	40,52 ± 3,24	0,002*
general health (GH)	36,26 ± 2,20	49,22 ± 3,92	0,006*
vitality (VT)	33,51 ± 2,62	47,83 ± 3,24	0,007*
social functioning (SF)	31,88 ± 2,54	58,12 ± 3,33	0,001*
role emotional functioning (RE)	27,03 ± 2,91	60,83 ± 3,61	0,001*
mental health (MH)	25,43 ± 3,04	47,28 ± 3,92	0,002*
physical component summary (PCS)	35,97 ± 3,26	42,68 ± 3,04	0,09

Note. * – significant difference between groups, $p < 0.05$.

In the analysis of correlation relationships, a dependence between disease activity and SF-36 PCS in patients from both cohorts was found (Table 18). Based on this, we established that disease activity significantly influences the quality of life of patients. A strong direct relationship was found between the HAQ-DI index and disease activity in patients with RA associated with *B. burgdorferi*, and a moderate direct correlation in individuals with isolated RA, which is explained by a higher degree of functional impairment in daily living activities in patients with higher disease activity (Figure 21, 22). No significant dependence of age on quality of life in isolated RA was established based on weak reverse correlation between SF-36 PCS indicators and weak direct correlation with the HAQ-DI index. Age in RA associated with *B. burgdorferi* is also not a significant factor for quality of life.

Table 18. Correlation between SF-36 PCS, SF-36 MCS, HAQ-DI, and clinical manifestations of disease in patients with rheumatoid arthritis associated with *B. burgdorferi* and isolated rheumatoid arthritis

Variable	PCS SF-36		MCS SF-36		HAQ-DI	
	Patients with RA associated with B. burgdorferi, n = 44 (48.9%)	Patients with isolated RA, n = 46 (51.1%)	Patients with RA associated with B. burgdorferi, n = 44 (48.9%)	Patients with isolated RA, n = 46 (51.1%)	Patients with RA associated with B. burgdorferi, n = 44 (48.9%)	Patients with isolated RA, n = 46 (51.1%)
Disease activity (DAS-28)	-0,80	-0,72	–	–	0,71	0,66
Age	–	-0,27	–	–	–	0,23
Total number of affected joints	–	-0,35	–	-0,25	–	0,47
Duration of the disease	-0,58	-0,40	-0,62	0,49	0,60	0,54

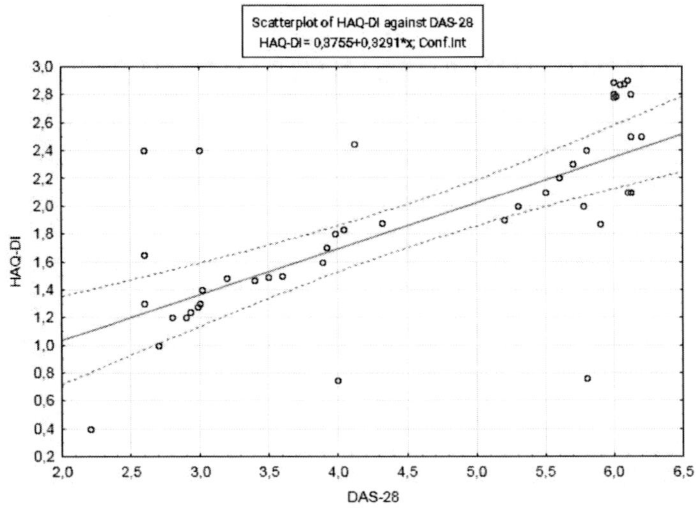

Figure 21. Scatter plot of HAQ-DI depending on DAS-28 index in patients with isolated rheumatoid arthritis.

As for the total number of affected joints, we have the following data: in patients with isolated RA, there is an average inverse correlation between this indicator and SF-36 PCS, and a moderate direct correlation with HAQ-DI, along with a weak inverse correlation with SF-36 MCS. Based on this, we can conclude that the greater the number of joints involved in the pathological process, the lower the patient's activity in daily life, and the poorer their physical and emotional condition. In contrast, patients with RA associated with *B. burgdorferi* showed no dependency between these indicators. Regarding the duration of the disease, there were moderate inverse correlations between disease duration and SF-36 PCS, and moderate direct correlations with HAQ-DI in patients from both examined cohorts. This indicator indicated that with increasing disease duration, the HAQ-DI index increases, thereby significantly reducing a person's ability to perform daily tasks and professional duties.

Also, a correlation was found between disease duration and the SF-36 MCS: in patients with isolated RA – both mean direct and mean inverse – in those with RA associated with *B. burgdorferi*. Thus, in patients with isolated RA, as disease duration increases, the MCS of SF-36 increases, which can be explained by the psychological adaptation of individuals to their perception of their illness and health status. Conversely, in individuals with RA associated with B. burgdorferi, as disease duration increases, the SF-36 MCS decreases, indicating anxiety and frequent depression.

Table 19. The relationship between SF-36 PCS, SF-36 MCS, HAQ-DI, and the most significant factors according to multiple regression analysis in patients with rheumatoid arthritis associated with *B. burgdorferi*

Variable	SF-36 PCS		SF-36 MCS		HAQ-DI	
	β	p	β	p	β	p
DAS-28	0,57	0,006	–	–	0,33	0,004
Age	–	–	–	–	–	–
Total number of affected joints	–	–	–	–	–	–
Duration of the disease	0,33	0,03	-0,45	0,004	0,40	0,009

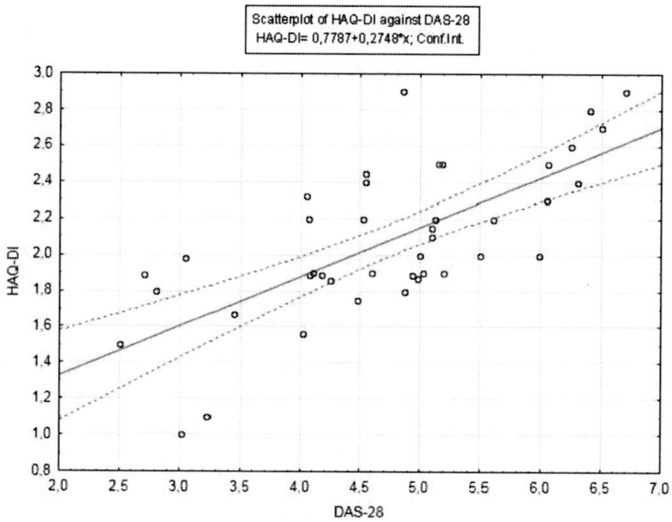

Figure 22. Scatter plot of HAQ-DI depending on DAS-28 index in patients with rheumatoid arthritis associated with *B. burgdorferi*.

To identify the most significant factors affecting quality of life in patients from both studied groups, multiple regression analysis was conducted (Tables 19, 20). It was found that disease activity and duration significantly influenced the quality of life in patients from both cohorts, while age and total number of affected joints affected only those with isolated RA.

The obtained data from the survey of patients with RA associated with *B. burgdorferi* and those with isolated RA indicate a negative impact of arthritis on all quality of life indicators according to SF-36 scales and the HAQ-DI index. Decreased physical functioning in patients from both groups was observed alongside increased inflammatory activity as measured by the DAS-28 index. However, during the study, we identified the following differences: patients with RA associated with *B. burgdorferi* showed significantly lower MCS scores, which can be explained by their difficult psychological adaptation to their condition, considering the current prevalence of Lyme borreliosis and its tendency to become chronic.

Factors influencing the quality of life in patients from both groups include disease activity and duration, while age and total number of affected joints are significant only for patients with isolated RA.

Table 20. The relationship between SF-36 PCS, SF-36 MCS, HAQ-DI, and the most significant factors according to multiple regression analysis in patients with isolated rheumatoid arthritis

Variable	SF-36 PCS		SF-36 MCS		HAQ-DI	
	β	p	β	p	β	p
DAS-28	-0,69	0,0001	–	–	0,33	0,002
Age	-0,28	0,06	–	–	–	–
Total number of affected joints	-0,38	0,01	–	–	0,42	0,003
Duration of the disease	-0,48	0,003	0,32	0,03	0,37	0,007

Studying the dynamics of pro-inflammatory and anti-inflammatory cytokines allows us to explore new aspects of the immunopathogenesis of Lyme borreliosis [178]. Cytokines are highly specific regulatory peptides produced by immune system cells and organs involved in the inflammatory process. They mediate signals between interacting cells [179]. When Borrelia enters the human body, multiple inflammatory mediators are released: in the early stages, first-line defence cells (fibroblasts, macrophages, endothelial cells, etc.) produce a specific set of cytokines crucial for the infection course. During this period, immune system activation occurs with the development of humoral and cellular immunity [178].

First-line cytokines include interleukin IL-1 and TNF-α, which are potent inducers of pro-inflammatory cytokines such as IL-1β, IL-6, and IL-8 [180]. IL-1 family cytokines promote inflammation and regulate T-cell responses, initiating proliferation of pre-activated antigen-specific T and B lymphocytes. Depending on the antigen characteristics, differentiation of Th1 or Th2 helper cells occurs: Th1 cells secrete IL-2, IFN-γ, and TNF-α, stimulating T-cell and macrophage functions, and promoting cellular immune response. In contrast, Th2 helper cell synthesis leads to production of IL-4, IL-10, and IL-13, predominantly stimulating B lymphocytes and the humoral immune response [178, 181]. IL-6 is known to regulate acute phase immune responses and haematopoiesis. Hyperproduction of this cytokine induces plasma cell production, thrombocytosis, and hypergammaglobulinemia. IL-6 is implicated in the pathogenesis of autoimmune diseases, endothelial cell dysfunction, and fibrogenesis [182]. One of the most important anti-inflammatory interleukins is IL-10, which also exhibits anti-cytokine action. It inhibits Th1 cytokine synthesis, chemokines, and adhesion molecules, suppresses monocyte-macrophage TNF-α, IL-1, IL-6, and IL-12 synthesis. IL-10 enhances natural killer cell growth, B-cell proliferation, and immunoglobulin secretion. Thus, IL-10's main function is to limit and resolve inflammatory processes [183].

The primary target of *B. burgdorferi* is the joints. Despite completing a course of antibiotic therapy, a significant number of patients experience recurrent or persistent Lyme arthritis. Immune response plays a crucial role in this chronic arthritic joint complication of infectious aaetiology. Patients with Lyme arthritis are prone to enhanced inflammatory responses and the development of pronounced immune reactions. In the serum of such patients, high concentrations of TNF-α, IFN-γ, IL-1β, IL-17, IL-10, IL-6, IL-8 are observed, which play an important role in disease progression [184].

In a study [185] that examined levels of 14 cytokines/chemokines in the serum and synovial fluid of 21 antibiotic-resistant Lyme arthritis patients and 9 patients with a positive antibiotic response, increased IL-6, IL-8, IL-10, IL-27, IFN were demonstrated in the synovial fluid, and IL-4, IL-8, IL-17A, IL-17F, IL-23, IFNγ in the serum, which were significantly higher in patients resistant to antibiotics.

Therefore, we found it appropriate to study the dynamics of pro-inflammatory cytokines TNF-α, IL-6, IL-8 and anti-inflammatory IL-10, IL-4 in the serum of patients with Lyme arthritis and RA. The study involved 92 patients undergoing outpatient or inpatient treatment at the rheumatology department of Ternopil University Hospital. There were 33 (35.9%) men and 59 (64.1%) women, with a mean age of (42.38±11.68) years. Patients were divided into three groups: the 1st group comprised 25 (27.2%) individuals with Lyme arthritis; the 2nd group comprised 34 (36.9%) patients with RA associated with B. burgdorferi; the 3rd group comprised 33 (35.9%) patients with isolated RA.

Table 21. The content of interleukins in the serum of patients in the study groups (Me (Lq; Uq))

Parameter	Group of patients			Significance of the indicators (p-value)
	with Lyme arthritis	with rheumatoid arthritis associated with B. burgdorferi	with isolated rheumatoid arthritis	
	1	2	3	
TNF-α	7,08 (2,67; 9,14)	11,34 (3,56; 20,12)	9,82 (3,54; 18,27)	p1 = 0,01 p2 = 0,42 p3 = 0,04
IL-8	6,78 (4,9;14,2)	9,43 (2,48;14,67)	8,23 (2,10;18,37)	p1 = 0,73 p2 = 0,60 p3 = 0,16
IL-6	5,31 (2,43; 8,84)	10,23 (4,23; 12,60)	9,05 (3,04; 13,72)	p1 = 0,01 p2 = 0,42 p3 = 0,04
IL-10	12,39 (3,08; 21,1)	5,92 (2,89; 9,05)	5,28 (1,94; 6,87)	p1 = 0,01 p2 = 0,002 p3 = 0,96
IL-4	6,87 (2,08; 6,92)	4,80 (4,20; 6,45)	3,26 (0,89; 6,25)	p1 = 0,09 p2 = 0,02 p3 = 0,26

Notes:
1. p1 – significance of indicators between patients of the 1st and 2nd groups.
2. p2 – significance of indicators between the 1st and 3rd groups.
3. p3 – significance of indicators between the 2nd and 3rd groups of patients.

Cytokine levels (TNF-α, IL-6, IL-10, IL-4, IL-8) in the serum of patients were determined using the ELISA method with test systems manufactured by Vector-Best LLC. Reference concentrations were as follows: for TNF-α – up to 6 pg/mL; for IL-6 – up to 10 pg/mL; for IL-10 – up to 31 pg/mL; IL-4 – up to 4 pg/mL; IL-8 – up to 10 pg/mL. For quantitative data with non-normal distribution, the median (Me) and lower (Lq) and upper (Uq) quartiles were calculated, and for qualitative indicators – absolute (n) and relative (%) quantities were used. Mann-Whitney criterion was used for comparison of non-normally distributed variables. Results were considered statistically significant at $p < 0.05$.

During the study of cytokine status in patients from three groups, the following results were obtained: individuals with Lyme arthritis showed elevated levels of anti-inflammatory cytokines IL-10 and IL-4 in their serum, which were significantly higher ($p < 0.05$) compared to patients with RA associated with *B. burgdorferi* and isolated RA (Table 21). This cohort predominantly included individuals with an acute course of the disease, leading us to conclude that the onset of inflammation in Borrelia infection is accompanied by the formation of an adequate immune response, characterized by the production of specific antibodies, proliferation of B-lymphocytes, T-lymphocytes, and plasma cells. Key stimulators of lymphocyte proliferation include IL-4 and IL-10. Elevated levels of IL-4 and IL-10 reduce macrophage activity, cytokine synthesis (TNF-α, IL-1, IL-6), creating conditions for transitioning the disease into a stage of limited inflammation and rapid resolution of the pathological process.

In the group of patients with RA associated with *B. burgdorferi* and those with isolated RA, we observed hyperproduction of IL-6, IL-8, TNF-α. Conversely, the deficiency of IL-10 and IL-4 in patients with RA associated with B. burgdorferi leads to bacteraemia and increased IL-6 release. Significant imbalance between anti-inflammatory and pro-inflammatory cytokines, with predominance of the latter, accompanies the progression of inflammatory processes in the joints. The high content of TNF-α in patients with isolated RA can be explained as follows: TNF-α is synthesized by cells found abundantly at the junction between the pannus and synovial cartilage, where joint destruction begins in RA. TNF-α acts as an inducer of another pro-inflammatory cytokine, IL-6, which leads to hyperproduction of acute phase proteins such as CRP and fibrinogen (K. Schroecksnadel et al., 2003). Studying the biological activity of TNF-α has confirmed that it is a key mediator of the immune-inflammatory process in RA (A. Verbruggen et al., 1998; C. A. Wise et al., 2000).

4.3. Gut Microbiota

Today, research aimed at studying the state of the gut microbiota under conditions of various pathologies appears quite modern. The gut microbiota functions as a metabolic "organ" that not only participates in food digestion but also synthesizes various biologically active substances, stimulates innate and acquired immune functions, prevents invasion by pathogenic microorganisms, and performs detoxification, anticancer, and synthetic functions [186, 187]. There is accumulating literature data on the interrelationship between gut microbiota and the pathology of the musculoskeletal system. The role of gut microbiota in the pathogenesis of autoimmune diseases, including inflammatory joint diseases such as RA, ankylosing spondylitis, and psoriatic arthritis, has been studied in detail [188, 189]. Experimental studies have elucidated the importance of gut microbiota in the genesis and maintenance of inflammatory cartilage damage [190]. One of the factors implicated in such damage is lipopolysaccharides produced by gut microbiota, specifically gram-negative bacteria. Under conditions of increased gut permeability, the level of lipopolysaccharides increases not only in the blood but also in the synovial fluid of arthritis patients, with their concentration correlating with the severity of joint involvement, intensity of pain syndrome, and degree of joint space narrowing [191].

What possible mechanism could explain the influence of gut microorganisms on joints? Gram-negative gut microbiota can produce and then release vesicles containing lipopolysaccharides and proteins. Particularly under conditions of increased gut permeability, these vesicles can be absorbed into the bloodstream and spread throughout the body, including penetrating into joint cavities. Depending on their composition, such vesicles can exert both pro-inflammatory and anti-inflammatory effects. The pro-inflammatory effect of lipopolysaccharides is largely mediated by lipid A bound to lipoprotein. This pro-inflammatory complex activates neutrophils and macrophages. Activated cells initiate an inflammatory cascade involving IL-1β, TNF-α, matrix metalloproteinases, and free radicals, which adversely affect joint structures [192].

The gut microbiota plays a crucial role in the activation of inflammatory processes in patients with RA. One such gut microorganism of significant importance is *Prevotella copri* [193]. *Prevotella* species possess a high pro-inflammatory potential and activate a Th17-mediated inflammatory mechanism. In this mechanism, stimulation of TLR2 is a key event, leading to increased synthesis of IL-23, IL-1, IL-6, and IL-8, which are associated with the development of RA induced by gut microbiota [194, 195]. Numerous studies have shown that *Prevotella copri* significantly increases in abundance during the preclinical stage in untreated RA patients compared to those receiving treatment and healthy individuals [196, 197]. In RA, immune response IgA against *Prevotella copri* correlates with innate (MIP-1), Th1 (IFN-γ and IL-12), Th17 (IL-23, IL-17), and anti-citrullinated peptide antibodies (ACPA) [198].

The activity of RA correlates with gut dysbiosis, which partially resolves during remission after treatment with traditional or biologic disease-modifying drugs [199, 200]. Among the causes contributing to disruptions in the normal gut microbiota, the impact of pharmacological agents holds a prominent place. Several studies have demonstrated the negative effect of antibiotic therapy on the gut microbiome, correlating with an increased risk of RA development. Repeated courses of antibiotic therapy pose significant challenges in restoring both the quantitative and qualitative composition of gut flora, leading to functional and metabolic disorders with a high likelihood of developing autoimmune diseases [201]. Additionally, besides antibiotics, disease-modifying anti-rheumatic drugs and immunobiological therapies also influence the state of the gut microbiota. According to some authors, 76% of RA patients treated with NSAIDs and methotrexate exhibited intestinal dysbiosis predominantly of grades III–IV [202].

The absence of information regarding the gut microbiota status in arthritis associated with *B. burgdorferi* served as impetus for studying this issue at the rheumatology clinic of I. Horbachevsky Ternopil National Medical University, in Ternopil University Hospital, where research was conducted to establish the peculiarities of gut microbiota in RA patients associated with *B. burgdorferi*. A total of 96 individuals were examined, including 52 (Group 1) with RA associated with *B. burgdorferi* and 44 (Group 2) with isolated RA. The patients ranged in age from 21 to 78 years [203]. Bacteriological examination of faeces was conducted for all patients. The qualitative and quantitative composition of the colon microflora was assessed using a tenfold dilution method (10-1–10-9) of feces on a standard set of selective and differential nutrient media for isolating aerobic and anaerobic microorganisms. The degree of colon dysbiosis was evaluated according to the classification of I. B. Kuvaieva and K. S. Ladodo (1991).

Table 22. Composition of gut microbiota in patients with rheumatoid arthritis associated with *B. burgdorferi* and isolated rheumatoid arthritis (M ± m)

Genus and species of microorganism, lgCFU/g	Group of patients		Significance of the indicators (p-value)
	with rheumatoid arthritis associated with B. burgdorferi, n = 52 (54,2%)	with isolated rheumatoid arthritis, n = 44 (45,8%)	
	1	2	
Bifidobacteria	5,25 ± 0,15	6,44 ± 0,17	0,012
Lactobacilli	4,96 ± 0,14	5,68 ± 0,20	0,013
Total number of Escherichia coli	5,15 ± 0,19	6,07 ± 0,22	0,004
Candida fungi	5,92 ± 0,16	4,68 ± 0,17	0,002
Staphylococci (S. aureus, S. epidermidis)	5,13 ± 0,15	4,41 ± 0,16	0,009
Opportunistic flora (Clostridium, Proteus mirabilis, Pseudomonas, Hemolytic E. coli, Enterococcus, Klebsiella pneumoniae)	6,07 ± 0,24	4,54 ± 0,19	0,007

Note. p – the difference is significant between groups.

During the course of this study, data were obtained indicating disruptions in both the qualitative and quantitative composition of both anaerobic and aerobic representatives of the microflora (Table 22).

Results of the analysis of faecal microbial composition in examined patients from both groups indicate pronounced changes in the qualitative and quantitative composition of the colonic microflora. Decreases in the levels of anaerobic flora representatives were observed: bifidobacteria were less than 10^7, as well as lactobacilli below 10^6 in all patients, accompanied by an increase in the quantity of opportunistic microflora representatives. Significant decreases in bifidobacteria ($p = 0.012$), lactobacilli ($p = 0.013$), and Escherichia coli ($p = 0.004$) were observed in patients of the 1st group compared to those in the 2nd group, indicating a more significant impact of *B. burgdorferi* on gut microbiota. Elevated levels of Staphylococcus and Candida species were diagnosed in almost every patient, yet the level of Candida in individuals with *B. burgdorferi* was nearly 1.5 times higher than in those of the 2nd group ($p = 0.002$). Increased amounts of other opportunistic pathogens were also observed in patients of both groups. *Proteus mirabilis* (36.8%) and *hemolytic E. coli* (31.6%) predominated in the 2nd group, while *Enterococcus faecium* (32.6%), *Klebsiella pneumoniae* (22.4%), and *haemolytic E. coli* (18.4%) showed significant growth above normal in the 1st group (Figure 23).

Upon bacteriological examination of feces from 96 patients, disturbances in the colonic dysbiosis were detected in 87 individuals from both groups. Grade III dysbiosis prevailed among patients with RA associated with *B. burgdorferi* (59.2%), whereas patients with isolated RA mostly showed Grade II dysbiosis (57.9%) (Figure 24). Grade IV dysbiosis was not detected in any examined patient of the 2nd group, while it was diagnosed in 3 patients (6.1%) of the 1st group. Grade I dysbiosis was more frequently registered in patients with isolated RA (23.7%) compared to the 1st group (8.2%) of the examined individuals.

Based on the analysis of the obtained data, it can be concluded that patients with RA associated with *B. burgdorferi* exhibited more pronounced disturbances in colonic microbiota prior to antibiotic therapy, resulting in a more severe degree of dysbiosis due to increased levels of opportunistic pathogens and significant reduction in normal microbiota compared to patients with isolated RA.

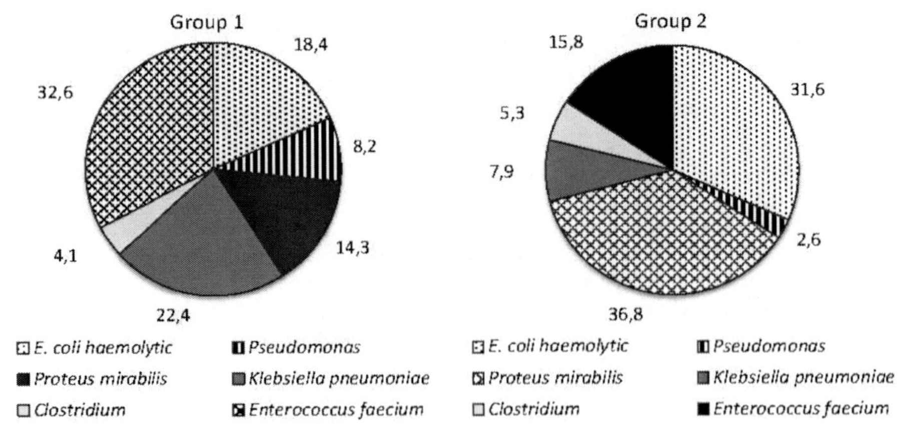

Figure 23. The frequency of detection of opportunistic microflora in patients from both groups with signs of dysbiosis, %.

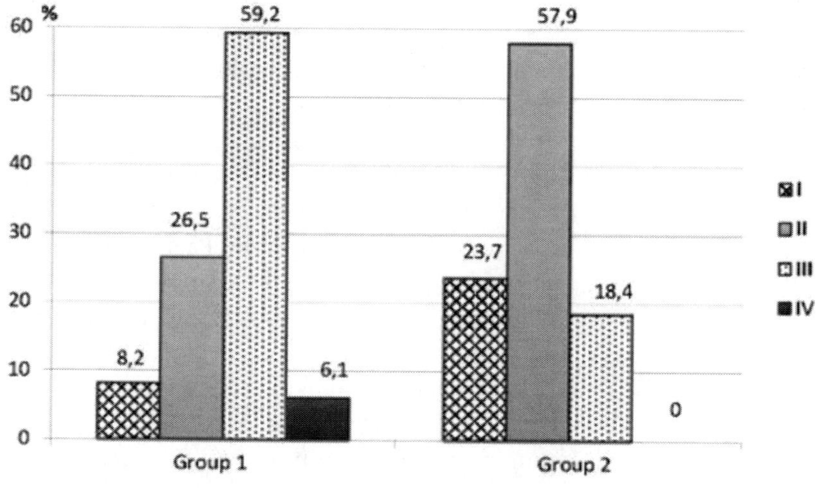

Figure 24. Severity grades of dysbiosis of the colon in examined patients (1st group – patients with rheumatoid arthritis associated with *B. burgdorferi*, 2nd – isolated RA).

4.4. Other Rheumatic Manifestations of Lyme Borreliosis

Despite the increased knowledge about LB over the past decades, the wide range of clinical manifestations of the disease and the limited informativeness of diagnostic methods mean that erroneous situations and delays in the correct diagnosis occur in medical practice with a certain frequency. To date, there are no universally agreed symptoms, laboratory, or instrumental data that are sensitive and specific enough to aid in the clinical assessment of patients with persistent LB-like symptoms mimicking connective tissue systemic diseases [204]. Prolonged subjective manifestations frequently reported in the context of LB (such as fatigue, headache, cognitive complaints, paresthesias, arthralgia, arthritis, and sleep disturbances) may also be present in all rheumatic diseases [205–207].

Fibromyalgia (FM) is the second most common "rheumatic" disease (after osteoarthritis), occurring in 2–8% of the general population. One of the possible triggering factors is LB. As early as 1995, M. Frey detected *B. burgdorferi* DNA in the muscle tissue of a patient with FM. Over the past years, several large-scale studies have been conducted, including during one study (4 years, 287 patients with verified LB diagnosis and no FM data at the onset of the main disease), FM was diagnosed in 37 patients (12.9%). It is worth noting that complete regression of symptoms after antibiotic therapy was achieved in only one (!) patient, while in others, despite negative serological test results, FM symptoms persisted. The lack of a clearer clinical picture after eliminating the pathogen, according to the authors, is associated with the presence of the so-called post-Lyme syndrome. Therefore, for a more detailed assessment, it is necessary to observe patients for a much longer period and exclude reinfection [208].

LB can induce complex dermatological conditions leading to autoimmune inflammatory dermatomyositis, including dermatopolymyositis (DM). It is known that 8 cases of DM manifestations associated with borreliae have been registered [209]. Unlike idiopathic DM, Lyme-associated DM is more common in men and is largely associated with other autoimmune diseases such as dermatitis herpetiformis, recurrent polychondritis, idiopathic pulmonary fibrosis, and cryoglobulinemia [210–213]. Although DM can occur in acute stages of the disease, most registered cases had chronic LB [214–218]. Perhaps this could be associated with the prolonged survival of *B. burgdorferi* in the reticuloendothelial system. Several attempts have been made to explain the development of DM in LB, but the actual mechanism remains unclear. Nevertheless, a multifactorial pathogenicity is possible, involving *B. burgdorferi* immunologically altering both cellular and humoral immunity, leading to lymphopenia, decreased suppressor cell activity, increased T-cell ratio, natural killer cell anomalies, increased polyclonal B-cells, and oligoclonal immunoglobulin synthesis [152].

Separate from immune dysfunction, mechanisms have been proposed that include inflammation due to direct invasion of *B. burgdorferi*, supported by the presence of spirochetes in skin or muscle biopsy samples. Taking this fact into account, Hoffmann et al., [219] described Lyme-associated DM as a variant of LB. In muscle biopsy samples, borreliae are present in perivascular zones and may release their antigens, contributing to the activation of antigenic inflammatory reactions as a mechanism of surrounding muscle trauma. These authors suggested the role of HLA-Cw3 haplotype susceptibility to borreliae-associated DM. While most cases are acquired DM during infection, Fraser et al., reported exacerbation of pre-existing DM after infection.

Based on the literature review [209], the link between DM and *B. burgdorferi* can be established directly or indirectly. Indirect evidence may include 1) positive results of ELISA or western blot for antibodies to borreliae in the presence of DM, 2) development of DM during or after LB, 3) exacerbation of DM caused by LB, 4) DM relapse correlated with borreliae reinfection, 5) recovery with DM correlating with recovery from LB, and 6) recovery with DM after antibiotic treatment.

Dermatomyositis associated with *B. burgdorferi* is one of the rare manifestations of DM. However, this possibility should be considered in patients with a new DM-like clinical picture living in endemic areas for LB or having acute or chronic forms of the disease. Lyme-associated DM is treatable and can be completely cured with appropriate therapy. Testing for Lyme-associated DM should include testing for LB, DM, and their etiological association.

Regarding the pathogenesis of skin lesions in LB and the potential involvement of *B. burgdorferi* in other fibrotic skin conditions, it is important to note the high affinity of borreliae with collagen and elastic fibres observed in histopathological studies of skin lesions in LB patients [220, 221].

First and foremost, it should be noted that *B. burgdorferi* has numerous adaptive properties that facilitate its penetration into the human body, especially into the musculoskeletal system [222]. There is evidence that the presence of decorin in ligaments and tendons plays a crucial role in bacterial infection. It has been noted that mice deficient in this enzyme were resistant to *B. burgdorferi* infection. Decorin is a proteoglycan localized within the cell or in the extracellular matrix. It is a connective tissue component that binds to collagen fibres of types I and II and plays a role in forming the extracellular matrix structure. There is a hypothesis that when the spirochete binds to decorin, its binding to collagen becomes impossible, leading to the breakdown of collagen. It is believed that the pathomechanism of this condition is complex, and its aaetiology is multifactorial, including disturbances in collagen synthesis, fibroblasts, and vessel damage, which together may influence the development of sclerosis. Endothelial damage is the first stage in its pathogenesis and may manifest as symptoms of Raynaud's phenomenon and microangiopathy. Genetic, environmental, and infectious factors may play a role in the pathomechanism of this condition [223].

It is believed that persistent infection with *B. burgdorferi* affects vascular endothelial cells, which can lead to their damage and the development of microvasculopathy and/or activation of skin fibroblasts. As early as 2005, A. Wackernagel described a patient with systemic scleroderma that developed only after *B. burgdorferi* infection [224]. In a 61-year-old woman with Raynaud's syndrome and capillaroscopic changes, sudden onset of erythema and induration of the skin of the face and upper trunk was noted. Laboratory studies, including ELISA, immunoblot, and PCR, detected *B. burgdorferi s. l.* infection. The patient was successfully treated with intravenous ceftriaxone. Within 14 days after completing the treatment, the skin became less stiff and dense. The author emphasizes that LB should be considered in atypical cases of skin sclerosis in patients predisposed to systemic scleroderma.

It is worth noting that while most patients who receive adequate treatment for LB recover, some individuals develop unexplained chronic conditions with persistent or recurrent symptoms post-treatment, similar to recently described "long-COVID-19," sharing many common characteristics [226]. The most frequent symptoms include fatigue, musculoskeletal pain, and cognitive dysfunction [85, 227, 228]. The Infectious Diseases Society of America (IDSA) has proposed the term "Post-Treatment Lyme Disease Syndrome" (PLDS) for this condition. However, patients with PLDS often report a wide range of other neurologic symptoms, sleep disturbances, mood disorders, eye involvement, and more [229–231]. Due to the lack of large-scale studies among PLDS patients, this diversity in clinical manifestations has not been thoroughly investigated. However, advancements in personalized medicine have identified clinically and/or biologically coherent subgroups [232, 233].

Moreover, similar to fibromyalgia, PLDS is likely a complex, multifactorial disease involving immunological, microbiological, genetic, and/or psychosocial factors that contribute to its development and severity [234, 235]. Alison W. Rebman et al., [236] studied the heterogeneity of clinical manifestations in PLDS patients and categorized them according to different demographic, clinical, laboratory, and psychosocial spheres. Research factor analysis classified 30 reported symptoms into 6 factors: "Cognitive Symptoms," "Eye Involvement," "Infection Type," "Mood," "Muscle and Skeletal Pain," and "Neurological." Hidden profile analysis identified 3 profiles of new symptoms, and all study participants were classified into respective subgroups: 1-59.0%, 2-18.9%, and 3-22.1%, respectively. Compared to the other two subgroups, subgroup 1 had lower scores across all factors for the overall sample and lower disability levels (1.6 vs. 10.0%, 12.8%; $q = 0.126$, $p = 0.035$) and higher perceived efficacy scores (median 7.5 vs. 6.0%, 5.3%; $q = 0.068$, $p < 0.001$). Subgroup 2 had the highest scores based on the "muscle-skeletal pain" factor ($q \leq 0.001$). Subgroup 3 was characterized by overall higher symptom factor scores and reported deeper depression ($q \leq 0.001$). This analysis identified 6 symptom factors and 3 potentially clinically relevant subgroups among PLDS patients, requiring further study.

During the LB study period, factors contributing to the increased risk of persistent symptoms post-treatment were identified [237]. These factors include: more severe initial disease presentation with a greater number of symptoms [238] and/or objective signs or symptoms (such as headache, photophobia, neck pain), nervous system involvement [239, 240], presence of comorbid conditions [241], delay in diagnosis and initiation of appropriate treatment [242], decreased immune response during acute infection [243], elevated levels of specific immune mediators such as IL-23 and CCL19 at disease onset and/or early convalescence [244, 245], and co-infection with *B. burgdorferi* and *Babesia microti* [246].

Therefore, LB based on clinical manifestations can present as a systemic connective tissue disease, acting as a triggering factor that initiates a complex cascade of reactions in the systemic inflammatory response. Patient B was under our observation (case described in collaboration with S. I. Smiyan, I. Y. Halaychuk, I. V. Zhulkevych, V. D. Nykoliuk, R. R. Komorovsky, S. R. Husak, I. I. Bilozetskyi [158]), who was referred for consultation to the rheumatology clinic from oncologists due to a leading syndrome of lymphadenopathy associated with intoxication syndrome and xerostomia. Regarding lymphadenopathy, she was examined at the oncology clinic, where histopathological and immunohistochemical examination of the left axillary lymph node was performed.

The results of the histopathological description indicated suspicion of follicular lymphoma, but immunohistochemical examination showed the following: CD3 (DAKO, polyclonal) – positive reaction in small lymphocytes of the paracortical zone and in scattered lymphocytes in the cortical zone, including germinal centres; CD3 (DAKO, clone L26) – positive reaction in small lymphocytes of cortical compartments and in cells of germinal centres, positive reaction in scattered lymphocytes in the paracortical zone; bcl-2 (DAKO, clone 124) – positive reaction in lymphocytes of the mantle, marginal, and paracortical zones, in scattered lymphocytes in germinal centres, negative reaction in most lymphocytes in germinal centres; CD30 (DAKO, clone Ber-H2) – positive reaction in scattered cells with immunoblast morphology located in germinal centres and in the paracortical zone; Ki-67 (DAKO, clone MIB-1) – positive reaction in nearly 100% of cells in germinal centres of secondary follicles, positive reaction in scattered cells in the paracortical zone. Capsid protein p24 of human immunodeficiency virus (DAKO, clone Kal-1) – negative reaction.

The pathomorphological conclusion confirmed the absence of cytological atypia in cells of the cortical and paracortical zones. Thus, immunohistochemical staining confirmed preservation of the overall structure of the lymph node, without evidence of lymphoproliferative processes. Changes in the lymph node were due to mixed (cortical and paracortical) hyperplasia (Figures 25–30).

Microslides (presented and described by I. Y. Halaychuk, I. V. Zhulkevych, and V. D. Nykoliuk) – addition to the histopathological conclusion CSD: there were pseudo-granulomas with homogeneous content and lymphogistiocytic infiltration around the granuloma (Figures 27–29), forming a fibrous pseudocapsule indicating specific granulomatous inflammation. Multiple macrophages were present in the pseudocapsule (Figure 30).

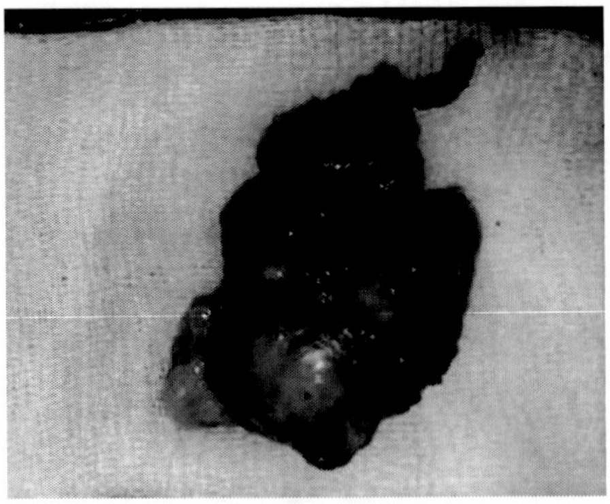

Figure 25. Surgical specimen of the excised left axillary lymph node conglomerate 4.5 × 4.0 × 3.5 cm.

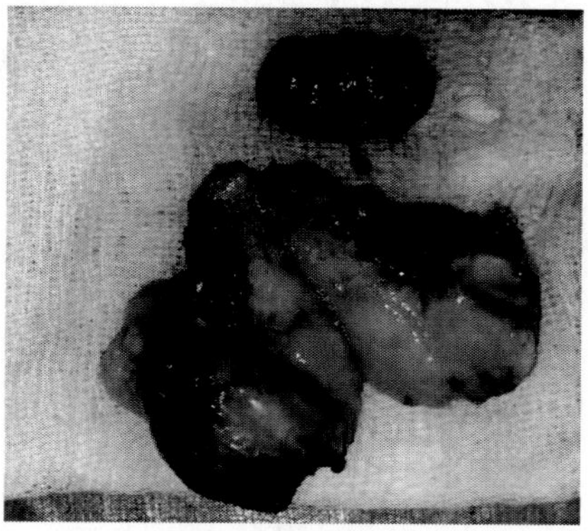

Figure 26. Yellow-grayish cut surface of the same (Figure 25) lymph node conglomerate.

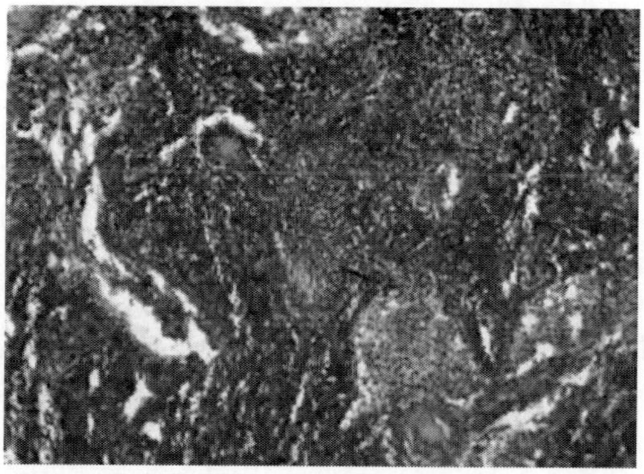

Figure 27. Light-microscopy appearance of an excised lymph node transverse section showing altered general architecture due to presence lymphoid cells of variable size and irregular shape arranged in follicle-like groups with lymphoid proliferation centers (arrowheads) and pseudogranulomas (arrows) (hematoxylin-eosin staining, 100×).

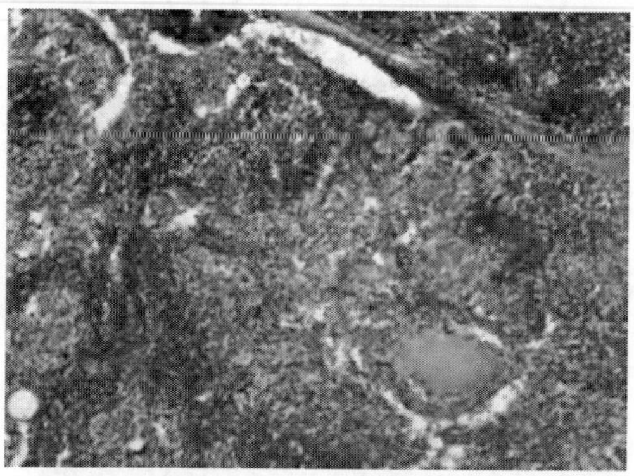

Figure 28. Histopathologic findings in a lymph node consistent with specific granulomatous inflammation: pseudogranuloma surrounded by lympho-histiocytic infiltration and forming connective tissue pseudocapsule (hematoxylin-eosin staining, 150×).

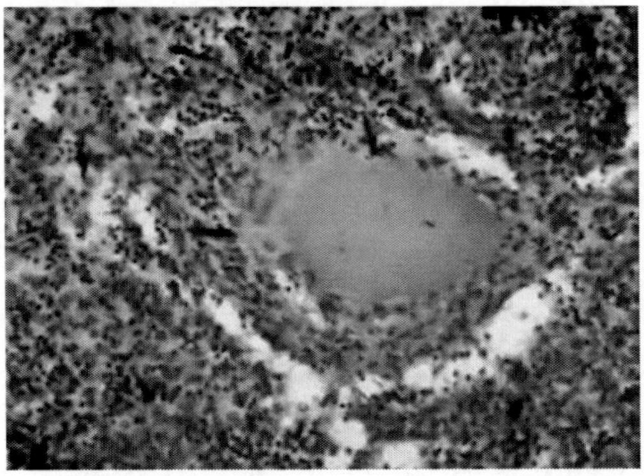

Figure 29. Histopathologic findings in a lymph node consistent with specific granulomatous inflammation: pseudogranuloma (asterisk) with homogeneous structure surrounded by lympho-histiocytic infiltration (arrow) and a forming connective tissue pseudocapsule (arrowhead) (hematoxylin-eosin staining, 200×).

Upon detailed questioning, it was determined that the patient had a history of tick attachment six months prior to the onset of symptoms. Upon examination, there were no rashes on the skin, but lymphadenopathy was noted in the cervical, submandibular, axillary, and inguinal regions. Examination of internal organs did not reveal any abnormalities. Routine laboratory tests were within normal limits.

Given the history of tick bite, the patient was tested for Lyme borreliosis (blot analysis): *B. burgdorferi* IgG and IgM antibodies were positive. Specific antibodies to VlsE, p41, p39, OspC Ba (*B. afzelii*), OspC Bb (*B. burgdorferi*), and OspC Bg (*B. garinii*) were not detected. Antibodies to IgG against VlsE (*B. burgdorferi, B. afzelii, B. garinii*), Lipid Ba (*B. afzelii*), and Lipid Bb (*B. burgdorferi*) were also not detected. Antibodies to IgG against p41, OspC (*B. afzelii*), p19, IgG, p83, p39, p58, p18 were not detected, while antibodies to p21 and p20 showed borderline results.

Systemic disease examination showed positive results for ANA-Screen, SS-A 52/60 IgG > 8, and SS-B IgG > 8.

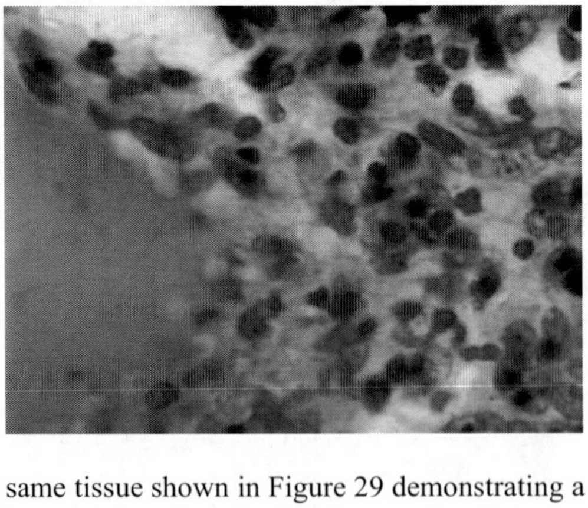

Figure 30. Fragment of the same tissue shown in Figure 29 demonstrating a part of pseudogranuloma (asterisk), a pseudocapsule (arrows), lymphocytes (white arrowhead), and macrophages (black arrowhead) (hematoxylin-eosin staining, 400×).

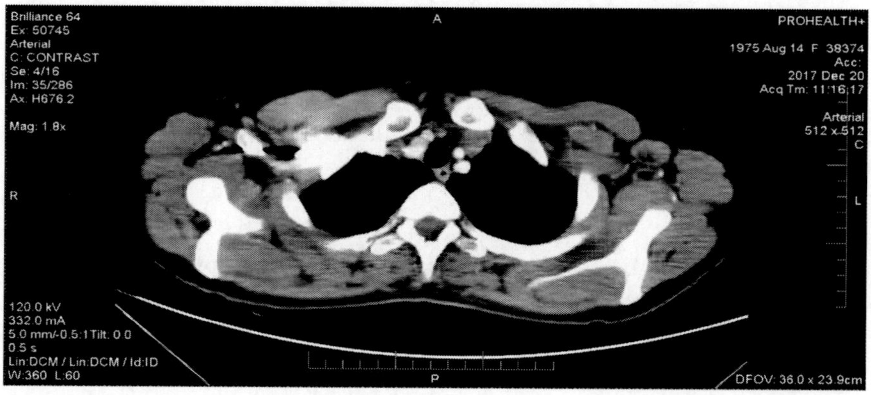

Figure 31. Computer tomogram of patient B., showing asymmetrically enlarged axillary lymph nodes.

CT scan performed at the oncology clinic (Figure 31) revealed bilaterally unevenly enlarged axillary lymph nodes (23/16 mm).

Consultations with an ophthalmologist revealed retinal angiopathy and dry eye syndrome. A dentist noted objective xerostomia.

Based on the above findings, the patient was diagnosed with Sjögren's syndrome associated with Lyme borreliosis.

Additionally, according to our data from the rheumatology clinic of Ternopil University Hospital, over the past four years (2017–2021), Lyme borreliosis with systemic manifestations, excluding arthritis, was diagnosed in 44 patients (Table 23). It is noteworthy that only 27 of them reported a history of tick attachment.

Most often, myalgic syndrome resembling fibromyalgia is noted in combination with chronic fatigue syndrome. Incorrect diagnosis could lead to systemic use of glucocorticoids, which in the case of *B. burgdorferi* infection would worsen patients' conditions.

Therefore, the rheumatological aspects of Lyme borreliosis and post-Lyme syndrome are currently inadequately studied, providing opportunities for further scientific developments. However, the issue of indications for examinations to exclude or verify these conditions in rheumatology practice is urgent and quite relevant.

Table 23. Systemic manifestations of Lyme borreliosis in the examined patients

Systemic changes	Number of patients	Peculiarities of the course of the disease
Lymphadenopathy	2	Previous diagnosis of lymphoma (histologically), ruled out by cytochemical method
Muscle pain (VAS – 90 mm)	23	No signs of arthritis, inflammatory changes. Fibromyalgia type
Localized scleroderma	3	No systemic manifestations
Sjögren's syndrome	2	Improvement after adequate treatment
Leukocytoclastic vasculitis	2	Continuous-relapsing course
Weber-Christian panniculitis	2	Complete regression after antibiotic therapy
Conditions resembling systemic lupus erythematosus	4	Regression of symptoms after antibiotic therapy in 2 patients, in others – onset of systemic lupus erythematosus
Antiphospholipid syndrome	2	Improvement after adequate treatment
Polyneuropathy (suspected systemic vasculitis) with signs of inflammatory syndrome	4	Improvement after adequate treatment

5. Lesions of Cardio-Vascular System

Serhii Andreychyn
Nataliia Bilkevych
Nataliia Kavetska
and Mariia Shkilna

Heart involvement in Lyme borreliosis (known as Lyme carditis) has been recognized since 1980 [257, 258]. During the acute phase of the disease, cardiovascular pathology ranks third in frequency among other manifestations, ranging from 0.2% to 25% depending on geographic zones [247, 250, 256, 257, 259, 260]. Specifically, in the United States, the frequency of Borrelia-induced myocarditis is approximately 8-10% among untreated adults with Lyme disease [256, 262, 263], though recent reports indicate a significant decrease [255, 256]. In this country, between 1985 and 2018, medical literature documented 9 cases of fatal Lyme carditis [256], and myocarditis occurs in about 10% of untreated Lyme disease cases [253].

In Europe, Lyme carditis is much less commonly reported compared to the United States, which may be attributed to differences in Borrelia genotypes on these continents [253, 256]. Statistical data on Lyme carditis in Europe correspond to 0.4–4% of all Lyme disease cases, approximately 1% in Northern Europe, and up to 8% in Southern Europe [248, 255–257]. Similar heterogeneity is observed in various geographic regions of Russia [250, 257], where cardiac involvement during the acute phase of Lyme disease is found in 43.2% of cases (mild carditis), and clinically significant chronic Lyme carditis is observed in 4.3% of cases, with mild chronic carditis in 22.7% of cases. Statistical data on paediatric cases also vary.

The problem of LB in Ukraine is significant due to its increasing incidence and the risk of complications, life-threatening in nature, as well as a high frequency of residual (residual) phenomena, which increases disability periods and worsens the quality of life of patients [253, 258]. The development of autoimmune reactions sometimes leads to LB presenting under the guise of rheumatic disease [249, 250].

The diagnostic challenge of Lyme carditis, particularly in Ukraine, lies in its mild symptomatic course during both acute and chronic phases, as reliable clinical signs can only be detected through additional diagnostic methods [249, 254, 264]. Therefore, the frequency of subclinical signs of cardiovascular system involvement, especially in the late stage, remains unknown [250]. There is a lack of vigilance among healthcare providers regarding the need for additional examinations for patients with mild symptomatic presentation of this “new” infection. In cases of prolonged disease progression, it is often difficult to trace the chronological connection between cardiovascular system involvement and the tick bite event. In some cases, heart involvement may be the sole manifestation of LB without accompanying changes in the skin, nervous system, or other organs [248, 250, 257].

According to research from the Scientific Research Institute of Epidemiology and Hygiene at Danylo Halytsky Lviv National Medical University, during 1995-2004, among individuals from 20 regions of Ukraine examined, 58.1% were seropositive for LD, with LD diagnosis confirmed in 37.2% of them. Cardiovascular system involvement was observed in 10.7% of diagnosed LD cases, and it was established that B. burgdorferi was the cause of etiologically undiagnosed rheumatological disorders in 20.7% of cases [249].

In the United States, the majority of Lyme carditis cases occur from June to December, with an incubation period ranging from 4 days to 7 months (average 21 days). There is a slight male predominance in incidence, and two age peaks are noted: 5-14 years and 44-59 years [10]. In Ukraine, the seasonal activity of *I. ricinus*, the main vector of infection, peaks notably in April-May and August-September. The majority (81.7%) of "new" cases are registered from May to September, predominantly during the spring-summer-autumn period [249]. Typically, cardiac manifestations occur 1-3 months (less commonly 6 months) after tick attachment and the appearance of erythema migrans [248].

There is conflicting data in studies evaluating the status of the cardiovascular system and interpreting data during different periods of LD. The scientific literature contains isolated descriptions of cardiac manifestations, which do not provide a unified view of the problem as a whole. According to some authors, signs of cardiovascular dysfunction manifest during the disseminated stage of the pathogen, on average 2-3 months after disease onset (while others argue they may appear within the first week of illness) [247, 250, 257]. Conversely, in later stages (after six months), cardiac symptoms observed in patients may no longer have a direct connection to Borrelia infection [257]. Results from other studies confirm Borrelia aaetiology cardiac involvement even in chronic LD, occurring later than two or more years after tick attachment [254, 265].

Cardiovascular involvement in acute Lyme borreliosis. Lyme carditis typically occurs during the early disseminated stage of the disease, often in conjunction with joint manifestations or symptoms of neurological involvement, although cardiac manifestations can dominate [250, 256]. Dissemination of the pathogen without a preceding erythema migrans phase is observed in approximately 20-45% of cases [254]. Borrelia bacteria have the ability to penetrate macrophages, endothelial cells, basophils, eosinophils, B cells, and other cell types [254]. Through the bloodstream, bacteria can invade cardiac tissues, including the conduction system around the atrioventricular node, the external or internal membranes of the heart, the myocardium, and less frequently, the heart vessels or valves [250, 256]. Histological studies of biopsies from the endo- and myocardium of patients and autopsy findings provide direct evidence of the infectious agent's damaging effects. In the interstitium of the myocardium, researchers have identified spirochetes, focal necrosis of cardiomyocytes, interstitial and perivascular lymphoplasmacytic infiltration. Using special silver staining, Borrelia can be observed freely lying within infiltrates and between muscle fibres, as well as within cardiomyocytes, as shown in Figure 3.32 [249, 258]. Living Borrelia have been detected in tissues even 10 years after infection [249, 258].

While residing in the patient's tissues, spirochetes elicit an immune response to the presence of antigens (including Osp antigens). This triggers activation of neutrophils, macrophages, stimulates cytokine production [254], increases levels of IL-1 and TNF-α with development of local and systemic immune responses, stimulates collagenase synthesis, interferons. The death of Borrelia is accompanied by the release of endotoxins [254]. The accumulation of specific immune complexes containing spirochaetal antigens in the body tissues, including the myocardium, is of significant importance in the pathogenesis [248].

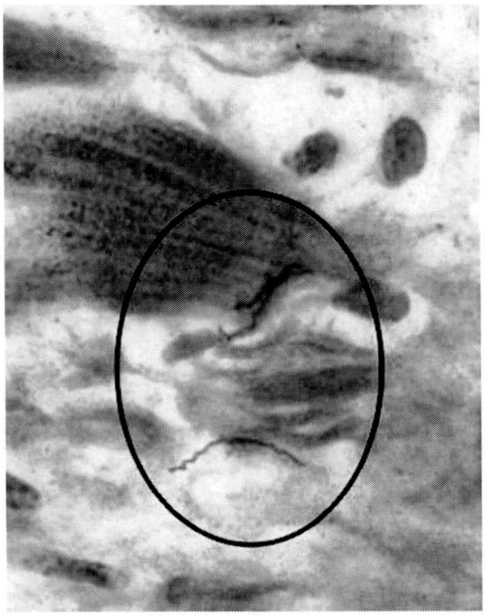

Figure 32. Spirochetes in the myocardium. Staining with Warthin – Starry (borrowed from A. Fish [258]).

The systemic nature of dissemination during the spirochete's spread to organs and tissues is explained by the development of endothelial dysfunction, vasculitis, which can become chronic (perivascular lymphocytic-histiocytic infiltrates in vessel walls were often found) [248, 250, 257]. The consequence of these pathological processes includes inflammatory changes, and later, dystrophic changes in the myocardium [248, 254–256], leading to myocarditis, pericarditis, or pancarditis [250, 252, 266], as well as myocytolysis and interstitial fibrosis, formation of focal or confluent scars [255, 256]. These significant pathological changes may cause diastolic dysfunction of the left ventricle (DDLV) in patients with Lyme carditis [248, 254]. Research data indicate myocardial damage, revealing increased levels of the MB fraction of creatine kinase and elevated concentrations of specific IgM immunoglobulins in the blood during the first two months of the disease in patients with Lyme carditis [248].

Experimental evidence has demonstrated the possibility of the spirochete's multiplication in endothelial cells [249]. Patients with Lyme carditis have shown productive vasculitis with vasodilation and leukocyte adhesion along the vascular intima [248].

In the acute phase of LB, there is an imbalance of immune-regulating cells with predominance of T-suppressors and intracellular parasitism of Borrelia, contributing to the recurrent course of the disease with spirochaetal persistence in the human body [254]. This can potentially trigger an autoimmune reaction against myocardial tissue, as the pathogen has antigenic similarity with host cells [254, 255]. It has been observed that systemic manifestations, particularly involving the cardiovascular system, are more common in early disseminated LB, possibly due to rapid spirochaetal dissemination and delayed medical intervention [257, 264].

More frequently, scientific literature reports on acute Lyme carditis and its complications, sometimes fatal [254, 262, 265], with disturbances in heart rhythm and conduction. Cardiac involvement can also manifest as myocarditis with or without circulatory insufficiency (typically affecting the left ventricle – LV), less commonly as pericarditis with pericardial friction rub or effusion detected by ultrasound or radiological examination. Endocarditis with heart valve defects is extremely rare [248, 254, 257]. Symptoms usually appear in the early stages of the disease, within several weeks or months [256, 263].

Clinical symptoms of carditis in LB include chest pain, palpitations, shortness of breath, dizziness, and brief syncopal episodes occurring alongside other manifestations of this infection [250, 264, 266]. Physical examination findings include bradycardia, weakened heart sounds, splitting of the first heart sound, and systolic murmurs at the apex or in the precordial area, explained by myocardial involvement, while pericardial friction rub indicates pericarditis [248, 257]. According to a study conducted in the United States [265], among 875 examined patients, cardiac manifestations were present in 10% of patients, 20% of whom were hospitalized. The following clinical signs were noted: palpitations – 6.6% of all examined, cardiac conduction disorders – 1.8%, myocarditis – 0.9%, signs of left ventricular failure – 0.5%, pericarditis – 0.2%.

We examined 90 patients with early disseminated LB who were treated on an outpatient and inpatient basis from 2015 to 2020 at the Ternopil Regional Dermatovenereological Dispensary, Infectious Diseases Department of Ternopil Municipal Emergency Hospital, Ternopil Regional Tuberculosis and Pulmonology Medical Centre of Ternopil Regional Council, Ternopil University Hospital. There were 33 (36.7%) men and 57 (63.3%) women ($p < 0.05$). The majority were of working age (86.7%), residents of urban areas (62.2%) rather than rural areas (37.8%) ($p < 0.05$). Their average age was (43.1 ± 14.3) years.

Intoxication syndrome was observed in 35 (38.9%) patients, cardiovascular system involvement in 23 (25.5%), nervous system (NS) involvement in 11 (12.2%), musculoskeletal system involvement in 46 (51.1%), skin involvement in 25 (27.8%), and eye involvement in 15 (16.6%) individuals (Table 24).

It was determined that the most common signs of cardiovascular system involvement in patients with early disseminated LB were rhythm disturbances in 33 (36.7%) individuals, predominantly due to heart rate disturbances (11; 33.3%), $p < 0.05$ (Table 25).

Cardiomyopathy, myocarditis, pericarditis, and mitral valve defects (prolapse, insufficiency) were significantly less noted in the examined patients.

Observations of patients in the acute period show that symptoms of cardiac involvement are secondary and depend on the severity of the disease course (intoxication) [248, 250]. Cardiac involvement is never isolated; other organs are always involved in the pathological process (lymphatic system, central and peripheral nervous system, skin, musculoskeletal system, etc.) [256, 257, 261, 266]. Combined involvement of different systems and organs is found in 62.7% of cases. Clinical examination results of patients with LB have shown a direct correlation between clinical symptoms of cardiac involvement and the presence of generalized lymphadenopathy, symptoms of infectious intoxication (prolonged periodic fever, weakness, chills, headache), peripheral and central nervous system involvement (radiculoneuritis, hyperesthesia, paresthesia, irritability, drowsiness, memory impairment), musculoskeletal system involvement (arthritis, myositis, arthralgia, myalgia), and specific dermatological manifestations (localized scleroderma, benign lymphocytoma of the skin, chronic atrophic acrodermatitis). Such polymorphism of clinical manifestations in various combinations with cardiovascular system involvement indicates systemic borrelial infection [250].

Table 24. Frequency of detection of main clinical syndromes in patients with non-erythema migrans form of Lyme borreliosis (n = 90)

Syndrome	Patients	
	Absolute number	%
Intoxication	35	38,9
Cardiovascular system involvement	23	25,5
Musculoskeletal system involvement	46	51,1
Nervous system involvement	11	12,2
Skin involvement	25	27,8
Eye involvement	15	16,6

Although the most common manifestations of Lyme carditis are disturbances in heart rhythm and conduction [20], changes interpreted as "hypoxic" (flattening and inversion of the T wave, prolongation of the QT interval) are often found on the electrocardiogram during the first 1-2 weeks of the disease in patients, which disappear with the resolution of the infectious intoxication syndrome [250, 257]. Later on, due to dystrophic changes in the myocardium, conduction disturbances may occur at various levels of the cardiac conduction system (atria, atrioventricular node, His bundle branches, Purkinje fibres), leading to the development of blocks of varying degrees. The frequency of conduction disturbances, according to various authors, ranges from 10-20-25% of all cardiac manifestations. Atrioventricular block is one of the most severe, sometimes fatal complications of Lyme borreliosis [256, 257, 263]. According to some studies, there is a high probability of developing first-degree atrioventricular block in almost all cases of Lyme carditis (98%), and the likelihood of complete heart block occurrence should be expected in about half of cases (58% according to [263]) with manifest heart involvement. Atrioventricular block in Lyme borreliosis is characterized by an intermittent nature, where the degree of block rapidly changes from minor to severe and back over several hours. At the same time, there is noted stability and duration of conduction disturbances along the His-Purkinje system [248, 258, 266]. Results of electrophysiological studies of the heart indicate the possibility of simultaneous development of blocks at multiple levels of the cardiac conduction system [256].

Table 25. Characterization of cardiovascular manifestations in patients with non-erythema migrans form of Lyme borreliosis (n = 90)

Manifestation	Patients	
	Absolute number	%
Discomfort in the chest area	12	13,3
Cardiac rhythm disturbances:	33	36,7
Sinus tachycardia (>90 beats per minute)	11	12,2
Sinus bradycardia (<60 beats per minute)	9	10,0
Extrasystoles	8	8,9
Atrial fibrillation	5	5,5
Cardiomyopathy	9	10,0
Myocarditis	12	13,3
Pericarditis	3	3,3
Mitral valve disorders (prolapse, insufficiency)	6	3,3

In addition to conduction disturbances, episodes of supraventricular and ventricular tachycardia, premature ventricular contractions from various sections of the heart up to bigeminy, episodes of atrial fibrillation, and migration of the pacemaker rhythm into the atria are often recorded on the ECG. Usually, rhythm disturbances are temporary, with clinical and electrocardiographic signs appearing and disappearing repeatedly within a day [257, 258]. Rhythm and conduction disturbances in Lyme borreliosis typically occur in combination with clinical signs of myopericarditis [256].

When rhythm and conduction disturbances develop, differential diagnosis of Lyme borreliosis includes consideration of conditions such as idiopathic cardiac fibrosis, acute or previously experienced myocardial infarction, hyperkalaemia, aortic valve endocarditis, severe calcification of the fibrous ring of the aortic valve, infiltrative cardiomyopathies (such as sarcoidosis, amyloidosis), iatrogenic influences (e.g., post-ablation), Chagas disease, increased vagal tone, Steinert's disease (myotonic dystrophy), as well as medication-related effects (such as β-blockers, calcium channel blockers, digoxin) [255].

It should be noted that clinically significant changes are not always detected in routine ECG examinations in all cases of the disease. The most characteristic manifestations of electrical instability in patients with LB are changes in the terminal part of the QRS complex, sinus tachycardia, and subsequently, conduction disturbances [250, 258].

Signs of disturbance in the processes of rapid terminal repolarization of the ventricular myocardium (flattening or inversion of the T wave) on days 1-3 of the disease were recorded in 8.1% of patients with *B. miyamotoi* infection [250]. Such repolarization disturbances, along with clinical manifestations (mild or stabbing precordial pain and discomfort in the apex of the heart without radiation, dyspnoea with minimal physical exertion, palpitations), were considered by the authors as nonspecific but early signs of inflammatory myocardial involvement [250].

In echocardiographic studies of the heart, specific changes were not found in a significant portion of patients with LB [263]. However, there is likely a certain peculiarity of heart involvement in LB induced by various pathogens. For instance, some researchers have identified impaired myocardial functional status with the development of left ventricular diastolic dysfunction (LVDD) in patients with LB [250, 265]. Signs of LVDD observed included reduced transmitral gradient, worsening of early diastolic filling, and compensatory increase in filling during atrial systole [250].

In acute and subacute courses of LB, alongside clinical and electrocardiographic signs of myocarditis, the appearance of pericarditis is sometimes noted. Echocardiography in most observations indicates a small pericardial effusion in the form of pericardial leaflet divergence in the apex and posterior wall of the left ventricle [257, 261].

The course of myocarditis in LB is generally benign with a tendency to regress within several weeks, although relapses may occur [257, 261]. Due to the mild symptomatic course of cardiopathy in LB, only the use of more sensitive studies reveals heart involvement, especially in the presence of electrical function disturbances [248]. The development of new ultrasound technologies, such as transthoracic visualization of coronary arteries and evaluation of intramural (myocardial) gradient using tissue Doppler, allows for the detection of the earliest signs of heart involvement, such as hidden areas of contractility impairment not visible on visual echocardiography. Increased coronary blood flow velocity has been detected in patients with LB, possibly due to increased resistive resistance resulting from inflammation in the vessel intima, vasculitis, and endothelial dysfunction [250, 265]. In another study, MRI and myocardial scintigraphy with indium-111-labeled myosin antibodies confirmed the diffuse nature of myocardial muscle damage with a decrease in its pumping function [257]. The use of gadolinium-enhanced MRI detected signs of myocarditis in patients with acute complete atrioventricular block in whom such changes were not seen during routine ultrasound examinations [255]. These data confirm changes in the heart and vessels in LB and highlight the importance of monitoring patients with LB for the risk of heart disease.

In addition to rhythm and conduction disturbances, myocarditis and pericarditis reveal changes in blood pressure (BP) during the acute period of LB, likely related to endothelial dysfunction. It was studied that the degree of increased BP depends on the activity of the infectious process, as the level of specific IgM immunoglobulins in serum correlated with indicators of daily BP monitoring in examined patients, namely, with minimal systolic BP and the index of diastolic BP. Worsening of the course of concomitant hypertension in patients with acute LB, in the form of more frequent hypertensive crises, was accompanied by an increase in C-reactive protein.

The possible presence of subclinical Lyme carditis in patients with acute LB and hypertension was confirmed by such correlation links: the level of specific IgM directly correlated with the presence of bradycardia ($r = 0.55$, $p = 0.0379$) and fever ($r = 0.35$, $p = 0.0448$) in patients, while C-reactive protein correlated directly with shortness of breath ($r = 0.64$, $p = 0.0455$). Thus, LB and concomitant hypertension occur as mutually exacerbating conditions, confirmed by correlations: specific IgM and the discomfort index in the morning (determined by variability and BP values in the morning hours), worsening of hypertension course, and enhanced subjective symptomatology with subfebrile body temperature ($r = 0.47$) and elevated C-reactive protein ($r = 0.66$).

Overall, the prognosis for conduction disturbances induced by LB is favourable [253, 262]. Atrioventricular node conduction typically recovers within a week, and minor disturbances resolve within 6 weeks [253, 256]. Over a 12-month observation period after completing antibiotic therapy, there is gradual disappearance of intraventricular conduction disorders [248]. However, the electrical activity instability of the heart during acute LB requires hospitalization and monitoring of such patients to provide timely urgent care, as illustrated by the case history excerpt below (excerpted from J. Van Hattem [253]).

A young male patient (36 years old) was admitted to the cardio-surgical department of the hospital following a syncopal episode. According to his medical history, there were no chronic illnesses, but two weeks prior to admission, he experienced pain and stiffness in the upper left calf, which resolved within 2 days. Over the past week, he intermittently experienced dizziness upon changing from a horizontal to vertical position, shortness of breath, and palpitations. Additionally, on the eve of hospitalization, he complained of pain in the large joints of his left arm. He had no harmful habits, no history of travel abroad, and no tick bites were detected.

Upon examination: arterial blood pressure, body temperature, and blood oxygen saturation were within normal limits, but his pulse was irregular at 48 beats per minute. There were no abnormalities detected upon auscultation of the lungs and heart; however, palpation revealed enlarged lymph nodes in the left groin area. There were no changes observed in the joints or skin during the initial examination.

An ECG upon admission showed complete atrioventricular block, and in the subsequent hours, second-degree atrioventricular block, Mobitz type 1 with progressive PR prolongation (Figure 33).

Considering the atypical clinical presentation of the disease, severe arrhythmias in a young person without a history of chronic pathology prompted an extensive diagnostic search. Acute myocardial infarction and abnormalities of the aortic valve were ruled out based on the absence of typical data from transthoracic echocardiography and deviations from normal levels of myocardial necrosis markers in laboratory tests.

Given the history of arthralgia, Lyme disease serology (ELISA) was performed on the day of admission. Elevated levels of specific IgG (498 IU/ml) and IgM (2.7 IU/ml) were detected, which were also confirmed by the presence of these antibodies in immunoblotting. The patient was prescribed intravenous ceftriaxone at a dose of 2000 mg daily for 7 days.

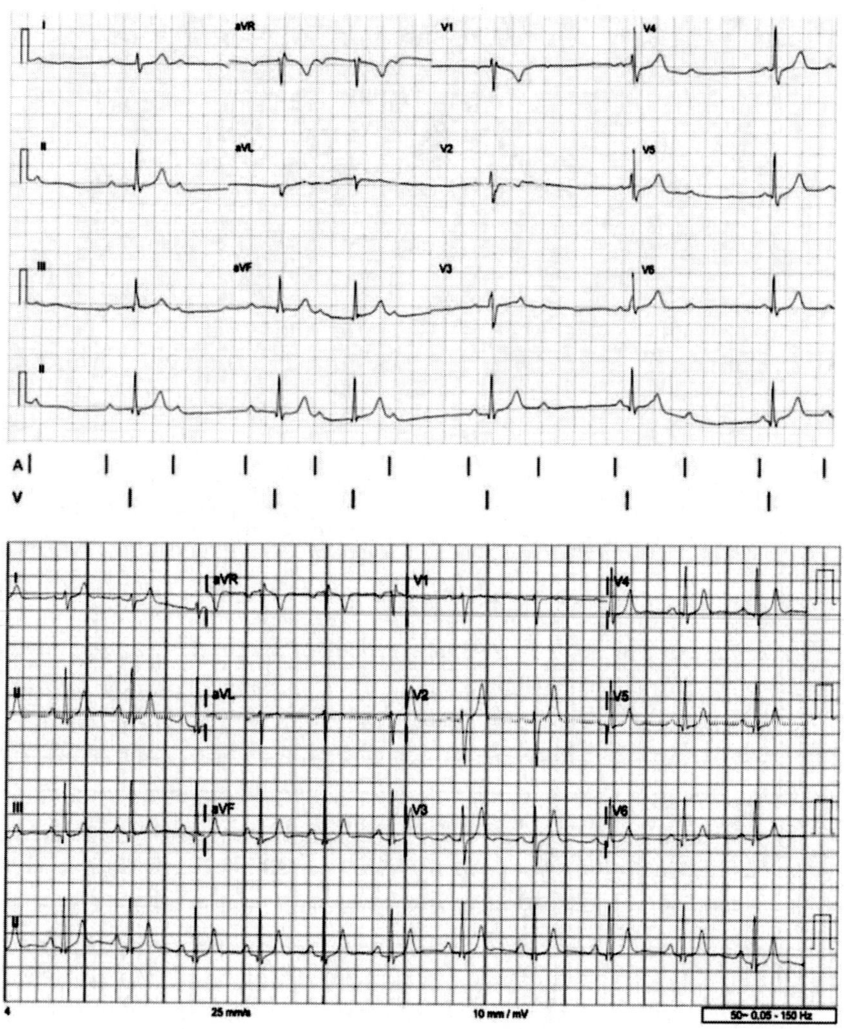

Figure 33. ECG of the patient in dynamics: a – atrioventricular block II degree, Mobitz type 1 with passive ventricular complexes, b – after normalization of cardiac conduction. Paper speed 25 mm/s [253].

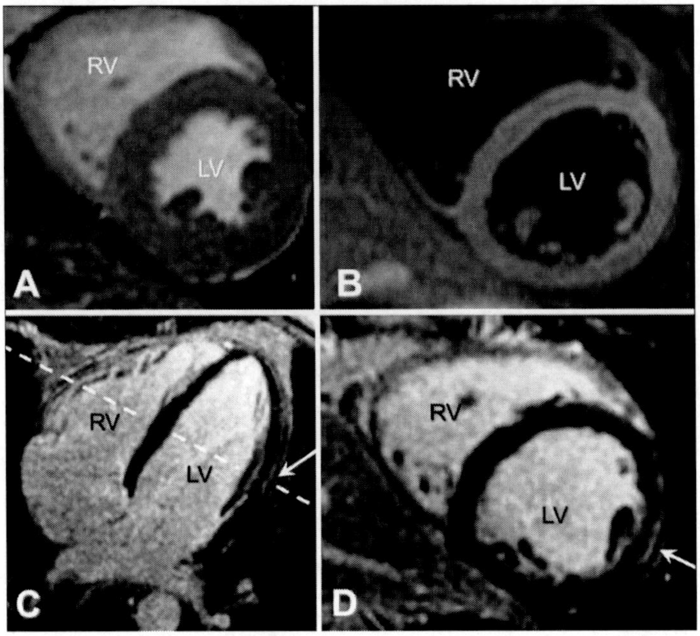

Note: LV – left ventricle, RV – right ventricle.

Figure 34. MRI data: A – normal systolic function of the left ventricle without wall motion abnormalities; B – T2-weighted image without high signal intensity in the myocardium, no evidence of acute myocardial inflammation; C, D – delayed enhancement images with small areas of epicardial thickening (marked by white arrow) [253].

Five days after hospitalization, a cardiovascular MRI was performed, which did not reveal any decrease in systolic function of the ventricles or any other abnormalities in the movement of the heart walls. T2-weighted visualization showed no signs of acute inflammation; however, delayed gadolinium-enhanced images demonstrated increased density of the mid-wall of the epicardium (Figure 34). These findings supported the diagnosis of myocarditis, the low activity of which likely explained the absence of deviations during the initial examination, with typical changes observable only through T2-weighted imaging. Thus, cardiovascular MRI findings and the presence of Borrelia IgM antibodies confirmed the diagnosis of Lyme carditis.

In the course of the disease, under the influence of the administered treatment, there was resolution of atrioventricular block and normalization of the PR interval duration. The patient was discharged home after 5 days of hospitalization, with a recommendation to continue treatment with oral doxycycline 100 mg twice daily for 2 weeks.

Next week, the patient returned to the doctor, this time with neurological symptoms (complaints of asymmetric facial deformation, headache, photophobia, and pain in the lower back and right thigh). Objectively, increased muscle tone, unilateral facial nerve paralysis, and symptoms of sciatic nerve irritation on the right side were observed. Laboratory examination of cerebrospinal fluid after lumbar puncture revealed elevated protein content and increased IgG levels. CSF ELISA showed elevated IgG levels with normal IgM levels for Borrelia. A diagnosis of neuroborreliosis with meningopolyradiculitis (Garin-Bujadoux-Bannwarth syndrome) was made. It should be noted that no changes were recorded on ECG amidst neurological symptoms. After adjusting antibiotic therapy (intravenous ceftriaxone 2000 mg daily for 2 weeks), the patient fully recovered.

The provided data confirm that:

- Lyme carditis should be suspected in young patients without chronic cardiac pathology in their medical history, especially if they present with acute atrioventricular conduction disturbances, even in the absence of a tick bite;
- The diagnosis of Lyme carditis should be based on a combination of clinical manifestations, Lyme borreliosis signs (such as EM), and laboratory data;
- Cardiac MRI is the most accurate tool for non-invasive assessment of myocardial inflammation in patients suspected of myocarditis, which can aid in the diagnosis of Lyme carditis [253, 266].

The cardiovascular system involvement in chronic LB is less studied. Conditions such as chronic LB and so-called post-Lyme disease (PLD) or consequences of previous LB are highlighted [248, 249, 257]. According to some data, chronic or residual Lyme borreliosis may develop in approximately one-third (up to 36.7%) of patients [253, 254]. Traditionally, the third stage of the disease manifests with changes in joints, skin, and the nervous system (Lyme arthritis, chronic atrophic acrodermatitis, or neuroborreliosis) [268].

In Ukraine, based on research from the Lviv Scientific Research Institute of Epidemiology and Hygiene, *B. burgdorferi* accounts for 16.7% of undiagnosed neurological and 20.7% of pseudorheumatic pathologies. Late-stage manifestations in various systems and organs due to delayed diagnosis and treatment lead to chronicity (3.5–10.6% of cases), long-term disability, invalidation, and sometimes fatal outcomes [249, 254]. In 15–53% of convalescents of previous LB within the first 2–3 months, post-Lyme syndrome (PLS) can develop, which is not associated with laboratory signs of Borrelia infection and, according to some reports, lacks signs of inflammation. However, clinical symptoms, including cardiac symptoms, may persist for several years [254, 262]. Currently, there are no universally accepted diagnostic criteria for PLS. The term is applied to patients experiencing subjective symptoms (general weakness, myalgia, arthralgia, memory impairment, depression, chest pain, etc.) for more than 6 months after completing antibiotic therapy. This condition is explained by slow resolution of the inflammatory process; however, studies have not shown an increase in inflammation markers in these patients [262]. Chronic progression of LB with significant organ and system involvement often occurs after a short incubation period, absence of fever, and general infectious manifestations at the onset of the disease. This is presumed to be related to local and systemic immune responses, suppression of cytokine synthesis during the acute phase of LB, and difficulty in Borrelia elimination. Additionally, chronic disease stages may result from inadequate (in terms of timing, duration, and prescribed doses) treatment during the acute phase or its absence, which often occurs in cases of early localized LB [257].

The association of predisposition to chronic disease progression with certain histocompatibility genes is well established [248, 257]. Specifically, carriage of the DRB107 allele is considered unfavourable for severe forms of the disease, while the DRB102 allele has a protective effect, defining the development compared to benign forms of LB [2].

In chronic persistence stage LB, the disease may have a recurrent course or progress gradually. Prolonged persistence of Borrelia often occurs without clinical manifestations of the disease (latent infection). Autoimmune reactions may sustain the pathological process even after eradication of the pathogen [248, 251].

The possibility of disease progression to the chronic stage in LB is attributed to the complexity of immunopathological processes that develop due to unique mechanisms of Borrelia adaptation within the human body [254]. Several authors explain prolonged persistence and formation of organic pathology through a number of reasons: potential transformation of Borrelia into L-forms, intracellular localization of the pathogen; marked variability of Borrelia surface antigens; increased resistance of certain pathogen genotypes to nonspecific host resistance factors; suppressive activity of T-cells in the early stages of the disease; inhibition of phagocytosis activity and its incompleteness; weak antigenic stimulation during slow Borrelia replication; insufficient activation of macrophages under conditions of weak Th1 response; slow and weak production of specific antibodies: IgM after 1-1.5 months and IgG after 2-3 months from the onset of the disease; Borrelia-triggered autoimmune reactions (molecular mimicry due to the presence of antigenic determinants shared with human cell and tissue proteins); accumulation of specific immune complexes containing spirochaetal antigens in the synovial membrane of joints, skin, kidneys, myocardium amidst impaired phagocyte elimination function [249, 257].

According to some authors, clinical manifestations of chronic LB are largely attributed to the development of autoimmune reactions rather than hematogenous spread of the pathogen. The chronicity of the process is exacerbated by the absence of EM in the acute phase, which often results in inadequate examination and lack of etiotropic treatment for these patients [264].

It has been proven that Borrelia can activate caspase synthesis, the direct executors of apoptosis, and induce synthesis of matrix metalloproteinases, which degrade collagen and consequently cause cardiomyocyte necrosis, leading to myocardial remodelling and potential cardiac damage in the chronic stage of the disease [248, 250].

Currently, it remains unclear whether patients with underlying heart disease have an increased risk of LB affecting or complicating their condition compared to the general population [256]. Some international authors consider it unlikely for Lyme aetiology to affect the heart more than 6 months after the appearance of EM, including the development of chronic cardiomyopathy due to LB [248, 256, 257, 269].

There are data suggesting that prolonged subclinical Lyme carditis can lead to morphofunctional myocardial remodelling with the formation of eccentric hypertrophy [250, 265]. In contrast to the acute stage of the disease, where echocardiography may reveal signs of relaxation impairment or no obvious changes, later stages may show signs of diffuse cardiac involvement: chamber enlargement, increased myocardial thickness, reduced contractile function, and ejection fraction [248, 250, 257]. Echocardiographic results in patients with chronic LB and clinical data indicate the likely development of specific Lyme myocarditis, which causes chamber dilation and reduced cardiac systolic function [248, 250, 265, 267].

In patients with non-coronary cardiomegaly examined for LB who resided in an endemic region, stage 3 LB was found in 37.5% of individuals, confirmed by diagnostic significant titres of specific antibodies. In individuals with non-coronary cardiomyopathy, an association was established in 28.1% of cases between tick exposure and heart failure, within (7.2 ± 1.6) months following inoculation, linking heart remodelling with a history of borrelial myocarditis. Among patients with cardiomegaly and concomitant IHD living in endemic areas, stage 3 LB was detected in 28.1% of cases, significantly more frequently than in patients with IHD but without cardiomegaly (6.3%). Heart damage in patients with coronary cardiomyopathy and chronic LB was associated with a higher frequency of repeated myocardial infarctions than in the examined control group [270].

There is a likelihood of Lyme disease playing a role in the development of coronary insufficiency and the progression of IHD. The described involvement of Borrelia in coronary artery damage with aneurysm formation during chronic LB [247, 252] is interpreted as transient vasculitis. Some authors point to the development of endothelial dysfunction as one of the causes of myocardial and vascular damage in LB. Endothelial dysfunction and myocardial remodelling are interconnected with autoimmune inflammation in both acute and chronic LB stages. Holter monitoring during the acute phase of the disease (1-3 days) identified episodes of painless myocardial ischemia, which were absent after 2 months, attributed by the authors to inflammatory changes in the cardiac muscle and coronary arteries during the acute phase of LB [248, 250].

The aforementioned vascular changes persist against a backdrop of sustained moderate elevation in markers of systemic inflammation [250, 265]. It has been established that elevated levels of high-sensitivity C-reactive protein (hs-CRP) in the blood are associated with a high risk of cardiovascular events [266]. Even after 12 months of observation, a small but significant increase in serum hs-CRP concentration, assessed by an ultra-sensitive method, was recorded in more than a quarter of LB patients [257].

Two months later, markers of systemic inflammatory reaction correlated with parameters of coronary blood flow: early diastolic filling velocity (E) with average velocity in diastole in the perforant artery correlated with the level of high-sensitivity CRP, suggesting an independent contribution of systemic inflammation to persistent coronary blood flow impairment. Such impairment in coronary blood flow may lead to decreased active diastolic relaxation of the left ventricle, as confirmed by correlation between diastolic function parameters of the left ventricle and coronary blood flow parameters [257, 265].

The role of Borrelia infection in the development of systemic atherosclerosis is discussed. According to coronary angiography data, atherosclerosis was found in 14% of cases among patients with more than 50% increase in specific IgG titres to Borrelia, whereas in individuals with normal coronary angiography findings, it was found in only 6% [250, 270]. Significant thickening of the intima-media complex of the internal carotid artery and increased frequency of atherosclerotic plaques in the carotid arteries were observed in patients with elevated IgG class antibodies to B. burgdorferi. Consequently, Lyme disease can be considered an additional risk factor for cardiovascular diseases. However, there is still no unified understanding of the impact of this infection on vascular walls. It is plausible to consider the possible role of Borrelia infection in the progression of atherosclerosis, pathogenetically linked to persistent systemic inflammation and dyslipidaemia [257, 270].

Several authors link the development of vascular lesions in LB with endothelial dysfunction [247, 250, 253, 258]. In patients during both acute and chronic phases of LB, there is a tendency towards decreased linear velocities and increased resistance in cerebral arteries, indicating increased stiffness of their vascular walls and potential impairment of blood flow in distal regions. An increase in the intima-media thickness index in carotid arteries of more than 0.9 mm was found in 61.1% and 59.0% of patients during acute and chronic phases of LB, respectively. Evidence supporting endothelial dysfunction includes a reduction in endothelium-dependent vasodilation of less than 10% in all examined patients in both phases of the disease [250, 270].

Thus, there is evidence that cardiovascular involvement in the chronic course of LB can manifest as symptoms of myocarditis, pericarditis, pancarditis, but more commonly as cardiomyosclerosis, which is more characteristic of individuals who did not receive treatment during the manifest acute period, as well as systemic vasculitis. The development of a chronic course of the disease more often occurs after erythema migrans and subclinical forms of the early period of LB [250, 257, 261]. It is important to note that according to international clinical guidelines on LB, severe or fulminant congestive heart failure or the development of valvular heart disease are not associated with Lyme disease [256, 266]. On the other hand, the possibility of reduced left ventricular contractile function due to pericarditis and myocarditis is confirmed by international authors [253]. Therefore, the issue of cardiovascular involvement in LB is insufficiently studied and requires further research.

6. Lesions of Nervous System

Vasyl Kopcha
and Svitlana Shkrobot

LB frequently involves the nervous system, a condition known as neuroborreliosis. This neurological complication is often associated with Borrelia garinii, although other genospecies of Borrelia can also cause similar pathology [274, 275]. In the pathogenesis of LB, infection plays a crucial role. Borreliae enter through the skin, causing local inflammatory processes, and later disseminate to other organs and tissues. Even in the early stages of the disease, these spirochetes can be found not only in the skin but also in the blood, cerebrospinal fluid (CSF), and in small quantities in the myocardium, retina, muscles, bones, liver, meninges, and brain. The body's defence response to infection begins with phagocytosis of the microorganisms. During phagocytosis, Borreliae die, leading to the activation of specific immune defence mechanisms [276, 277].

Cellular immunity responds early to *B. burgdorferi* antigens, aiming to destroy spirochetes. However, in patients with LB, there is a noted decrease in suppressor and natural killer cell activity, which may be a significant mechanism allowing Borrelia to disseminate, including into the nervous system. One of the immune response peculiarities in LB is the delayed onset of the humoral response to *B. burgdorferi* antigens. The peak of the immune response occurs between the 3rd and 6th weeks after the onset of the disease [277]. As the disease progresses, there is an expanded synthesis of antibodies against numerous Borrelia proteins, indicating possible cross-reactivity of the immune system with Borrelia antigens and subsequent formation of autoimmune mechanisms. These antibodies, directed against *B. burgdorferi* proteins and nervous tissue proteins, contribute to inflammation and demyelination [278–281]. There are hypotheses suggesting the potential involvement of Borrelia in initiating autoimmune processes due to activation of myelin-specific T-cells and detection of auto-reactive antibodies to myelin and its components in LB [282]. The prolonged persistence of the pathogen in tissues and its intracellular localization play a key role in these processes.

The dysfunction of the blood-brain barrier (BBB), particularly endothelial cell activation or damage, likely facilitates the penetration of Borrelia and lymphocytes, including various T-cell populations, into the central nervous system (CNS). Evidence supporting this includes increased levels of von Willebrand factor antigen – a marker of endothelial cell activation/destruction – in the serum of 35.7% of patients with neuroborreliosis [283]. Experimental *in vivo* studies on mice have shown that Borrelia circulating in the blood during the early stages of the disease can later penetrate organs and tissues through sites of junction between endothelial cells or even through these cells themselves. This process involves endothelial activation and expression of adhesion molecules on their surface, which significantly facilitates the spirochete's transmigration into deeper vascular structures [284]. Conversely, significant increases in the soluble form of intercellular adhesion molecule-1 (ICAM-1), a major cellular adhesion molecule, have been observed in the cerebrospinal fluid (CSF) of patients with neuroborreliosis, further indicating increased permeability of the BBB.

It is evident that molecular mimicry and the accumulation of T-cell clones that recognize specific Borrelia antigens, which cross-react with human tissue components, play an important role in the development of both chronic arthritis and chronic nervous system involvement in LB. Genetic factors, including carriage of specific HLA system antigens like DR4 and DR2, are also crucial in these reactions.

Over time, the infectious agent itself may play a lesser role, although the inflammatory process persists and is maintained by complex cellular and humoral disturbances involving autoimmune mechanisms. Today, knowledge about auto-reactivity in LB remains controversial [278–281]. It is believed that in both early and late stages of LB, damage to elements of the CNS parenchyma occurs. For instance, in patients with neuroborreliosis (meningoradiculitis and encephalopathy), increased levels of markers of nerve tissue damage and astrocyte cells are detected in the CSF during the early stage of the disease before the start of antibiotic treatment. Their concentration decreases after the initiation of active antibiotic therapy.

The pathogenesis of LB involving the nervous system is complex and multifaceted. During the development of the disease, both humoral and cellular immune responses are triggered, involving inflammatory mediators. In some patients, the engagement of these defence mechanisms is effective, leading to recovery. However, there is evidence that *B. burgdorferi* possesses properties that help them survive by evading the host's immune defences, persisting even in the presence of specific antibodies. These mechanisms include gene recombination of immunodominant surface proteins of Borrelia, resulting in changes to their antigenic determinants. Gene conversion and point mutations contribute to the emergence of new genetic variants of Borrelia capable of evading previously formed immune responses of the host. There is a feedback loop between the humoral response that develops during infection and the expression of various surface antigens of Borrelia [285].

Histologically, affected tissues in LB show lymphocytic and plasma cell infiltration, as well as vasculopathy, vasculitis, and vessel occlusions by proliferating cells. Biopsies of nerves reveal cellular infiltrates along the endoneurium [285].

Neurological involvement, or neuroborreliosis, occurs in 10–60% of LB patients depending on the geographical region [284, 285]. These significant variations in the frequency of neurological manifestations are associated with the peculiarities of Borrelia genospecies and the insufficient study of this problem in certain regions. The highest frequency of nervous system involvement is observed in the north-western and central regions of Russia, ranging from 43% to 64% [283]. Differences in frequency and clinical manifestations of neurological involvement are primarily linked to genetic and antigenic differences among LB pathogens.

To date, specific reliable clinical and laboratory criteria for late forms of LB are under discussion worldwide. It is considered that the diagnosis of these forms of the disease is often both mistaken and insufficiently established. This is primarily due to the lack of universally accepted diagnostic criteria and identification methods for Borrelia that are widely accessible. Furthermore, in cases of chronic LB with neurological involvement, there is often a loss of connection between the development of neurological symptoms and the history of tick attachment, especially in cases of LB without EM [286, 287].

The most challenging aspect in diagnosis involves cases of chronic neuroborreliosis that mimic other nosological forms clinically, such as multiple sclerosis (MS), cerebral vasculitis, amyotrophic lateral sclerosis (ALS), extrapyramidal disorders, and others. The contribution of Borrelia infection to the development of these forms remains inadequately studied. LB has been dubbed the "new great imitator" due to these diagnostic challenges [288]. There is a lack of differential diagnostic criteria for the main manifestations of chronic neuroborreliosis, such as encephalomyelitis, radiculopathy, and encephalopathy.

Questions regarding the pathogenetic mechanisms and risk factors for the development of neurological pathology in chronic LB, as well as the role of autoimmune mechanisms in the development of chronic neuroborreliosis, remain open. Dysfunction of the blood-brain barrier (BBB) is also discussed in foreign literature as playing a role in these processes [289].

We examined 92 patients, divided into 3 groups (Figure 35):

- 15 individuals with acute Lyme borreliosis were examined at disease onset and followed up after 3-4 months from the beginning of the illness to detect disease progression, including 6 (40.0%) males and 9 (60.0%) females aged 18 to 68 years, with a mean age of (48.2 ± 9.4) years.
- 47 patients with possible chronic neuroborreliosis were under observation by the Department of Neurological Diseases of TNMU, including 29 (61.7%) males and 18 (38.3%) females aged 18 to 70 years, with a mean age of (51.0 ± 10.4) years.
- 30 patients with confirmed diagnosis of LD, who were also observed by the Department of Neurological Diseases to study the prevalence of antibodies to B. burgdorferi and to identify cases of LD previously undiagnosed, included 8 (26.7%) males and 22 (73.3%) females aged 19 to 56 years, with a mean age of (36.6 ± 10.3) years.

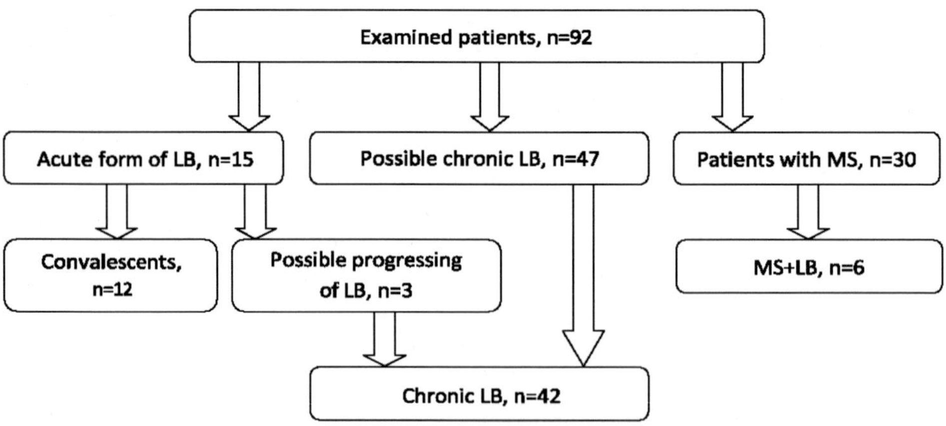

Figure 35. Research design.

The diagnosis of chronic neuroborreliosis was established based on the following criteria:

- Presence of clinical signs of nervous system involvement typical for late stages of LB.

- Development of neurological symptoms more than 6 months after the onset of EM and/or tick bite, or persistence of symptoms for more than 6 months.
- Detection of diagnostic titres of antibodies to *B. burgdorferi* in serum by indirect immunofluorescence assay (IIFA), as well as presence of IgG to Borrelia in immunoblotting.
- Exclusion of other aetiologies of pathological processes in the nervous system that could account for the patient's clinical symptoms.

As a result of clinical and serological examinations, chronic stage of LB with nervous system involvement was diagnosed in 42 patients. The frequency of detection of the main diagnostic criteria for LB is presented in Table 26.

All patients underwent clinical therapeutic and neurological examinations, taking into account epidemiological data (tick bite, stay in forested areas), and the presence of typical LB manifestations in the medical history.

Cognitive functions were assessed using Schulz tables, Luria's "10 words" test, Mini-Mental State Examination (MMSE), Frontal Assessment Battery, and clock drawing test.

Lumbar puncture was performed in 28 (66.7%) neuroborreliosis patients to detect inflammatory changes in the cerebrospinal fluid (CSF).

Electroneuromyography (ENMG) was conducted using a two-channel electromyograph "Neuro-MVP." Fibres of median, ulnar, tibial, and peroneal nerves were examined. Bipolar skin electrodes were used for stimulation during ENMG, measuring parameters of M-response, conduction velocity, residual latency, and conduction blocks.

To assess cerebral blood flow, we measured the lumen and linear (systolic) velocities of the common carotid, internal carotid, and middle cerebral arteries, as well as the Pourcelot resistance index. We determined the lumen of the vertebral arteries and the permeability of the cerebral arteries, and assessed the type of atherosclerotic plaques using the "ACUSON SEQU1A-512" device.

To detect statistical differences in quantitative parameters between patient groups with a normal distribution of features, we used Student's t-test. For features that did not follow a normal distribution and for small sample sizes, we applied the non-parametric Mann-Whitney U test. For all tests, a two-sided significance level of 5% ($p < 0.05$) was chosen to consider group differences statistically significant.

Table 26. Frequency of detection of diagnostic signs of chronic stage Lyme borreliosis in patients with nervous system involvement (n = 42)

Diagnostic criterion	Number of patients	
	Absolute number	%
History of EM + positive serological tests for LB	19	45,2
Acute period of LB without EM + positive serological tests for LB	6	14,3
Absence of acute period of Lyme borreliosis with positive serological tests	17	40,5
Total	42	100,0

When comparing groups based on qualitative characteristics, we used the Pearson's chi-squared test. In cases of small sample sizes (where the frequency in at least one element of the expected frequency table was less than or equal to 5), we employed Fisher's exact test.

Statistical analysis of the study results was conducted using the statistical software Statistica 6.0 (Statsoft Inc., USA).

As known, the acute phase of Lyme disease corresponds to a period of 1–3 months from the onset of the disease, the subacute phase from 3 to 6 months, and the chronic phase involves symptoms persisting for more than 6 months. Severity of the disease is noted to be dependent on its duration. Chronic infection may exhibit both continuous and recurrent courses.

Early involvement of the nervous system in the disease is primarily characterized by syndromes such as cranial neuropathy (most commonly facial), less frequently by radiculopathy, lymphocytic meningitis, and encephalitis (encephalopathy). Often, multiple levels of the nervous system are affected. Any of these symptoms of nervous system involvement may present as the sole clinical manifestation of Lyme borreliosis, without erythema or clear signs of systemic intoxication.

In the early stages of neuroborreliosis, symptoms of involvement are identified in segments located near the EM or the site of tick attachment in 30–50% of cases [290, 291].

All 15 patients with acute neuroborreliosis that we examined were treated in the neurological department for unilateral cranial nerve neuritis: facial nerve in 12 (80.0%) individuals and vestibulocochlear nerve in 3 (20.0%) patients. Due to delayed presentation, antibiotic treatment was expedited. Despite this, 12 patients recovered, although convalescence continued for another 3 months.

We present a clinical case.

Patient O. M., 59 years old (hospital record of inpatient No. 008330), an accountant at PJSC "Ternopil Quarry," was admitted on August 28, 2019, to the Neurology Department No. 1 of Ternopil Regional Clinical Psychoneurological Hospital with complaints of left-sided facial asymmetry, difficulty in puffing out the left cheek, and a sensation of "fullness of tears" in the left eye.

She considers herself ill since August 28, 2019, when facial asymmetry on the left appeared "after spending time outdoors." Due to the nature of her work, she was frequently exposed to tick bites but did not use antibiotics preventively. She does not recall having had any instances of erythema migrans. Blood pressure at onset was 200/100 mmHg.

Examination revealed the following: general condition relatively satisfactory. Skin and visible mucous membranes of normal colour, clean. Tongue moist, clean. Heart sounds rhythmic, tones weakened. Pulse – 76 beats per minute, blood pressure – 170/100 mmHg. Vesicular breathing over the lungs. Abdomen soft, non-tender.

Neurological status: conscious, alert, oriented. Palpebral fissures S > D, pupils D = S. No nystagmus or diplopia. Slight weakness of the left m. orbicularis oculi. Bell's sign (+), lagophthalmos on the left. Trigeminal and occipital points non-tender. Moderately smoothed forehead folds on the left. Flattened left nasolabial fold (Figure 36). Moderate weakness of m. orbicularis oris, m. buccalis on the left. Tongue midline. Speech, voice, swallowing preserved. Muscle strength in limbs – 5 points. Tendon and periosteal reflexes D = S from hands, brisk, from legs: absent right knee reflex, Achilles D = S, brisk, plantar D = S, brisk. No sensory disturbances. Coordination tests performed satisfactorily. No signs of meningeal irritation. Strümpell's sign (+) bilaterally, clearer on the right.

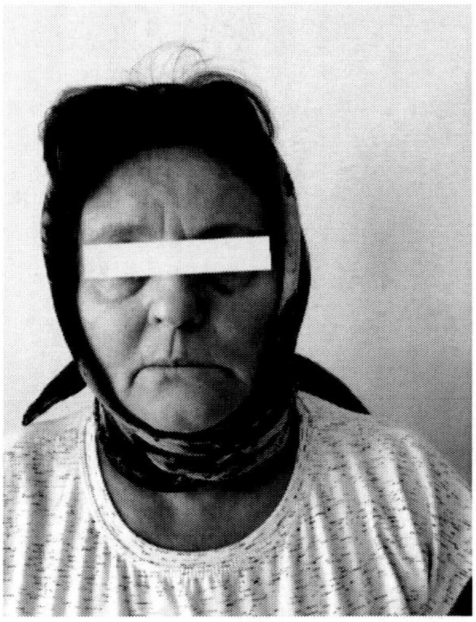

Figure 36. Patient O. M., suffering from acute left-sided facial neuropathy (August 28, 2019) of borrelial aetiology with pronounced prosoparesis on the left (noticeable moderate smoothing of the left forehead fold and significant smoothing of the left nasolabial fold, causing facial asymmetry).

Complete blood count: RBC 4.0 T/L, Hb 128 g/L, leukocytes 13.4 G/L, segmented neutrophils 3%, band neutrophils 86%, lymphocytes 8%, monocytes 3%, ESR 25 mm/hour. Biochemical blood analysis: glucose 5.8 mmol/L, bilirubin 12.0 µmol/L, urea 7.8 mmol/L, total protein 79.8 g/L. RW negative. General urine analysis, stool for helminth eggs and protozoa without peculiarities.

Serological blood tests (September 9, 2019): IgM to B. burgdorferi – 14.277 (norm 0-0.9), IgG to B. burgdorferi – 9.033 (norm 0-1). Immunoblot method (September 16, 2019): IgM and IgG to B. burgdorferi detected.

Thyroid gland hormones (September 23, 2019): TSH 1.88 µIU/mL (norm 0.3-4.0 µIU/mL), free T3 5.74 pmol/L (norm 4.0-8.6 pmol/l), free T4 24.43 pmol/L (norm 10.0-24.5 pmoL/L).

Chest X-ray (August 30, 2019), ECG (August 29, 2019) – within normal limits. EEG (August 29, 2019): signs of diffuse brain irritation with emphasis on brainstem structures. Doppler ultrasound of neck vessels (September 2, 2019): angiospasm with decreased blood flow in vertebral arteries by 20-25% on the right and by 15-20% on the left. Slowed venous outflow in veins causing 5% congestion bilaterally. No vessel patency disorders, haemodynamics, congenital vascular defects, or AVM (arteriovenous malformation) detected. MRI of the brain (August 29, 2019): solitary small foci in both hemispheres of the brain, likely of vascular origin. Cystic formation (cyst?) of the pineal gland. Thyroid ultrasound (September 23, 2019): echosigns of autoimmune thyroiditis.

Consultations: gynaecologist (August 30, 2019) – no pathologies found; ophthalmologist (September 9, 2019; September 16, 2019) – lagophthalmos OS. Swelling of the cornea of the left eye; infectious disease specialist (September 17, 2019) – based on history, clinical and serological evidence, the patient has acute left-sided facial neuropathy (August 28, 2019) of borrelial aetiology with pronounced prosoparesis on the left.

Treatment: ceftriaxone 2 g/day intramuscularly for 14 days, dexamethasone, euphyllin, renalgin, furosemide, actovegin, platyphyllin, nimesulide, diacore, blockades with dexamethasone, iontophoresis with hydrocortisone ointment on the left auricular area.

In a significantly improved clinical condition on October 2, 2019, the patient was discharged home.

Among the remaining 3 patients with acute neuroborreliosis, the clinical manifestations of neuropathy subsided very sluggishly, and soon signs of infection dissemination appeared, which we interpreted as possible progression of Lyme borreliosis.

One of the characteristic features of Lyme borreliosis in the subacute stage is Bannwarth's syndrome, characterized by a combination of meningeal involvement and peripheral nervous system (meningoradiculoneuritis). The meningeal syndrome is notable for mild clinical signs of meningitis. Bannwarth's syndrome is typical primarily for European Lyme borreliosis.

Remote manifestations of the nervous system, which appear months and years after the onset of the disease, often following a prolonged latent period, also include signs of involvement of all parts of the nervous system. Chronic forms of neuroborreliosis include progressive encephalomyelitis, cerebral vasculitis, encephalopathy, radiculopathy, and polyneuropathy [292–294].

Unlike acute manifestations of neuroborreliosis, its late forms are characterized by a slow progressive course, mimicking various diseases such as multiple sclerosis, discirculatory encephalopathy, spinal dystrophic lesions, and others. Moreover, during the prolonged course of the disease, the connection between nervous system damage and tick attachment is often lost, especially in cases of European Lyme borreliosis. Therefore, diagnosing nervous system involvement in Lyme borreliosis is often delayed.

Overall, the frequency of chronic forms of neuroborreliosis is not high and ranges, according to various authors, from 4 to 20% of all cases of Lyme borreliosis. However, there is data indicating that after a tick bite fever (Lyme borreliosis), this figure can reach 85% [295, 296].

Through dynamic clinical and serological examination, we managed to diagnose chronic Lyme borreliosis with nervous system involvement in 42 individuals. In the main group with chronic Lyme borreliosis, there were 28 (66.7%) men and 14 (33.3%) women aged 19 to 70 years, with an average age of (49.3 ± 9.8) years.

We found that the presence of tick bites and the development of typical clinical manifestations in the acute phase of Lyme borreliosis, including symptoms of early dissemination, are characteristic of patients with subsequent development of late forms of Lyme borreliosis. On the other hand, the absence of a documented tick bite history in patients with chronic neuroborreliosis may be due to the fact that bites by male and immature ticks often go unnoticed by people [297].

In a comparative analysis of patients with chronic neuroborreliosis and convalescents from the acute stage, it was found that multiple tick bites and symptoms of early infection dissemination were significantly more frequent in the group with chronic Lyme borreliosis, namely 9 (21.4%) vs. 1 (8.3%) patient ($p < 0.05$) and 27 (64.3%) vs. 2 (16.7%) patients ($p < 0.01$), respectively.

The presence of erythema migrans was significantly more observed in the convalescent group from the acute stage of Lyme borreliosis, while systemic inflammatory syndrome without erythema migrans was more common in patients with subsequent chronicization of the disease. The absence of erythema migrans as a pathognomonic sign of Lyme borreliosis may have led to delayed diagnosis and treatment of the disease (in 14.3% of patients), with subsequent disease progression.

In patients with chronic LB, statistically significantly more often than in the convalescent group, antibiotic treatment was delayed (initiated more than 2 weeks after the onset of the disease) – in 10 (23.8%) and 1 (8.3%) patients, respectively ($p < 0.01$); in 4 (9.5%) individuals with chronic LB, treatment was conducted with a short course.

Thus, in 3 (7.1%) individuals with clinically manifest early disseminated LB in the acute stage and in 18 (42.9%) patients without EM, the diagnosis was established in the late stages of the disease during the development of infection dissemination. It should be noted that according to scientific literature, the frequency of EM-less LB is lower and ranges from 2 to 20% of cases [298].

Nervous system involvement in chronic LB in the patients we examined was presented with various syndromes, the main ones being peripheral nervous system involvement – radiculopathy in 19 (45.2%) patients and polyneuropathy in 8 (19.0%), and central nervous system (CNS) involvement – encephalopathy in 21 (50.0%) and encephalomyelitis in 3 (7.1%) patients. Combined involvement of the peripheral and central nervous systems was observed in 9 (21.4%) individuals. These syndromes are typical for chronic neuroborreliosis [299].

The initial signs of infection chronicization from the moment of tick bite were observed from 6 months to 15 years, with an average of (23.6 ± 14.3) months. According to scientific literature, the latent period in late neuroborreliosis can range from 1.5 to 17 years [300]. Such a prolonged latent course of the disease may be associated with the transition of *B. burgdorferi* into inactive forms (L-forms, cysts) with subsequent reactivation [301].

The onset of chronic forms of neuroborreliosis in the majority (36; 85.7%) of patients was monosymptomatic. The disease most often started with signs of nervous system involvement (in 23; 54.8%), less frequently with joint and muscle symptoms (8; 19.0%), or another organ involvement (5; 11.9%).

At the time of the study, the duration of LB ranged from 6 months to 18 years, with an average of 34.3 months. Despite almost half of the patients experiencing an acute stage of LB, almost all patients were seen in general medical practice networks with other diagnoses.

In most patients (36; 85.7%) who did not receive treatment, there was relentless progression of the pathological process. Less frequently (in 6; 14.3%), there were periods of improvement and worsening.

General infectious syndrome in the late period of LB was observed in almost half of the patients (45.2%). Generalized lymphadenopathy was diagnosed in 6 (14.3%) individuals. Among 5 patients in whom a diagnosis of chronic LB was excluded, general infectious syndrome was observed in 2 individuals, with no lymphadenopathy. Therefore, these manifestations should be taken into account in the differential diagnosis of LB.

Nervous system involvement in the late stage of LB was isolated in 18 (42.9%) patients and combined with extraneural manifestations typical for the chronic course of the disease in 24 (57.1%). Most commonly, the musculoskeletal system was affected in 12 (50.0%) individuals presenting with arthritis, arthralgia, myalgia, less frequently the heart and skin in 1 (8.3%) case each.

Chronic radiculopathy (RP) occurs in approximately 30-60% of patients in the late stages of LB [303]. The course of RP in LB can be recurrent or continuously progressive. Isolated RP without other characteristic signs of the disease is often interpreted by physicians as a manifestation of degenerative spinal disorders.

Patients with RP often complain of radicular pain or distal paresthesias in the limbs. They note a constant pain syndrome refractory to non-steroidal anti-inflammatory drugs (NSAIDs).

Compared to acute LB, these individuals more frequently exhibit symptoms of radicular involvement such as motor or sensory disturbances. Additionally, there is typically a mild intensity of symptoms of muscle fixation and limited range of motion in the spine. RP caused by LB is also characterized by frequent combinations of these clinical manifestations with systemic inflammatory and asthenic syndromes, often accompanied by depression and symptoms of LB progression, predominantly affecting the musculoskeletal system (arthritis, arthralgia, myalgia).

According to our data, RP in the late period of LB was found in 19 (45.2%) patients. Multilevel involvement predominated – 12 (63.2%) individuals had pathology affecting nerve roots and peripheral nerves. Pain syndrome dominated the clinical picture of the disease, with gradual progression noted, as indicated by other researchers [304, 305]. In 7 (16.7%) patients, the pain localization coincided with the tick bite site, which is more typical for early stages of the disease [306]. There was no clear correlation of the pain syndrome intensity with body position and physical load; the pain intensity was moderate at (6.5 ± 2.3) points on the VAS scale, with nocturnal exacerbation of back pain in one person, indicative of an inflammatory nature of the pain syndrome. In most cases, the pain was radiating (69.0%), with bilateral radiation noted in half of the patients (52.4%). The effectiveness of NSAIDs in LB patients was modest, with only 16.7% reporting relief.

Vertebral syndrome was registered in more than half of the patients, characterized as mild or moderate. Isolated painful variant of RP in LB, described by European and predominantly Russian researchers, was not observed [307, 308]. Objectively, sensory disturbances were diagnosed in all patients, limb paresthesias in 29 (69.0%) cases. Most frequently (24 individuals; 82.8%), a combination of radicular and polyneuritic disorders was noted. Peripheral distal paresis was observed in only a quarter of the patients, which is typical for Russian and American variants of LB course [286]. A gradual development of clinical manifestations was noted: the onset of radicular pain, sensory disturbances, followed by paralysis, typical for this condition in LB.

Table 27. Comparative characteristics of radicular pain syndrome in patients with radiculopathy caused by Lyme borreliosis and of vertebral origin

Signs	Patients with RP			
	caused by Lyme borreliosis		vertebrogenic	
	Absolute number, n = 23	%	Absolute number, n = 25	%
Acute onset of the disease with periods of exacerbations and remissions	6	26,1 ± 9,2	15	60,0 ± 9,8*
Gradual progression	17	73,9 ± 9,2	9	36,0 ± 9,6*
Presence of pain	23	100,0 ± 0,0	25	100,0 ± 0,0
Intensity of pain, according to VAS, average score	6,5 ± 2,3		7,0 ± 0,3	
Dependence of pain on body position, physical exertion	6	26,1 ± 9,2	24	96,0 ± 3,9*
Radiation of pain	16	69,6 ± 9,6	17	68,0 ± 9,3
Bilateral radiation	12	52,2 ± 10,4	3	12,0 ± 6,5*
Pain relief with NSAIDs	4	17,4 ± 7,9	20	80,0 ± 8,0*
Pain relief after a course of antibiotics	17	73,9 ± 9,2	Was not applied	

Note (hereafter). * – the difference is significant compared to the group of patients with LB, $p < 0.05$-0.01.

Table 28. Comparative characteristics of vertebral and radicular syndromes in radiculopathy caused by Lyme borreliosis and of vertebral origin

Signs	Patients with RP			
	caused by Lyme borreliosis		vertebrogenic	
	Absolute number, n = 23	%	Absolute number, n = 25	%
Pain upon palpation of paravertebral points and spinous processes	15	65,2 ± 9,9	25	100,0 ± 0,0*
Tonic tension of paravertebral muscles	16	69,6 ± 9,6	25	100,0 ± 0,0*
Restriction of movements in spinal segments: – moderate – pronounced	15 10 5	65,2 ± 9,9 43,5 ± 10,3 21,7 ± 8,6	25 14 11	100,0 ± 0,0* 56,0 ± 9,9 44,0 ± 9,9*
Signs of tension	13	56,5 ± 10,3	25	100,0 ± 0,0*
Combination of radicular and polyneuropathic sensory disorders	19	82,6 ± 7,9	0	0,0 ± 0,0*
Sensory disorders of radicular type	4	17,4 ± 7,9	25	100,0 ± 0,0*
Presence of paresthesia in the limbs	16	69,6 ± 9,6	17	68,0 ± 9,3
Motor disturbances in distal parts of the limbs	5	21,7 ± 8,6	3	12,0 ± 6,5

Given that most patients with RP were diagnosed with osteochondrosis before LB diagnosis, we compared the clinical manifestations of chronic RP in LB (main group, n = 23) with vertebral RP (comparison group, n = 25) to identify differential diagnostic criteria for these conditions. The groups were comparable in terms of gender and age composition. The study results (Tables 27, 28) showed that in LB, the disease more often had a gradual progressive course – in (73.9 ± 9.2%) of cases, while vertebral RP was characterized by periods of remission and exacerbation – in (60.0 ± 9.8%) of cases. Multilevel involvement with multiple root and nerve involvement was significantly more common ($p < 0.01$) in the LB group.

The intensity of pain assessed by VAS was nearly the same in both groups. In LB patients with RP, pain syndrome depended only slightly on body position and physical load – in (26.1 ± 9.2%) of cases, whereas in vertebral RP, this dependence was significantly more pronounced – in (96.0 ± 3.9%) ($p < 0.01$). Only LB patients reported nocturnal pain. In most cases in both groups, the pain was radiating; however, bilateral radiation was significantly more common in LB patients – (52.2 ± 10.4%) versus (12.0 ± 6.5%) in the comparison group ($p < 0.01$).

The symptoms of paravertebral muscle tension and limited range of motion in the spine with LB were weaker and observed significantly less frequently compared to vertebral radiculopathy (VRP) ($p < 0.01$ and $p < 0.05$, respectively). The combination of radicular and polyneuritic sensory disorders was typical for LB, occurring in (82.6 ± 7.9%) of cases, while radicular type sensory disorders were characteristic of vertebral radiculopathy, present in all (100%) patients ($p < 0.01$).

General infectious syndrome and generalized lymphadenopathy were observed only in patients with chronic LB, in (26.1 ± 9.2%) and (13.0 ± 7.0%) respectively. Extraneural manifestations were significantly more frequent ($p < 0.05$) in LB compared to degenerative spine disorders. The use of NSAIDs for pain relief in patients with LB and VRP was significantly less frequent compared to vertebral radiculopathy, in (17.4 ± 7.9%) versus (80.0 ± 8.0%) of cases ($p < 0.01$).

Isolated cranial nerve involvement at late stages of LB was detected in only 2 patients: one with facial nerve neuropathy 6 months after tick bite associated with LB, and another with retrobulbar neuritis 7 months after acute LB. Generally, isolated cranial neuropathies are more characteristic of early stages of the disease [309].

In chronic polyneuropathy (PNP), patients commonly complain of moderate pain, paresthesia, or weakness in distal parts of the limbs. Sensory disturbances are typically mosaic or can be localized distally, asymmetrically or symmetrically. Often, there is a reduction in tendon reflexes to their absence, or mild limb paresis.

Electroneuromyography usually reveals predominantly axonal damage to peripheral nerves with possible partial demyelination of proximal and distal segments. Studies have shown mosaic changes in parameters, indicating multiple mononeuropathy that may remain subclinical without clinical signs [309, 310].

Nerve biopsy shows perivascular lymphocytic and plasma cell infiltration around small and medium-calibre epineural vessels and in epineural tissues. Additionally, disseminated loss of myelinated fibres due to axonal degeneration is observed [311].

According to researchers [283], all 30 examined patients with chronic radiculopolyneuropathy experienced sensory disorders, with radicular type observed in 5 (16.7%) cases, and a combination of radicular and polyneuritic in 25 (83.3%) patients. 21 (70.0%) individuals reported limb paresthesia, while 3 (10.0%) had pain along nerve tracts. Symptoms of muscle tension and limited range of motion in the affected spinal segment were noted in 22 (73.3%) patients. Importantly, vertebral syndromes were mild. Motor disturbances in the form of mild distal paresis were found in 7 (23.3%) patients, and moderate in 3 (10.0%). Muscle atrophy of the affected limb and disturbances in muscle tone were recorded in isolated cases. Bannwarth's syndrome was diagnosed in 3 patients. The absence of pronounced inflammatory changes in cerebrospinal fluid distinguishes neuroborreliosis in Russia from the European variant. Nervous system involvement was isolated in only 9 (30.0%) patients, and combined with other systemic manifestations typical for chronic LB in 21 (70.0%) cases [283].

According to our data, chronic neuroborreliosis was significantly more often diagnosed in patients with PNP compared to those without LB, as well as in cases of combined encephalopathy and radiculopathy ($p < 0.05$), and significantly less frequently in isolated cranial nerve neuropathies ($p < 0.05$) and encephalomyelitis ($p < 0.05$).

We diagnosed chronic mono- or polyneuropathies of the limbs in 1 (2.4%) and 5 (11.9%) out of 42 patients, respectively. In one patient with multiple mononeuropathy, disturbances in superficial and deep sensitivity of upper and lower limbs were detected in the mononeuritic type, without diagnosed motor disturbances.

Upon objective examination, most patients with PNP exhibited disturbances in superficial and deep sensitivity of the polyneuritic type. Distal peripheral limb paresis was diagnosed in 3 out of 5 such individuals, and segmental vegetative disturbances in 1 patient. In another patient, polyneuritic disorders were subclinical and diagnosed only through electroneuromyographic examination, as noted in other studies [286].

Thus, the clinical picture of poly- and mononeuropathies was characterized by a predominance of sensory disorders over motor and vegetative disturbances.

According to electroneuromyography findings, patients with LB exhibiting signs of peripheral nervous system involvement showed decreased M-response amplitudes, indicating predominant axonal nerve degeneration. According to several researchers, the process in chronic LB is often generalized, despite clinically isolated nerve involvement [312].

Against the background of antibacterial therapy, a significant increase in M-response amplitudes and conduction velocity of affected nerves was observed, indirectly indicating the infectious aetiology of peripheral nervous system pathology in LB.

Encephalopathy (EP) is one of the characteristic manifestations of late LB, often dominating the clinical picture of the disease. The frequency of encephalopathy varies from 7–15% to 76% in different regions of the world [313].

The manifestations of EP in LB mainly include cognitive impairments, evidenced by reduced concentration of attention and memory, speech disturbances such as difficulty in word finding, and focal neurological symptoms. Psychological symptoms such as depression, irritability, or paranoia may also occur. Neurocognitive tests show statistically significant declines in verbal and visual memory. These disorders, along with sleep disturbances, significantly reduce the quality of life of patients and can lead to persistent loss of workability. In some cases, memory disturbances are secondary to depression or chronic pain in patients with LB. Often, clinical symptoms of EP are not accompanied by inflammatory changes in the cerebrospinal fluid. MRI examination can reveal multifocal lesions in the white matter of the brain.

According to some authors, the structure of EP in LB highlights tendon hyperreflexia, mild to moderate cerebellar disorders, asthenic syndrome, and concurrent peripheral nerve involvement [313, 314].

Due to the nonspecificity of clinical manifestations, EP in LB often mimics chronic fatigue syndrome, depression, normal aging with slight memory decline, early stages of Alzheimer's disease, and chronic cerebral ischemia. According to researchers [313, 315], signs of EP in the late stages of LB were found in 50.0% of patients with neuroborreliosis. Cognitive impairments were noted: mild in 24.1% of patients, moderate in 48.3%, and severe in 27.6%. In 86.0% of patients, cognitive impairments were combined with vestibulo-atactic syndrome and pyramidal insufficiency, and 65.5% had asthenic syndrome, with varying degrees of depression in 92.8%.

The mechanism of EP development in LB is not yet fully understood. It remains unclear whether it is a manifestation of direct spirochaetal infection, the action of Borrelia exotoxins, or related to dysfunction of the central nervous system due to a previously acquired infection. Perhaps different mechanisms are involved, as in some cases, these manifestations regress with antibiotic therapy, while in some patients, they persist or appear after treatment [316]. In the chronic period of LB, we identified EP in 21 (50.0%) patients, including 15 (71.4%) men and 6 (28.6%) women aged 19 to 68 years, with a mean age of (44.2 ± 6.3) years.

In the development of EP in the late stages of LB, patients complained of memory and attention deficits, sleep disturbances, irritability, mood decline, and speech disturbances such as "difficulty in word finding." Combined disturbances were observed in the majority of patients (85.7%), consistent with findings in other studies [317].

Disorders in the function of the first functional block of the brain, identified using Shulte's tables and Luria's "10 Words" test, were found in the majority (80.9%) of patients, manifesting as nonspecific memory and attention disorders, slowed task execution, fatigue, and decreased cognitive performance. In 3 (14.3%) patients, complaints of attention and memory disturbances were rather subjective, accompanied by pronounced depression, which could mimic cognitive impairments. Other authors also suggest that memory disturbances in chronic LB may be secondary to depression or chronic pain [318].

The results of the MMSE test in 66.7% of patients showed mild cognitive decline, moderate cognitive deficit in 14.3%, and normal values in 19.0%. No severe cognitive impairments were noted in any of the examined individuals. Frontal lobe test batteries diagnosed mild cognitive impairments in 47.6% of cases. Using the clock drawing test, mild cognitive impairments were found in 57.1% of patients and moderate impairments in 4.7%.

Thus, patients with chronic EP in LB predominantly exhibited mild to moderate impairments in various types of cognitive operations (praxis, gnosis, and language disorders) based on neuropsychological testing.

According to several foreign authors, neuropsychological tests in patients with EP in LB typically reveal impairments in verbal and visual memory, and sometimes moderate depression [319]. In the patients we examined, various cognitive impairments were predominantly observed.

All patients with EP exhibited focal neurological symptoms. Pyramidal tract involvement syndrome was noted in 17 (81.0%) patients, atactic syndrome in 15 (71.4%), cranial nerve involvement in 2 (9.5%), and extrapyramidal syndrome in 1 (4.8%). Some authors also highlight tendon hyperreflexia (24–39%) and mild to moderate cerebellar disorders (8–44%), although less frequently compared to our patient group [320].

MRI of the brain before antibiotic therapy revealed periventricular punctate changes and mild ventriculomegaly in 14 (66.7%) patients, with no pathology detected in 1 (4.8%) case. Post-antibiotic therapy, 3 (14.3%) individuals were diagnosed with post-infectious focal gliosis in the white matter of the cerebral hemispheres.

One of the late manifestations of LB is progressive encephalomyelitis. Chronic borrelial encephalomyelitis (CBEM) was first described in 1985 by R. Ackermann et al., in 8 LB patients. Subsequently, a group of 44 patients was examined, presenting predominantly cerebral manifestations resembling multifocal encephalitis or spinal symptoms typical of MS. Currently, the frequency of encephalomyelitis detection in LB averages 4–5% [281], although other authors report rates ranging from 4 to 20% of LB cases involving the nervous system [321, 322].

Borrelial progressive encephalomyelitis is usually observed in patients aged 40–60 years, equally affecting men and women, with cases among children being rare. The duration of the disease until diagnosis can range from 6 months to 25 years, sometimes developing within the first year after EM. Typically, there is a slow progression of nervous system involvement, gradual worsening of the pathological process mimicking other nosological forms, including MS, disseminated encephalomyelitis. Most patients do not report a preceding EM or tick bite. This contributes to delayed diagnosis.

Unlike acute CNS involvement, progressive encephalomyelitis rarely presents with a previous root syndrome, headache, or clinical signs of infection. A more typical presentation involves a slow progressive course without pain syndrome, occasionally noted during exacerbations. There are usually no asymptomatic periods. Similar to neurosyphilis, both spinal and cerebral types of lesions can occur. The main symptoms of borrelial encephalomyelitis in LB include spastic paraparesis and tetraparesis, ataxia, dysfunction of pelvic organs, and cognitive impairments such as memory and attention deficits. These manifestations resemble MS symptoms. However, in early neuroborreliosis, unlike MS, intellectual-memory disorders dominate the clinical picture. Additionally, the depth of paresis, ataxia, and pelvic disorders is usually less severe compared to MS. Encephalomyelitis symptoms in LB often accompany the involvement of spinal root or cranial nerves, diagnosed in approximately a quarter of patients. Vestibulocochlear nerve involvement is more frequent (15–80% of cases). Polyorgan involvement, including the heart, joints, and eyes, is possible. The most characteristic combination involves chronic nervous system and joint damage.

Similar to acute Lyme neuroborreliosis, progressive encephalomyelitis is characterized by involvement of cranial nerves, but predominantly affects the vestibulocochlear nerve (in 15 to 80% of cases) and the optic nerve in 5–10% [323].

Instrumental and laboratory methods significantly aid in diagnosing progressive borrelial encephalomyelitis. For instance, electroencephalography (EEG) often reveals pathological changes confirming multifocal involvement. MRI detects inflammatory changes in the substance of the brain and spinal cord in half of the cases. Borrelial infection may act as a trigger for pathological changes, explaining the occasional presence of large foci of white matter involvement. MRI findings sometimes include nonspecific multiple periventricular foci in the white matter of the brain, similar to those seen in MS. However, these changes are not obligatory. Autopsy data of a patient with chronic progressive encephalomyelitis described chronic basal leptomeningitis, ependymitis, and leptomeningeal obliterative inflammatory vasculopathy with infarctions in the myelencephalon [281].

According to most authors, the diagnostic criteria for borrelial encephalomyelitis include finding inflammatory changes in cerebrospinal fluid (CSF) such as lymphocytic pleocytosis, elevated protein levels, and intrathecal synthesis of IgM, IgG, and IgA antibodies against Borrelia. Additional evidence supporting borrelial aetiology includes partial or complete regression of symptoms following specific antibiotic therapy.

According to the National Multiple Sclerosis Society of the USA, two studies in endemic Lyme areas investigated cases of neuroborreliosis among patients with a suspected diagnosis of MS. In one study, based on the detection of antibodies to *B. burgdorferi* in blood and CSF, atypical MRI changes, and absence of oligoclonal bands, the diagnosis of MS was excluded in favour of Lyme disease. The second study showed that encephalomyelitis in patients with a likely diagnosis of MS may be due to neuroborreliosis only in isolated cases.

According to N. S. Baranova [283], among 18 patients with a positive titre of antibodies to Borrelia in blood serum, borrelial aetiology of developed encephalomyelitis was found only in 1 (5.6%) patients with a history of acute Lyme disease. In 6 (33.3%) seropositive patients with moderate response to etiotropic treatment and absence of intrathecal antibody synthesis to *B. burgdorferi*, a combination of MS and chronic Lyme disease could be considered. Positive results in 11 (61.1%) patients with MS and positive serologic testing for Lyme disease were interpreted as pseudo-positive upon dynamic serological testing.

Typically, a specific antibody immune response can be detected in both CSF and blood serum, facilitating differential diagnosis from other systemic inflammatory diseases involving the nervous system (e.g., sarcoidosis, systemic lupus erythematosus).

However, sometimes unexpected combinations of diseases arise, which need to be excluded during differential diagnosis. Here is a clinical case.

Patient L., born in 1975. History of the disease: considers himself ill since May 2017, when, without an objective cause, body temperature rose to 37.5°C, initial signs of weakness primarily in the muscles of the shoulder girdle, periorbital swelling, fatigue. Upon examination (June 2017), complete blood count showed: haemoglobin – 134 g/L, ESR – 12 mm/hr, leukopenia – 2.68 G/L, thrombocytopenia – 112 G/L, hypertransaminasaemia – AST 80.3 U/L, ALT 59.5 U/L. Albumin content and protein fractions were within normal limits. Urinalysis was unremarkable.

Since August 2017, increased periorbital swelling with bluish discolouration, facial muscle atrophy resembling a mask, erythema on the exposed parts of the body ("décolleté" symptom), increasing fatigue were noted. At this time, laboratory tests for the first time showed elevated levels of creatine phosphokinase (CPK) up to 628 U/L (normal range 20-200 U/L), lactate dehydrogenase (LDH) – up to 542 U/L (normal range 135-225 U/L), creatinine – up to 134 μmol/L (normal range 71-106 μmol/L), with persistent thrombocytopenia (110 G/L) and leukopenia (2.6 G/L).

Considering typical manifestations such as "dermatomyositis oculi" symptom, erythema on exposed skin areas ("décolleté" symptom), proximal muscle weakness, facial muscle atrophy resembling a mask, and elevated CPK levels, dermatomyositis was diagnosed. Intravenous methylprednisolone therapy was started at a dose of 60 mg/day. During this treatment, body temperature normalized, periorbital swelling significantly decreased, CPK, AST, ALT levels decreased, and leukocyte and platelet counts returned to normal. However, after 2 weeks, likely due to rapid tapering of corticosteroid dose, fever recurred, periorbital swelling worsened, and signs of vasculitis on exposed skin areas intensified. Cyclophosphamide 1000 mg in combination with intravenous methylprednisolone 500 mg monthly was added to therapy.

During the observation period, oncological screening was performed, including CT of the chest organs, MRI of the brain, and consultations with specialists, which did not reveal pathology.

The mentioned therapy provided rapid positive dynamics: body temperature normalized, skin erythema subsided, muscle strength increased, and CPK levels decreased to 152 U/L, LDH to 224 U/L, AST to 36 U/L, ALT to 32 U/L. Haematological parameters remained within normal limits.

However, during this period (since October 2017), signs of focal CNS involvement rapidly developed: bilateral facial nerve paresis (with preserved sensitivity), ptosis of lower eyelids leading to incomplete eyelid closure and corneal drying, unilateral auditory nerve neuritis accompanied by almost complete deafness in the affected ear, dizziness upon orthostasis. Due to progressing leg muscle weakness, the patient became unable to walk independently.

It was unlikely that the mentioned focal symptoms were caused by dermatomyositis. Therefore, they were interpreted as manifestations of polyneuropathy, which was later confirmed by EMG.

A repeat MRI of the brain in December 2017 revealed signs of brain ooedema and multiple infiltrative foci in the cortical layer of both frontal lobes and in the right temporal lobe.

To search for the cause of activated latent neuroinfection, additional serological studies were performed, excluding syphilis, HIV infection, herpes infections (anti-IgM to HSV, VZV, CMV not detected, corresponding anti-IgG within reference ranges). However, ELISA indicated a high titre of anti-IgG to B. burgdorferi – 4.33 R (reference values: R < 0.8 – negative, R≥1.1 – positive result) in the absence of anti-IgM. Analysis of the cerebrospinal fluid showed an even higher titre of anti-IgG to B. burgdorferi – 6.12 R (CSF-serum index (CSI) = 1.41), with CSI for all antigens of herpes, rubella, measles, and other immunoglobulins <0.8, reliably indicating neuroborreliosis. Immunoblotting was used to confirm the ELISA findings regarding Lyme disease: anti-IgM to B. burgdorferi – borderline result (anti-IgM: detected to p41, to OspC Bb, OspC Bg – borderline result), anti-IgG to B. burgdorferi – detected (anti-IgG: to VlsE B. garinii, to p41 – detected, to p21, p18 – borderline result). Infection with Ehrlichia and Anaplasma was excluded during laboratory examination.

Thus, considering the clinical (focal demyelinating CNS lesions), serological (presence of anti-IgG to B. burgdorferi in cerebrospinal fluid and serum), and instrumental (MRI – multiple infiltrative lesions and brain ooedema) findings, as well as after excluding other causes of pathological processes in the nervous system that could explain the current clinical symptoms, Lyme borreliosis was diagnosed in the patient at the late stage of infection: CNS involvement manifested as encephalomyelitis (focal changes in the cortical layer of both frontal lobes and the right temporal lobe), cranial nerve involvement, peripheral polyneuropathy, myopathic syndrome, and high seropositivity of anti-IgG to Borrelia.

Refining the diagnosis required appropriate treatment adjustments: cyclophosphamide was discontinued, the dose of glucocorticoids was reduced, and antibacterial therapy was initiated – ceftriaxone 2.0 g/day intravenously for 3 weeks. Additionally, neurotropin 10 mg twice daily for 1 month, berlithion 600 mg/day, and vitamin E 400 mg/day were prescribed.

In January 2018, against the background of the mentioned antibacterial therapy, prednisolone 40 mg/day, and discontinuation of cytostatics, the clinical picture stabilized, and symptoms of leg polyneuropathy slowly began to diminish – the patient could sit independently and walk with the help of walkers.

The diagnostic and therapeutic management complexity was driven by the difficulty in differential diagnosis. On one hand, the presence of vasculitis, fever, leukopenia, and thrombocytopenia in the clinical picture before glucocorticoid treatment required excluding systemic lupus erythematosus and systemic vasculitis primarily. However, negative results of laboratory tests for rheumatic diseases (anti-DNA, antinuclear factor, anti-Sm, etc.) did not allow a definitive diagnosis of these conditions. On the other hand, considering the progressive multifocal brain involvement, differential diagnosis included multiple sclerosis and progressive multifocal leukoencephalopathy. The latter is a progressive demyelinating CNS disorder caused by reactivation of the latent JC virus of the Papovaviridae family and manifests against the background of immunosuppression: HIV infection, lymphoproliferative diseases, malignant tumours, etc.

Analysis of medical history, clinical picture, laboratory, and instrumental data justified excluding the mentioned neurological pathologies. Instead, clear positive dynamics of the neurological status with antibacterial therapy confirmed the diagnosis of Lyme borreliosis.

Therefore, in this patient, the onset of dermatomyositis against the background of active immunosuppressive therapy was accompanied by subsequent manifestation of latent Lyme borreliosis.

Isolated myelopathy occurs in 5-10% of cases of chronic Lyme borreliosis. It is characterized by moderate conductive disorders of superficial and deep sensitivity, and urinary dysfunction of the central type [297].

According to our data, CBEM was detected in 3 (7.1%) patients. Two of them had asthenia, as well as cognitive disorders such as memory impairment and concentration difficulties; one patient also had a systemic infectious syndrome combined with headache, arthralgia, and myalgia.

CBEM is characterized by a primary progressive course of the disease. All three patients showed signs of combined central and peripheral nervous system involvement. Predominantly observed were pyramidal, cerebellar, and sensory disturbances, signs of cranial nerve involvement; dysfunction of pelvic organs, which is generally characteristic of this condition [288], was not observed.

On MRI examination of the brain, foci of demyelination were found in 1 out of 3 cases. These findings are consistent with the views of other researchers who believe that some patients with neuroborreliosis exhibit focal lesions mainly in the white matter of the brain [324, 325].

All mentioned patients with CBEM were treated with antibiotics. The time of initiation of antibiotic therapy from the onset of neurological symptoms ranged from 1 to 8 months. Clinical improvement along with a decrease in antibody titres to Borrelia in serum was observed in 2 patients. Lack of effect after treatment could be associated with a prolonged course of the disease and predominance of autoimmune processes over infectious ones. The scientific literature has repeatedly suggested the possible involvement of *B. burgdorferi* in initiating autoimmune processes [326]. As the disease progresses, the spectrum of antibodies to many Borrelia proteins expands, which may be a risk factor for cross-reactivity of the immune system with Borrelia and host antigens. Prolonged persistence of the pathogen in tissues and its intracellular localization are given a leading role in this process [275].

Based on their clinical manifestations, CBEM most closely resembles MS, which prompted a comparative characterization of these two conditions to identify differential diagnostic features. A comparison group was composed of 24 patients with clinically definite MS according to the McDonald criteria (2005), without antibodies to B. burgdorferi in serum. Comparative analysis of the MS and CBEM groups identified tentative differential diagnostic features (Table 29).

A history of tick attachment, the presence of EM, systemic infectious syndrome, asthenia, and arthralgia are predominantly characteristic for patients with CBEM. At the same time, in endemic areas for Lyme borreliosis, large segments of the population may be exposed to tick bites, explaining a history of tick bites in 4 (16.7%) patients with MS.

Table 29. Comparative characterization of neurological status at the time of examination in multiple sclerosis and chronic borrelial encephalomyelitis

Syndrome	Characteristics of the syndrome		Group of patients	
			MS, n = 24	CBEM, n = 3
Signs of cranial nerve involvement	Optic nerve neuropathy		1	0
	Oculomotor nerve neuropathy		3	2
	Vestibulocochlear nerve neuropathy		1	0
	Facial nerve neuropathy		3	0
	Trigeminal nerve neuropathy		1	0
	Total		9 (37,5%)	2 з 3
Pyramid disturbances	Pyramid insufficiency without paresis		9	0
	Spastic paraparesis		6	1
	Central hemiparesis		3	0
	Spastic tetraparesis		0	1
	Spastic monoparesis		3	1
	Total		21 (87,5%)	3 з 3
Cerebellar symptoms			22 (91,7%)	2 з 3
Sensory disturbances	PNS involvement	Polyneuropathy	4	1
		Radiculopathy	0	2
	CNS + PNS involvement	Conduction type + polyneuropathy	1	0
	CNS involvement	Conduction type	6	0
	Total		11 (45,8%)	3 з 3

The onset of the disease with an isolated syndrome, particularly involving optic, vestibulocochlear, facial, or trigeminal nerves, was observed only in patients with MS and not in patients with CBEM. Therefore, the debut of the disease with retrobulbar, vestibulocochlear, facial, and trigeminal neuritis more strongly supports a diagnosis of MS rather than Lyme borreliosis. Overall, the frequency of optic nerve involvement in chronic neuroborreliosis is low (5-10%) and is more of an exclusion diagnosis [286].

Cranial nerve involvement in MS was predominantly associated with brainstem involvement, while in CBEM it was associated with nerve roots. Sensory disturbances were less frequently observed in the MS group – 11 (45.8%) patients compared to the CBEM group (all 3 patients).

Pyramidal insufficiency without paresis was noted only in the MS group (9 out of 24 individuals) and none in the CBEM group. Spastic paraparesis and monoparesis were observed in both groups. However, central hemiparesis developed in only 3 individuals with MS and none with CBEM. Additionally, spastic tetraparesis was observed in only 1 patient with CBEM and none with MS.

In MS, sensory disorders due to CNS pathway involvement were characteristic, whereas CBEM typically involved the peripheral nervous system with the development of polyneuritic or radicular types of sensory disorders.

Foci of demyelination in the brain were detected only in the MS group upon MRI examination. Conversely, all 3 patients with CBEM showed clinical symptoms indicating focal brain substance involvement.

Upon MRI examination of the spinal cord, foci of demyelination were found in 16 (66.7%) MS patients and none in CBEM patients. Scientific literature also indicates a more typical presence of lesions at the spinal cord level in MS compared to neuroborreliosis [325].

Thus, the main distinctive clinical manifestations of encephalomyelitis in Lyme borreliosis (CBEM) compared to MS include: a primary progressive course of the disease, involvement of the peripheral nervous system with root pathology, absence of involvement of the optic, vestibulocochlear, facial, and trigeminal nerves, and multi-organ manifestations.

In all 30 patients with a confirmed diagnosis of MS, the presence of antibodies to *B. burgdorferi* in serum was determined to detect undiagnosed cases of Lyme borreliosis. According to serological studies, antibodies to B. burgdorferi were not detected in 24 (80.0%) MS patients, and a combination of confirmed MS and probable Lyme borreliosis was diagnosed in 6 (20.0%) cases. Several studies also noted a statistically significant association between MS and the presence of antibodies to *B. burgdorferi* in serum [325, 326].

Differences in the MS+LB group compared to the MS group were related to epidemiological peculiarities and the addition of extraneural clinical manifestations of LB to the overall disease picture. Tick attachment was significantly more frequent in patients from the MS+LB group compared to the isolated MS group – in 4 out of 6 (66.7%) and 4 out of 24 (16.7%) cases, respectively, $p < 0.05$.

Sensory disturbances and polyneuropathy were diagnosed in 5 out of 6 individuals (83.3%) in the MS+LB group. In contrast, such disorders were only found in 10 (41.6%) patients with isolated MS ($p < 0.05$). All 6 MS+LB patients complained of pain in large joints, which was three times more frequent than in the group of patients with only MS. Antibacterial therapy was administered to all 6 patients in the MS+LB group. During follow-up, a decrease in antibody titres to *B. burgdorferi* in serum was observed. Clinical improvement, manifested by reduced general weakness and ataxia, was noted in 3 (50.0%) patients after the course of antibacterial therapy.

Thus, in 20% of patients with confirmed MS, its combination with LB was observed. Lyme infection contributed to a polysymptomatic debut of MS, more frequent involvement of the sensory sphere, development of polyneuropathy, and arthralgia. The observed positive effect after the course of antibacterial therapy for LB in MS+LB patients indirectly indicated the activity of the Borrelia-induced infectious process.

The dynamics of IgM and IgG antibody levels to B. burgdorferi in serum at the late stages of neuroborreliosis were assessed using the ELISA in 28 patients. The mean values and interquartile range of anti-IgM to *B. burgdorferi* before treatment were 1.33 (0.50; 1.70) units, and after therapy, they were 0.86 (0.30; 1.10) units, significantly lower ($p < 0.05$). The mean values and interquartile range of anti-IgG to *B. burgdorferi* in patients before treatment were 2.18 (0.30; 2.70) units, and after therapy, they were 0.92 (0.20; 0.80) units, which were also significantly lower ($p < 0.05$).

In total, after treatment, diagnostically significant antibody titres were not detected in 23 out of 28 patients (82.1%). Diagnostically significant titres of anti-IgM and/or anti-IgG to *B. burgdorferi* persisted in 5 (17.9%) patients, with only anti-IgM in 1 (3.6%), only anti-IgG in 2 (7.1%), and both anti-IgM and anti-IgG in 2 (7.1%) individuals. Moreover, in all patients, there was no increase in antibody titres or progression of the disease during the study period.

Therefore, in the majority of patients with chronic neuroborreliosis undergoing therapy, there was a noted decrease in antibody titres to non-diagnostic levels. In some patients, however, these titres remained elevated, which, in the absence of new clinical signs, does not indicate progression of Lyme borreliosis.

CSF examinations were conducted in 11 out of 42 patients with chronic neuroborreliosis, all prior to the initiation of antibacterial therapy. Lymphocytic pleocytosis was found in only 2 (18.2%) patients, and elevated protein levels were observed in 3 (27.2%) patients. No dependence on the timing of illness onset was established for the detection of inflammatory changes in the CSF.

Thus, in the study group, inflammatory changes in the CSF were diagnosed in only a quarter of patients, which may be associated with the specific features of neuroborreliosis in our patient population, including immune deficiency and the addition of autoimmune processes during prolonged disease course. It was noted that in the development of a protracted and chronic course, there was suppression of specific antibody production [327].

According to scientific literature sources, nervous system involvement in Lyme borreliosis occurs in approximately 10-25% of patients. Signs of such involvement are observed in both acute (subacute) and chronic disease courses.

B. burgdorferi s. l. can affect all parts of the nervous system, manifesting with a wide range of clinical symptoms and syndromes:

- Mono(poly)neuritis
- Lymphocytic meningitis
- Chorioretinitis
- Meningoradiculoneuritis
- Myelitis with paraplegia
- Myeloradiculoneuritis

- Focal or diffuse encephalitis with manifestations:
  - Extrapyramidal, pyramidal, psychotic symptoms
  - Paroxysmal disorders of consciousness
  - Epileptic seizures
  - Cerebral vasculitis with brain infarctions
  - Progressive encephalomyelitis.

All these syndromes can occur in isolation or in various combinations. However, the presence of only one syndrome is quite rare (in 8% of patients). Initially, nervous system involvement predominantly has an inflammatory character. As the disease progresses, manifestations of degenerative changes in nervous tissue become more distinct [321].

In 85% of cases, the first sign of the disease is EM, accompanied by moderate symptoms of general infectious intoxication (fever, often subfebrile, body aches, and headache). Another common symptom is radicular and pseudoradicular pain, noted in up to 70% of patients with nervous system involvement, with 40% experiencing these symptoms at the onset of the disease. In certain cases, neuroborreliosis starts with cranial nerve involvement (12%), headache (10%), myalgia (7%), or fever (5%) [328, 329].

It is important to note a certain stage-wise appearance of symptoms in the involvement of the nervous system.

1. Tick attachment.
2. Development of EM (in case of tick attachment) after an incubation period averaging 12 days.
3. Onset of radicular pain on average 10-15 days (range from 0 to 95 days) after the development of EM.
4. Appearance of other neurological symptoms on average 40 days after the onset of EM (range from 0 to 150 days).

As is known, organic lesions of borrelial aetiology are accompanied by an inflammatory reaction. Its main mechanisms are only partially studied today and relate to the process of interaction between Borrelia, non-specific, and specific factors of organism resistance. The reactions of Borrelia interaction with components of the humoral (antibodies and complement system) and cellular (activated T-lymphocytes) links of the immune system determine the further mechanism of not only local but also general inflammation. Inflammatory reactions persist until specific and non-specific factors of organism resistance completely eliminate the pathogens.

Lesions of internal organs and systems in the chronic course of the disease are accompanied by pronounced clinical manifestations. Often the disease acquires a recurrent course, where exacerbations alternate with asymptomatic periods of varying duration. In other cases, the disease progresses gradually. There are known cases when initial clinical manifestations of organ and system damage appear months or even years after the primary infection, indicating the possibility of a latent (asymptomatic) period of borrelial infection. Such a wide spectrum of clinical course variants of chronic infection points to a certain inadequacy of the immune system, which is unable to completely immobilize the infectious process. Persistence of Borrelia over a long period is characterized by the formation of an unstable balance between the pathogen and the patient's organism. Each exacerbation is accompanied by an increase in the number of Borrelia and intensification of inflammatory reactions aimed at bringing relations to a new equilibrium state. Specific mechanisms that enable prolonged persistence of Borrelia under conditions of evident immune response can only be hypothesized.

The cause of organic lesions in acute or chronic LB can largely be attributed to the variability of factors that induce inflammation. Under the influence of various factors of organism resistance, Borrelia form membranous protrusions containing lipoproteins (OspA, OspB, OspC). These lipoproteins are potent inducers of inflammatory reactions, particularly characteristic of OspA. Persisting on the surface of Borrelia, they can activate both non-specific resistance cells (macrophages) and polyclonal cells of the immune system (B- and T-lymphocytes). Activation of polyclonal B-lymphocytes leads to the synthesis of antibodies that induce inflammatory reactions in the corresponding organ. In this process, the produced antibodies have cross-immune activity both against Borrelia antigens and tissue proteins (such as axonal proteins of nervous tissue, proteins of the synovial membrane, etc.). Thus, autoimmune mechanisms with predominant impairment of the humoral response (intrathecal synthesis of anti-Borrelia monoclonal antibodies, some of which resemble myelin) contribute to myelin breakdown and secondary axonal damage of the nervous system, resembling a mechanism of "molecular mimicry" [330]. There are suggestions about the possible involvement of Borrelia in initiating an autoimmune process through activation of myelin-specific T-cells and detection of auto-reactive antibodies to myelin and its components in LB [331].

The development of inflammation in Borrelia infection is not the sole mechanism of pathogenic action on the macroorganism. In *B. burgdorferi*, a gene responsible for synthesizing an exotoxin protein called Bbtox1 has been identified. Its action is similar to botulinum toxin C2, and certain pathological changes in the nervous system are associated with its production [332].

The case we described is interesting not only as a clinical observation - a manifestation of previously latent LB in the form of rapidly progressing neuroinfection against the background of immunosuppressive therapy. The breadth of differential-diagnostic search is also intriguing, complicated by some atypical features of onset and course of dermatomyositis, and the initiation of patient observation already amidst glucocorticoid treatment.

Within the structure of neuroborreliosis, rare nervous system impairments have been described, such as isolated cerebellar disorders, psychiatric, extrapyramidal disorders like chorea, Parkinsonism syndrome, Brown-Sequard syndrome. Cases are known of bilateral optic nerve involvement, retrobulbar neuritis, isolated hypoglossal nerve neuropathy, myasthenia-like syndrome. Some patients exhibit symptoms of autonomic ganglia irritation and a wide spectrum of autonomic reactions [333].

The diagnosis of LB is based on epidemiological features, clinical presentation, and confirmed by direct or indirect laboratory methods to detect B. burgdorferi infection [27, 60]. Tests for detecting Borrelia antigens have not yet found widespread use in diagnostic practice. PCR for examining cerebrospinal fluid in patients with neuroborreliosis, while specific, is less sensitive compared to serological testing. PCR sensitivity in early LB is 25-30%, and in chronic neuroborreliosis, it is 10%. The main drawback of PCR is a high number of false-negative results [283].

Today, the frequency of detecting antibodies to *B. burgdorferi* in cerebrospinal fluid (CSF) of LB patients with signs of nervous system involvement remains an open question. The presence of *B. burgdorferi* in CSF usually stimulates an intrathecal immune response starting from the second week of neurological manifestations, which according to most Western European scientists [274], is one of the main diagnostic criteria for neuroborreliosis.

Determining a high concentration of specific IgG in CSF allows for better diagnosis of persistent neuroinfections. However, in cases of pathologically increased blood-brain barrier permeability, a high content of such antibodies in CSF may not indicate local immune response but rather result from diffusion of immunoglobulins from serum [334]. Normally, the blood-brain barrier is nearly impermeable to immunoglobulin molecules, hence the concentration of IgG in CSF of healthy individuals is only 0.2% compared to serum levels [335]. However, in infectious-inflammatory CNS diseases, epilepsy, and under the influence of certain medications, blood-brain barrier permeability can significantly increase.

Overcoming the diagnostic challenge associated with difficulties in detecting persistent neuroinfections is facilitated by comparative serological studies, initially developed and tested for diagnosing cerebral vessel vasculitis caused by herpes simplex virus type 3 (VZV) [336].

It is necessary to perform the collection of cerebrospinal fluid (CSF) and blood on the same day. The calculation of the cerebrospinal fluid-serum index (CSF-SI) is carried out using the formula (1):

$$\text{CSF-SI} = \frac{\text{specific IgG (CSF)} \times \text{total IgG (serum)}}{\text{total IgG (CSF)} \times \text{specific IgG (serum)}} \tag{1}$$

when using ELISA, an index value of greater than 2 is considered a positive result, indicating the presence of intrathecal synthesis of antibodies to Borrelia in the central nervous system (CNS); an index of 1.5–2 is borderline. When using indirect immunofluorescence assay (IIFA) to determine specific antibodies, index values greater than 4 are considered positive, 2–3 are borderline, and less than 2 are negative [261].

However, there is another perspective that the absence of pleocytosis and intrathecal synthesis of antibodies to B. burgdorferi does not exclude neuroborreliosis even in the later stages of the disease. This is more typical for American patients, in whom intrathecal synthesis of antibodies to *B. burgdorferi* is inconsistent and non-consecutive [337]. Such a situation seems logical, considering that chronic forms of LB typically develop under conditions of immune deficiency in patients and/or weak immunogenicity of certain Borrelia genovariants.

Thus, the acute form of neuroborreliosis manifests as unilateral cranial nerve involvement: facial nerve in 80.0% of individuals and vestibulocochlear nerve in 20.0% of patients. In the structure of chronic LB with neurological involvement, the predominant syndromes are encephalopathy (50.0%), radiculopathy (45.2%), polyneuropathy (19.0%), and encephalomyelitis (7.1%). Combined peripheral and central nervous system involvement is noted in 21.4% of patients. The acute phase of LB precedes the development of chronic forms of neuroborreliosis in only 59.5% of cases; in other cases (40.5%), a primary-chronic course of the disease is observed. Risk factors for chronic LB include multiple tick bites, absence of primary erythema migrans, early signs of dissemination, and delayed and/or incomplete course of antibiotic therapy during the acute phase of the disease.

Chronic LB is characterized by progressive neurological impairment in 45.2% of cases, accompanied by systemic infectious syndrome in 45.2%, lymphadenopathy in 14.3%, and extra-neural syndromes in 57.1%, predominantly myalgia (50.0%) and arthralgia/arthritis. Radiculopathy in chronic LB is characterized by multilevel involvement in 63.2% of patients, moderate constant pain syndrome independent of body position and physical activity, combination of radicular and polyneuritic disorders (82.8%), predominantly bilateral pain radiation (52.4%), mild vertebral syndrome, and poor response to nonsteroidal anti-inflammatory drugs.

The main manifestations of encephalopathy in chronic LB are mild to moderate cognitive impairment (90.5%) in combination with ataxic syndrome (71.4%) and pyramidal insufficiency (80.9%). Unlike Lyme neuroborreliosis, chronic Lyme encephalomyelitis is characterized by a primary-progressive course, peripheral nerve involvement with root pathology, absence of optic, vestibulocochlear, facial, and trigeminal nerve involvement, and multi-organ manifestation. Combined Lyme disease and Lyme borreliosis are observed in 20.0% of cases, characterized by frequent polysymptomatic onset, marked sensitive disorders, development of polyneuropathy, and arthralgia.

Antibiotic therapy in patients with chronic LB leads to a statistically significant decrease in titres of anti-IgM and anti-IgG antibodies to *B. burgdorferi* in serum. In 17.9% of patients, antibody titres to Borrelia remain above normal values despite the absence of clinical signs of disease progression. In chronic LB, inflammatory changes in CSF are mainly detected in combined peripheral and central nervous system involvement, manifested by elevated protein levels (27.2%) and lymphocytic pleocytosis (18.2%). A positive clinical and laboratory effect after a course of antibiotic therapy in patients with chronic LB should be considered as an additional criterion for the presence of active infectious processes in them.

7. Influence of Non-Erythematous Form of Lyme Borreliosis on the Course of Pulmonary Tuberculosis

Mykhaylo Andreychyn
and Larysa Melnyk

Tuberculosis (TB) continues to be a significant medical and social issue for humanity. According to the World Health Organization (WHO), it is the leading cause of death among infectious diseases worldwide, surpassing HIV infection, and due to the COVID-19 pandemic, TB incidence may increase by more than 1 million cases annually [338]. In recent years, the TB situation in Ukraine has shown improvement due to a decrease in incidence; however, worsening epidemiological indicators are expected due to the COVID-19 pandemic [338–340].

The effectiveness of treatment depends not only on the rational use of etiotropic and pathogenetic agents but also on the presence of concomitant diseases, including those of infectious aetiology [341–345]. The prevalence of TB remains high in regions endemic for parasitic and blood infections, which may lead to their co-occurrence [345].

Literature data indicates that in Ethiopia [343], among 91 TB patients examined via coproscopy, intestinal parasitoses were found in 20 individuals (22%), most commonly Giardia lamblia in 8 (33.3%), followed by Ascaris lumbricoides and Hymenolepis nana in 4 each (16.7%). In India, among 118 pulmonary TB patients, bacterial infections were diagnosed in 84 (71.18%) individuals [344]. After three coproscopic examinations, helminths were found in 28 (87.5%) patients, and protozoal invasions in 4 (12.5%). Hookworm infection was the most prevalent helminthiasis (66.6%). Notably, parasitosis prevalence was higher among bacteriologically positive TB patients compared to those without it, at 31.0% versus 17.0%, respectively. It has been established that in endemic regions of Russia, infection rates with trematodes range from 47.3% to 60.3%. Among 189 TB patients with concurrent trematodiasis (clonorchiasis, nanophyetiasis, metagonimiasis), mycobacteria were detected in 80.5% of patients, compared to 69.8% in the group without trematodiasis [345].

Despite anti-tuberculosis measures, the prevalence of TB remains high worldwide, including in Ukraine, especially in regions endemic for blood and parasitic infections, such as LB and lambliasis [346–350]. However, the scientific literature currently lacks data on the impact of LB on the course of pulmonary tuberculosis.

The aim of the study was to investigate the impact of LB, lambliasis, and their combination on the course of pulmonary TB.

Ninety-nine patients with newly diagnosed pulmonary tuberculosis (NDPTB) were included in the study: 77 (77.8%) males and 22 (22.2%) females, aged between 21 and 76 years. The majority (76.8%) were residents of rural areas.

Based on the presence of concomitant asymptomatic LB (AsyLB) and lambliasis, NDPTB patients were divided into three groups: Group 1 consisted of 21 patients with NDPTB and concomitant AsyLB and lambliasis; Group 2 included 43 patients with NDPTB and diagnosed lambliasis as a concomitant disease; Group 3 comprised 35 patients with NDPTB only.

Statistical analysis of the data was conducted using the Mann-Whitney U-test and Wilcoxon T-test. Based on complaints and physical examination data, the following syndromes were identified in NDPTB patients, with or without concomitant AsyLB and lambliasis: bronchopulmonary syndrome in 67.8% of the examined, intoxication syndrome in 50.5%, cardiovascular system involvement in 41.4%, gastrointestinal system in 38.4%, and respiratory system involvement in 16.2%. The frequency of these syndromes in patient groups is depicted in Figure 37.

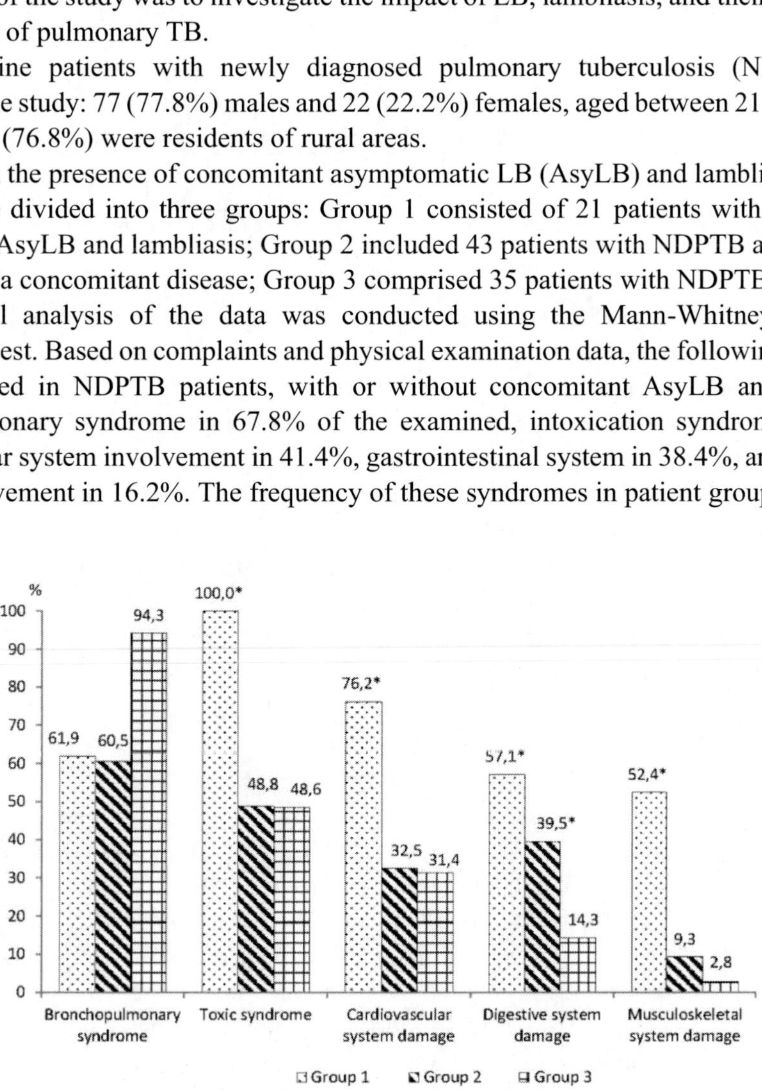

Note. * – significance of the difference between groups within one syndrome, $p < 0.05$.

Figure 37. Comparative characterization of syndromes in patients: newly diagnosed pulmonary tuberculosis with concomitant Lyme borreliosis and lambliasis (Group 1, n = 21); newly diagnosed pulmonary tuberculosis and lambliasis (Group 2, n = 43); solely with newly diagnosed pulmonary tuberculosis (Group 3, n = 35).

Table 30. Comparison of the frequency of clinical manifestations of bronchopulmonary syndrome in patients with newly diagnosed pulmonary tuberculosis (n = 99)

Symptom	Group of patients					
	1 (n = 21)		2 (n = 43)		3 (n = 35)	
	Absolute number	%	Absolute number	%	Absolute number	%
Complaints						
Cough	13	61,9	21	48,8	33	94,3
Shortness of breath	12	57,1	15	34,9	29	82,5*
Night sweats	9	42,8	18	41,9	16	45,7
Results of physical examination						
Reduced breath sounds	9	42,8*	7	16,3	6	17,1
Harsh breathing	12	57,1	34	79,1	26	74,3
Rales	16	76,2	21	48,8	15	42,8
Use of accessory muscles in respiration	6	28,6*	3	7,0	5	14,3
Increased respiratory rate	11	53,4	15	34,9	17	48,6
Increased heart rate	7	33,3	11	25,6	24	68,6*

Note. Here and in Tables 3.30–3.32: * – significance of the difference in indicators of one group compared to the other two, $p < 0.05$.

Bronchopulmonary syndrome was most frequently diagnosed in patients with NDPTB only (Group 3) – 94.3% ($p > 0.05$). Intoxication syndrome was found in all patients with both bacterial infections and lambliasis (Group 1), compared to Groups 2 and 3 (100.0 versus 48.8% ($p < 0.05$) and 100.0 versus 48.6%) ($p < 0.05$). Clinical manifestations of gastrointestinal system involvement were more frequently diagnosed in patients with concomitant LB and lambliasis (Groups 1 and 2), compared to those with NDPTB only (Group 3) (57.1 versus 14.3% and 39.5 versus 14.3%) ($p < 0.05$). It is noteworthy that respiratory system involvement was more commonly found in Group 1 patients compared to patients in the other two groups (52.4 versus 2.8% and 52.4 versus 9.3%, respectively) ($p < 0.05$).

The analysis of clinical manifestations of bronchopulmonary syndrome showed that dyspnoea significantly more often bothered patients with NDPTB only compared to those with NDPTB and concomitant lambliasis – 82.5% versus 34.9% ($p < 0.05$). However, night sweats were equally troubling for patients in all three groups.

When analysing the results of physical (objective) examination, significant differences regarding auscultation of coarse breathing sounds and rales were not found among patients in all three groups. Weakened breathing was more frequent in patients with both bacterial infections and lambliasis (Group 1) compared to Groups 3 and 2 (42.8% versus 17.1% and 42.8% versus 16.3%) ($p < 0.05$). The involvement of accessory respiratory muscles was more frequently noted in patients of Group 1 compared to Groups 3 and 2 (28.6% versus 14.3% and 28.6% versus 7.0%, respectively) ($p < 0.05$). At the same time, increased heart rate was more frequently observed in patients of Group 1 compared to those in Group 2 (68.6% versus 25.6%) ($p < 0.05$) and Group 3 (68.6% versus 33.3%) ($p < 0.05$) (Table 30).

The results of the analysis of clinical manifestations of the intoxication syndrome showed that fever was more frequently noted in patients with newly diagnosed pulmonary tuberculosis (NDPTB) combined with Lyme borreliosis and lambliasis (Group 1) compared to those in Groups 2 and 3 (100.0% versus 48.6%) ($p < 0.05$) and (100.0% versus 48.8%) ($p < 0.05$). Patients with NDPTB and concomitant lambliasis (Group 2) and NDPTB with concomitant

Lyme borreliosis and lambliasis (Group 1) most commonly complained of general weakness – 83.7% and 90.5% respectively ($p < 0.05$). Complaints of loss/reduced appetite were also more prevalent in patients with both bacterial infections and lambliasis (Group 1), with significant differences noted only compared to Group 3 ($p < 0.05$) (Table 31).

Table 31. Comparative characterization of clinical manifestations of the intoxication syndrome in patients with newly diagnosed pulmonary tuberculosis (n = 99)

Criterion	Group of patients					
	1 (n = 21)		2 (n = 43)		3 (n = 35)	
	Absolute number	%	Absolute number	%	Absolute number	%
Fever	21	100,0*	21	48,8	17	48,6
General weakness	19	90,5	36	83,7	21	60,0
Loss/Decrease of appetite	12	57,1*	19	44,2	8	22,8
Weight loss	13	61,9	23	51,5	18	51,4

The results of the analysis of clinical manifestations of cardiovascular system involvement showed that complaints of heart rhythm disturbances were significantly more common in patients with both bacterial infections and lambliasis (Group 1) compared to patients with only NDPTB (Group 3) and NDPTB with lambliasis (Group 2) ($p < 0.05$). Additionally, weakened heart tones (at auscultation) were more prevalent in patients with NDPTB and Lyme borreliosis and lambliasis compared to patients with only NDPTB or NDPTB with lambliasis (76.2% versus 31.4% and 76.2% versus 32.5%) ($p < 0.05$). Chest discomfort, however, was equally common among patients in all groups (Table 32).

Table 32. Comparative characterization of clinical manifestations of cardiovascular system involvement in patients with newly diagnosed pulmonary tuberculosis (n = 99)

Criterion	Group of patients					
	1 (n = 21)		2 (n = 43)		3 (n = 35)	
	Absolute number	%	Absolute number	%	Absolute number	%
Complaints						
Irregular heart rhythm	15	71,4*	11	25,6	12	34,3
Chest discomfort	7	33,3	10	23,2	8	22,8
Results of physical examination						
Diminished heart sounds	16	76,2*	14	32,5	11	31,4

Table 33. Comparative characterization of clinical manifestations of gastrointestinal system involvement in patients with newly diagnosed pulmonary tuberculosis (n = 99)

Complaints	Group of patients					
	1 (n = 21)		2 (n = 43)		3 (n = 35)	
	Absolute number	%	Absolute number	%	Absolute number	%
Bitter taste in the mouth	16	76,2*	21	48,8*	4	11,4
Heaviness in the right hypochondrium	13	61,9*	19	44,2*	5	14,3
Nausea	12	57,1*	13	30,2*	5	14,3

Table 34. Comparative characterization of clinical manifestations of musculoskeletal system involvement syndrome in patients with newly diagnosed pulmonary tuberculosis (n = 99)

Criterion		Group of patients					
		1 (n = 21)		2 (n = 43)		3 (n = 35)	
		Absolute number	%	Absolute number	%	Absolute number	%
Complaints:	joint pain	11	52,4**	4	9,3**	1	2,8
	muscle pain	1	4,8	0	0	0	0
VAS, mm		41,21 ± 1,09		–		–	
number of swollen joints		2	9,5	0	0	0	0
number of painful joints		11	52,4	0	0	0	0

Note. Here and in Tables 34 and 35: ** – significance of the difference between indicators of two groups for one, $p < 0.05$.

In the analysis of clinical manifestations of gastrointestinal involvement, patients with concomitant lambliasis were found to frequently complain of a heaviness in the right hypochondrium, in contrast to patients with only newly diagnosed pulmonary tuberculosis (44.2% versus 14.3% and 61.9% versus 14.3% respectively) ($p < 0.05$). Nausea was more commonly reported by individuals with accompanying infections compared to those with only newly diagnosed pulmonary tuberculosis (30.2% versus 14.3%) ($p < 0.05$) and (57.1% versus 14.3%) ($p < 0.05$). A similar difference was found in patients complaining of unstable bowel movements (constipation, diarrhoea): 39.5% versus 17.1% and 38.1% versus 17.1%, $p < 0.05$ (Table 33).

Table 35. Comparative characterization of data from radiological examination of patients with newly diagnosed pulmonary tuberculosis (n = 99)

X-ray examination results		Group of patients					
		1 (n = 21)		2 (n = 43)		3 (n = 35)	
		Absolute number	%	Absolute number	%	Absolute number	%
Clinical form of tuberculosis	Focal	0	0	2	4,6	1	2,8
	Infiltrative	11	52,4	15	34,9	18	51,4
	Disseminated	12	57,1	16	37,2	12	34,3
	Presence of pleurisy	2	9,5	6	13,9	4	11,4
Presence of destruction cavities		12	57,1**	26	60,5**	10	28,6

The analysis of clinical manifestations of joint involvement showed that patients experiencing joint pain were four times more frequent in those with concomitant lambliasis alone and eleven times more frequent in those with both bacterial infections and lambliasis compared to patients with only newly diagnosed pulmonary tuberculosis ($p < 0.05$). Additionally, in patients with newly diagnosed pulmonary tuberculosis and concomitant Lyme borreliosis and lambliasis (group 1), complaints of joint pain were more common than muscle pain (52.4% versus 4.8%) ($p < 0.05$). Patients with only newly diagnosed pulmonary tuberculosis and those with newly diagnosed pulmonary tuberculosis and concomitant lambliasis did not report muscle pain. It is important to note that swelling and tenderness of the joints were diagnosed exclusively in patients in group 1 ($p < 0.05$) (Table 34).

Further, we analysed in detail the results of radiological examination of patients with newly diagnosed pulmonary tuberculosis (Table 35).

The results of the analysis of these indicators showed that among patients with only pulmonary tuberculosis (Group 3), the infiltrative form of lung tuberculosis was slightly more common at 51.4% ($p > 0.05$), while among patients with accompanying infections, the disseminated form was slightly more prevalent at 37.2% and 57.1%, respectively ($p > 0.05$). Interestingly, among patients with both bacterial infections and giardiasis, no one exhibited a focal form of lung tuberculosis. The presence of cavity destruction was more prevalent among patients with accompanying infections compared to those with only pulmonary tuberculosis (60.5% vs. 28.6% and 57.1% vs. 28.6%, respectively) ($p < 0.05$).

In the analysis of bacteriological examination of sputum from patients with pulmonary tuberculosis, it was found that patients with the mentioned bacterial infections and giardiasis (Group 1) and pulmonary tuberculosis with accompanying giardiasis (Group 2) more frequently isolated Mycobacterium tuberculosis (MTB) compared to patients with only pulmonary tuberculosis (Group 3) ($p < 0.05$). Conversely, MTB in sputum was less frequently observed in patients with only pulmonary tuberculosis compared to patients with accompanying infections ($p < 0.05$) (Table 36).

Patients with pulmonary tuberculosis and Lyme-borreliosis (VTBCL) received a standard chemotherapy regimen according to the Unified Clinical Protocol "Tuberculosis" (categories 1, 2, 3): "Isoniazid," "Rifampicin," "Ethambutol," "Pyrazinamide" – for 2-3 months of intensive treatment phase (not less than 60 and not more than 90 doses), followed by 4 months of "Isoniazid" and "Rifampicin" (120 doses) in the maintenance phase of chemotherapy [351]. Treatment effectiveness was assessed using commonly accepted indicators – cessation of bacterial isolation and healing of destructive lung changes dynamically throughout the disease: before treatment, after 2 and 6 months of the main course of chemotherapy (MCT) [338, 344]. The dynamics of mycobacterial isolation in examined patients were as follows (Figure 38).

Table 36. Comparison of results of bacteriological examination of sputum from patients in three groups ($n = 99$)

Bacterial discharge	Group of patients					
	1 (n = 21)		2 (n = 43)		3 (n = 35)	
	Absolute number	%	Absolute number	%	Absolute number	%
MTB+	16	76,2 ± 9,3**	31	72,1 ± 6,8**	18	51,4 ± 8,4
MTB-	5	23,8 ± 9,3	12	27,9 ± 6,8	17	48,6 ± 8,4**

After 2 months of MCT, patients with concurrent infections (Groups 1 and 2) remained more likely to have mycobacterial isolation compared to those with only VTBCL (Group 3) (41.9% vs. 17.1% and 42.8% vs. 17.1%) ($p < 0.05$). Similar differences were found after 6 months of treatment ($p < 0.05$), with significant differences noted between patients in Group 1 compared to those in Group 2 (8.6% vs. 11.6%) ($p < 0.05$).

Analysing the results of destructive changes in the examined patients showed that after 2 months of MCT, the closure of destruction cavities in the lungs of patients with only VTBCL (Group 3) occurred twice as fast compared to those with concurrent infections (Groups 1 and 2) ($p < 0.05$). After 6 months of treatment, destructive changes persisted significantly more often in patients in Groups 1 and 2 compared to Group 3 (28.6% vs. 5.7% and 11.6% vs. 5.7%) ($p < 0.05$) (Figure 39).

The effectiveness of treatment in patients with only VTBCL (Group 3) was higher than in patients with concurrent infections (Groups 1 and 2), particularly achieving cessation of mycobacterial isolation in 88.8% of patients with only VTBCL and in 62.5% of individuals in Group 1 and 61.3% in Group 2. A similar trend was observed regarding the closure of destruction cavities in lung tissue – in 80.0% of patients in Group 3 and 50.0% and 61.5% of patients in Groups 1 and 2, respectively ($p < 0.05$).

According to several authors, respiratory organ involvement is not typical in the clinical presentation of LB, although scientific literature contains isolated reports of pleural effusion syndrome as a manifestation of LB [352, 353]. At the same time, no data was found on the peculiarities of tuberculosis and LB co-occurrence, as well as the influence of borrelia and lamblia on the destructive process in pulmonary tuberculosis.

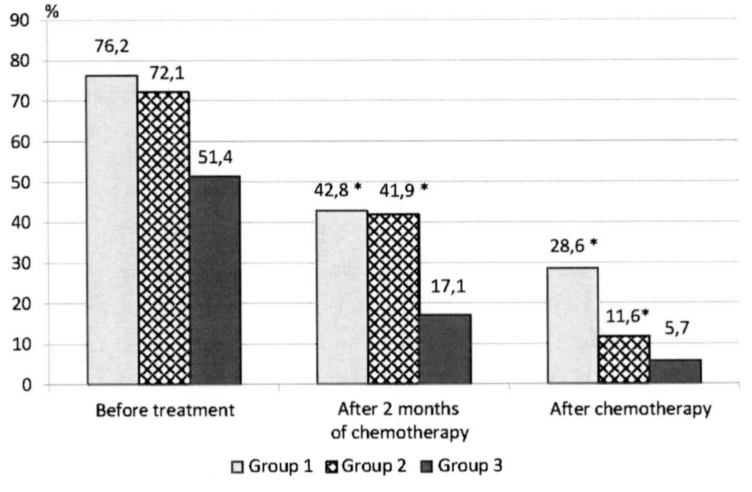

Note. Here and in Figure 38: * – significance of the difference between groups within the same indicator, $p < 0.05$.

Figure 38. Dynamics of mycobacterial isolation in patients: initially diagnosed pulmonary tuberculosis with concurrent Lyme borreliosis and giardiasis (Group 1, $n = 21$); initially diagnosed pulmonary tuberculosis and giardiasis (Group 2, $n = 43$); solely with initially diagnosed pulmonary tuberculosis (Group 3, $n = 35$).

Intoxication syndrome, according to authors' findings, accompanies all infectious diseases, including tuberculosis (TB), LB, and giardiasis [339, 349, 354], which can explain its significantly more frequent manifestations in patients with a combination of these infections. Heart involvement, according to researchers, is registered in 1-10% of LB patients [3, 355]. Patients with tuberculosis may also experience cardiovascular disorders caused by tuberculosis intoxication and pronounced pathological changes in the lungs; the frequency of these disorders' symptoms decreases under the influence of anti-tuberculosis treatment [356].

According to observations by some scientists, symptoms of gastrointestinal and hepatobiliary system involvement are characteristic for both LB [357], giardiasis [349], and tuberculosis [358], but in tuberculosis, they develop mainly from the 2nd to 3rd month of treatment. Therefore, the detected complaints from the gastrointestinal system in our patients before starting tuberculosis chemotherapy can be explained by the combined influence of LB and giardiasis. Disorders of the musculoskeletal system in the examined patients, in our opinion, can be attributed to the predominant influence of borreliosis and giardiasis, as they were recorded before the start of treatment, and only in patients with these concurrent infections [3, 357, 359].

Thus, we have established a significant impact of LB and giardiasis on the clinical course of pulmonary tuberculosis: in the case of concurrent giardiasis, more frequent clinical manifestations of gastrointestinal involvement ($p < 0.05$); LB and giardiasis in combination – intoxication syndrome, musculoskeletal system involvement ($p < 0.05$), cardiovascular system ($p < 0.05$). In patients with tuberculosis, destructive lung changes and mycobacterial isolation are significantly more often detected with concurrent LB and giardiasis than in their absence. The effectiveness of treatment in patients with only pulmonary tuberculosis based on the indicators of cessation of mycobacterial isolation and healing of lung cavity destruction was higher compared to patients with concurrent LB and giardiasis ($p < 0.05$).

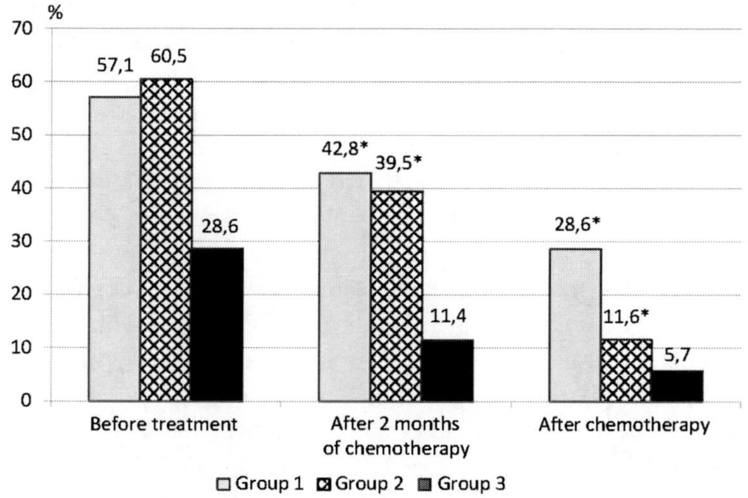

Figure 39. Dynamics of destructive changes in the lungs of patients: initially diagnosed pulmonary tuberculosis with concurrent Lyme borreliosis and giardiasis (Group 1, n = 21); initially diagnosed pulmonary tuberculosis and giardiasis (Group 2, n = 43); solely with initially diagnosed pulmonary tuberculosis (Group 3, n = 35).

8. Features of the Combination of Lyme Disease with Epstein-Barr Virus and the Vitamin D Levels in the Blood Serum of Patients

Mariia Shkilna
Oleh Ivakhiv
and Mariana Huk

It is evident that the course of LB may be influenced by potential comorbidities, including Epstein-Barr virus infection (EBVI), which is observed in the majority of people in our population (about 90-95% of adults and 50-80% of children) [360, 361]. Epstein-Barr virus (EBV) causes diseases of the immune system, leading to lymphoproliferative syndromes and immune deficiencies, and possesses opportunistic and oncogenic properties [362].

Chronic EBVI can manifest in both latent (asymptomatic) and active phases. Chronic active EBVI is usually defined as a condition lasting at least 6 months, characterized by elevated EBV levels in the patient's tissues or blood in the absence of other diseases causing immune deficiency. Such patients often exhibit fever, lymphadenopathy, splenomegaly, hepatitis, or pancytopenia, and over time, develop progressive immune deficiency, opportunistic infections, hemophagocytic syndrome, multiple organ failure, or specific lymphoma [360-362].

Vitamin D is a group of biologically active fat-soluble compounds (over 6 vitamers and 50 metabolites) that are produced in the skin under the influence of ultraviolet B rays or obtained from food [363]. The most biologically active forms of vitamin D in the human body are vitamins D2 (ergocalciferol or ergosterol) and D3 (cholecalciferol). The hormonally active form of vitamin D is 1α,25-dihydroxyvitamin D (1α,25(OH)2 D), formed from vitamin D vitamers through 25-hydroxyvitamin D (25(OH)D), which includes 25(OH)D2 and 25(OH)D3 and is measured in blood serum as total 25(OH)D to assess vitamin D status [364].

In 2011, the Endocrinology Association proposed considering vitamin D deficiency (VDD) in children and adults as a clinical syndrome caused by low levels of 25(OH)D in the blood serum [365]. In 2023, the First Ukrainian Consensus on Vitamin D Management established criteria for assessing vitamin D sufficiency [366].

VDD is extremely widespread globally. It is found in approximately 20% of the population in Northern Europe, and even more frequently in Western, Southern, and Eastern Europe – 30-60% [367].

In recent decades, Ukraine has conducted a number of epidemiological studies on vitamin D status [368-374]. The first major epidemiological study (2011) involving 1,575 people aged 20 to 89 from various regions of the country found a significant proportion of individuals (81.8%) with VDD in the Ukrainian population. Adequate levels of 25(OH)D in blood serum were found in only 4.6% of the participants, and insufficiency in 13.6%. The average level of 25(OH)D in patients' blood was 34.49 nmol/L (13.80 ng/mL) [368].

Numerous epidemiological studies have found an increased incidence of oncological, infectious, autoimmune, and cardiovascular diseases in individuals with VDD [372].

The relationship between VDD and adequate immune response is particularly noteworthy. The obvious positive effect of vitamin D on immune system reactivity is further supported by the fact that, before the advent of antibacterial drugs, vitamin D was successfully used to treat tuberculosis [373].

Currently, scientific literature includes several publications on the relationship between retrovirus activity associated with multiple sclerosis, EBV, and vitamin D status in patients with relapsing multiple sclerosis [374]. It has been established that the amount of EBV in the blood of patients is significantly higher with lower levels of 25(OH)D3 [375]. An integrative analysis of transcriptomic data with micro-RNAs revealed that VDD promotes EBV replication, which, in turn, contributes to the development of multiple sclerosis by disrupting gene expression regulation at the post-transcriptional level [376].

Considering the immunomodulatory properties of vitamin D, researchers suggest that it may influence antiviral immune responses [377].

At the Centre for Lyme Borreliosis and Other Tick-Borne Diseases Research, which operates at I. Horbachevsky Ternopil National Medical University, 81 patients aged 19 to 76 with clinical manifestations of LB and EBV infection were examined. There were 26 men (32.1%), and the majority of the examined were women –55 (67.9%).

Patients reported joint and muscle pain, headaches, swollen lymph nodes, throat discomfort, periodic fever, nasal congestion, skin rashes (morphea), increased fatigue/general weakness, and cognitive impairments, particularly during mental tasks, as well as insomnia and/or chronic sleep deprivation. These symptoms had been noted by patients for more than 6 months.

To investigate the epidemiological features of potential Lyme borreliosis in patients with swollen lymph nodes, a standardized questionnaire developed by scientists at the John Paul II University of Applied Sciences (Biała Podlaska, Poland) and adapted for Ukrainian patients by the Department of Infectious Diseases, Epidemiology, Dermatology and Venereology at I. Horbachevsky Ternopil National Medical University was used. Patients answered questions about the number and timing of tick bites, the area where they occurred, the site of tick attachment, and the method of tick removal, among other details.

Serological confirmation of LB diagnosis was performed in two stages. At the first stage, enzyme-linked immunosorbent assay (ELISA) was used to detect antibodies to *B. burgdorferi s. l.* antigens in patients' blood serum. For identifying IgM and IgG antibodies, the test systems "*Anti-Borrelia burgdorferi* ELISA (IgM)" and "*Anti-Borrelia* plus VIsE ELISA (IgG)" from Euroimmun AG (Germany) were used. At the second stage, positive and intermediate results obtained from ELISA were confirmed by immunoblotting using the EUROLINE *Borrelia RN-AT* test system from Euroimmun AG (Germany).

To diagnose EBV infection, a multiplex immunoassay with BIOCHIP technology was employed. The test system "BIOCHIP Sequence EBV (with avidity determination)" (EUROIMMUN, Germany) was used, allowing the simultaneous detection of specific IgM and IgG antibodies to viral capsid antigens (VCA) and its proteins: gp125 (native antigen) and p19 (recombinant protein), as well as IgG antibodies to nuclear antigens (EBNA) and early antigens (EBV-EA).

To determine the active or latent phase of chronic EBV infection, real-time PCR was used to detect EBV DNA in plasma and saliva samples. Active chronic EBV infection was diagnosed based on the presence of EBV DNA in blood and saliva (in both or one of the samples; detection range – 10^3–10^7 copies/mL). In the absence of viral DNA in blood or saliva, latent chronic EBV infection was established.

Additionally, vitamin D levels were measured in the blood serum of patients with LB and chronic EBV infection, both separately and in combination. Vitamin D sufficiency was assessed based on the level of 25(OH)D in serum. Blood samples were taken in the morning after fasting for 10–12 hours post-last meal. Patients were examined from September to May to minimize the seasonal impact of ultraviolet rays on serum 25(OH)D levels. The 25(OH)D content was measured using chemiluminescent immunoassay (CMIA) on the Alinity I analyzer (Abbott, USA) and Cobas 6000/Cobas 8000 test systems from Abbott (USA).

The diagnosis of VDD and insufficiency was verified according to the recommendations of the First Ukrainian Consensus on Vitamin D Management. The following criteria were used: < 20 ng/mL (< 50 nmol/L) – VDD; ≥ 20 ng/mL (≥ 50 nmol/L) and < 30 ng/mL (< 75 nmol/L) – vitamin D insufficiency (VDI); > 30-50 ng/mL (75-125 nmol/L) – adequate vitamin D level (AVDL); > 50-60 ng/mL (125-150 nmol/L) – safe but non-target vitamin D level; > 60-100 ng/mL (150-250 nmol/L) – zone of uncertainty with potential benefits or risks; > 100 ng/mL (> 250 nmol/L) – excess/toxic zone of vitamin D.

It was found that most individuals (57; 70.3%) experienced joint pain, nearly half (40; 49.4%) reported insomnia and/or chronic sleep deprivation, 37 (45.7%) had swollen lymph nodes (lymphadenopathy), and 33 (40.7%) had periodic fever. Additionally, more than a third of patients (32; 39.5%) noted increased fatigue/general weakness, and a third (27; 33.3%) reported impaired memory and cognitive functions, particularly during mental tasks. Only 21 (25.9%) reported muscle pain, and 19 (23.4%) had headaches. Notably, 14 (17.9%) patients who visited the Centre for Lyme Borreliosis and Other Tick-Borne Diseases Research were diagnosed with skin disease in the form of morphea. Complaints of throat discomfort and nasal congestion were the least common, reported by only 11 (13.6%) patients.

Upon examination, the localization of enlarged lymph nodes was determined. It was found that 77.8% of patients had regional lymph nodes enlarged, specifically: submandibular and anterior cervical nodes in 35.7% each, axillary nodes in 32.2%, posterior cervical nodes in 17.9%, and groin nodes in 10.7%. Meanwhile, generalized lymphadenopathy was observed in 22.2% of patients.

The two-stage serological diagnostic approach for LB using sequential ELISA and immunoblotting identified positive or intermediate results for antibodies of classes M and/or G to *B. burgdorferi s. l.* in the serum of 69.4% of patients, with 33.3% having both classes of antibodies simultaneously.

A detailed analysis of serological results showed that in 15 patients, only IgM antibodies to *B. burgdorferi s. l.* were found. Notably, no seroconversion occurred during the 6-month observation period – specific IgM remained, and specific IgG did not appear, which can be interpreted as a false-positive result. Thus, overall, Lyme borreliosis was diagnosed in 41 (50.6%) of the 81 patients through the two-stage serological testing.

Chronic EBV infection was diagnosed using two methods: immunoassay and real-time PCR. The first method, BIOCHIP technology, detected IgM and IgG antibodies to several EBV antigens simultaneously in patients' serum. The presence of IgG antibodies to viral capsid antigen (EBV-CA) and its highly specific recombinant protein (p19), native antigen (gp125), and their combination with specific IgM and IgG antibodies to other viral antigens led to the diagnosis of chronic EBV infection in all examined patients.

Using PCR, EBV DNA was detected in 43 (53.1%) patients with chronic EBV infection. Moreover, viral nucleic acid was found more frequently in saliva than in blood – 36 (83.7%) vs. 7 (16.3%) of the 43 patients, $p < 0.05$.

Thus, among the 81 patients with chronic EBV infection, 43 (53.1%) were diagnosed with the active phase, and the remaining 38 (46.9%) had the latent phase.

Based on laboratory-confirmed LB and chronic EBV infection phases, all patients were divided into 4 groups. Group 1 included 22 patients with LB and chronic EBV infection in the active phase, Group 2 included 21 patients with only active chronic EBV infection, Group 3 had 19 patients with LB and chronic EBV infection in the latent phase, and Group 4 included 21 patients with only latent chronic EBV infection.

Vitamin D levels were measured in the serum of all patients. It was found that only 21 (25.9%) had adequate vitamin D levels (30-50 ng/mL), 17 (21.0%) had insufficient levels (≥ 20 ng/mL and < 30 ng/mL), 3 (3.7%) had safe but non-target levels (> 50-60 ng/mL), and almost half of the patients (40; 49.4%) had deficiency (< 20 ng/mL).

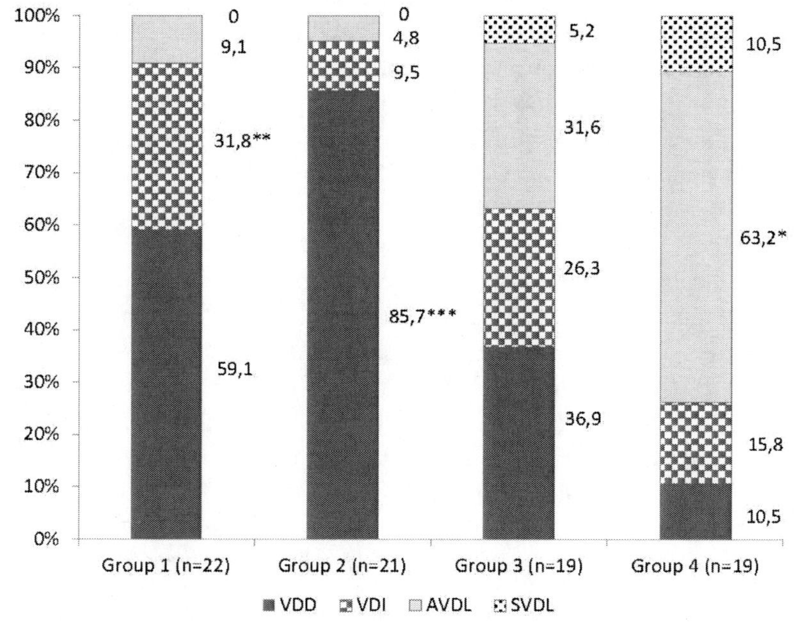

Notes:
* – The difference is statistically significant between Group 4 and Groups 1, 2, and 3, $p < 0.05$.
** – The difference is statistically significant between Group 1 and Groups 2 and 4, $p < 0.05$.
*** – The difference is statistically significant between Group 2 and Groups 3 and 4, $p < 0.05$.

Figure 40. Percentages of patients with different levels of 25(OH)D in blood serum in the groups: 1 – Group 1 (Lyme borreliosis with chronic Epstein-Barr virus infection in the active phase); 2 – Group 2 (chronic Epstein-Barr virus infection in the active phase only); 3 – Group 3 (Lyme borreliosis and chronic Epstein-Barr virus infection in the latent phase); 4 – Group 4 (chronic Epstein-Barr virus infection in the latent phase only).

Subsequent analysis of 25(OH)D levels in serum of patients from different groups (Figure 40) revealed that safe vitamin D levels were found only in the serum of patients with latent phase of EBV infection – 1 (5.2%) in Group 3 (with LB) and 2 (10.5%) in Group 4 (only EBV infection). Patients with AVDL were least common among those with active EBV infection – 2 (9.1%) in Group 1 (with LB) and 1 (5.0%) in Group 2 (only EBV). Nearly a third of such patients (6; 31.6%) were found in Group 3 (LB and EBV in the latent phase). Meanwhile, among patients in Group 4 (only EBV in the latent phase), those with AVDL were significantly more frequent (12; 63.2%) than in other groups ($p < 0.05$).

It was found that the highest percentage of patients with VDI was in Group 1 (Lyme borreliosis with chronic EBV infection in the active phase), with 7 patients (31.8%), which was significantly higher than in Groups 2 and 4, $p < 0.05$. Meanwhile, Group 2 (chronic EBV infection in the active phase only) had the highest number of patients with vitamin D deficiency compared to patients in Groups 3 and 4-18 patients (85.7%) versus 7 (36.9%) and 24 (10.5%), $p < 0.05$.

Thus, in groups where the active phase of chronic EBV infection was present together with Lyme borreliosis (Group 1) and EBV mono-infection (Group 2), the highest percentage of individuals with low vitamin D levels in blood serum (VDD and VDI) was observed, compared to the groups where chronic EBV infection was in the latent phase – 90.9% and 95.2% versus 26.3% in Group 4 (chronic EBV infection only), $p < 0.05$, and 63.2% in Group 3 (Lyme borreliosis with chronic EBV infection). At the same time, the number of individuals with adequate vitamin D levels in blood serum (AVDL and SVDL) was significantly higher in the groups with chronic EBV infection in the latent phase with Lyme borreliosis (Group 3) and EBV mono-infection (Group 4) compared to the groups that included patients with chronic EBV infection in the active phase with Lyme borreliosis (Group 1) and EBV mono-infection (Group 2) – 36.8% and 73.8% versus 9.1% and 4.8%, $p < 0.05$.

The mean levels of 25(OH)D in the blood serum of patients in each group were also calculated (see Table 37).

The results indicate that for chronic EBV infection in the active phase (groups 1 and 2), the level of 25(OH)D in the blood serum is significantly lower compared to chronic Epstein-Barr virus monoinfection in the latent phase (group 4) – specifically, (18.69 ± 1.71) and (15.53 ± 1.16) versus (35.01 ± 1.96) ng/mL ($p < 0.05$). Moreover, the vitamin D level in the serum of patients with only active-phase chronic EBV infection (group 2) was even lower than in the group with Lyme disease and chronic EBV infection in the latent phase (group 3), $p < 0.05$.

Table 37. The level of 25(OH)D in the blood serum of patients of different groups (M ± m), ng/mL

Indicator	Group			
	1, n = 22	2, n = 21	3, n = 19	4, n = 19
25(OH) D content	18,69 ± 1,71	15,53 ± 1,16	24,26 ± 2,65***	35,01 ± 1,96*,**

Notes:
* – The difference is significant between groups 4 and 1, $p < 0.05$;
** – The difference is significant between groups 4 and 2, $p < 0.05$;
*** – The difference is significant between groups 3 and 2, $p < 0.05$.

The results for diagnosing chronic EBV infection in the active phase in 53.1% of patients with enlarged lymph nodes exceed the figures reported by Japanese researchers, who found a prevalence of 40.0% among individuals with enlarged lymph nodes, and are lower than the 70.0% reported by researchers in the USA who observed enlarged lymph nodes in such patients [378].

Additionally, our findings are similar to those of Spanish researchers who studied the relationship between 25(OH)D levels and the quantity of EBV and human herpesvirus type 6 in the blood serum of patients with multiple sclerosis [375]. The researchers identified an inverse proportional relationship between the number of DNA copies of the above viruses and the concentration of vitamin D in the patients' serum. In our study, the concentration of 25(OH)D in the serum of patients with chronic EBV infection, whether in the active phase alone or in combination with Lyme disease, was significantly lower than in patients with this viral disease in the latent phase.

In summary, patients with Lyme disease and chronic EBV infection more frequently reported joint pain, insomnia and/or chronic sleep deprivation, enlarged lymph nodes, periodic fever, and increased fatigue/general weakness. The multiplex indirect immunofluorescence method using BIOCHIP technology (which detects antibodies of classes M and G to the EBV capsid antigen and its proteins gp125 and p19, as well as class G antibodies to the viral nuclear and early antigens in one serum sample) allowed for the diagnosis of chronic EBV infection in all patients with enlarged lymph nodes. Low levels of vitamin D (deficiency and insufficiency combined) in the blood serum were more frequently recorded in patients with chronic EBV infection in the active phase, whether combined with Lyme disease or alone, compared to patients with only this viral infection in the latent phase ($p < 0.05$) or in combination with Lyme disease.

A safe but non-target level of vitamin D was noted only in the serum of patients with chronic EBV infection in the latent phase alone or in combination with Lyme disease. Adequate levels of vitamin D (sufficient and safe but non-target levels combined) in the serum were mostly found in patients with only chronic EBV infection in the latent phase or in combination with Lyme disease, compared to patients with this viral disease in the active phase, whether combined with Lyme disease or alone ($p < 0.05$). Patients with chronic EBV infection in the latent phase had a significantly higher average level of 25(OH)D in the serum compared to those with the disease in the active phase, whether combined with Lyme disease or not ($p < 0.05$). At the same time, the vitamin D content in the serum of patients with chronic EBV infection in the latent phase combined with Lyme disease was also higher than in those with only the active phase of the viral infection ($p < 0.05$).

Conclusion

The pathogenesis of Lyme borreliosis encompasses three main stages: localized, disseminated, and organ-specific involvement. The initial stage corresponds to cutaneous manifestations (observed in 80-90%), with erythema migrans at the tick bite site being the pathognomonic sign in 60-90% of patients.

The disseminated stage of early infection, occurring 1-3 months after disease onset, primarily affects the nervous and cardiovascular systems, skin, and joints. Neurological manifestations commonly include encephalomyelitis, peripheral radiculopathy, meningitis, flaccid paresis of the facial nerve or limbs. Cardiovascular involvement is characterized by symptoms of myocarditis with varying degrees of atrioventricular block, pericarditis, and rarely, pancarditis. Cutaneous manifestations during the disseminated stage may include rashes on areas distant from the bite site, resembling capillaritis, diffuse erythema, or benign lymphocytoma of the skin. Joint involvement, predominantly affecting large and medium joints, may present as arthralgia or arthritis.

The late stage of Lyme borreliosis is characterized by a chronic continuous or relapsing course, with predominant involvement of the joints, skin, and nervous system. Articular pathology may manifest as persistent arthralgia, benign recurrent arthritis, or chronic progressive arthritis. Cutaneous changes at this stage are typified by chronic atrophic acrodermatitis and localized skin atrophy (morphea). Neurological involvement may include encephalopathy, encephalitis, encephalomyelitis, cerebrovascular neuroborreliosis, and meningoradiculoneuritis.

Patients with concurrent Lyme borreliosis and chronic Epstein-Barr virus infection more frequently reported joint pain, insomnia and/or chronic sleep deprivation, lymphadenopathy, periodic fever, and increased fatigue/general weakness. Serum levels of vitamin D (deficiency and insufficiency combined) were significantly lower in patients with chronic active-phase Epstein-Barr virus infection, both with and without coexisting Lyme borreliosis, compared to those with latent-phase infection ($p < 0.05$) or in combination with Lyme borreliosis.

Lyme borreliosis and giardiasis complicate the clinical course of pulmonary tuberculosis by exacerbating intoxication symptoms, increasing involvement of the musculoskeletal and cardiovascular systems, and significantly increasing the incidence of destructive lung changes and Mycobacterium tuberculosis shedding, while reducing the effectiveness of anti-tuberculosis therapy ($p < 0.05$).

References

[1] Pacian, A., Kulik, T., Szwedo, E. Lyme borreliosis as a current health problem of the 21st century. *Health Problems of Civilization.* 2017;11(2):66-70. doi: doi: 10.5114/hpc.2017.69019.

[2] Bhate, C., Schwartz, R. A. Lyme disease: Part I. Advances and perspectives. *J Am Acad Dermatol.* 2011;64(4):619-36; quiz 637-8. doi: 10.1016/j.jaad.2010.03.046.

[3] Zinchuk, O. M. Lyme Borreliosis. In: Malyi VP, Andreychyn MA, eds. *Infectious Diseases: Textbook in 2 Vol.* Vol 2. Lviv: Magnolia-2006; 2018. c. 400-5. [in Ukrainian].

[4] Kulias, S. M. Current opinion on peculiarities of specific diagnostics, treatment and prevention of Lyme borreliosis [Internet]. *Biomedical and biosocial anthropology.* 2013 [cited 2025 Feb 3];(20):245-51. Available from: http://nbuv.gov.ua/UJRN/bba_2013_20_62. [in Ukrainian].

[5] Glatz, M., Resinger, A., Semmelweis, K., Ambros-Rudolph, C. M., Müllegger, R. R. Clinical spectrum of skin manifestations of Lyme borreliosis in 204 children in Austria. *Acta Derm Venereol.* 2015 May;95(5):565-71. doi: 10.2340/00015555-2000.

[6] Wilhelmsson, P., Fryland, L., Lindblom, P., Sjöwall, J., Ahlm, C., Berglund, J., Haglund, M., Henningsson, A. J., Nolskog, P., Nordberg, M., Nyberg, C., Ornstein, K., Nyman, D., Ekerfelt, C., Forsberg, P., Lindgren, P. E. A prospective study on the incidence of Borrelia burgdorferi sensu lato infection after a tick bite in Sweden and on the Åland Islands, Finland (2008-2009). *Ticks Tick Borne Dis.* 2016;7(1):71-79. doi: 10.1016/j.ttbdis.2015.08.009.

[7] Hofmann, H., Fingerle, V., Hunfeld, K. P., Huppertz, H. I., Krause, A., Rauer, S., Ruf, B.; Consensus group. Cutaneous Lyme borreliosis: Guideline of the German Dermatology Society. *Ger Med Sci.* 2017;15:Doc14. doi: 10.3205/000255.

[8] Radolf, J. D., Strle, K., Lemieux, J. E., Strle, F. Lyme Disease in Humans. *Curr Issues Mol Biol.* 2021;42:333-384. doi: 10.21775/cimb.042.333.

[9] Maraspin, V., Lusa, L., Blejec, T., Ružić-Sabljić, E., Pohar Perme, M., Strle, F. Course and Outcome of Erythema Migrans in Pregnant Women. *J Clin Med.* 2020;9(8):2364. doi: 10.3390/jcm9082364.

[10] Sprong, H., Azagi, T., Hoornstra, D., Nijhof, A. M., Knorr, S., Baarsma, M. E., Hovius, J. W. Control of Lyme borreliosis and other Ixodes ricinus-borne diseases. *Parasit Vectors.* 2018;11(1):145. doi: 10.1186/s13071-018-2744-5.

[11] Chemych, M., Lutai, I. Lyme disease. Modern issue condition. *East Ukr Med J.* 2020;8(2):230-41. doi: 10.21272/eumj.2020;8(2):230-41.

[12] Svintsitskyi, A. S. Lyme disease as a current integrated problem of modern internal medicine. *Health of Ukraine* [Internet]. Thematic issue "Cardiology. Rheumatology. Cardiac Surgery". 2012 [cited 2025 Feb 3];(5):84–87. Available from: http://ir.librarynmu.com/handle/123456789/4113. [in Ukrainian].

[13] Yehudina, Y., Trypilka, S. Lyme borreliosis as a trigger for autoimmune disease. *Cureus.* 2021 Oct 10;13(10):e18648. doi: 10.7759/cureus.18648.

[14] Iliopoulou, B. P., Huber, B. T. Infectious arthritis and immune dysregulation: lessons from Lyme disease. *Curr Opin Rheumatol.* 2010;22(4):451–455. doi: 10.1097/BOR.0b013e328338f73f.

[15] Casjens, S. R., Gilcrease, E. B., Vujadinovic, M., Mongodin, E. F., Luft, B. J., Schutzer, S. E., et al., Plasmid diversity and phylogenetic consistency in the Lyme disease agent Borrelia burgdorferi. *BMC Genomics.* 2017;18(1):165. doi: 10.1186/s12864-017-3553-5.

[16] Casjens, S. R., Mongodin, E. F., Qiu, W. G., Luft, B. J., Schutzer, S. E., Gilcrease, E. B., et al., Genome stability of Lyme disease spirochetes: comparative genomics of Borrelia burgdorferi plasmids. *PLoS One.* 2012;7(3):e33280. doi: 10.1371/journal.pone.0033280.

[17] Qiu, W. G., Martin, C. L. Evolutionary genomics of *Borrelia burgdorferi* sensu lato: findings, hypotheses, and the rise of hybrids. *Infect Genet Evol.* 2014;27:576–593. doi: 10.1016/j.meegid.2014.03.025.

[18] Eggers, C. H., Gray, C. M., Preisig, A. M., Glenn, D. M., Pereira, J., Ayers, R. W., et al., Phage-mediated horizontal gene transfer of both prophage and heterologous DNA by ϕBB-1, a bacteriophage of *Borrelia burgdorferi*. *Pathog Dis*. 2016;74(9):ftw107. doi: 10.1093/femspd/ftw107.

[19] Stanek, G. Lyme borreliosis, ticks and *Borrelia* species. *Wien Klin Wochenschr*. 2018;130(15–16):459–462. doi: 10.1007/s00508-018-1376-2.

[20] Mavrutenkov, V. V. Lyme disease. General issues (Part I). *Child Health*. 2014;(2):106–110. [in Russian].

[21] Figoni, J., Chirouze, C., Hansmann, Y., Lemogne, C., Hentgen, V., Saunier, A., et al., Lyme borreliosis and other tick-borne diseases. Guidelines from the French Scientific Societies (I): prevention, epidemiology, diagnosis. *Med Mal Infect*. 2019;49(5):318–334. doi: 10.1016/j.medmal.2019.04.381.

[22] Grążlewska, W., Holec-Gąsior, L. Antibody cross-reactivity in serodiagnosis of Lyme disease. *Antibodies (Basel)*. 2023;12(4):63. doi: 10.3390/antib12040063.

[23] Strnad, M., Rudenko, N., Rego, R. O. M. Pathogenicity and virulence of *Borrelia burgdorferi*. *Virulence*. 2023;14(1):2265015. doi: 10.1080/21505594.2023.2265015.

[24] Weiss, T., Zhu, P., White, H., Posner, M., Wickiser, J. K., Washington, M. A., et al., Latent Lyme disease resulting in chronic arthritis and early career termination in a United States Army officer. *Mil Med*. 2019;184(7–8):e368–e370. doi: 10.1093/milmed/usz026.

[25] Anderson, C., Brissette, C. A. The brilliance of *Borrelia*: mechanisms of host immune evasion by Lyme disease-causing spirochetes. *Pathogens*. 2021;10(3):281. doi: 10.3390/pathogens10030281.

[26] Volokha, A. P. Lyme Disease (Tick-Borne Borreliosis) in Children. *Infectious Diseases*. 2014;(1):80–87. doi: 10.11603/1681-2727.2014.1.4739 [in Ukrainian].

[27] Djokic, V., Primus, S., Akoolo, L., Chakraborti, M., Parveen, N. Age-Related Differential Stimulation of Immune Response by *Babesia microti* and *Borrelia burgdorferi* During Acute Phase of Infection Affects Disease Severity. *Front Immunol*. 2018;9:2891. doi: 10.3389/fimmu.2018.02891.

[28] Woitzik, P., Linder, S. Molecular Mechanisms of *Borrelia burgdorferi* Phagocytosis and Intracellular Processing by Human Macrophages. *Biology (Basel)*. 2021 Jun 22;10(7):567. doi: 10.3390/biology 10070567.

[29] Rudenko, N., Golovchenko, M., Grubhoffer, L., Oliver, J. H. Jr. Updates on *Borrelia burgdorferi* sensu lato complex with respect to public health. *Ticks Tick Borne Dis*. 2011;2(3):123–8. doi: 10.1016/j.ttbdis.2011.04.002.

[30] Klitgaard, K., Kjær, L. J., Isbrand, A., Hansen, M. F., Bødker, R. Multiple infections in questing nymphs and adult female *Ixodes ricinus* ticks collected in a recreational forest in Denmark. *Ticks Tick Borne Dis*. 2019;10(5):1060–65. doi: 10.1016/j.ttbdis.2019.05.016.

[31] Stanek, G., Wormser, G. P., Gray, J., Strle, F. Lyme borreliosis. *Lancet*. 2012 Feb 4;379(9814):461–73. doi: 10.1016/S0140-6736(11)60103-7.

[32] Coipan, E. C., Jahfari, S., Fonville, M., Oei, G. A., Spanjaard, L., Takumi, K., Hovius, J. W., Sprong, H. Imbalanced presence of *Borrelia burgdorferi* s.l. multilocus sequence types in clinical manifestations of Lyme borreliosis. *Infect Genet Evol*. 2016;42:66–76. doi: 10.1016/j.meegid.2016.04.019.

[33] Sprong, H., Azagi, T., Hoornstra, D., Nijhof, A. M., Knorr, S., Baarsma, M. E., Hovius, J. W. Control of Lyme borreliosis and other *Ixodes ricinus*-borne diseases. *Parasit Vectors*. 2018;11(1):145. doi: 10.1186/s13071-018-2744-5.

[34] Strnad, M., Hönig, V., Růžek, D., Grubhoffer, L., Rego, R. O. M. Europe-Wide Meta-Analysis of *Borrelia burgdorferi* Sensu Lato Prevalence in Questing *Ixodes ricinus* Ticks. *Appl Environ Microbiol*. 2017;83(15):e00609-17. doi: 10.1128/AEM.00609-17.

[35] Malyi, V. P., Shepileva, N. V. Tick-borne infections (Lyme disease, granulocytic anaplasmosis, and monocytic ehrlichiosis) in Kharkiv region. *Clinical Immunology* [Internet]. *Allergy. Infectious Diseases*. 2013 [cited 2025 Feb 3];(2):49–52. Available from: https://kiai.com.ua/ua/archive/2013/2%2861%29/pages-49-52/klishchovi-infekciyi-hvoroba-layma-granulocitarniy-anaplazmoz-i-monocitarniy-erlihioz-u-harkivskiy-oblasti [in Ukrainian].

[36] Özdemir, D., İnce, N. Lyme Disease. *Journal of Microbiology and Infectious Diseases*. 2014;4(5):32–40. doi: 10.5799/ahinjs.02.2014.S1.0139.

[37] Dandashi, J. A., Nizamutdinov, D., Dayawansa, S., Fonkem, E., Huang, J. H. Texas Occurrence of Lyme Disease and Its Neurological Manifestations. *J Neuroinfect Dis*. 2016;7(2):217. doi: 10.4172/2314-7326.1000217.

[38] British Infection Association. The epidemiology, prevention, investigation and treatment of Lyme borreliosis in United Kingdom patients: a position statement by the British Infection Association. *J Infect*. 2011;62(5):329–38. doi: 10.1016/j.jinf.2011.03.006.

[39] Trevisan, G., Bonin, S., Ruscio, M. A Practical Approach to the Diagnosis of Lyme Borreliosis: From Clinical Heterogeneity to Laboratory Methods. *Front Med (Lausanne)*. 2020;7:265. doi: 10.3389/fmed.2020.00265.

[40] Sharma, A., Guleria, S., Sharma, R., Sharma, A. Lyme Disease: A Case Report with Typical and Atypical Lesions. *Indian Dermatol Online J*. 2017;8(2):124–127. doi: 10.4103/2229-5178.202271.

[41] Pedrycz-Wieczorska, A. Analysis of the methods for diagnosing borreliosis − Lyme disease. *Health Problems of Civilization*. 2017;11(2):80–86. doi: 10.5114/hpc.2017.69022.

[42] Lindsay, L. R., Bernat, K., Dibernardo, A. Laboratory diagnostics for Lyme disease. *Can Commun Dis Rep*. 2014;40(11):209–217. doi: 10.14745/ccdr.v40i11a02.

[43] Ang, C. W., Brandenburg, A. H., van Burgel, N. D., Bijlmer, H. A., Herremans, T., Stelma, F., Lunel, F. V., van Dam, A. P.; Dutch Working Group on Diagnosis of Lyme Borreliosis. A Dutch nationwide evaluation of serological assays for detection of *Borrelia* antibodies in clinically well-defined patients. *Diagn Microbiol Infect Dis*. 2015;83(3):222–8. doi: 10.1016/j.diagmicrobio.2015.07.007.

[44] Di Meo, N., Retrosi, C., Corneli, P., Trevisan, G. Multiple erythema migrans due to borreliosis. *G Ital Dermatol Venereol*. 2019;154(5):599–600. doi: 10.23736/S0392-0488.18.05888-1.

[45] Arnež, M., Ružić-Sabljić, E. *Borrelia burgdorferi* sensu lato bacteremia in Slovenian children with solitary and multiple erythema migrans. *Pediatr Infect Dis J*. 2011;30(11):988–90. doi: 10.1097/INF.0b013e318225b8c3.

[46] Liveris, D., Schwartz, I., McKenna, D., Nowakowski, J., Nadelman, R. B., DeMarco, J., Iyer, R., Cox, M. E., Holmgren, D., Wormser, G. P. Quantitation of cell-associated borrelial DNA in the blood of Lyme disease patients with erythema migrans. *Eur J Clin Microbiol Infect Dis*. 2012;31(5):791–5. doi: 10.1007/s10096-011-1376-x.

[47] Eriksson, P., Schröder, M. T., Niiranen, K., Nevanlinna, A., Panelius, J., Ranki, A. The many faces of solitary and multiple erythema migrans. *Acta Derm Venereol*. 2013;93(6):693–700. doi: 10.2340/00015555-1549.

[48] Stanek, G., Reiter, M. The expanding Lyme Borrelia complex--clinical significance of genomic species? *Clin Microbiol Infect*. 2011;17(4):487–93. doi: 10.1111/j.1469-0691.2011.03492.x.

[49] Shkilna, M. I. Clinical and epidemiological features of erythema migrans in residents of the Ternopil region. *Dermatology and Venereology*. 2019;(1):37–41. doi: 10.33743/2308-1066-2019-1-37-41 [in Ukrainian].

[50] Shkilna, M. I. Epidemiological features and some etiological agents of erythema migrans [Internet]. *Current Infectology*. 2019 [cited 2025 Feb 3];7(2):84–85. Available from: http://www.mif-ua.com/archive/article/47321 [in Ukrainian].

[51] Aberer, E., Wutte, N. Atrophosclerodermic manifestations of Lyme borreliosis. *The Open Dermatology Journal*. 2016;10(1):27–43. doi: 10.2174/1874372201610010027.

[52] Verberkt, R. M., Janssen, M., Wesseling, J. A boy with a tight skin: Borrelia-associated early-onset morphea. *Clin Exp Rheumatol*. 2014;32(1):121–2.

[53] Zinchuk, O. M., Kalyuzhna, L. D. Skin lesions in patients with late-stage Lyme borreliosis. *Dermatology, Cosmetology, Sexopathology*. 2016;(1–2):10–14. [in Ukrainian].

[54] Gade, A., Matin, T., Rubenstein, R., Robinson, C. A. Acrodermatitis Chronica Atrophicans. 2023. In: StatPearls [Internet]. Treasure Island (FL): StatPearls Publishing; 2025.

[55] Farhangdoost, F. The role of infection in morphea disease. *Reviews in Clinical Medicine*. 2015;2(4):187–189. doi: https://doi.org/10.17463/RCM.2015.04.006.

[56] Santos, M., Haddad Júnior, V., Ribeiro-Rodrigues, R., Talhari, S. Lyme borreliosis. *A Bras Dermatol*. 2010;85(6):930–8. doi: 10.1590/s0365-05962010000600029.

[57] Romanenko, K. V., Gritsay, O. D. About the role of *Borrelia burgdorferi* in the development of localized scleroderma. *The questions of experimental and clinical medicine: a collection of articles.* 2010;14(2):161–164.

[58] Zinchuk, A. N., Kalyuzhna, L. D., Pasichna, I. A. Is Localized Scleroderma Caused by *Borrelia burgdorferi*? *Vector Borne Zoonotic Dis.* 2016;16(9):577–80. doi: 10.1089/vbz.2016.2004.

[59] Choi, M. S., Seong, G. H., Park, M. J., Park, M., Hong, S. P., Park, B. C., Kim, M. H. Rapidly Progressing Generalized Morphea with High Lyme Disease Titer. *Indian J Dermatol.* 2020 Sep–Oct;65(5):432–434. doi: 10.4103/ijd.IJD_279_18.

[60] Şandru, F., Popa, A., Petca, A., Miulescu, R. G., Constantin, M. M., Petca, R. C., Constantin, T., Dumitraşcu, M. C. Etiologic role of *Borrelia burgdorferi* in morphea: A case report. *Exp Ther Med.* 2020;20(3):2373–2376. doi: 10.3892/etm.2020.8815.

[61] Shkilna, M. I. Morphea and Lyme borreliosis. Diagnostics and therapy of infectious diseases at various levels of medical care. In: Viral diseases. HIV infection; 29–30 September 2016; Vinnytsia. Vinnytsia: [publisher unknown]; 2016. pp. 196–7. [in Ukrainian].

[62] Shkilna, M. I., Yavorska, K. B. Localized scleroderma, associated with Lyme disease. *J Dermat Cosmetol.* 2018;2(4):191. doi: 10.15406/jdc.2018.02.00075.

[63] Litaiem, N., Idoudi, S. Atrophoderma of Pasini and Pierini. [cited 2025 Feb 3]. In: *StatPearls* [Internet]. Treasure Island (FL): StatPearls Publishing; 2025. Available from: https://www.ncbi.nlm.nih.gov/books/NBK519069.

[64] Czupryna, P., Moniuszko-Malinowska, A., Pancewicz, S., Garkowski, A., Gościk, J., Siemieniako, A., Zajkowska, J. Lyme disease in Poland - A serious problem? *Adv Med Sci.* 2016;61(1):96–100. doi: 10.1016/j.advms.2015.10.007.

[65] Stricker, R. B., Fesler, M. C. Chronic Lyme disease: A working case definition. *Chronic Dis Int.* 2017;4(1):96–100. doi: 10.3844/ajidsp.2018.1.44.

[66] Malawista, S. E., Steere, A. C., Hardin, J. A. Lyme disease: a unique human model for an infectious etiology of rheumatic disease. *Yale J Biol Med.* 1984;57(4):473–7.

[67] Zinchuk, O. M. Detection of Lyme borreliosis among patients with reactive arthritis. Clinical and diagnostic aspects. *Infectious Diseases*. 2008;(2):28–31. doi: 10.11603/1681-2727.2008.2.999.

[68] Justin, D. R. Lyme Disease in Humans. *Current issues in molecular biology.* 2021;42:333-84. doi: 10.21775/cimb.042.333.

[69] Benach, J. L., Bosler, E. M., Hanrahan, J. P., Coleman, J. L., Habicht, G. S., Bast, T. F., Cameron, D. J., Ziegler, J. L., Barbour, A. G., Burgdorfer, W., Edelman, R., Kaslow, R. A. Spirochetes isolated from the blood of two patients with Lyme disease. *N Engl J Med.* 1983;308(13):740–2. doi: 10.1056/NEJM198303313081302.

[70] Steere, A. C., Grodzicki, R. L., Kornblatt, A. N., Craft, J. E., Barbour, A. G., Burgdorfer, W., Schmid, G. P., Johnson, E., Malawista, S. E. The spirochetal etiology of Lyme disease. *N Engl J Med.* 1983;308(13):733–40. doi: 10.1056/NEJM198303313081301.

[71] Wormser, G. P. Clinical practice. Early Lyme disease. *N Engl J Med.* 2006;354(26):2794–801. doi: 10.1056/NEJMcp061181.

[72] Steere, A. C., Strle, F., Wormser, G. P., Hu, L. T., Branda, J. A., Hovius, J. W., Li, X., Mead, P. S. Lyme borreliosis. *Nat Rev Dis Primers.* 2016;2:16090. doi: 10.1038/nrdp.2016.90.

[73] Molins, C. R., Ashton, L. V., Wormser, G. P., Andre, B. G., Hess, A. M., Delorey, M. J., Pilgard, M. A., Johnson, B. J., Webb, K., Islam, M. N., Pegalajar-Jurado, A., Molla, I., Jewett, M. W., Belisle, J. T. Metabolic differentiation of early Lyme disease from southern tick-associated rash illness (STARI). *Sci Transl Med.* 2017;9(403):eaal2717. doi: 10.1126/scitranslmed.aal2717.

[74] Zhou, Y., Qin, S., Sun, M., Tang, L., Yan, X., Kim, T. K., Caballero, J., Glusman, G., Brunkow, M. E., Soloski, M. J., Rebman, A. W., Scavarda, C., Cooper, D., Omenn, G. S., Moritz, R. L., Wormser, G. P., Price, N. D., Aucott, J. N., Hood, L. Measurement of Organ-Specific and Acute-Phase Blood Protein Levels in Early Lyme Disease. *J Proteome Res.* 2020;19(1):346–359. doi: 10.1021/acs.jproteome.9b00569.

[75] Comstock, L. E., Thomas, D. D. Penetration of endothelial cell monolayers by *Borrelia burgdorferi*. *Infect Immun.* 1989;57(5):1626–8. doi: 10.1128/iai.57.5.1626-1628.1989.

[76] Szczepanski, A., Furie, M. B., Benach, J. L., Lane, B. P., Fleit, H. B. Interaction between *Borrelia burgdorferi* and endothelium *in vitro*. *J Clin Invest*. 1990;85(5):1637–47. doi: 10.1172/JCI114615.

[77] Moriarty, T. J., Norman, M. U., Colarusso, P., Bankhead, T., Kubes, P., Chaconas, G. Real-time high resolution 3D imaging of the Lyme disease spirochete adhering to and escaping from the vasculature of a living host. *PLoS Pathog*. 2008;4(6):e1000090. doi: 10.1371/journal.ppat.1000090.

[78] Norman, M. U., Moriarty, T. J., Dresser, A. R., Millen, B., Kubes, P., Chaconas, G. Molecular mechanisms involved in vascular interactions of the Lyme disease pathogen in a living host. *PLoS Pathog*. 2008;4(10):e1000169. doi: 10.1371/journal.ppat.1000169.

[79] Quintero, J. A., Attah, R., Khianey, R., Capitle, E., Schutzer, S. E. Arthritis and Diagnostics in Lyme Disease. *Trop Med Infect Dis*. 2021;6(1):18. doi: 10.3390/tropicalmed6010018.

[80] Steere, A. C., Schoen, R. T., Taylor, E. The clinical evolution of Lyme arthritis. *Ann Intern Med*. 1987;107(5):725–731. doi: 10.7326/0003-4819-107-5-725.

[81] Herzer, P. Joint manifestations of Lyme borreliosis in Europe. *Scand J Infect Dis Suppl*. 1991;77:55–63.

[82] Bockenstedt, L. K., Wormser, G. P. Review: unraveling Lyme disease. *Arthritis Rheumatol*. 2014;66(9):2313–23. doi: 10.1002/art.38756.

[83] Stanek, G., Strle, F. Lyme borreliosis - from tick bite to diagnosis and treatment. *FEMS Microbiol Rev*. 2018;42(3):233–258. doi: 10.1093/femsre/fux047.

[84] Akin, E., McHugh, G. L., Flavell, R. A., Fikrig, E., Steere, A. C. The immunoglobulin (IgG) antibody response to OspA and OspB correlates with severe and prolonged Lyme arthritis and the IgG response to P35 correlates with mild and brief arthritis. *Infect Immun*. 1999;67(1):173–81. doi: 10.1128/IAI.67.1.173-181.1999.

[85] Wormser, G. P., Dattwyler, R. J., Shapiro, E. D., Halperin, J. J., Steere, A. C., Klempner, M. S., Krause, P. J., Bakken, J. S., Strle, F., Stanek, G., Bockenstedt, L., Fish, D., Dumler, J. S., Nadelman, R. B. The clinical assessment, treatment, and prevention of Lyme disease, human granulocytic anaplasmosis, and babesiosis: clinical practice guidelines by the Infectious Diseases Society of America. *Clin Infect Dis*. 2006;43(9):1089–134. doi: 10.1086/508667.

[86] Gryczyńska, A., Welc-Falęciak, R. Long-term study of the prevalence of *Borrelia burgdorferi* s.l. infection in ticks (Ixodes ricinus) feeding on blackbirds (Turdus merula) in NE Poland. *Exp Appl Acarol*. 2016;70(3):381–394. doi: 10.1007/s10493-016-0082-x.

[87] Kmieciak, W., Ciszewski, M., Szewczyk, E. M. Tick-borne diseases in Poland: Prevalence and difficulties in diagnostics. *Med Pr*. 2016;67:73–87. doi: 10.13075/mp.5893.00264. [in Polish]

[88] Cerar, T., Strle, F., Stupica, D., Ruzic-Sabljic, E., McHugh, G., Steere, A. C., Strle, K. Differences in Genotype, Clinical Features, and Inflammatory Potential of *Borrelia burgdorferi* sensu stricto Strains from Europe and the United States. *Emerg Infect Dis*. 2016;22(5):818–27. doi: 10.3201/eid2205.151806.

[89] de Taeye, S. W., Kreuk, L., van Dam, A. P., Hovius, J. W., Schuijt, T. J. Complement evasion by *Borrelia burgdorferi*: it takes three to tango. *Trends Parasitol*. 2013;29(3):119–28. doi: 10.1016/j.pt.2012.12.001.

[90] Kraiczy, P., Stevenson, B. Complement regulator-acquiring surface proteins of *Borrelia burgdorferi*: Structure, function and regulation of gene expression. *Ticks Tick Borne Dis*. 2013;4(1–2):26–34. doi: 10.1016/j.ttbdis.2012.10.039.

[91] Rogovskyy, A. S., Bankhead, T. Variable VlsE is critical for host reinfection by the Lyme disease spirochete. *PLoS One*. 2013;8(4):e61226. doi: 10.1371/journal.pone.0061226.

[92] Russell, T. M., Johnson, B. J. Lyme disease spirochaetes possess an aggrecan-binding protease with aggrecanase activity. *Mol Microbiol*. 2013;90(2):228–40. doi: 10.1111/mmi.12276.

[93] Arvikar, S. L., Steere, A. C. Diagnosis and treatment of Lyme arthritis. *Infect Dis Clin North Am*. 2015;29(2):269–80. doi: 10.1016/j.idc.2015.02.004.

[94] Orczyk, K., Świdrowska-Jaros, J., Smolewska, E. When a patient suspected with juvenile idiopathic arthritis turns out to be diagnosed with an infectious disease—a review of Lyme arthritis in children. *Pediatr Rheumatol Online J*. 2017;15(1):35. doi: 10.1186/s12969-017-0166-0.

[95] Enkelmann, J., Böhmer, M., Fingerle, V., Siffczyk, C., Werber, D., Littmann, M., Merbecks, S. S., Helmeke, C., Schroeder, S., Hell, S., Schlotthauer, U., Burckhardt, F., Stark, K., Schielke, A., Wilking,

H. Incidence of notified Lyme borreliosis in Germany, 2013–2017. *Sci Rep*. 2018;8(1):14976. doi: 10.1038/s41598-018-33136-0.

[96] Kuo, J., Warner, T. F., Schell, R. F. *Borrelia*-primed and -infected mice deficient of interleukin-17 develop arthritis after neutralization of gamma-interferon. *Pathog Dis*. 2017;75(2). doi: 10.1093/femspd/ftx014.

[97] Oosting, M., ter Hofstede, H., van de Veerdonk, F. L., Sturm, P., Kullberg, B. J., van der Meer, J. W., Netea, M. G., Joosten, L. A. Role of interleukin-23 (IL-23) receptor signaling for IL-17 responses in human Lyme disease. *Infect Immun*. 2011;79(11):4681–7. doi: 10.1128/IAI.05242-11.

[98] Crowley, J. T., Strle, K., Drouin, E. E., Pianta, A., Arvikar, S. L., Wang, Q., Costello, C. E., Steere, A. C. Matrix metalloproteinase-10 is a target of T and B cell responses that correlate with synovial pathology in patients with antibiotic-refractory Lyme arthritis. *J Autoimmun*. 2016;69:24–37. doi: 10.1016/j.jaut.2016.02.005.

[99] Hammond, E. M., Baumgarth, N. CD4 T cell responses in persistent *Borrelia burgdorferi* infection. *Curr Opin Immunol*. 2022;77:102187. doi: 10.1016/j.coi.2022.102187.

[100] Sahay, B., Patsey, R. L., Eggers, C. H., Salazar, J. C., Radolf, J. D., Sellati, T. J. CD14 signaling restrains chronic inflammation through induction of p38-MAPK/SOCS-dependent tolerance. *PLoS Pathog*. 2009;5(12):e1000687. doi: 10.1371/journal.ppat.1000687.

[101] Strle, K., Shin, J. J., Glickstein, L. J., Steere, A. C. Association of a Toll-like receptor 1 polymorphism with heightened Th1 inflammatory responses and antibiotic-refractory Lyme arthritis. *Arthritis Rheum*. 2012;64(5):1497–507. doi: 10.1002/art.34383.

[102] Steere, A. C., Glickstein, L. Elucidation of Lyme arthritis. *Nat Rev Immunol*. 2004;4(2):143–52. doi: 10.1038/nri1267.

[103] Nardelli, D. T., Callister, S. M., Schell, R. F. Lyme arthritis: current concepts and a change in paradigm. *Clin Vaccine Immunol*. 2008;15:2134. doi: 10.1128/CVI.00330-07.

[104] Swidrowska-Jaros, J., Orczyk, K., Smolewska, E. Macrophages – silent enemies in juvenile idiopathic arthritis. *Postepy Hig Med Dosw (Online)*. 2016;70:743–50. doi: 10.5604/17322693.1208887.

[105] Jin, C., Roen, D. R., Lehmann, P. V., Kellermann, G. H. An enhanced ELISPOT assay for sensitive detection of antigen-specific T cell responses to *Borrelia burgdorferi*. *Cells*. 2013;2:607–20. doi: 10.3390/cells2030607.

[106] Sonderegger, F. L., Ma, Y., Maylor-Hagan, H., Brewster, J., Huang, X., Spangrude, G. J., Zachary, J. F., Weis, J. H., Weis, J. J. Localized production of IL-10 suppresses early inflammatory cell infiltration and subsequent development of IFN-γ-mediated Lyme arthritis. *J Immunol*. 2012;188(3):1381–93. doi: 10.4049/jimmunol.1102359.

[107] Kuo, J., Warner, T. F., Munson, E. L., Nardelli, D. T., Schell, R. F. Arthritis is developed in Borrelia-primed and -infected mice deficient of interleukin-17. *Pathog Dis*. 2016;74(7):ftw077. doi: 10.1093/femspd/ftw077.

[108] Burchill, M. A., Nardelli, D. T., England, D. M., DeCoster, D. J., Christopherson, J. A., Callister, S. M., Schell, R. F. Inhibition of interleukin-17 prevents the development of arthritis in vaccinated mice challenged with *Borrelia burgdorferi*. *Infect Immun*. 2003;71(6):3437–42. doi: 10.1128/IAI.71.6.3437-3442.2003.

[109] Nardelli, D. T., Burchill, M. A., England, D. M., Torrealba, J., Callister, S. M., Schell, R. F. Association of CD4+ CD25+ T cells with prevention of severe destructive arthritis in *Borrelia burgdorferi*-vaccinated and challenged gamma interferon-deficient mice treated with anti-interleukin-17 antibody. *Clin Diagn Lab Immunol*. 2004;11(6):1075–84. doi: 10.1128/CDLI.11.6.1075-1084.2004.

[110] Infante-Duarte, C., Horton, H. F., Byrne, M. C., Kamradt, T. Microbial lipopeptides induce the production of IL-17 in Th cells. *J Immunol*. 2000;165(11):6107–15. doi: 10.4049/jimmunol.165.11.6107.

[111] Katchar, K., Drouin, E. E., Steere, A. C. Natural killer cells and natural killer T cells in Lyme arthritis. *Arthritis Res Ther*. 2013;15:R183. doi: 10.1186/ar4373.

[112] Sjöwall, J., Fryland, L., Nordberg, M., Sjögren, F., Garpmo, U., Jansson, C., Carlsson, S. A., Bergström, S., Ernerudh, J., Nyman, D., Forsberg, P., Ekerfelt, C. Decreased Th1-type inflammatory cytokine expression in the skin is associated with persisting symptoms after treatment of erythema migrans. *PLoS One*. 2011 Mar 31;6(3):e18220. doi: 10.1371/journal.pone.0018220.

[113] Vudattu, N. K., Strle, K., Steere, A. C., Drouin, E. Dysregulation of CD4+CD25(high) T cells in the synovial fluid of patients with antibiotic-refractory Lyme arthritis. *Arthritis Rheum.* 2013;65:1643–53. doi: 10.1002/art.37910.

[114] Kinjo, Y., Tupin, E., Wu, D., Fujio, M., Garcia-Navarro, R., Benhnia, M. R., Zajonc, D. M., Ben-Menachem, G., Ainge, G. D., Painter, G. F., Khurana, A., Hoebe, K., Behar, S. M., Beutler, B., Wilson, I. A., Tsuji, M., Sellati, T. J., Wong, C. H., Kronenberg, M. Natural killer T cells recognize diacylglycerol antigens from pathogenic bacteria. *Nat Immunol.* 2006;7(9):978–86. doi: 10.1038/ni1380.

[115] Philipp, M. T., Aydintug, M. K., Bohm, R. P. Jr, Cogswell, F. B., Dennis, V. A., Lanners, H. N., Lowrie, R. C. Jr, Roberts, E. D., Conway, M. D., Karaçorlu, M., Peyman, G. A., Gubler, D. J., Johnson, B. J., Piesman, J., Gu, Y. Early and early disseminated phases of Lyme disease in the rhesus monkey: a model for infection in humans. *Infect Immun.* 1993;61(7):3047–59. doi: 10.1128/iai.61.7.3047-3059.1993.

[116] Munson, E., Nardelli, D. T., Du Chateau, B. K., Callister, S. M., Schell, R. F. Hamster and murine models of severe destructive Lyme arthritis. *Clin Dev Immunol.* 2012;2012:504215. doi: 10.1155/2012/504215.

[117] Tang, T. T., Zhang, L., Bansal, A., Grynpas, M., Moriarty, T. J. The Lyme Disease Pathogen *Borrelia burgdorferi* Infects Murine Bone and Induces Trabecular Bone Loss. *Infect Immun.* 2017;85(2):e00781-16. doi: 10.1128/IAI.00781-16.

[118] Steere, A. C., Gibofsky, A., Patarroyo, M. E., Winchester, R. J., Hardin, J. A., Malawista, S. E. Chronic Lyme arthritis. Clinical and immunogenetic differentiation from rheumatoid arthritis. *Ann Intern Med.* 1979;90(6):896–901. doi: 10.7326/0003-4819-90-6-896.

[119] Duray, P. H., Steere, A. C. The spectrum of organ and systems pathology in human Lyme disease. *Zentralbl Bakteriol Mikrobiol Hyg A.* 1986;263(1-2):169–78. doi: 10.1016/s0176-6724(86)80120-1.

[120] Jones, K. L., Muellegger, R. R., Means, T. K., Lee, M., Glickstein, L. J., Damle, N., Sikand, V. K., Luster, A. D., Steere, A. C. Higher mRNA levels of chemokines and cytokines associated with macrophage activation in erythema migrans skin lesions in patients from the United States than in patients from Austria with Lyme borreliosis. *Clin Infect Dis.* 2008;46(1):85–92. doi: 10.1086/524022.

[121] Strle, K., Sulka, K. B., Pianta, A., Crowley, J. T., Arvikar, S. L., Anselmo, A., Sadreyev, R., Steere, A. C. T-Helper 17 Cell Cytokine Responses in Lyme Disease Correlate With *Borrelia burgdorferi* Antibodies During Early Infection and With Autoantibodies Late in the Illness in Patients With Antibiotic-Refractory Lyme Arthritis. *Clin Infect Dis.* 2017;64(7):930–938. doi: 10.1093/cid/cix002.

[122] Murphy, G., Nagase, H. Progress in matrix metalloproteinase research. *Mol Aspects Med.* 2008;29(5):290–308. doi: 10.1016/j.mam.2008.05.002.

[123] Hu, L. T., Eskildsen, M. A., Masgala, C., Steere, A. C., Arner, E. C., Pratta, M. A., Grodzinsky, A. J., Loening, A., Perides, G. Host metalloproteinases in Lyme arthritis. *Arthritis Rheum.* 2001;44(6):1401–10. doi: 10.1002/1529-0131(200106)44:6<1401::AID-ART234>3.0.CO;2-S.

[124] Lin, B., Kidder, J. M., Noring, R., Steere, A. C., Klempner, M. S., Hu, L. T. Differences in synovial fluid levels of matrix metalloproteinases suggest separate mechanisms of pathogenesis in Lyme arthritis before and after antibiotic treatment. *J Infect Dis.* 2001;184(2):174–80. doi: 10.1086/322000.

[125] Behera, A. K., Thorpe, C. M., Kidder, J. M., Smith, W., Hildebrand, E., Hu, L. T. *Borrelia burgdorferi*-induced expression of matrix metalloproteinases from human chondrocytes requires mitogen-activated protein kinase and Janus kinase/signal transducer and activator of transcription signaling pathways. *Infect Immun.* 2004;72(5):2864–71. doi: 10.1128/IAI.72.5.2864-2871.2004.

[126] Gebbia, J. A., Coleman, J. L., Benach, J. L. Selective induction of matrix metalloproteinases by *Borrelia burgdorferi* via toll-like receptor 2 in monocytes. *J Infect Dis.* 2004;189;(1):113–9. doi: 10.1086/380414.

[127] Snydman, D. R., Schenkein, D. P., Berardi, V. P., Lastavica, C. C., Pariser, K. M. *Borrelia burgdorferi* in joint fluid in chronic Lyme arthritis. *Ann Intern Med.* 1986;104(6):798–800. doi: 10.7326/0003-4819-104-6-798.

[128] Schmidli, J., Hunziker, T., Moesli, P., Schaad, U. B. Cultivation of *Borrelia burgdorferi* from joint fluid three months after treatment of facial palsy due to Lyme borreliosis. *J Infect Dis.* 1988;158(4):905–6. doi: 10.1093/infdis/158.4.905.

[129] Nocton, J. J., Dressler, F., Rutledge, B. J., Rys, P. N., Persing, D. H., Steere, A. C. Detection of *Borrelia burgdorferi* DNA by polymerase chain reaction in synovial fluid from patients with Lyme arthritis. *N Engl J Med.* 1994;330(4):229–34. doi: 10.1056/NEJM199401273300401.

[130] Barthold, S. W., Persing, D. H., Armstrong, A. L., Peeples, R. A. Kinetics of *Borrelia burgdorferi* dissemination and evolution of disease after intradermal inoculation of mice. *Am J Pathol.* 1991;139(2):263–73.

[131] Steere, A. C., Angelis, S. M. Therapy for Lyme arthritis: strategies for the treatment of antibiotic-refractory arthritis. *Arthritis Rheum.* 2006;54(10):3079–86. doi: 10.1002/art.22131.

[132] Singh, S. K., Girschick, H. J. Lyme borreliosis: from infection to autoimmunity. *Clin Microbiol Infect.* 2004;10(7):598–614. doi: 10.1111/j.1469-0691.2004.00895.x.

[133] Shin, J. J., Glickstein, L. J., Steere, A. C. High levels of inflammatory chemokines and cytokines in joint fluid and synovial tissue throughout the course of antibiotic-refractory Lyme arthritis. *Arthritis Rheum.* 2007;56(4):1325–35. doi: 10.1002/art.22441.

[134] Steere, A. C., Dwyer, E., Winchester, R. Association of chronic Lyme arthritis with HLA-DR4 and HLA-DR2 alleles. *N Engl J Med.* 1990;323(4):219–23. doi: 10.1056/NEJM199007263230402.

[135] Bolz, D. D., Weis, J. J. Molecular mimicry to *Borrelia burgdorferi*: pathway to autoimmunity? *Autoimmunity.* 2004;37(5):387–92. doi: 10.1080/08916930410001713098.

[136] Gross, D. M., Forsthuber, T., Tary-Lehmann, M., Etling, C., Ito, K., Nagy, Z. A., Field, J. A., Steere, A. C., Huber, B. T. Identification of LFA-1 as a candidate autoantigen in treatment-resistant Lyme arthritis. *Science.* 1998;281(5377):703–6. doi: 10.1126/science.281.5377.703.

[137] Steere, A. C., Klitz, W., Drouin, E. E., Falk, B. A., Kwok, W. W., Nepom, G. T., Baxter-Lowe, L. A. Antibiotic-refractory Lyme arthritis is associated with HLA-DR molecules that bind a *Borrelia burgdorferi* peptide. *J Exp Med.* 2006;203(4):961–71. doi: 10.1084/jem.20052471.

[138] Sigal, L. H., Zahradnik, J. M., Lavin, P., Patella, S. J., Bryant, G., Haselby, R., Hilton, E., Kunkel, M., Adler-Klein, D., Doherty, T., Evans, J., Molloy, P. J., Seidner, A. L., Sabetta, J. R., Simon, H. J., Klempner, M. S., Mays, J., Marks, D., Malawista, S. E. A vaccine consisting of recombinant *Borrelia burgdorferi* outer-surface protein A to prevent Lyme disease. Recombinant Outer-Surface Protein A Lyme Disease Vaccine Study Consortium. *N Engl J Med.* 1998;339(4):216–22. doi: 10.1056/NEJM 199807233390402.

[139] Plotkin, S. A. Correcting a public health fiasco: The need for a new vaccine against Lyme disease. *Clin Infect Dis.* 2011;52(3):s271–275. doi: 10.1093/cid/ciq119.

[140] Willyard, C. Resurrecting the "yuppie vaccine." *Nat Med.* 2014;20(7):698–701. doi: 10.1038/nm0714-698.

[141] Drouin, E. E., Seward, R. J., Strle, K., McHugh, G., Katchar, K., Londoño, D., Yao, C., Costello, C. E., Steere, A. C. A novel human autoantigen, endothelial cell growth factor, is a target of T and B cell responses in patients with Lyme disease. *Arthritis Rheum.* 2013;65(1):186–96. doi: 10.1002/art.37732.

[142] Chen, J., Field, J. A., Glickstein, L., Molloy, P. J., Huber, B. T., Steere, A. C. Association of antibiotic treatment-resistant Lyme arthritis with T cell responses to dominant epitopes of outer surface protein A of *Borrelia burgdorferi. Arthritis Rheum.* 1999 Sep;42(9):1813–22. doi: 10.1002/1529-0131 (199909)42:9<1813::AID-ANR4>3.0.CO;2-0.

[143] Steere, A. C. Posttreatment Lyme disease syndromes: distinct pathogenesis caused by maladaptive host responses. *J Clin Invest.* 2020;130(5):2148–51. doi: 10.1172/JCI138062.

[144] Lochhead, R. B., Arvikar, S. L., Aversa, J. M., Sadreyev, R. I., Strle, K., Steere, A. C. Robust interferon signature and suppressed tissue repair gene expression in synovial tissue from patients with postinfectious, *Borrelia burgdorferi*-induced Lyme arthritis. *Cell Microbiol.* 2019;21(2):e12954. doi: 10.1111/cmi.12954.

[145] Lochhead, R. B., Ordoñez, D., Arvikar, S. L., Aversa, J. M., Oh, L. S., Heyworth, B., Sadreyev, R., Steere, A. C., Strle, K. Interferon-gamma production in Lyme arthritis synovial tissue promotes differentiation of fibroblast-like synoviocytes into immune effector cells. *Cell Microbiol.* 2019;21(2):e12992. doi: 10.1111/cmi.12992.

[146] Jutras, B. L., Lochhead, R. B., Kloos, Z. A., Biboy, J., Strle, K., Booth, C. J., Govers, S. K., Gray, J., Schumann, P., Vollmer, W., Bockenstedt, L. K., Steere, A. C., Jacobs-Wagner, C. *Borrelia burgdorferi*

peptidoglycan is a persistent antigen in patients with Lyme arthritis. *Proc Natl Acad Sci U S A*. 2019;116(27):13498–507. doi: 10.1073/pnas.1904170116.

[147] Bockenstedt, L. K., Gonzalez, D. G., Haberman, A. M., Belperron, A. A. Spirochete antigens persist near cartilage after murine Lyme borreliosis therapy. *J Clin Invest*. 2012;122(7):2652–60. doi: 10.1172/JCI58813.

[148] Smith, B. G., Cruz, A. I. Jr., Milewski, M. D., Shapiro, E. D. Lyme disease and the orthopaedic implications of Lyme arthritis. *J Am Acad Orthop Surg*. 2011;19(2):91–100. doi: 10.5435/00124635-201102000-00004.

[149] Bachur, R. G., Adams, C. M., Monuteaux, M. C. Evaluating the child with acute hip pain ("irritable hip") in a Lyme endemic region. *J Pediatr*. 2015;166(2):407–11.e1. doi: 10.1016/j.jpeds.2014.09.040.

[150] Cruz, A. I. Jr., Aversano, F. J., Seeley, M. A., Sankar, W. N., Baldwin, K. D. Pediatric Lyme Arthritis of the Hip: The Great Imitator? *J Pediatr Orthop*. 2017;37(5):355–361. doi: 10.1097/BPO.0000000000000664.

[151] Collins, K. A., Gotoff, J. R., Ghanem, E. S. Lyme Disease: A Potential Source for Culture-negative Prosthetic Joint Infection. *J Am Acad Orthop Surg Glob Res Rev*. 2017;1(5):e023. doi: 10.5435/JAAOSGlobal-D-17-00023.

[152] Czupryna, P., Moniuszko, A., Czeczuga, A., Pancewicz, S., Zajkowska, J. Ultrasonographic evaluation of knee joints in patients with Lyme disease. *Int J Infect Dis*. 2012;16(4):e252–5. doi: 10.1016/j.ijid.2011.12.004.

[153] Lochhead, R. B., Strle, K., Arvikar, S. L., Weis, J. J., Steere, A. C. Lyme arthritis: linking infection, inflammation and autoimmunity. *Nat Rev Rheumatol*. 2021;17(8):449–461. doi: 10.1038/s41584-021-00648-5.

[154] Lantos, P. M., Rumbaugh, J., Bockenstedt, L. K., Falck-Ytter, Y. T., Aguero-Rosenfeld, M. E., Auwaerter, P. G., Baldwin, K., Bannuru, R. R., Belani, K. K., Bowie, W. R., Branda, J. A., Clifford, D. B., DiMario, F. J. Jr., Halperin, J. J., Krause, P. J., Lavergne, V., Liang, M. H., Cody Meissner, H., Nigrovic, L. E., Nocton, J. J. J., Osani, M. C., Pruitt, A. A., Rips, J., Rosenfeld, L. E., Savoy, M. L., Sood, S. K., Steere, A. C., Strle, F., Sundel, R., Tsao, J., Vaysbrot, E. E., Wormser, G. P., Zemel, L. S. Clinical Practice Guidelines by the Infectious Diseases Society of America (IDSA), American Academy of Neurology (AAN), and American College of Rheumatology (ACR): 2020 Guidelines for the Prevention, Diagnosis, and Treatment of Lyme Disease. *Arthritis Rheumatol*. 2021;73(1):12–20. doi: 10.1002/art.41562.

[155] Smiyan, S. I., Shkilna, M. I., Regaliuk, V. V., Makhovska, O. S., Zadorozhna, L. V., Makhovsky, V. P., Grubar, Y. Yu. Modern aspects of the etiology, pathogenesis, clinical course, and treatment of Lyme arthritis (literature review, personal observations) [Internet]. *Ukrainian Rheumatology Journal*. 2018 [cited 5 Feb 2025];72(2):40–5. Available at: https://www.rheumatology.kiev.ua/wp/wp-content/uploads/2018/07/1085.pdf?upload= [in Ukrainian].

[156] DAS28 [Internet]. *DAS28 Disease activity score calculator for rheumatoid arthritis* [cited 5 Feb 2025]. Available at: https://www.das28.nl/das28/DAScalculators/dasculators.html.

[157] Arvikar, S. L., Steere, A. C. Lyme Arthritis. *Infect Dis Clin North Am*. 2022 Sep;36(3):563–577. doi: 10.1016/j.idc.2022.03.006.

[158] Smiyan, S., Galaychuk, I., Zhulkevych, I., Nykolyuk, V., Komorovsky, R., Gusak, S., Bilozetsky, I. Sjögren's syndrome and lymphadenopathy unraveling the diagnosis of Lyme disease. *Reumatologia*. 2019;57(1):59–62. doi: 10.5114/reum.2019.83242.

[159] Galaychuk, I. Y., Zhulkevych, I. V., Smiyan, S. I., Nykolyuk, V. D., Komorovsky, R. R. Borrelious Lymphadenopathy in Oncology Practice (Clinical Observations). *Oncology*. 2019;21(3):251–53. doi: 10.32471/oncology.2663-7928.t-21-3-2019-g.7896.

[160] Shapiro, E. D., Gerber, M. A. Lyme disease. *Clin Infect Dis*. 2000;31(2):533–42. doi: 10.1086/313982.

[161] Brouwer, M. A. E., van de Schoor, F. R., Vrijmoeth, H. D., Netea, M. G., Joosten, L. A. B. A joint effort: The interplay between the innate and the adaptive immune system in Lyme arthritis. *Immunological Reviews*. 2020;294:63–79. doi: 10.1111/imr.12837.

[162] Steere, A. C., Brinckerhoff, C. E., Miller, D. J., Drinker, H., Harris, E. D. Jr, Malawista, S. E. Elevated levels of collagenase and prostaglandin E2 from synovium associated with erosion of cartilage and

bone in a patient with chronic Lyme arthritis. *Arthritis Rheum.* 1980;23(5):591–9. doi: 10.1002/art.1780230511.

[163] Miller, J. R., Dunn, K. W., Braccia, D., Ciliberti, L. J. Jr, Becker, D. K., Hollinger, J. K., Brand, S. M. Lyme Disease Manifestations in the Foot and Ankle: A Retrospective Case Series. *J Foot Ankle Surg.* 2016;55(6):1241–4. doi: 10.1053/j.jfas.2015.06.006.

[164] Aiyer, A., Hennrikus, W., Walrath, J., Groh, B., Ostrov, B. Lyme arthritis of the pediatric lower extremity in the setting of polyarticular disease. *J Child Orthop.* 2014;8(4):359–65. doi: 10.1007/s 11832-014-0602-3.

[165] Smiyan, S. I., Yuskevych, V. V. Features of the clinical course of rheumatoid arthritis associated with *Borrelia burgdorferi. Achievements of Clinical and Experimental Medicine.* 2019;(4):111–16. doi: 10.11603/1811-2471.2019.v.i4.10810 [in Ukrainian].

[166] Kuzmina, H. P., Lazarenko, O. M. Quality of life and functional status indicators of patients with arterial hypertension and comorbid gout [Internet]. *Family Medicine.* 2019 [cited 5 Feb 2025];2:89–93. Available at: https://repo.dma.dp.ua/id/eprint/4234 [in Ukrainian].

[167] Stepanenko, A. M., Bibliva, I. I., Monastyrsky, O. V., Onyshchenko, K. I., Podstriganova, Y. U., Tkachenko, M. O. Quality of life in patients with rheumatoid arthritis during treatment with tumor necrosis factor inhibitors [Internet]. In: *Current Issues in Clinical Medicine*; 23 May 2019 [cited 5 Feb 2025]; Poltava. Poltava; 2019. p. 90–2. Available at: https://repository.pdmu.edu.ua/handle/123456789/10918 [in Ukrainian].

[168] Vansovych, O. S. Articular form of borreliosis in the practical activities of a rheumatologist [Internet]. In: *International medical students' conference in Poltava*; April 2–3, 2020 [cited 5 Feb 2025]; Poltava. Poltava; 2020. p. 10–1. Available at: https://repository.pdmu.edu.ua/handle/123456789/13443 [in Ukrainian].

[169] Svitlytska, O. A., Fedorova, O. P., Dudko, O. V., Gorbatkova, N. G. A case of severe rheumatoid arthritis in the structure of chronic Lyme borreliosis [Internet]. In: *Current Issues in the Diagnosis and Treatment of Internal Diseases*; March–May 2018 [cited 5 Feb 2025]; Kharkiv. Kharkiv: KhNMU, 2018. P. 45–46. Available at: http://dspace.zsmu.edu.ua/handle/123456789/8175 [in Ukrainian].

[170] Ponyk, R. M., Korytko, Z. I. Incidence and features of rehabilitation in patients with rheumatoid arthritis in the present day. *Achievements of Clinical and Experimental Medicine.* 2019;3:18387. doi: 10.11603/1811-2471.2019.v.i3.10504 [in Ukrainian].

[171] Frikha, F., Maazoun, F., Ben Salah, R., Snoussi, M., Masmoudi, J., Nabil Mhiri, M., Bahloul, Z. Sexual function in married women with rheumatoid arthritis. *Presse Med.* 2011 Dec;40(12 Pt 1):e521–7. doi: 10.1016/j.lpm.2011.04.015. [in French]

[172] Buitinga, L., Braakman-Jansen, L. M., Taal, E., van de Laar, M. A. Future expectations and worst-case future scenarios of patients with rheumatoid arthritis: a focus group study. *Musculoskeletal Care.* 2012;10(4):240–7. doi: 10.1002/msc.1026.

[173] Hill, E. M., Frost, A. Illness perceptions, coping, and health-related quality of life among individuals experiencing chronic Lyme disease. *Chronic Illn.* 2022;18(2):426–438. doi: 10.1177/1742395320983875.

[174] Vallerand, I. A., Patten, S. B., Barnabe, C. Depression and the risk of rheumatoid arthritis. *Curr Opin Rheumatol.* 2019;31(3):279–84. doi: 10.1097/BOR.0000000000000597.

[175] Więdłocha, M., Marcinowicz, P., Krupa, R., Janoska-Jaździk, M., Janus, M., Dębowska, W., Mosiołek, A., Waszkiewicz, N., Szulc, A. Effect of antidepressant treatment on peripheral inflammation markers – A meta-analysis. *Prog Neuropsychopharmacol Biol Psychiatry.* 2018;80(Pt C):217–226. doi: 10.1016/j.pnpbp.2017.04.026.

[176] Johnson, L., Wilcox, S., Mankoff, J., Stricker, R. B. Severity of chronic Lyme disease compared to other chronic conditions: a quality of life survey. *PeerJ.* 2014;2:e322. doi: 10.7717/peerj.322.

[177] Arvikar, S. L., Crowley, J. T., Sulka, K. B., Steere, A. C. Autoimmune Arthritides, Rheumatoid Arthritis, Psoriatic Arthritis, or Peripheral Spondyloarthritis Following Lyme Disease. *Arthritis Rheumatol.* 2017;69(1):194–202. doi: 10.1002/art.39866.

[178] Kondo, N., Kuroda, T., Kobayashi, D. Cytokine Networks in the Pathogenesis of Rheumatoid Arthritis. *Int J Mol Sci.* 2021;22(20):10922. doi: 10.3390/ijms222010922.

[179] Hirano, T. IL-6 in inflammation, autoimmunity and cancer. *Int. Immunol.* 2021;33:127–48. doi: 10.1093/intimm/dxaa078.

[180] Tokarska-Rodak, M., Pańczuk, A., Kozioł-Montewka, M., Plewik, D., Szepeluk, A. Monoinfections caused by *Borrelia burgdorferi* and *Borrelia burgdorferi/Anaplasma phagocytophilum* co-infections in forestry workers and farmers. *Med. Pr.* 2015;66(5):645–651. doi: 10.13075/mp.5893.00226. [in Polish].

[181] Shkilna, M. I., Andreychyn, M. A., Ivakhiv, O. L., Iosyk, I. I., Zavidniuk, N. H., Tvorko, M. S., et al., Dynamics of interleukins in patients with Lyme borreliosis. *Med. Clin. Chem.* 2020;22(1):17–22. doi: 10.11603/mcch.2410-681X.2020.v.i1.11051 [in Ukrainian].

[182] Barnes, T. C., Anderson, M. E., Moots, R. J. The many faces of interleukin-6: the role of IL-6 in inflammation, vasculopathy, and fibrosis in systemic sclerosis. *Int. J. Rheumatol.* 2011;2011:721608. doi: 10.1155/2011/721608.

[183] Kaya, F. Ö., Ceylan, Y., İpek, B. Ö., Özünal, Z. G., Sezgin, G., Nalbant, S. Can cytokines be used as an activation marker in rheumatoid arthritis? *Endocr. Metab. Immune Disord. Drug Targets.* 2021;21(8):1459–1465. doi: 10.2174/1871530320666201019115030.

[184] Brouwer, M. A. E., van de Schoor, F. R., Vrijmoeth, H. D., Netea, M. G., Joosten, L. A. B. A joint effort: the interplay between the innate and the adaptive immune system in Lyme arthritis. *Immunol. Rev.* 2020;294(1):63–79. doi: 10.1111/imr.12837.

[185] Sulka, K. B., Strle, K., Crowley, J. T., Lochhead, R. B., Anthony, R., Steere, A. C. Correlation of Lyme disease-associated IgG4 autoantibodies with synovial pathology in antibiotic-refractory Lyme arthritis. *Arthritis Rheumatol.* 2018;70(11):1835–1846. doi: 10.1002/art.40566.

[186] Zhao, T., Wei, Y., Zhu, Y., Xie, Z., Hai, Q., Li, Z., Qin, D. Gut microbiota and rheumatoid arthritis: from pathogenesis to novel therapeutic opportunities. *Front. Immunol.* 2022;13:1007165. doi: 10.3389/fimmu.2022.1007165.

[187] Rowland, I., Gibson, G., Heinken, A., Scott, K., Swann, J., Thiele, I., Tuohy, K. Gut microbiota functions: metabolism of nutrients and other food components. *Eur. J. Nutr.* 2018;57(1):1–24. doi: 10.1007/s00394-017-1445-8.

[188] Picchianti-Diamanti, A., Rosado, M. M., D'Amelio, R. Infectious agents and inflammation: the role of microbiota in autoimmune arthritis. *Front. Microbiol.* 2018;8:2696. doi: 10.3389/fmicb.2017.02696.

[189] Zhong, D., Wu, C., Zeng, X., Wang, Q. The role of gut microbiota in the pathogenesis of rheumatic diseases. *Clin. Rheumatol.* 2018;37(1):25–34. doi: 10.1007/s10067-017-3821-4.

[190] Hernandez, C. J. The microbiome and bone and joint disease. *Curr. Rheumatol. Rep.* 2017;19(12):77. doi: 10.1007/s11926-017-0705-1.

[191] Huang, Z. Y., Stabler, T., Pei, F. X., Kraus, V. B. Both systemic and local lipopolysaccharide (LPS) burden are associated with knee OA severity and inflammation. *Osteoarthritis Cartilage.* 2016;24(10):1769–1775. doi: 10.1016/j.joca.2016.05.008.

[192] Lorenz, W., Buhrmann, C., Mobasheri, A., Lueders, C., Shakibaei, M. Bacterial lipopolysaccharides form procollagen-endotoxin complexes that trigger cartilage inflammation and degeneration: implications for the development of rheumatoid arthritis. *Arthritis Res. Ther.* 2013;15(5):R111. doi: 10.1186/ar4291.

[193] Maeda, Y., Takeda, K. Role of gut microbiota in rheumatoid arthritis. *J. Clin. Med.* 2017;6(6):60. doi: 10.3390/jcm6060060.

[194] Larsen, J. M. The immune response to *Prevotella* bacteria in chronic inflammatory disease. *Immunology.* 2017;151(4):363–374. doi: 10.1111/imm.12760.

[195] Sakkas, L. I., Bogdanos, D. P. Multiple hit infection and autoimmunity: the dysbiotic microbiota–ACPA connection in rheumatoid arthritis. *Curr. Opin. Rheumatol.* 2018;30(4):403–409. doi: 10.1097/BOR.0000000000000503.

[196] Maeda, Y., Kurakawa, T., Umemoto, E., Motooka, D., Ito, Y., Gotoh, K., et al., Dysbiosis contributes to arthritis development via activation of autoreactive T cells in the intestine. *Arthritis Rheumatol.* 2016;68(11):2646–2661. doi: 10.1002/art.39783.

[197] Alpizar-Rodriguez, D., Lesker, T. R., Gronow, A., Gilbert, B., Raemy, E., Lamacchia, C., et al., *Prevotella copri* in individuals at risk for rheumatoid arthritis. *Ann. Rheum. Dis.* 2019;78(5):590–593. doi: 10.1136/annrheumdis-2018-214514.

[198] Pianta, A., Arvikar, S. L., Strle, K., Drouin, E. E., Wang, Q., Costello, C. E., Steere, A. C. Two rheumatoid arthritis-specific autoantigens correlate microbial immunity with autoimmune responses in joints. *J. Clin. Invest.* 2017;127(8):2946–2956. doi: 10.1172/JCI93450.

[199] Chen, J., Wright, K., Davis, J. M., Jeraldo, P., Marietta, E. V., Murray, J., et al., An expansion of rare lineage intestinal microbes characterizes rheumatoid arthritis. *Genome Med.* 2016;8(1):43. doi: 10.1186/s13073-016-0299-7.

[200] Picchianti-Diamanti, A., Panebianco, C., Salemi, S., Sorgi, M. L., Di Rosa, R., Tropea, A., et al., Analysis of gut microbiota in rheumatoid arthritis patients: disease-related dysbiosis and modifications induced by etanercept. *Int. J. Mol. Sci.* 2018;19(10):2938. doi: 10.3390/ijms19102938.

[201] Merkulova, A. Antibiotic therapy, dysbiosis, and potential risks [Internet]. *Health of Ukraine — XXI Century.* 2017;(4):72–73 [cited 2025 Feb 6]. Available from: https://health-ua.com/article/25955-antibiotikoterapiya-disbakterioz-i-vozmozhnye-riski [in Ukrainian].

[202] Lysenko, H. I., Bilko, I. P., Nikolska, O. I., Tesliuk, L. V. *Diagnosis and treatment of intestinal dysbiosis in rheumatology patients*. Kyiv: Znania; 1999. 22 p. [in Ukrainian].

[203] Smiyan, S. I., Yuskevych, V. V., Makhovska, O. S. The state of microbiota of the large intestine in patients with rheumatoid arthritis associated with *Borrelia burgdorferi*. *Ukrainian Journal of Rheumatology.* 2020;80(2):9–13. doi: 10.32471/rheumatology.2707-6970.80.15262 [in Ukrainian].

[204] Wills, A. B., Spaulding, A. B., Adjemian, J., Prevots, D. R., Turk, S. P., Williams, C., Marques, A. Long-term follow-up of patients with Lyme disease: longitudinal analysis of clinical and quality-of-life measures. *Clin. Infect. Dis.* 2016;62(12):1546–1551. doi: 10.1093/cid/ciw189.

[205] Wessely, S. Chronic fatigue: symptom and syndrome. *Ann. Intern. Med.* 2001;134(9 Pt 2):838–843. doi: 10.7326/0003-4819-134-9_part_2-200105011-00007.

[206] Murphy, K. R., Han, J. L., Yang, S., Hussaini, S. M., Elsamadicy, A. A., Parente, B., et al., Prevalence of specific types of pain diagnoses in a sample of United States adults. *Pain Physician.* 2017;20(2):E257–E268.

[207] Luck, T., Roehr, S., Rodriguez, F. S., Schroeter, M. L., Witte, A. V., Hinz, A., et al., Memory-related subjective cognitive symptoms in the adult population: prevalence and associated factors - results of the LIFE-Adult-Study. *BMC Psychol.* 2018;6(1):23. doi: 10.1186/s40359-018-0236-1.

[208] Dinerman, H., Steere, A. C. Lyme disease associated with fibromyalgia. *Ann. Intern. Med.* 1992;117(4):281–285. doi: 10.7326/0003-4819-117-4-281.

[209] Novitch, M., Wahab, A., Kakarala, R., Mukerji, R. The emergence of a forgotten entity: dermatomyositis-like presentation of Lyme disease in rural Wisconsin. *Cureus.* 2018;10(5):e2608. doi: 10.7759/cureus.2608.

[210] Doskaliuk, B., Zimba, O. *Borrelia burgdorferi* and autoimmune mechanisms: implications for mimicry, misdiagnosis, and mismanagement in Lyme disease and autoimmune disorders. *Rheumatol. Int.* 2024;44(11):2265–2271. doi: 10.1007/s00296-024-05580-x.

[211] Yehudina, Y., Trypilka, S. Lyme borreliosis as a trigger for autoimmune disease. *Cureus.* 2021;13(10):e18648. doi: 10.7759/cureus.18648.

[212] Nguyen, H., Le, C., Nguyen, H. Acute Lyme infection presenting with amyopathic dermatomyositis and rapidly fatal interstitial pulmonary fibrosis: a case report. *J. Med. Case Rep.* 2010;4:187. doi: 10.1186/1752-1947-4-187.

[213] Waton, J., Pinault, A. L., Pouaha, J., Truchetet, F. Lyme disease could mimic dermatomyositis. *Rev. Med. Interne.* 2007;28(5):343–345. doi: 10.1016/j.revmed.2007.01.002. [in French].

[214] Horowitz, H. W., Sanghera, K., Goldberg, N., Pechman, D., Kamer, R., Duray, P., et al., Dermatomyositis associated with Lyme disease: case report and review of Lyme myositis. *Clin. Infect. Dis.* 1994;18(2):166–171. doi: 10.1093/clinids/18.2.166.

[215] Fraser, D. D., Kong, L. I., Miller, F. W. Molecular detection of persistent *Borrelia burgdorferi* in a man with dermatomyositis. *Clin. Exp. Rheumatol.* 1992;10(4):387–390.

[216] Nguyen, H., Le, C., Nguyen, H. Acute Lyme infection presenting with amyopathic dermatomyositis and rapidly fatal interstitial pulmonary fibrosis: a case report. *J. Med. Case Rep.* 2010;4(1). doi: 10. 1186/1752-1947-4-187.

[217] Detmar, U., Maciejewski, W. Borrelial dermatomyositis-like syndrome. In: Weber, K., Burgdorfer, W., Schierz, G., eds. *Aspects of Lyme Borreliosis* [Internet]. Berlin: Springer-Verlag; 1993 [cited 2025 Feb 08]. p. 259–265. Available from: doi: 10.1007/978-3-642-77614-4_20.

[218] Cadavid, D., Bai, Y., Dail, D., Hurd, M., Narayan, K., Hodzic, E., et al., Infection and inflammation in skeletal muscle from nonhuman primates infected with different genospecies of the Lyme disease spirochete *Borrelia burgdorferi*. *Infect. Immun.* 2003;71(12):7087–7098. doi: 10.1128/IAI.71.12.7087-7098.2003.

[219] Hoffmann, J. C., Stichtenoth, D. O., Zeidler, H., Follmann, M., Brandis, A., Stanek, G., et al., Lyme disease in a 74-year-old forest owner with symptoms of dermatomyositis. *Arthritis Rheum.* 1995;38(8):1157–1160. doi: 10.1002/art.1780380820.

[220] Smoleńska, Ż., Masiak, A., Strzelecki, A., Zbigniew, Z. The role of *Borrelia burgdorferi* infection in scleroderma. *Reumatologia.* 2014;52(5):326–331. doi: 10.5114/reum.2014.46671.

[221] Müller, K. E. Damage of collagen and elastic fibres by *Borrelia burgdorferi* — known and new clinical and histopathological aspects. *Open Neurol. J.* 2012;6:179–186. doi: 10.2174/1874205X01206010179.

[222] Berndtson, K. Review of evidence for immune evasion and persistent infection in Lyme disease. *Int. J. Gen. Med.* 2013;6:291–306. doi: 10.2147/IJGM.S44114.

[223] Mayes, M. D., Whittum-Hudson, J. A., Oszust, C., Gérard, H. C., Hudson, A. P. Lack of evidence for bacterial infections in skin in patients with systemic sclerosis. *Am. J. Med. Sci.* 2009;337(4):233–235. doi: 10.1097/maj.0b013e3181891612.

[224] Wackernagel, A., Bergmann, A. R., Aberer, E. Acute exacerbation of systemic scleroderma in *Borrelia burgdorferi* infection. *J. Eur. Acad. Dermatol. Venereol.* 2005;19(1):93–96. doi: 10.1111/j.1468-3083.2004.01074.x.

[225] Hickie, I., Davenport, T., Wakefield, D., Vollmer-Conna, U., Cameron, B., Vernon, S. D., Reeves, W. C., Lloyd, A.; Dubbo Infection Outcomes Study Group. Post-infective and chronic fatigue syndromes precipitated by viral and non-viral pathogens: prospective cohort study. *BMJ.* 2006;333(7568):575. doi: 10.1136/bmj.38933.585764.AE.

[226] Nath, A. Long-Haul COVID. *Neurology.* 2020;95:559–560. doi: 10.1212/WNL.0000000000010640.

[227] Aucott, J. N. Posttreatment Lyme disease syndrome. *Infect. Dis. Clin. North Am.* 2015;29:309–323. doi: 10.1016/j.idc.2015.02.012.

[228] Geebelen, L., Lernout, T., Devleesschauwer, B., Kabamba-Mukadi, B., Saegeman, V., Belkhir, L., De Munter, P., Dubois, B., Westhovens, R.; Humtick Hospital Group; Van Oyen, H., Speybroeck, N., Tersago, K. Non-specific symptoms and post-treatment Lyme disease syndrome in patients with Lyme borreliosis: a prospective cohort study in Belgium (2016–2020). *BMC Infect. Dis.* 2022;22(1):756. doi: 10.1186/s12879-022-07686-8.

[229] Lobraico, J., Butler, A., Petrini, J., Ahmadi, R. New insights into stages of Lyme disease symptoms from a novel hospital-based registry. *J. Prim. Care Community Health.* 2014;5(4):284–287. doi: 10.1177/2150131914540693.

[230] Zomer, T. P., Barendregt, J. N. M., van Kooten, B., van Bemmel, T., Landman, G. W., van Hees, B. C., Vermeeren, Y. M. Non-specific symptoms in adult patients referred to a Lyme centre. *Clin. Microbiol. Infect.* 2019;25(1):67–70. doi: 10.1016/j.cmi.2018.09.016.

[231] Rebman, A. W., Bechtold, K. T., Yang, T., Mihm, E. A., Soloski, M. J., Novak, C. B., Aucott, J. N. The Clinical, Symptom, and Quality-of-Life Characterization of a Well-Defined Group of Patients with Posttreatment Lyme Disease Syndrome. *Front. Med. (Lausanne).* 2017;4:224. doi: 10.3389/fmed.2017.00224.

[232] Curtis, C., Shah, S. P., Chin, S. F., Turashvili, G., Rueda, O. M., Dunning, M. J., Speed, D., Lynch, A. G., Samarajiwa, S., Yuan, Y., Gräf, S., Ha, G., Haffari, G., Bashashati, A., Russell, R., McKinney, S.; METABRIC Group; Langerød, A., Green, A., Provenzano, E., Wishart, G., Pinder, S., Watson, P., Markowetz, F., Murphy, L., Ellis, I., Purushotham, A., Børresen-Dale, A. L., Brenton, J. D., Tavaré, S., Caldas, C., Aparicio, S. The genomic and transcriptomic architecture of 2,000 breast tumours reveals novel subgroups. *Nature.* 2012;486(7403):346–352. doi: 10.1038/nature10983.

[233] Mukherjee, S., Mez, J., Trittschuh, E. H., Saykin, A. J., Gibbons, L. E., Fardo, D. W., Wessels, M., Bauman, J., Moore, M., Choi, S. E., Gross, A. L., Rich, J., Louden, D. K. N., Sanders, R. E., Grabowski, T. J., Bird, T. D., McCurry, S. M., Snitz, B. E., Kamboh, M. I., Lopez, O. L., De Jager, P. L., Bennett,

D. A., Keene, C. D., Larson, E. B.; EPAD Study Group; Investigators from ACT; Investigators from ROS; Investigators from MAP; Investigators from ADNI; Investigators from the University of Pittsburgh ADRC; Crane, P. K. Genetic data and cognitively defined late-onset Alzheimer's disease subgroups. *Mol. Psychiatry.* 2020;25(11):2942–2951. doi: 10.1038/s41380-018-0298-8.

[234] Bellato, E., Marini, E., Castoldi, F., Barbasetti, N., Mattei, L., Bonasia, D. E., Blonna, D. Fibromyalgia syndrome: etiology, pathogenesis, diagnosis, and treatment. *Pain Res. Treat.* 2012;2012:426130. doi: 10.1155/2012/426130.

[235] Nemeth, J., Bernasconi, E., Heininger, U., Abbas, M., Nadal, D., Strahm, C., Erb, S., Zimmerli, S., Furrer, H., Delaloye, J., Kuntzer, T., Altpeter, E., Sturzenegger, M., Weber, R., For The Swiss Society For Infectious Diseases And The Swiss Society For Neurology. Update of the Swiss guidelines on post-treatment Lyme disease syndrome. *Swiss Med. Wkly.* 2016;146:w14353. doi: 10.4414/smw.2016.14353. PMID: 27922168.

[236] Rebman, A. W., Yang, T., Aucott, J. N. Symptom heterogeneity and patient subgroup classification among US patients with post-treatment Lyme disease: an observational study. *BMJ Open.* 2021;11(1):e040399. doi: 10.1136/bmjopen-2020-040399.

[237] Rebman, A. W., Aucott, J. N. Post-Treatment Lyme disease as a model for persistent symptoms in Lyme disease. *Front. Med.* 2020;7:57. doi: 10.3389/fmed.2020.00057.

[238] Nowakowski, J., Nadelman, R. B., Sell, R., McKenna, D., Cavaliere, L. F., Holmgren, D., Gaidici, A., Wormser, G. P. Long-term follow-up of patients with culture-confirmed Lyme disease. *Am. J. Med.* 2003;115(2):91–96. doi: 10.1016/s0002-9343(03)00308-5.

[239] Shadick, N. A., Phillips, C. B., Sangha, O., Logigian, E. L., Kaplan, R. F., Wright, E. A., Fossel, A. H., Fossel, K., Berardi, V., Lew, R. A., Liang, M. H. Musculoskeletal and neurologic outcomes in patients with previously treated Lyme disease. *Ann. Intern. Med.* 1999;131(12):919–926. doi: 10.7326/0003-4819-131-12-199912210-00003.

[240] Kalish, R. A., Kaplan, R. F., Taylor, E., Jones-Woodward, L., Workman, K., Steere, A. C. Evaluation of study patients with Lyme disease, 10-20-year follow-up. *J. Infect. Dis.* 2001;183(3):453–460. doi: 10.1086/318082.

[241] Wills, A. B., Spaulding, A. B., Adjemian, J., Prevots, D. R., Turk, S. P., Williams, C., Marques, A. Long-term Follow-up of Patients with Lyme Disease: Longitudinal Analysis of Clinical and Quality-of-life Measures. *Clin. Infect. Dis.* 2016;62(12):1546–1551. doi: 10.1093/cid/ciw189.

[242] Hirsch, A. G., Herman, R. J., Rebman, A., Moon, K. A., Aucott, J., Heaney, C., Schwartz, B. S. Obstacles to diagnosis and treatment of Lyme disease in the USA: a qualitative study. *BMJ Open.* 2018;8(6):e021367. doi: 10.1136/bmjopen-2017-021367.

[243] Blum, L. K., Adamska, J. Z., Martin, D. S., Rebman, A. W., Elliott, S. E., Cao, R. R. L., Embers, M. E., Aucott, J. N., Soloski, M. J., Robinson, W. H. Robust B Cell Responses Predict Rapid Resolution of Lyme Disease. *Front. Immunol.* 2018;9:1634. doi: 10.3389/fimmu.2018.01634.

[244] Aucott, J. N., Soloski, M. J., Rebman, A. W., Crowder, L. A., Lahey, L. J., Wagner, C. A., Robinson, W. H., Bechtold, K. T. CCL19 as a Chemokine Risk Factor for Posttreatment Lyme Disease Syndrome: a Prospective Clinical Cohort Study. *Clin. Vaccine Immunol.* 2016;23(9):757–766. doi: 10.1128/CVI.00071-16.

[245] Strle, K., Stupica, D., Drouin, E. E., Steere, A. C., Strle, F. Elevated levels of IL-23 in a subset of patients with post-lyme disease symptoms following erythema migrans. *Clin. Infect. Dis.* 2014;58(3):372–380. doi: 10.1093/cid/cit735.

[246] Krause, P. J., Telford, S. R. 3rd, Spielman, A., Sikand, V., Ryan, R., Christianson, D., Burke, G., Brassard, P., Pollack, R., Peck, J., Persing, D. H. Concurrent Lyme disease and babesiosis. Evidence for increased severity and duration of illness. *JAMA.* 1996;275(21):1657–1660.

[247] Dzyga, S. V., Bakalets, O. V., Behosh, N. B., Maksiv, K. Ya. Clinical case of borreliosis infection as a possible cause of heart damage and syncope. *Bulletin of Medical and Biological Research.* 2020;(1):83–85. doi: 10.11603/bmbr.2706-6290.2020.1.10959. [in Ukrainian].

[248] Radesich, C., Del Mestre, E., Medo, K., Vitrella, G., Manca, P., Chiatto, M., Castrichini, M., Sinagra, G. Lyme Carditis: From Pathophysiology to Clinical Management. *Pathogens.* 2022 May 15;11(5):582. doi: 10.3390/pathogens11050582.

[249] Methodological recommendations on the epidemiology, diagnosis, and prevention of tick-borne borreliosis (Lyme disease) in Ukraine, Order of the Ministry of Health of Ukraine from №. 218, May 16, 2005, *Zakon Online* [Internet], [cited 4 Feb 2025] (Ukraine). Available at: https://zakononline.com.ua/documents/show/83937___83937. [in Ukrainian].

[250] Young, S., Omair Arshad, O., Arikan, Y., Mirzanejad, Y. Lyme carditis: A can't miss diagnosis [Internet]. *BCMJ.* 2020 [cited 4 Feb 2025];62(10):368-72. Available at: https://bcmj.org/articles/lyme-carditis-cant-miss-diagnosis.

[251] Zinchuk, O. M. Features of antimicrobial treatment of Lyme borreliosis [Internet]. *Zaporizhzhia Medical Journal.* 2011 [cited 4 Feb 2025]; 13(5):109–111. Available at: http://nbuv.gov.ua/UJRN/Zmzh_2011_13_5_31 [in Ukrainian].

[252] Maly, V. P., Shepileva, N. V., Volobueva, V. A., Grinenko, V. A. Lyme borreliosis: current state of the problem. *International Medical Journal.* 2009;(1):123–126. [in Russian].

[253] van Hattem, J. M., Keijer, J. T., Nijveldt, R. A man with cardiac Lyme borreliosis. *CMAJ.* 2015;187(14):1071–1073. doi: 10.1503/cmaj.141468.

[254] Popovych, O. Lyme borreliosis: current problem of infectiology (Clinical Lecture). *Actual Infectology.* 2022;(3.12):114–122. doi: 10.22141/2312-413x.3.12.2016.81725. [in Ukrainian].

[255] Krause, P. J., Linda, K. B. Lyme Disease and the Heart. *Circulation.* 2013;127(7):451–454. doi: 10.1161/CIRCULATIONAHA.112.101485.

[256] Wormser, G. P., Dattwyler, R. J., Shapiro, E. D., Halperin, J. J., Steere, A. C., Klempner, M. S., Krause, P. J., Bakken, J. S., Strle, F., Stanek, G., Bockenstedt, L., Fish, D., Dumler, J. S., Nadelman, R. B. The clinical assessment, treatment, and prevention of lyme disease, human granulocytic anaplasmosis, and babesiosis: clinical practice guidelines by the Infectious Diseases Society of America. *Clin. Infect. Dis.* 2006;43(9):1089–1134. doi: 10.1086/508667.

[257] Scheffold, N., Herkommer, B., Kandolf, R., May, A. E. Lyme carditis–diagnosis, treatment and prognosis. *Dtsch Arztebl Int.* 2015;112(12):202–208. doi: 10.3238/arztebl.2015.0202.

[258] Fish, A. E., Pride, Y. B., Pinto, D. S. Lyme carditis. *Infectious Disease Clinics of North America.* 2008;22(2):275–288. doi: 10.1016/j.idc.2007.12.008.

[259] Radesich, C., Del Mestre, E., Medo, K., Vitrella, G., Manca, P., Chiatto, M., Castrichini, M., Sinagra, G. Lyme Carditis: From Pathophysiology to Clinical Management. *Pathogens.* 2022;11(5):582. doi: 10.3390/pathogens11050582.

[260] Steere, A. C., Sikand, V. K., Meurice, F., Parenti, D. L., Fikrig, E., Schoen, R. T., Nowakowski, J., Schmid, C. H., Laukamp, S., Buscarino, C., Krause, D. S. Vaccination against Lyme disease with recombinant Borrelia burgdorferi outer-surface lipoprotein A with adjuvant. Lyme Disease Vaccine Study Group. *N Engl J Med.* 1998;339(4):209–215. doi: 10.1056/NEJM199807233390401.

[261] Osadchy, O. Lyme disease: treatment and prevention guidelines. *Ukrainian Medical Journal.* 2020 [cited 4 Feb 2025]. Available from: https://umj.com.ua/uk/publikatsia-195683-hvoroba-lajma-nastanovi-z-likuvannya-ta-profilaktiki [in Ukrainian].

[262] Bratton, R. L., Whiteside, J. W., Hovan, M. J., Engle, R. L., Edwards, F. D. Diagnosis and treatment of Lyme disease. *Mayo Clin Proc.* 2008;83(5):566–571. doi: 10.4065/83.5.566.

[263] Goldberg, N. Healio [Internet]. Cardiologists: Know the signs of Lyme disease; April 14, 2014 [cited 4 Feb 2025]. Available at: www.healio.com/news/cardiology/20140414/cardiologists-know-the-signs-of-lyme-disease.

[264] Kozlovska, A. Lyme disease: Clinical presentation, diagnosis, and treatment [Internet]. *Ukrainian Medical Journal.* 2019 [cited 4 Feb 2025];(6):10. Available from: https://www.umj.com.ua/article/158253/hvoroba-lajma-klinichna-kartina-diagnostika-ta-likuvannya. [in Ukrainian].

[265] Linden, H. UpToDate [Internet]. Lyme carditis; 2023 [cited 5 Feb 2025]. Available at: https://www.uptodate.com/contents/lyme-carditis.

[266] Pinto, D. S. Cardiac manifestations of Lyme disease. *Med Clin North Am.* 2002;86(2):285–296. doi: 10.1016/s0025-7125(03)00087-7.

[267] Motamed, M., Liblik, K., Miranda-Arboleda, A. F., Wamboldt, R., Wang, C. N., Cingolani, O., Rebman, A. W., Novak, C. B., Aucott, J. N., Farina, J. M., Baranchuk, A. Disseminated Lyme disease and dilated cardiomyopathy: A systematic review. *Trends Cardiovasc Med.* 2023;33(8):531–536. doi: 10.1016/j.tcm.2022.05.010.

[268] Kozlovska, A. Lyme borreliosis: modern principles of treatment from A to Z [Internet]. *Clinical Immunology. Allergology. Infectology.* 2020 [cited 4 Feb 2025];5:34–39. Available from: https://kiai.com.ua/ua/archive/2020/5%28126%29/pages-34-39/laym-borelioz-suchasni-principi-likuvannya-vid-a-do-ya. [in Ukrainian].

[269] Karkkonen, K., Stiernstedt, S. H., Karlsson, M. Follow-up of patients treated with oral doxycycline for Lyme neuroborreliosis. *Scand J Infect Dis.* 2001;33(4):259–262. doi: 10.1080/003655401300077225.

[270] Völzke, H., Wolff, B., Lüdemann, J., Guertler, L., Kramer, A., John, U., Felix, S. B. Seropositivity for anti-Borrelia IgG antibody is independently associated with carotid atherosclerosis. *Atherosclerosis.* 2006;184(1):108–112. doi: 10.1016/j.atherosclerosis.2004.10.048.

[271] Scheffold, N., Sucker, C., Bergler-Klein, J., Kaag, N., Cyran, J. Acute myocarditis and cardiomyopathy in Lyme borreliosis. *Z Kardiol.* 2000;89(11):1046–1052. doi: 10.1007/s003920070158. [in German]

[272] Burrascano, J. J. Diagnostic hints and treatment guidelines for Lyme and other tick-borne illnesses. 15th ed. New York; 2005. 33 p.

[273] Renaud, I., Cachin, C., Gerster, J. C. Good outcomes of Lyme arthritis in 24 patients in an endemic area of Switzerland. *Joint Bone Spine.* 2004;71(1):39–43. doi: 10.1016/S1297-319X(03)00160-X.

[274] Nguyen, C. T., Cifu, A. S., Pitrak, D. Prevention and Treatment of Lyme Disease. *JAMA.* 2022;327(8):772–773. doi: 10.1001/jama.2021.25302.

[275] Mygland, A., Ljøstad, U., Fingerle, V., Rupprecht, T., Schmutzhard, E., Steiner, I.; European Federation of Neurological Societies. EFNS guidelines on the diagnosis and management of European Lyme neuroborreliosis. *Eur J Neurol.* 2010;17(1):8–16, e1–e4. doi: 10.1111/j.1468-1331.2009.02862.x.

[276] Djukic, M., Schmidt-Samoa, C., Lange, P., Spreer, A., Neubieser, K., Eiffert, H., Nau, R., Schmidt, H. Cerebrospinal fluid findings in adults with acute Lyme neuroborreliosis. *J Neurol.* 2012 Apr;259(4):630–636. doi: 10.1007/s00415-011-6221-8.

[277] Ogrinc, K., Lusa, L., Lotrič-Furlan, S., Bogovič, P., Stupica, D., Cerar, T., Ružić-Sabljić, E., Strle, F. Course and Outcome of Early European Lyme Neuroborreliosis (Bannwarth Syndrome): Clinical and Laboratory Findings. *Clin Infect Dis.* 2016;63(3):346–353. doi: 10.1093/cid/ciw299.

[278] Ljostad, U., Mygland, A. Remaining complaints 1 year after treatment for acute Lyme neuroborreliosis; frequency, pattern, and risk factors. *European Journal of Neurology.* 2010;17(1):118–123. doi: 10.1111/j.1468-1331.2009.02756.x.

[279] Eikeland, R., Ljøstad, U., Mygland, A., Herlofson, K., Løhaugen, G. C. European neuroborreliosis: neuropsychological findings 30 months post-treatment. *Eur J Neurol.* 2012;19(3):480–487. doi: 10.1111/j.1468-1331.2011.03563.x.

[280] Skripuletz, T., Schwenkenbecher, P., Pars, K., Stoll, M., Conzen, J., Bolat, S., Pul, R., Vonberg, R. P., Sedlacek, L., Wurster, U., Stangel, M., Trebst, C. Importance of follow-up cerebrospinal fluid analysis in cryptococcal meningoencephalitis. *Dis Markers.* 2014;2014:162576. doi: 10.1155/2014/162576.

[281] Schwenkenbecher, P., Pul, R., Wurster, U., Conzen, J., Pars, K., Hartmann, H., et al., Common and uncommon neurological manifestations of neuroborreliosis leading to hospitalization. *BMC Infect Dis.* 2017;17(1):90. doi: 10.1186/s12879-016-2112-z.

[282] Kinzel, S., Lehmann-Horn, K., Torke, S., Häusler, D., Winkler, A., Stadelmann, C., et al., Myelin-reactive antibodies initiate T cell-mediated CNS autoimmune disease by opsonization of endogenous antigen. *Acta Neuropathol.* 2016;132(1):43–58. doi: 10.1007/s00401-016-1559-8.

[283] Vaysbrot, E. E., Bannuru, R. R., Christopher, M. C., Osani, M. C., Halperin, J. J. Papilledema secondary to neurologic Lyme borreliosis: a meta-case series. *J Neuroophthalmol.* 2021;41(4):e498–e508. doi: 10.1097/WNO.0000000000000983.

[284] Dersch, R., Sarnes, A. A., Maul, M., Hottenrott, T., Baumgartner, A., Rauer, S., Stich, O. Quality of life, fatigue, depression and cognitive impairment in Lyme neuroborreliosis. *J Neurol.* 2015;262(11):2572–7. doi: 10.1007/s00415-015-7891-4.

[285] Cox, M. G., Wolfs, T. F., Lo, T. H., Kappelle, L. J., Braun, K. P. Neuroborreliosis causing focal cerebral arteriopathy in a child. *Neuropediatrics.* 2005;36(2):104–7. doi: 10.1055/s-2005-837573.

[286] Halperin, J. J. Nervous system Lyme disease. *Infect Dis Clin North Am.* 2015;29(2):241–53. doi: 10.1016/j.idc.2015.02.002.

[287] Stanek, G., Wormser, G. P., Gray, J., Strle, F. Lyme borreliosis. *Lancet.* 2012;379(9814):461–73. doi: 10.1016/S0140-6736(11)60103-7.

[288] Schwenkenbecher, P., Sarikidi, A., Wurster, U., Bronzlik, P., Sühs, K. W., Raab, P., et al., McDonald Criteria 2010 and 2005 compared: persistence of high oligoclonal band prevalence despite almost doubled diagnostic sensitivity. *Int J Mol Sci.* 2016;17(9):1592. doi: 10.3390/ijms17091592.

[289] Skripuletz, T., Wurster, U., Worthmann, H., Heeren, M., Schuppner, R., Trebst, C., et al., Blood-cerebrospinal fluid barrier dysfunction in patients with neurological symptoms during the 2011 Northern German E. coli serotype O104:H4 outbreak. *Brain.* 2013;136(Pt 8):e241. doi: 10.1093/brain/aws361.

[290] Schwenkenbecher, P., Chacko, L. P., Wurster, U., Pars, K., Pul, R., Sühs, K. W., et al., Intrathecal synthesis of anti-Hu antibodies distinguishes patients with paraneoplastic peripheral neuropathy and encephalitis. *BMC Neurol.* 2016;16(1):136. doi: 10.1186/s12883-016-0657-5.

[291] Rey, V., Du Pasquier, R., Muehl, A., Péter, O., Michel, P. Multiple ischemic strokes due to *Borrelia garinii* meningovasculitis. *Rev Neurol (Paris).* 2010;166(11):931–4. doi: 10.1016/j.neurol.2010.03.010. [in French]

[292] Rauer, S., Kastenbauer, S., Fingerle, V., Hunfeld, K. P., Huppertz, H. I., Dersch, R. Lyme neuroborreliosis. *Dtsch Arztebl Int.* 2018;115(45):751–6. doi: 10.3238/arztebl.2018.0751.

[293] Van Snick, S., Duprez, T. P., Kabamba, B., Van De Wyngaert, F. A., Sindic, C. J. Acute ischaemic pontine stroke revealing Lyme neuroborreliosis in a young adult. *Acta Neurol Belg.* 2008;108(3):103–6.

[294] Lebas, A., Toulgoat, F., Saliou, G., Husson, B., Tardieu, M. Stroke due to Lyme neuroborreliosis: changes in vessel wall contrast enhancement. *J Neuroimaging.* 2012;22(2):210–2. doi: 10.1111/j.1552-6569.2010.00550.x.

[295] Back, T., Grünig, S., Winter, Y., Bodechtel, U., Guthke, K., Khati, D., von Kummer, R. Neuroborreliosis-associated cerebral vasculitis: long-term outcome and health-related quality of life. *J Neurol.* 2013;260(6):1569–75. doi: 10.1007/s00415-013-6831-4.

[296] Aboul-Enein, F., Kristoferitsch, W. Normal pressure hydrocephalus or neuroborreliosis? *Wien Med Wochenschr.* 2009;159(1–2):58–61. doi: 10.1007/s10354-008-0581-4.

[297] Topakian, R., Artemian, H., Metschitzer, B., Lugmayr, H., Kühr, T., Pischinger, B. Dramatic response to a 3-week course of ceftriaxone in late neuroborreliosis mimicking atypical dementia and normal pressure hydrocephalus. *J Neurol Sci.* 2016;366:146–8. doi: 10.1016/j.jns.2016.05.002.

[298] Castaldo, J. E., Griffith, E., Monkowski, D. H. Pseudotumor cerebri: early manifestation of adult Lyme disease. *Am J Med.* 2008;121(7):e5–6. doi: 10.1016/j.amjmed.2008.02.032.

[299] Bremell, D., Hagberg, L. Clinical characteristics and cerebrospinal fluid parameters in patients with peripheral facial palsy caused by Lyme neuroborreliosis compared with facial palsy of unknown origin (Bell's palsy). *BMC Infect Dis.* 2011;11:215. doi: 10.1186/1471-2334-11-215.

[300] Henningsson, A. J., Malmvall, B. E., Ernerudh, J., Matussek, A., Forsberg, P. Neuroborreliosis - an epidemiological, clinical and healthcare cost study from an endemic area in the south-east of Sweden. *Clin Microbiol Infect.* 2010;16(8):1245–51. doi: 10.1111/j.1469-0691.2009.03059.x.

[301] Rupprecht, T. A., Lechner, C., Tumani, H., Fingerle, V. CXCL13: a biomarker for acute Lyme neuroborreliosis: investigation of the predictive value in the clinical routine. *Nervenarzt.* 2014;85(4):459–64. doi: 10.1007/s00115-014-4020-z. [in German].

[302] Moniuszko, A., Czupryna, P., Pancewicz, S., Rutkowski, K., Zajkowska, O., Swierzbińska, R., Grygorczuk, S., Kondrusik, M., Owłasiuk, P., Zajkowska, J. Evaluation of CXCL8, CXCL10, CXCL11, CXCL12 and CXCL13 in serum and cerebrospinal fluid of patients with neuroborreliosis. *Immunol Lett.* 2014;157(1–2):45–50. doi: 10.1016/j.imlet.2013.11.002.

[303] Roux, F., Boyer, E., Jaulhac, B., Dernis, E., Closs-Prophette, F., Puéchal, X. Lyme meningoradiculitis: prospective evaluation of biological diagnosis methods. *Eur J Clin Microbiol Infect Dis.* 2007;26(10):685–93. doi: 10.1007/s10096-007-0347-8.

[304] Picha, D., Moravcova, L., Smiskova, D. Prospective study on the chemokine CXCL13 in neuroborreliosis and other aseptic neuroinfections. *J Neurol Sci.* 2016;368:214–20. doi: 10.1016/j.jns.2016.05.059.

[305] Dersch, R., Toews, I., Sommer, H., Rauer, S., Meerpohl, J. J. Methodological quality of guidelines for management of Lyme neuroborreliosis. *BMC Neurol.* 2015;15:242. doi: 10.1186/s12883-015-0501-3.

[306] Rauer, S., Kastenbauer, S., Fingerle, V., Hunfeld, K. P., Huppertz, H. I., Dersch, R. Neuroborreliosis, S3 guideline, 2018 [Internet]; in: German Society of Neurology (ed.), Guidelines for diagnostics and therapy in neurology [cited 6 Feb 2025]. Available at: www.dgn.org/leitlinien.

[307] Coiffier, G., Tattevin, P. Lyme disease: "End of the debate?." *Joint Bone Spine.* 2021;88(4):105181. doi: 10.1016/j.jbspin.2021.105181.

[308] Babbar, S., Galati, J., Corona, J., Zahid, S. Acute hemiplegia and ataxia from Lyme disease. *Cooper Rowan Med J.* 2022;4(1):131. doi: 10.31986/issn.2578.3343_vol4iss1.11.

[309] Mygland, A., Skarpaas, T., Ljøstad, U. Chronic polyneuropathy and Lyme disease. *Eur J Neurol.* 2006;13(11):1213–5. doi: 10.1111/j.1468-1331.2006.01395.x.

[310] Rothermel, H., Hedges, T. R. 3rd, Steere, A. C. Optic neuropathy in children with Lyme disease. *Pediatrics.* 2001;108(2):477–81. doi: 10.1542/peds.108.2.477.

[311] López-Alberola, R. F. Neuroborreliosis and the pediatric population: a review. *Rev Neurol.* 2006;42 Suppl 3:S91–6.

[312] Bontemps-Gallo, S., Lawrence, K. A., Richards, C. L., Gherardini, F. C. Genomic and phenotypic characterization of *Borrelia afzelii* BO23 and *Borrelia garinii* CIP 103362. *PLoS ONE.* 2018;13:e0199641. doi: 10.1371/journal.pone.0199641.

[313] Fallon, B. A., Keilp, J. G., Corbera, K. M., Petkova, E., Britton, C. B., Dwyer, E., Slavov, I., Cheng, J., Dobkin, J., Nelson, D. R., Sackeim, H. A. A randomized, placebo-controlled trial of repeated IV antibiotic therapy for Lyme encephalopathy. *Neurology.* 2008;70(13):992–1003. doi: 10.1212/01.WNL.0000284604.61160.2d.

[314] Logigian, E. L., Johnson, K. A., Kijewski, M. F., Kaplan, R. F., Becker, J. A., Jones, K. J., Garada, B. M., Holman, B. L., Steere, A. C. Reversible cerebral hypoperfusion in Lyme encephalopathy. *Neurology.* 1997;49(6):1661–70. doi: 10.1212/wnl.49.6.1661.

[315] Kieslich, M., Fiedler, A., Driever, P. H., Weis, R., Schwabe, D., Jacobi, G. Lyme borreliosis mimicking central nervous system malignancy: the diagnostic pitfall of cerebrospinal fluid cytology. *Brain Dev.* 2000;22(6):403–6. doi: 10.1016/s0387-7604(00)00165-0.

[316] Agosta, F., Rocca, M. A., Benedetti, B., Capra, R., Cordioli, C., Filippi, M. MR imaging assessment of brain and cervical cord damage in patients with neuroborreliosis. *AJNR Am J Neuroradiol.* 2006;27(4):892–4.

[317] Massengo, S. A., Bonnet, F., Braun, C., Vital, A., Beylot, J., Bastard, J. Severe neuroborreliosis: the benefit of prolonged high-dose combination of antimicrobial agents with steroids – an illustrative case. *Diagn Microbiol Infect Dis.* 2005;51(2):127–30. doi: 10.1016/j.diagmicrobio.2004.04.022.

[318] Steinbach, J. P., Melms, A., Skalej, M., Dichgans, J. Delayed resolution of white matter changes following therapy of *Borrelia burgdorferi* encephalitis. *Neurology.* 2005;64(4):758–9. doi: 10.1212/01.WNL.0000152048.34121.E1.

[319] Wormser, G. P., McKenna, D., Carlin, J., Nadelman, R. B., Cavaliere, L. F., Holmgren, D., Byrne, D. W., Nowakowski, J. Brief communication: hematogenous dissemination in early Lyme disease. *Ann Intern Med.* 2005;142(9):751–5. doi: 10.7326/0003-4819-142-9-200505030-00011.

[320] Ljøstad, U., Økstad, S., Topstad, T., Mygland, A., Monstad, P. Acute peripheral facial palsy in adults. *J Neurol.* 2005;252(6):672–6. doi: 10.1007/s00415-005-0715-1.

[321] Pachner, A. R., Steiner, I. Lyme neuroborreliosis: infection, immunity, and inflammation. *Lancet Neurol.* 2007;6(6):544–52. doi: 10.1016/S1474-4422(07)70128-X.

[322] Zinchuk, O. M. Lyme Borreliosis: Clinical-Immunopathogenetic Features and Emergency Preventive Treatment [Author's Abstract]. Kyiv; 2010. 41 c. [in Ukrainian].

[323] Cabello, F. C., Embers, M. E., Newman, S. A., Godfrey, H. P. *Borreliella burgdorferi* antimicrobial-tolerant persistence in Lyme disease and posttreatment Lyme disease syndromes. *mBio.* 2022;13(3):e0344021. doi: 10.1128/mbio.03440-21.

[324] Hoppa, E., Bachur, R. Lyme disease update. *Curr Opin Pediatr.* 2007;19(3):275–80. doi: 10.1097/MOP.0b013e3280e1269a.

[325] Triulzi, F., Scotti, G. Differential diagnosis of multiple sclerosis: contribution of magnetic resonance techniques. *J Neurol Neurosurg Psychiatry.* 1998;64 Suppl 1:S6–14.

[326] Martin, R., Gran, B., Zhao, Y., Markovic-Plese, S., Bielekova, B., Marques, A., Sung, M. H., Hemmer, B., Simon, R., McFarland, H. F., Pinilla, C. Molecular mimicry and antigen-specific T cell responses in multiple sclerosis and chronic CNS Lyme disease. *J Autoimmun.* 2001;16(3):187–92. doi: 10.1006/jaut.2000.0501.

[327] Peltomaa, M., Pyykkö, I., Seppälä, I., Viljanen, M. Lyme borreliosis and facial paralysis – a prospective analysis of risk factors and outcome. *Am J Otolaryngol.* 2002;23(3):125–32. doi: 10.1053/ajot.2002.123434.

[328] Feder, H. M. Jr., Johnson, B. J., O'Connell, S., Shapiro, E. D., Steere, A. C., Wormser, G. P.; Ad Hoc International Lyme Disease Group; Agger, W. A., Artsob, H., Auwaerter, P., Dumler, J. S., Bakken, J. S., Bockenstedt, L. K., Green, J., Dattwyler, R. J., Munoz, J., Nadelman, R. B., Schwartz, I., Draper, T., McSweegan, E., Halperin, J. J., Klempner, M. S., Krause, P. J., Mead, P., Morshed, M., Porwancher, R., Radolf, J. D., Smith, R. P. Jr, Sood, S., Weinstein, A., Wong, S. J., Zemel, L. A critical appraisal of "chronic Lyme disease." *N Engl J Med.* 2007;357(14):1422–30. doi: 10.1056/NEJMra072023.

[329] Wormser, G. P., Shapiro, E. D. Implications of gender in chronic Lyme disease. *J Womens Health (Larchmt).* 2009;18(6):831–4. doi: 10.1089/jwh.2008.1193.

[330] Rupprecht, T. A., Koedel, U., Fingerle, V., Pfister, H. W. The pathogenesis of Lyme neuroborreliosis: from infection to inflammation. *Mol Med.* 2008;14(3–4):205–12. doi: 10.2119/2007-00091.

[331] Kesteman, T., Rossi, C., Bastien, P., Brouillard, J., Avesani, V., Olive, N., Martin, P., Delmée, M. Prevalence and genetic heterogeneity of *Borrelia burgdorferi* sensu lato in *Ixodes* ticks in Belgium. *Acta Clin Belg.* 2010;65(5):319–22. doi: 10.1179/acb.2010.069.

[332] Usova, N. N. *Borreliosis In Vivo* [Internet]. Neurological complications of Lyme borreliosis 1.0; 2 Dec. 2014 [cited 6 Feb 2025]. Available at: https://borrelioz.com/forum/resources/nevrologicheskie-oslozhnenija-lajm-borre-lioza.101

[333] Harrer, T., Geissdörfer, W., Schoerner, C., Lang, E., Helm, G. Seronegative Lyme neuroborreliosis in a patient on treatment for chronic lymphatic leukemia. *Infection.* 2007;35(2):110–3. doi: 10.1007/s15010-007-6121-0.

[334] Maltsev, D. V., Kazmirchuk, V. Ye. Modified method of comparative serological studies for diagnosing persistent herpesvirus neuroinfection. *Laboratory Diagnostics.* 2011;3(57):24–30. [in Ukrainian].

[335] Saunders, N. R., Knott, G. W., Dziegielewska, K. M. Barriers in the immature brain. *Cell Mol Neurobiol.* 2000;20(1):29–40. doi: 10.1023/a:1006991809927.

[336] Gilden, D., Cohrs, R. J., Mahalingam, R., Nagel, M. A. Varicella zoster virus vasculopathies: diverse clinical manifestations, laboratory features, pathogenesis, and treatment. *Lancet Neurol.* 2009;8(8):731–40. doi: 10.1016/S1474-4422(09)70134-6.

[337] Ljostad, U., Skarpaas, T., Mygland, A. Clinical usefulness of intrathecal antibody testing in acute Lyme neuroborreliosis. *Eur J Neurol.* 2007;14:873–6. doi: 10.1111/j.1468-1331.2007.01799.x.

[338] World Health Organization. *Global Tuberculosis Report 2020* [Internet]. Andreychyn, M. A., editor. Geneva; 2007. 232 p. Available at: https://www.who.int/publications/i/item/9789240013131

[339] Todoriko, L. D., Ostrovskyi, M. M., Semianiv, I. O., Shevchenko, O. S. Features of tuberculosis course during the COVID-19 pandemic. *Tuberculosis, Pulmonary Diseases, HIV Infection.* 2020;(4):52–63. doi: 10.30978/TB2020-4-52 [in Ukrainian].

[340] Tuberculosis [Internet]. Public Health Centre of the Ministry of Health of Ukraine; [cited 6 Feb 2025]. Available at: https://phc.org.ua/kontrolzakhvoryuvan/tuberkuloz [in Ukrainian].

[341] Ashkin, A., Alexis, A., Ninneman, M., Tresgallo, R. R., Ashkin, D., Peloquin, C. A. Concomitant treatment of tuberculosis and hepatitis C virus in coinfected patients using serum drug concentration monitoring. *Open Forum Infect Dis.* 2023;10(6):ofad237. doi: 10.1093/ofid/ofad237.

[342] Feshchenko, Yu. I. Modern trends in studying tuberculosis problems [Internet]. *Ukrainian Pulmonological Journal.* 2019;(1):8–24 [cited 6 Feb 2025]. Available at: http://www.ifp.kiev.ua/doc/journals/upj/19/pdf19-1/8.pdf [in Ukrainian].

[343] Alemu, A., Kebede, A., Dagne, B., Amare, M., Diriba, G., Yenew, B., Tesfaye, E., Tadesse, M., Sinshaw, W., Challa, D., Desta, K. Intestinal parasites co-infection and associated factors among active pulmonary tuberculosis patients in selected health centers, Addis Ababa, Ethiopia: unmatched case control study. *BMC Infect Dis.* 2019;19(1):407. doi: 10.1186/s12879-019-4009-0.

[344] Panigrahi, K., Jena, A., Singh, P., Mohapatra, I., Lenka, P. R., Jena, J. Prevalence of intestinal parasitic infections among pulmonary tuberculosis patients in a tertiary care hospital, Bhubaneswar, Odisha, India. *J Clin Diagn Res.* 2019;13(8):DC12–15. doi: 10.7860/JCDR/2019/41590.13067.

[345] Gilmour, B., Alene, K. A., Clements, A. The prevalence of tuberculosis and malaria in minority indigenous populations of South-East Asia and the Western Pacific Region: a systematic review and meta-analysis. *Pathog Glob Health.* 2022;116(4):201–19. doi: 10.1080/20477724.2021.2011579.

[346] Andreychyn, M. A., editor. *Infectious diseases in general practice and family medicine.* Ternopil: TSMU: Ukrmedknyga; 2007. 500 p. [in Ukrainian].

[347] Sovkich, A. L., Pańczuk, A., Kozioł-Montewka, M., Tsyrkunov, M. V., Tokarska-Rodak, M., Hutko, A. R. Epidemiological situation of Lyme borreliosis in the Polish-Belarusian borderland in the years 2012–2016 (Podlasie Province and Grodno Region). *Health Probl Civiliz.* 2017;11(2):71–9. doi: 10.5114/hpc.2017.69021.

[348] Shkilna, M. I., Andreychyn, M. A., Korda, M. M., Klishch, I. M., Zaporozhan, S. Y., Morochkovskyi, R. S. The frequency of seropositive individuals to the complex *B. burgdorferi* sensu lato among forestry workers of Zhytomyr, Khmelnytskyi and Volyn region. *Infect Dis (Ukr).* 2018;(3):18–25. doi: 10.11603/1681-2727.2018.3.9408 [in Ukrainian].

[349] Malyi, V. P. Giardiasis. Clinical immunology [Internet]. *Allergology. Infectology.* 2014;(3):35–43 [cited 6 Feb 2025]. Available at: https://kiai.com.ua/ua/archive/2014/3%2872%29 [in Ukrainian].

[350] Buczek, A., Rudek, A., Bartosik, K., Szymanska, J., Wojcik-Fatla, A. Seroepidemiological study of Lyme borreliosis among forestry workers in southern Poland. *Ann Agric Environ Med.* 2009;16(2):257–61.

[351] Unified clinical protocol for primary, secondary (specialized), and tertiary (highly specialized) medical care for adults. Tuberculosis, Order of the Ministry of Health of Ukraine No. 620 [Internet], 4 Sept. 2014 [cited 6 Feb 2025]. Available at: https://zakon.rada.gov.ua/rada/show/v0620282-14#Text [in Ukrainian].

[352] Carranza-Tamayo, C. O., Costa, J. N., Bastos, W. M. Lyme disease in the state of Tocantins, Brazil: report of the first cases. *Braz J Infect Dis.* 2012;16(6):586–9. doi: 10.1016/j.bjid.2012.07.013.

[353] Duzhyi, I. D., Oleshchenko, H. P., Hresko, I. Ya., Yurchenko, A. V. Pleural effusion syndrome and Lyme disease. *Tuberculosis, pulmonary diseases, HIV infection.* 2016;(2):79–84 [in Ukrainian].

[354] Coburn, J., Garcia, B., Hu, L. T., Jewett, M. W., Kraiczy, P., Norris, S. J., Skare, J. Lyme disease pathogenesis. *Curr Issues Mol Biol.* 2021;42:473–518. doi: 10.21775/cimb.042.473.

[355] Besant, G., Wan, D., Yeung, C., Blakely, C., Branscombe, P., Suarez-Fuster, L., Redfearn, D., Simpson, C., Abdollah, H., Glover, B., Baranchuk, A. Suspicious index in Lyme carditis: systematic review and proposed new risk score. *Clin Cardiol.* 2018;41(12):1611–16. doi: 10.1002/clc.23102.

[356] Kornaga, S. I. Hemodynamics and myocardial function in patients with pulmonary tuberculosis during anti-mycobacterial therapy: clinical significance and correction methods [dissertation abstract]. Kyiv: State Institution "National Institute of Physiology and Pulmonology named after F.H. Yanovsky of the National Academy of Medical Sciences of Ukraine"; 2012. 30 p. [in Ukrainian].

[357] Zinchuk, O. M. Features of clinical manifestations and diagnostics of disseminated forms of Lyme borreliosis. *Practical Medicine.* 2008;(2):204–9 [in Ukrainian].

[358] Marchenko, H. V. Liver function in patients with newly diagnosed pulmonary tuberculosis combined with hepatitis B and/or C. *Tuberculosis, pulmonary diseases, HIV infection.* 2015;(1):30–4 [in Ukrainian].

[359] Painter, J. E., Collier, S. A., Gargano, J. W. Association between Giardia and arthritis or joint pain in a large health insurance cohort: could it be reactive arthritis? *Epidemiol Infect.* 2017;145(3):471–7. doi: 10.1017/S0950268816002120.

[360] Damania, B., Kenney, S. C., Raab-Traub, N. Epstein-Barr virus: biology and clinical disease. *Cell.* 2022;185(20):3652–70. doi: 10.1016/j.cell.2022.08.026.

[361] Atton, O. L., Harris-Arnold, A., Schaffert, S., Krams, S. M., Martinez, O. M. The interplay between Epstein-Barr virus and B lymphocytes: implications for infection, immunity, and disease. *Immunol Res.* 2014;58(2–3):268–76. doi: 10.1007/s12026-014-8496-1.

[362] Andreychyn, M. A., Huk, M. T., Shkilna, M. I., Shtokaylo, K. Ya., Korda, M. M. Study of blood serum of patients with lymphadenopathy for antibodies to tick-borne and other pathogens. *Zaporizhzhya medical journal.* 2022;24(1):38–43. doi: 10.14739/2310-1210.2022.1.238413 [in Ukrainian].

[363] Zmijewski, M. A. Vitamin D and human health. *Int J Mol Sci.* 2019;20(1):145. doi: 10.3390/ijms 20010145.

[364] Alonso, N., Zelzer, S., Eibinger, G., Herrmann, M. Vitamin D metabolites: analytical challenges and clinical relevance. *Calcif Tissue Int.* 2023;112(2):158–77. doi: 10.1007/s00223-022-00961-5.

[365] Holick, M. F., Binkley, N. C., Bischoff-Ferrari, H. A., Gordon, C. M., Hanley, D. A., Heaney, R. P., Murad, M. H., Weaver, C. M. Endocrine Society. Evaluation, treatment, and prevention of vitamin D deficiency: an Endocrine Society clinical practice guideline. *J Clin Endocrinol Metab.* 2011;96(7):1911–30. doi: 10.1210/jc.2011-0385.

[366] Grygorieva, N., Tronko, M., Kovalenko, V., Komisarenko, S., Tatarchuk, T., Dedukh, N., Veliky, M., Strafun, S., Komisarenko, Y., Kalashnikov, A., Orlenko, V., Pankiv, V., Shvets, O., Gogunska, I., Regeda, S. Diagnosis, prevention and treatment of vitamin D deficiency in adults: Ukrainian experts consensus statement. *Pain, Joints, Spine.* 2023;13(2):60–76. doi: 10.22141/pjs.13.2.2023.368 [in Ukrainian].

[367] Amrein, K., Scherkl, M., Hoffmann, M., Neuwersch-Sommeregger, S., Köstenberger, M., Tmava Berisha, A., Martucci, G., Pilz, S., Malle, O. Vitamin D deficiency 2.0: an update on the current status worldwide. *Eur J Clin Nutr.* 2020;74(11):1498–513. doi: 10.1038/s41430-020-0558-y.

[368] Povorozniuk, V. V., Pludovski, P. *Vitamin D deficiency and insufficiency: epidemiology, diagnosis, prevention, and treatment.* Donetsk: Publisher Zaslavskyi O. Yu; 2014. 262 p. [in Ukrainian].

[369] Povorozniuk, V., Balatska, N., Muts, V., Vdovina, O. Vitamin D deficiency and insufficiency in residents of Ukraine. *Pain. Joints. Spine* [Internet]. 2011 [cited 2025 Feb 6];4(4):5–13. Available from: http://www.mif-ua.com/archive/article/27747 [in Ukrainian].

[370] Povorozniuk, V., Pankiv, I. Vitamin D status in the population of Bukovina and Prykarpattia depending on the place of residence above sea level. *Pain. Joints. Spine.* 2021;22(02):7–10. doi: 10.22141/2224-1507.2.22.2016.75755 [in Ukrainian].

[371] Hryhorieva, N. V., Solonenko, T. Yu., Musiienko, A. S. Vitamin D deficiency during the COVID-19 pandemic and the war in Ukraine. *Pain. Joints. Spine*, 2023;13(1):7–14. doi: 10.22141/pjs.13.1. 2023.352 [in Ukrainian].

[372] Bouillon, R., Marcocci, C., Carmeliet, G., Bikle, D., White, J. H., Dawson-Hughes, B., Lips, P., Munns, C. F., Lazaretti-Castro, M., Giustina, A., Bilezikian, J. Skeletal and Extraskeletal Actions of Vitamin D: Current Evidence and Outstanding Questions. *Endocr Rev.* 2019;40(4):1109–1151. doi: 10.1210/er.2018-00126.

[373] Cai, L., Wang, G., Zhang, P., Hu, X., Zhang, H., Wang, F., Tong, Y. The Progress of the Prevention and Treatment of Vitamin D to Tuberculosis. *Front Nutr.* 2022;9:873890. doi: 10.3389/fnut. 2022.873890.

[374] Mostafa, A., Jalilvand, S., Shoja, Z., Nejati, A., Shahmahmoodi, S., Sahraian, M. A., Marashi, S. M. Multiple sclerosis-associated retrovirus, Epstein-Barr virus, and vitamin D status in patients with relapsing remitting multiple sclerosis. *J Med Virol.* 2017;89(7):1309–13. doi: 10.1002/jmv.24774.

[375] Pérez-Pérez, S., Domínguez-Mozo, M. I., García-Martínez, M. Á., Aladro, Y., Martínez-Ginés, M., García-Domínguez, J. M., López de Silanes, C., Casanova, I., Ortega-Madueño, I., López-Lozano, L., Torrejón, M. J., Arroyo, R., Álvarez-Lafuente, R. Study of the possible link of 25-hydroxyvitamin D with Epstein-Barr virus and human herpesvirus 6 in patients with multiple sclerosis. *Eur J Neurol.* 2018;25(12):1446–1453. doi: 10.1111/ene.13749.

[376] Teymoori-Rad, M., Mozhgani, S. H., Zarei-Ghobadi, M., Sahraian, M. A., Nejati, A., Amiri, M. M., Shokri, F., Marashi, S. M. Integrational analysis of miRNAs data sets as a plausible missing linker between Epstein-Barr virus and vitamin D in relapsing remitting MS patients. *Gene.* 2019;689:1–10. doi: 10.1016/j.gene.2018.12.004.

[377] Bivona, G., Scazzone, C., Sasso, B. L., Giglio, R. V., Gambino, C. M., Agnello, L., Ciaccio, M. Multiple Sclerosis Pathogenesis: Possible Interplay between Vitamin D Status and Epstein Barr Virus Infection. *J Integr Neurosci.* 2023;22(1):7. doi: 10.31083/j.jin2201007.

[378] Kimura, H., Cohen, J. I. Chronic Active Epstein-Barr Virus Disease. *Front Immunol.* 2017;8:1867. doi: 10.3389/fimmu.2017.01867.

Chapter 4

Diagnosis of Lyme Borreliosis

Mykhaylo Andreychyn[1]
Mykhaylo Korda[2]
Mariia Shkilna[3]
Oleh Ivakhiv[4]
Mariana Huk[5]
Roksolana Humenna[6]
Inna Ishchuk[7]
Ivan Klishch[8]
Vasyl Kopcha[9]
and Olga Marchuk[10]

[1]Academician of the National Academy of Medical Sciences of Ukraine,
Honoured Master of Sciences and Technologies of Ukraine, DSc in Medicine, Professor,
Head of the Department of Infectious Diseases with Epidemiology, Dermatology and Venerology,
I. Horbachevsky Ternopil National Medical University, Ternopil, Ukraine
[2]Corresponding Member of the National Academy of Medical Sciences of Ukraine,
Honoured Master of Sciences and Technologies of Ukraine, DSc in Medicine, Professor,
Department of Medical Biochemistry, I. Horbachevsky Ternopil National Medical University,
Ternopil, Ukraine
[3]DSc in Medicine, Professor, Department of Infectious Diseases with Epidemiology,
Dermatology and Venerology, I. Horbachevsky Ternopil National Medical University, Ternopil, Ukraine
[4]Honoured Doctor of Ukraine, PhD in Medicine, Associate Professor,
Department of Infectious Diseases with Epidemiology, Dermatology and Venerology,
I. Horbachevsky Ternopil National Medical University, Ternopil, Ukraine
[5]PhD in Medicine, Assistant Professor, Department of Infectious Diseases with Epidemiology,
Dermatology and Venerology, I. Horbachevsky Ternopil National Medical University, Ternopil, Ukraine
[6]PhD Student, Department of Microbiology, Virology and Immunology,
I. Horbachevsky Ternopil National Medical University, Ternopil, Ukraine
[7]PhD in Medicine, Associate Professor, Department of Infectious Diseases with Epidemiology,
Dermatology and Venerology, I. Horbachevsky Ternopil National Medical University, Ternopil, Ukraine
[8]Honoured Master of Sciences and Technologies of Ukraine, DSc in Biology, Professor,
Department of Functional and Laboratory Diagnostics,
I. Horbachevsky Ternopil National Medical University, Ternopil, Ukraine

In: Lyme Borreliosis
Editors: Mykhaylo Andreychyn, Mykhaylo Korda, Maria Shkilna and Oleh Ivakhiv
ISBN: 979-8-89530-657-4

[9]DSc in Medicine, Professor, Department of Infectious Diseases with Epidemiology, Dermatology and Venerology, I. Horbachevsky Ternopil National Medical University, Ternopil, Ukraine
[10]Leading Specialist of the Interdepartmental Educational and Research Laboratory, I. Horbachevsky Ternopil National Medical University, Ternopil, Ukraine

Abstract

The chapter presents contemporary specific and non-specific laboratory and instrumental methods for the diagnosis of Lyme borreliosis. It includes up-to-date data on the direct identification of the pathogen in ticks (via dark-field microscopy and polymerase chain reaction (PCR), as well as in the blood of pregnant women with a complicated obstetric history (PCR method). The results of screening for specific antibodies to Lyme borreliosis pathogens in the serum of forestry workers from various regions of Ukraine are shown. Specific IgM and/or IgG antibodies to B. burgdorferi s. l. were detected by ELISA in 474 (44.3%) of the 1,070 individuals tested, with the lowest prevalence among forestry workers in Chernivtsi region (29.0%) and the highest in Zhytomyr region (58.0%). The study also presents ELISA data from patients at various stages of Lyme borreliosis.
A clinical evaluation is provided for the multiplex indirect immunofluorescence assay utilizing BIOCHIP technology, which enables the simultaneous detection of IgM or IgG antibodies to multiple infectious and parasitic pathogens in a single blood sample. Western blot and line immunoblot techniques are described in detail, along with the outcomes of two-step serological diagnostics (ELISA and immunoblot) of Lyme borreliosis among patients and forestry workers from different regions of Ukraine. The EUROLINE Borrelia RN-AT adv IgM test system was shown to expand the spectrum of detectable pathogens in both erythema and non-erythema migrans forms of Lyme borreliosis, particularly in patients with predominant musculoskeletal involvement. It identified anti-IgM antibodies against OspC of B. spielmanii, B. burgdorferi s. s., B. garinii, and B. afzelii in 78.9% of patients with the erythema migrans form and in 64.7% with the non-erythema form.
A list of instrumental diagnostic methods is also provided. The diagnostic utility of remote thermography for sub-erythema forms of the disease is described for the first time.

Keywords: Lyme borreliosis, diagnostics, polymerase chain reaction, serological reactions, indirect immunofluorescence assay, BIOCHIP technology, thermography

1. Introduction

The diagnosis of Lyme borreliosis is based on characteristic clinical signs, the patient's epidemiological history, and laboratory findings. A two-tiered serological testing algorithm is widely accepted in Europe and the United States. In the first step, either ELISA or an indirect immunofluorescence assay is used. If the result is positive or equivocal, confirmation is performed via immunoblotting, which constitutes the second step.

Most available ELISA kits include antigens of the three main *B. burgdorferi s. l.* genospecies pathogenic to humans (*B. afzelii*, *B. garinii*, and *B. burgdorferi s. s.*). Immunoblot is used to eliminate false-positive results from ELISA. European immunoblot kits are prepared using lysates of spirochetes and/or purified antigens from different *B. burgdorferi s. l.*species. The choice of antigens is based on the prevalence of Borrelia genospecies in the specific region. Results are interpreted according to the manufacturer's recommendations.

The search for additional, especially instrumental, diagnostic methods for skin lesions caused by infectious diseases is ongoing. One such method is remote thermography, which is widely used across various medical fields. This technique provides insight into physiological and pathological processes by registering and interpreting temperature distribution on different body regions. It evaluates temperature differences (ΔT) between affected and symmetrical or unaffected areas. Local temperature increases typically indicate inflammation or infection, while decreases may suggest vascular or neoplastic conditions. The key advantages of remote thermography include high sensitivity, non-invasiveness, painlessness, and contactless application, as well as rapid and objective image analysis.

2. General Clinical and Biochemical Methods

Ivan Klishch
and Oleh Ivakhiv

Laboratory diagnosis of LB includes general clinical, biochemical, and specific methods [1–3]. Typically, in the initial period of the disease, there may not be significant changes in the complete blood count; during disseminated borrelia infection, moderate leucocytosis, anaemia, decreased platelet count, and significantly increased ESR (up to 40 mm/hour or more) are noted.

Non-specific markers of inflammation such as CRP, sialic acids, and CICs are elevated in the blood. Monitoring CICsconcentration is advisable to assess the effectiveness of etiotropic treatment in LB patients. CICs levels decrease during therapy and may persist in the development of late manifestations of borreliosis after EM [1]. It has also been established that specific antibodies to borrelia can circulate freely in the blood, rather than as immune complexes, and this is observed more commonly than previously thought.

In cases of cardiovascular system involvement, the activity of lactate dehydrogenase "heart" fractions may increase in the blood, although creatine kinase levels always remain within normal limits.

In 5–30% of LB cases, the liver is affected, indicated by increased serum aminotransferase activity. Although severe hepatitis does not occur, in some cases, the activity of these liver enzymes may increase by 100 times. Approximately one in ten LB patients experiences a slight increase in alpha-amylase activity, indicating pancreatic involvement.

Results of other biochemical blood tests show unchanged kidney function tests; rheumatoid factor remains normal or slightly elevated [3]. Urine examination reveals microhaematuria and proteinuria. In cases of joint involvement, synovial fluid shows significantly increased polymorphonuclear leukocytes and protein content [4].

3. Specific Diagnostics

Mykhaylo Korda
Mykhaylo Andreychyn
Ivan Klishch
Mariia Shkilna
Olga Marchuk
Roksolana Humenna
and Mariana Huk

Specific methods of laboratory diagnosis of LB are based on detecting the causative agent either through bacterioscopic and bacteriological methods or its DNA, as well as antibodies to it (serological) [3, 5, 6]. The detection of the agent in various biological materials (blood, skin biopsy, cerebrospinal fluid, synovial fluid, urine) can be achieved using direct microscopic methods. Unstained agents are visible in dark-field microscopy or phase contrast microscopy and resemble spirals (Figure 1). Borrelia can be stained in velvet-black colour using the Levaditi or Warthin silver staining methods [7]. Fluorescent and electron microscopy are also possible [8]. Dark-field microscopy is used to establish both tick infection, removed from the patient (examining hemolymph and gut content), and its degree. However, such diagnostics do not allow determining the species of borrelia and assessing its pathogenicity for humans [3, 5, 6, 9].

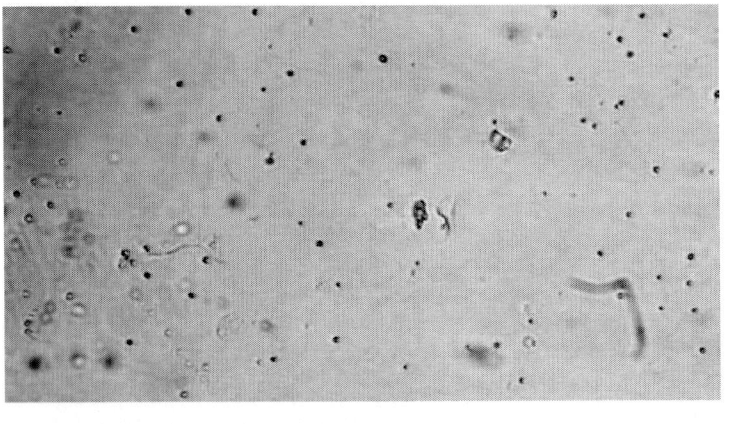

Figure 1. Borreliae in dark field of a light optical microscope.

According to Ternopil Regional Laboratory Centre of the Ministry of Health of Ukraine, from 2015 to 2020, tick infections with borrelia ranged from 17.6 to 23.4%.

Since the concentration of borrelia in tissues and biological fluids of infected individuals is very low, direct microscopic methods often fail to detect them in the studied material even after centrifugation enrichment. Therefore, negative results of microscopic examination do not exclude the presence of the agent in the patient's body. Regarding the bacteriological method of diagnosis, borrelia are very demanding in terms of culture conditions, requiring at least 3 weeks for isolation and identification [3, 10].

The most promising diagnostic method for LB is PCR, which detects fragments of borrelia DNA in various biological materials [11]. The sensitivity of the method varies from 20% to

80% depending on the substrate and duration of the disease [12]. This method can detect patient infection as early as 7-14 days after tick attachment, even during the incubation period of the disease [1, 2]. PCR is used in cases of meningitis, meningoencephalitis, atypical erythema, and arthritis to determine the aetiology of the disease. Another advantage of the method is that it allows identification of the borrelia species. PCR can be performed on all biological materials (blood, urine, tissue biopsies, cerebrospinal fluid, synovial fluid of patients, as well as ticks). This method enables the diagnosis of borrelial co-infections, detects cases of recurrent infections, and monitors treatment efficacy [5, 13, 14].

For obtaining more reliable PCR results, it is advisable to use several diagnostic systems. The European group studying tick-borne infections notes regarding the use of PCR in Lyme borreliosis diagnostics that a negative result cannot be considered an absolute criterion for absence of Borrelia [4], and exclusive reliance on this method is not recommended for daily practice [3]. At the same time, according to the literature [15], a positive PCR result does not necessarily indicate active infection.

We observed 43 pregnant women aged 19 to 43 years who were hospitalized in the gynaecological department of Ternopil Municipal Hospital No. 2 during 2018-2019. They were examined at 22-27 weeks of pregnancy. Using ultrasound examination, a range of pathological changes was found, often multiple in a single pregnant woman (Table 1).

Pregnant women were also screened for tick-borne pathogens. Blood testing was conducted at the laboratory of Centre for Lyme Borreliosis and Other Tick-Borne Diseases Research, functioning at the I. Horbachevsky Ternopil National Medical University.

DNA of *B. burgdorferi s. l.* (B. burgdorferi sensu stricto (s. s.), B. afzelii, and B. garinii), *A. phagocytophilum,* and *Babesia sp.* was detected using real-time PCR with the following kits: "RealBest DNA Borrelia burgdorferi s. l.," "RealBest DNA Anaplasma phagocytophilum/Ehrlichia muris, Ehrlichia chaeensis," and "RealBest RNA Babesia species." Results were processed using the "RealBest Diagnostics" service program by Vector-Best Ltd.

Table 1. Pathological changes in the examined pregnant women

Diagnosis	Pregnant women (n = 43)	
	Absolute number	%
Placental dysfunction	26	60,5
Polyhydramnios	14	32,6
Complicated obstetric history	7	16,3
Intrauterine infection	5	11,6
Threatened miscarriage	5	11,6
Oligohydramnios	4	9,3
Placental hyperplasia	3	6,9
Gestational oedema	3	6,9
Fetal growth restriction	3	6,9

For RNA/DNA extraction from clinical samples and tick suspensions, the "RealBest extraction 100" kit was used. Amplification for RNA/DNA detection was carried out using the real-time PCR amplifier "Rotor Gene-6000" (Corbett Research, Australia) and the following reagent kits: "RealBest DNA *Borrelia burgdorferi s. l.*" [16], "RealBest DNA *Anaplasma phagocytophilum/Ehrlichia muris*, *Ehrlichia chaffeensis*" [17], DNA *Borrelia miyamotoi* [18], and "RealBest DNA *Babesia species*" [19]. Results were analysed using the "RealBest Diagnostics" service program.

In the blood testing of pregnant women, DNA of *B. burgdorferi s. l.* was found in 5 (11.6%) out of 43 individuals; DNA of *A. phagocytophilum* was found in 3 (6.9%), and DNA of *Babesia sp.* was found in 2 (4.7%). No nucleic acids of any of the tick-borne pathogens tested were detected in the blood of 36 (83.7%) out of 43 expectant mothers (Figure 2).

It is worth noting that 4 (9.3%) pregnant women concurrently tested positive for both antibodies to Borrelia and DNA of *B. burgdorferi s. l.*, indicating a positive result. Thus, Borrelia DNA was detected in the blood of nearly every eleventh pregnant woman [20–22].

In EM LB, Borrelia can be isolated from skin biopsies (approximately 50–80%) using culture on BSK-II medium (Barbour-Stoenner-Kelly). Positive results from culturing Borrelia are less frequent in synovial fluid and cerebrospinal fluid (10–15%) and blood (1–3%). While the method's clinical diagnostic value is limited due to its complexity and high cost, it remains essential for scientific research on microbial properties of the pathogen and in the development of diagnostic test systems [23, 24].

Serological methods detect antibodies to the antigens of the pathogen in blood serum, cerebrospinal fluid (intrathecal), and synovial fluid using indirect hemagglutination reaction orELISA, IIFR, and immunoblot (specific antibodies to individual Borrelia antigens are determined) [25–29].

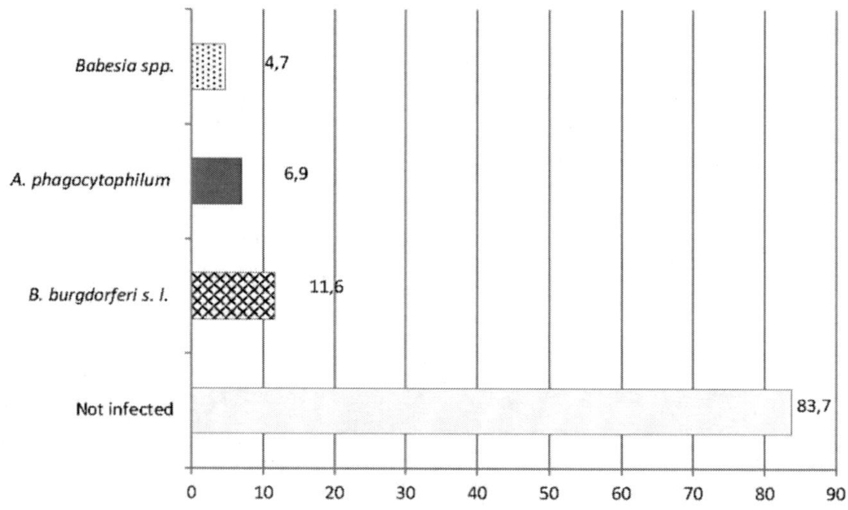

Figure 2. The frequency of detecting nucleic acids of causative agents of certain tick-borne infections in the blood of pregnant women (n = 43).

Antibodies to the antigens of the *B. burgdorferi s. l.* complex in blood serum are determined by enzyme-linked immunosorbent assay (ELISA) using Euroimmun AG test systems (Germany): IgM antibodies with the *Anti-Borrelia burgdorferi* ELISA (IgM) [30], IgG antibodies with the *Anti-Borrelia* plus VIsE ELISA (IgG) [31].

The determination of these antibodies is based on an optimized mixture of lysates from the most significant pathogenic strains of Borrelia (*B. burgdorferi s. s.*, *B. afzelii*, *B. garinii*). The Anti-Borrelia plus VIsE ELISA (IgG) test system additionally contains recombinant VIsE – a variable major protein, similar in sequence to *B. burgdorferi* (variable major protein-like sequence, expressed), a recently identified surface protein of Borrelia that is expressed exclusively *in vivo* and contains highly immunogenic epitopes.

In the first stage, diluted samples are incubated in wells. Specific IgM antibodies (as well as IgA and IgG classes) to Borrelia present in positive samples bind to antigens. A second incubation is conducted to detect bound antibodies. The intensity of staining is directly proportional to the concentration of Borrelia antibodies in the samples.

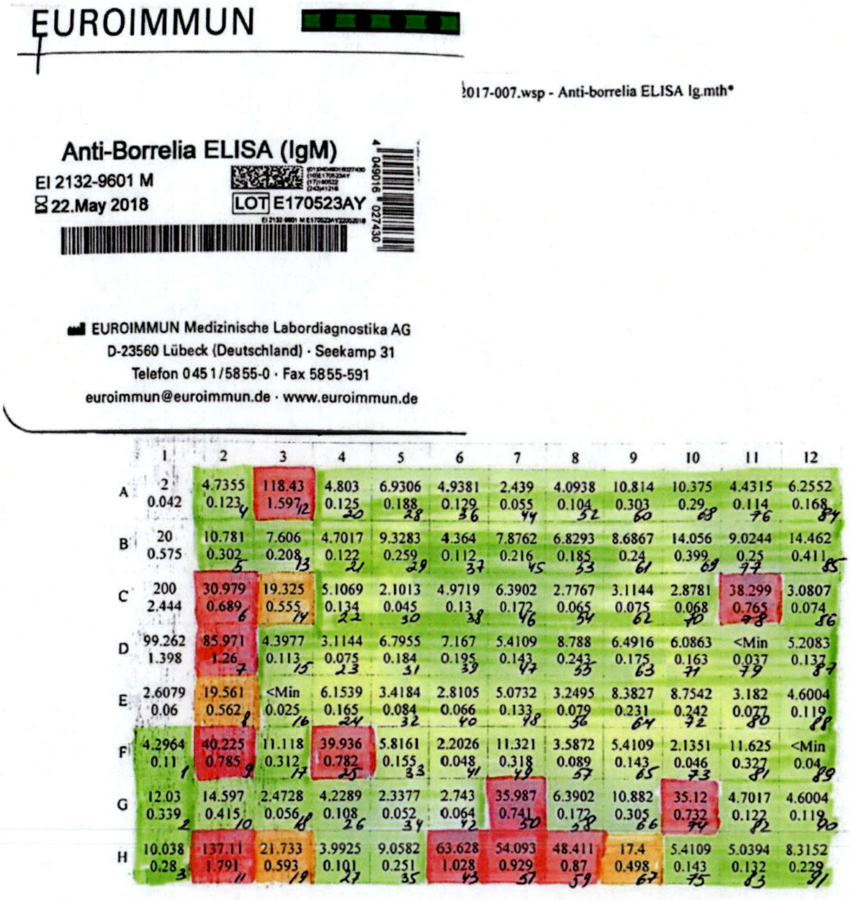

	1	2	3	4	5	6	7	8	9	10	11	12
A	2 0.042	4.7355 0.123	118.43 1.597	4.803 0.125	6.9306 0.188	4.9381 0.129	2.439 0.055	4.0938 0.104	10.814 0.303	10.375 0.29	4.4315 0.114	6.2552 0.168
B	20 0.575	10.781 0.302	7.606 0.208	4.7017 0.122	9.3283 0.259	4.364 0.112	7.8762 0.216	6.8293 0.185	8.6867 0.24	14.056 0.399	9.0244 0.25	14.462 0.411
C	200 2.444	30.979 0.689	19.325 0.555	5.1069 0.134	2.1013 0.045	4.9719 0.13	6.3902 0.172	2.7767 0.065	3.1144 0.075	2.8781 0.068	38.299 0.765	3.0807 0.074
D	99.262 1.398	85.971 1.26	4.3977 0.113	3.1144 0.075	6.7955 0.184	7.167 0.195	5.4109 0.143	8.788 0.243	6.4916 0.175	6.0863 0.163	<Min 0.037	5.2083 0.137
E	2.6079 0.06	19.561 0.562	<Min 0.025	6.1539 0.165	3.4184 0.084	2.8105 0.066	5.0732 0.133	3.2495 0.079	8.3827 0.231	8.7542 0.242	3.182 0.077	4.6004 0.119
F	4.2964 0.11	40.225 0.785	11.118 0.312	39.936 0.782	5.8161 0.155	2.2026 0.048	11.321 0.318	3.5872 0.089	5.4109 0.143	2.1351 0.046	11.625 0.327	<Min 0.04
G	12.03 0.339	14.597 0.415	2.4728 0.056	4.2289 0.108	2.3377 0.052	2.743 0.064	35.987 0.741	6.3902 0.172	10.882 0.305	35.12 0.732	4.7017 0.122	4.6004 0.119
H	10.038 0.28	137.11 1.791	21.733 0.593	3.9925 0.101	9.0582 0.251	63.628 1.028	54.093 0.929	48.411 0.87	17.4 0.498	5.4109 0.143	5.0394 0.132	8.3152 0.229

Figure 3. Data from wells of a plate with samples of serum or plasma from patients.

Patient serum or plasma samples are diluted 1:100 with sample buffer coloured green. The mixture is incubated for at least 10 minutes at room temperature (18–25°C). Subsequently, samples are added to the plate wells according to the reagent addition scheme (Figure 3). Results are evaluated quantitatively. Values $\geq$ 22 U/mL are considered positive, 16–22 U/mL are considered borderline, and $\leq$ 16 U/mL are considered negative.

The linear range of the *Anti-Borrelia* ELISA (IgM) test is 3–177 U/mL. The linear range of the *Anti-Borrelia* plus VIsE ELISA (IgG) test is 8–124 U/mL. The measurement ranges of both tests are 0–200 U/mL. The lowest detection level for the *Anti-Borrelia* ELISA (IgM) test is 1.3 U/mL, and for the *Anti-Borrelia* plus VIsE ELISA (IgG) test, it is 0.7 U/mL.

The specificity and sensitivity for EUROIMMUN *Anti-Borrelia* ELISA (IgM) are 96.4% and 100%, respectively; for EUROIMMUN *Anti-Borrelia* plus VIsE ELISA (IgG), they are 90.2% and 100%, respectively [30, 31].

This method was used for screening antibody diagnostics to LB pathogens among forestry workers in several regions of Ukraine.

Laboratory examination was conducted on 1070 forestry workers from seven regions: Volyn, Zhytomyr, Transcarpathian, Ternopil, Khmelnytskyi, Chernivtsi, and Chernihiv regions. There were significantly more men than women – 972 versus 98. The age of those examined ranged from 20 to 69 years. Forestry workers aged 69 years were only found in the Khust forestry of Transcarpathian region. The average age of those examined varied from (37.96 ± 0.79) years in Chernivtsi region to (45.26 ± 11.10) years in Chernihiv region ($p > 0.05$).

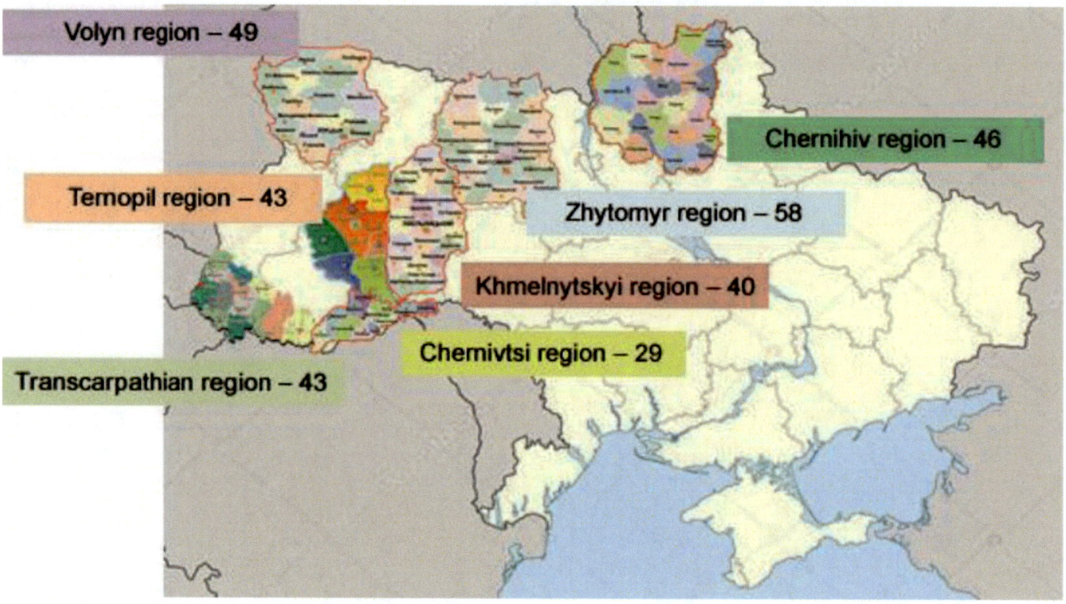

Figure 4. The frequency of detection of specific anti-IgM and anti-IgG antibodies by the ELISA to *B. burgdorferi s. l.* in the serum samples of 1070 forestry workers from seven regions of Ukraine.

The examined group included: foresters, assistant foresters, forest masters, lumberjacks, timber workers, machine operators, sorters, tractor drivers, laborers, administrative staff, gamekeepers, as well as mechanics, auto electricians, and machinists. Forest masters constituted the largest share (65.9%) in Chernihiv region, foresters (42.3%) in Ternopil, and administrative staff (38.4%) in Chernivtsi region.

The results of blood serum tests among forestry workers for the presence of specific IgM and IgG antibodies to *B. burgdorferi s. l.* using ELISA showed positive or borderline results for antibodies of at least one class in 474 (44.3%) of those examined: these antibodies were least frequently detected among forestry workers in Chernivtsi region (29.0%) and most frequently in Zhytomyr region (58.0%) (Figure 4).

Next, the dependency of specific IgM and IgG antibodies to *B. burgdorferi s. l.* in the blood serum of forestry workers from different regions on the natural zones of Ukraine (Polissia, Forest-Steppe, and Carpathians) where they work was investigated (Table 2, Figure 5).

It is known that these zones differ significantly in terms of forest vegetation conditions, forestry management methods, utilization of forest resources, and beneficial forest properties. Forestry workers from state forestry enterprises in Chernihiv and Zhytomyr regions worked in the mixed forest zone (Polissia); those from Volyn, Ternopil, and Khmelnytskyi regions worked in the forest-steppe zone; and those from Transcarpathian and Chernivtsi regions worked in the Carpathian zone.

Most frequently, positive results (positive and/or intermediate) for specific IgM and IgG antibodies to *B. burgdorferi s. l.* were found in the serum of forestry workers from Chernihiv and Zhytomyr regions (Ukrainian Polissia) – in 114 (51.8%) out of 220 examined (Table 2, Figure 5).

The least frequent presence of specific antibodies was found in the serum of forestry workers from Chernivtsi and Transcarpathian regions (Ukrainian Carpathians) – in 82 (38.3%) out of 214 examined (Table 2, Figure 5).

Table 2. The presence of IgM and IgG antibodies to *B. burgdorferi s. l.* in the serum samples of foresters from various landscape-geographical zones of Ukraine, using the ELISA test (n = 1070)

Landscape-geographical zone	Region	Number of the examined patients	Positive result	
			Absolute number	%
Polissia	Chernihiv	120	56	46,7
	Zhytomyr	100	58	58,0
Overall		220	114	51,8
Forest-steppe	Volyn	147	72	48,9
	Ternopil	339	146	43,1
	Khmelnytskyi	150	60	40,0
Overall		636	278	43,7
Carpathians	Chernivtsi	73	21	28,8
	Transcarpathian	141	61	43,3
Overall		214	82	38,3
Total		1070	474	44,3

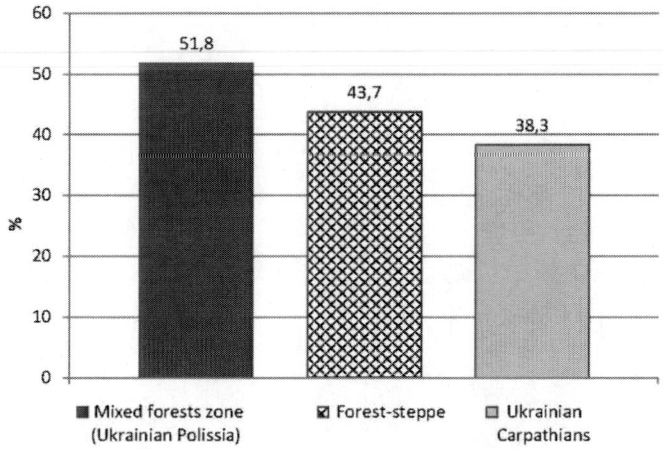

Figure 5. The presence of IgM and IgG antibodies to *B. burgdorferi s. l.* in the serum of forestry workers from various landscape-geographical zones, tested using ELISA (n = 1070).

Furthermore, we used the ELISA to detect specific IgM and IgG antibodies to the agents of Lyme borreliosis in patients with EM [32].

Laboratory examination was conducted on 146 patients with EM who were treated on an outpatient and inpatient basis at Ternopil Regional Skin and Venereal Diseases Dispensary and the infectious diseases department of the Ternopil City Municipal Emergency Hospital during 2015-2020. The patients ranged in age from 19 to 79 years, with a mean age of (43.09 ± 14.29) years. There were 63 males (43.2%) and 83 females (56.8%). Blood samples for testing were taken 3-4 weeks after the appearance of EM.

Analysis of the serological test results of patients' serum using IFA for the presence of specific IgM and IgG antibodies to the *B. burgdorferi s. l.* complex revealed that positive results for IgM antibodies to Borrelia were found in 65 (44.5%) individuals, intermediate results in 18 (12.3%), and negative results in 63 (43.2%). Meanwhile, positive results for IgG antibodies were found in 49 (33.6%) individuals, intermediate results in 8 (5.5%), and negative results in 89 (60.9%) (Figure 6).

Subsequently, the concentration of IgM and IgG antibodies to *B. burgdorferi s. l.* (*B. burgdorferi s. s.*, *B. garinii*, *B. afzelii*) in the serum of patients with EM was determined. This included studying the relationship between the levels of specific IgM and IgG antibodies in the serum of individuals with EM based on their gender (Table 3, Figure 7). No significant differences were found in the quantity of specific IgM antibodies based on gender. However, the concentration of IgG antibodies to *B. burgdorferi s. l.* in the serum of females was higher than in males ($p < 0.05$).

Table 3. Content of specific IgM and IgG in serum samples of patients of different genders with erythema migrans form of Lyme borreliosis (ELISA test; Me (Lq; Uq)), U/ml

Immunoglobulin class	Males	Females	Significance level of the Mann–Whitney U test, p
M	12,77 (6,79; 28,02)	19,99 (7,24; 57,21)	p = 0,108
G	5,17 (3,66; 17,09)	15,60 (4,96; 61,60)	p = 0,006*

Note. * – the difference is significant, $p < 0.05$.

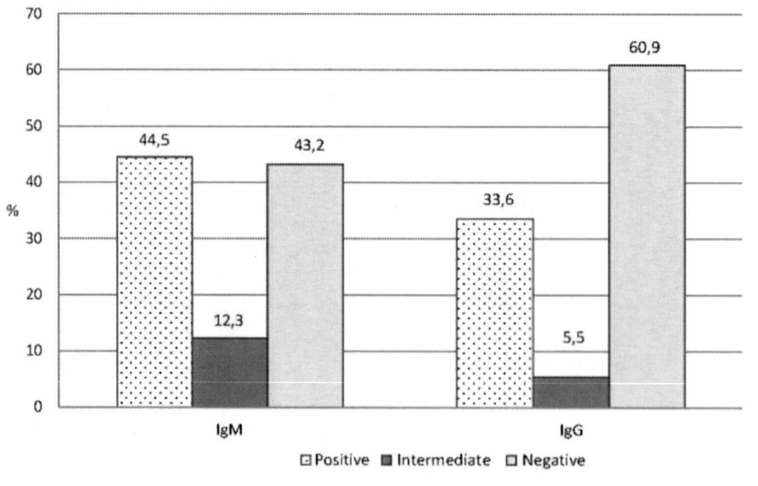

Figure 6. The results of the study of serum samples from patients with erythema migrans form of Lyme borreliosis for the presence of IgM and IgG antibodies to *B. burgdorferi s. l.* using the ELISA (n = 146).

We also investigated the levels of IgM and IgG antibodies to *B. burgdorferi s. l.* (*B. burgdorferi s. s.*, *B. garinii*, *B. afzelii*) in the serum of individuals with different clinical variants of EM (Table 4). It was found that the quantity of IgM antibodies was significantly higher in patients with atypical forms of EM LB compared to those with typical erythema, 35.59 vs. 11.14 AU/mL, $p < 0.001$.

These methods are indispensable in routine diagnostics of LB, especially in cases of atypical, latent, and chronic forms of the disease. Seroconversion is noted in 20-50% of patients with acute LB. The IgM antibody titre reaches its highest level at 4-6 weeks after the onset of illness, and these antibodies can persist for up to 1 year if clinical symptoms are present. The dynamics of antibody titres in patients are assessed at 3-4 weeks. False-negative results may occur due to the absence or low levels of antibodies in the early stages of the disease ("serological window"), various immunosuppressive conditions, antigenic heterogeneity of the pathogen, or insufficient sensitivity of the test systems [33]. After effective treatment and elimination of the pathogen, antibody levels can decrease rapidly, which is used to monitor treatment effectiveness. Decreasing antibody levels always indicate a favourable prognosis [5].

Table 4. Content of specific IgM and IgG in the serum of patients with various variants of erythema migrans in Lyme borreliosis (ELISA test; Me (Lq; Uq)), U/mL

Immunoglobulin class	EM		Significance level of the Mann–Whitney U test, p
	typical	atypical	
M	11,14 (4,01; 20,17)	35,59 (12,96; 101,00)	p = 0,001*
G	16,51 (4,55; 40,80)	14,32 (4,85; 49,60)	p = 0,739

Note. * – the difference is significant, $p < 0.05$.

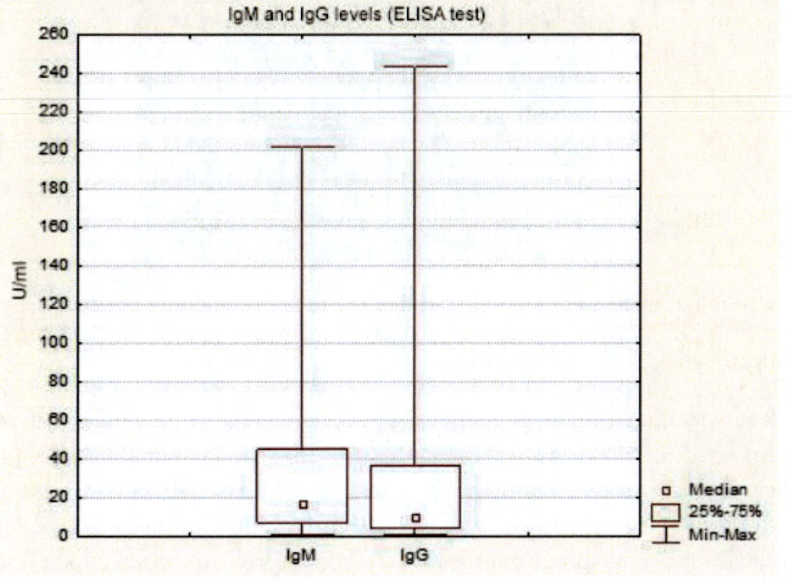

Figure 7. Concentration of specific IgM and IgG in the serum of patients with erythema migrans form of Lyme borreliosis (ELISA test), U/mL.

In cases where a patient consistently shows elevated IgM titres without seroconversion in repeated tests, the result should be considered as potentially false positive (the reasons often remain unclear) [3, 5, 6]. This can occur in patients with other spirochaetal infections (syphilis, leptospirosis, relapsing fever), rheumatoid arthritis of non-borrelial aetiology, systemic lupus erythematosus, as well as in patients with infections caused by cytomegalovirus or *Epstein-Barr virus*, or in pregnant women [2, 33].

Conversely, there are situations where specific antibodies against Borrelia may not be detectable in peripheral blood. False-negative results in serological testing may occur due to early specimen collection before antibodies reach detectable levels according to the diagnostic sensitivity of the method used, early initiation of antibiotic treatment in adequate or inadequate doses, which suppresses the immune response [5].

To detect specific anti-Borrelia antibodies, indirect immunofluorescence assay (IIFA) is also used. A new method of multiplex indirect immunofluorescence with BIOCHIP technology has been developed, allowing simultaneous detection of specific IgM or IgG antibodies to pathogens of many infectious and parasitic diseases in a single sample. The slide for these studies contains 5 fields, each with 4 chips coated with substrates of bacteria, infected cells, or tissues. The first field also includes a verification chip to assess the accuracy of the reaction and display the class of immunoglobulins involved in the reaction.

Results for antibodies against the mentioned pathogens are evaluated under an Olympus IX70 fluorescence microscope at approximately ×10, ×20, and ×40 magnifications, observing bright green fluorescence of the antigen-antibody complexes labelled with fluorescein. The distinctive bright green fluorescence outlining the spirochetes in each field is particularly evident in Lyme borreliosis (Figure 8).

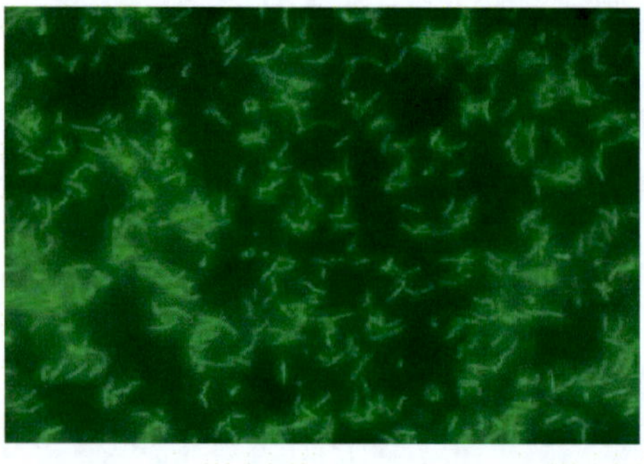

Figure 8. Detection of antibodies to *B. burgdorferi s. l.* using the indirect immunofluorescence in the serum of patient S., 42 years old. Diagnosis: non-erythema migrans form of Lyme borreliosis predominantly affecting the musculoskeletal system, acute course.

To detect specific antibodies to pathogens that could be the cause of musculoskeletal disorders, we used the "Mosaic for Infectious Serology, Infections arthritis profile 1 (IgM)" and "Mosaic for Infectious Serology, Infections arthritis profile 1 (IgG)" test systems from EUROIMMUN, Germany. These test systems include fluorescein-labelled antigens of pathogens causing various infectious diseases: Lyme borreliosis, chickenpox, influenza, enteric yersiniosis, toxoplasmosis, and chlamydia.

We examined 26 patients aged 19 to 68 years who were treated both as outpatients and inpatients at Ternopil Regional Clinical Dermatovenereological Dispensary and Ternopil

University Hospital TOR due to musculoskeletal disorders. There were 17 female and 9 male patients.

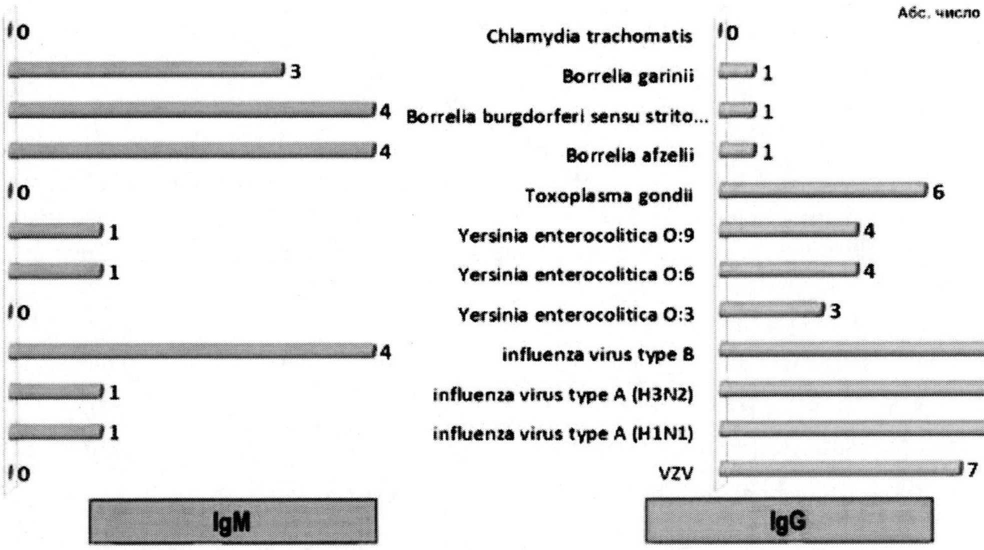

Figure 9. Presence of specific IgM and IgG antibodies to 11 pathogens of infectious diseases in the serum of 26 patients with musculoskeletal system involvement.

Specific anti-IgM and anti-IgG antibodies to 11 pathogens causing infectious diseases, including Lyme borreliosis, were detected in the patients, often in various combinations that could be related to the development of the mentioned pathology (Figure 9). Specifically, anti-IgM antibodies to *B. garinii* were present in the blood serum of 3 (11.5%) patients, to *B. burgdorferi s. s.* in 4 (15.4%), and to *B. afzelii* in 4 (15.4%); anti-IgG antibodies to *B. burgdorferi s. s.* were found in 1 (3.8%) patient, to *B. garinii* in 1 (3.8%), and to B. afzelii in 1 (3.8%) of those examined.

In the blood serum of the examined patients, specific antibodies of both classes to pathogens of other infectious diseases, where joint involvement is possible, were also detected, often in various combinations. Thus, the multiplex indirect immunofluorescence assay using BIOCHIP technology in patients with arthritis allows simultaneous detection of specific antibodies to twelve pathogens of various infectious diseases, including Lyme borreliosis.

Western blotting is a highly informative method for detecting specific antibodies to certain pathogen proteins, characterized by higher sensitivity and specificity compared to other methods. Recombinant proteins such as r83-100, r58, r41 (flagellin), VmpA (r39), OspC (r20-25), r17 (Dbp A), BVC32, and VlsE are primarily used as antigens, obtained for two or sometimes three species of Borrelia. Western blotting allows for differential diagnosis between antibody responses to specific and nonspecific Borrelia proteins, but it cannot identify the types of Borrelia responsible for the clinical features of the disease [3].

In addition, according to the recommendations of the Second National Conference on Serological Diagnosis of Lyme Disease [35], detection of IgM in blot analysis can be confirmed only when at least 2 out of 3 Borrelia antigens applied to the strips are present. Conversely, IgG in blot analysis is considered present when 5 out of 10 bacterial antigens are detected [35]. A positive Western blot result against a background of negative ELISA is not considered diagnostically significant [2].

However, such interpretation can only be used for detecting antibodies to *B. burgdorferi s. s.*, which are prevalent in the USA [2, 36], as Europe also encounters four other causative agents besides this species: *B. garinii*, *B. afzelii*, *B. spielmanii*, and *B. bavariensis*. Moreover, there is considerable heterogeneity among strains within each Borrelia species, including antigens crucial for serodiagnosis [37].

Therefore, European immunoblots are prepared from spirochete lysates and/or purified antigens from various species of *B. burgdorferi s. l.*, according to the region where the test systems are used. Additionally, criteria for interpreting immunoblots should be specifically defined by the Borrelia species selected for the particular test system, excluding universal interpretation recommendations similar to those of the Centres for Disease Control and Prevention (CDC) used in the USA [37].

Thus, laboratory testing for Lyme borreliosis in patients is conducted in two stages: the first stage involves screening with ELISAor indirect immunofluorescence assay; the second stage excludes false-positive results from the initial stage and identifies specific antibodies to certain pathogen antigens using immunoblotting [38-40], less frequently by determining the pathogen's DNA using PCR [6, 35]. Unfortunately, all the aforementioned specific research methods do not prevent obtaining both false-positive and false-negative results, so in doubtful cases, patient examination should be comprehensive, prolonged, and conducted dynamically [2, 4].

Table 5. Number of foresters in Ternopil region with NEM Lyme borreliosis affecting various organs and systems (n = 54)

Nature of lesions	Patients	
	Absolute number	%
Intoxication syndrome	20	37,0
Predominantly musculoskeletal system	26	48,1
Predominantly cardiovascular system	8	14,9
Total	54	100,0

There are several types of immunoblot reactions: Western blot (WB), EUROLINE-WB, EUROLINE Borrelia RN-AT, which differ in the number of available antigens and consequently in the interpretation of the results obtained.

Anti-Borrelia EUROLINE-WB allows for the detection of IgM and IgG antibodies against various antigens of one Borrelia genospecies. We diagnosed specific antibodies to the following *B. burgdorferi s. l.* antigens: p83 (late immune response antibodies, typical for neuroborreliosis), p41 (early immune response antibodies), p39/BmpA (late immune response antibodies, characteristic of disseminated Lyme disease, often associated with Lyme arthritis), p31/OspA (late immune response antibodies, typical for neuroborreliosis), p30 (mostly late immune response antibodies), p25/OspC (early immune response antibodies), p21 (early and late immune response antibodies), p17, p19, and membrane chip with recombinant antigen VlsE (variable major protein antigen).

Using this type of immunoblot, we examined the blood sera of 54 forestry workers in Ternopil region, who obtained positive and intermediate results regarding the presence of antibodies to the *B. burgdorferi s. l.* complex in ELISA tests. Table 5 outlines the nature of injuries to various organs and systems in these foresters.

According to the manufacturer's recommendations of the test systems from Euroimmun AG (Germany), the IgM indicator was considered positive, indeterminate, or negative depending on the combinations of the OspC antigen and p83, p39, p31, p30, p21, p19, p17 (Table 6).

Positive results for the presence of specific IgM antibodies to Borrelia were found in 28 (51.9%) individuals, indeterminate results in 2 (3.7%), and negative results in 24 (44.4%). Additionally, using the immunoblot method in serum samples of foresters, the presence of IgG antibodies to Borrelia was determined.

According to the manufacturer's recommendations, IgG test results were considered positive or negative depending on combinations of the VlsE antigen and the following antigens: p83, p39, p31, p30, p21, p19, p17 (Table 7).

Table 6. Criteria for evaluating IgM antibodies to antigens of the *B. burgdorferi s. l.* complex

OspC band	Specific antigens bands: p83, p39, p31, p30, p21, p19, p17	
	1 band is positive	no positive bands
The antigen band is positive	Positive	Positive
The antigen band is weakly positive	Positive	Intermediate
The antigen band is negative	Positive	Negative

Table 7. Criteria for evaluating IgG antibodies to antigens of the B. *burgdorferi s. l.* complex

VlsE band	Specific antigens bands: p83, p39, p31, p30, p21, p19, p17		
	2 or more bands are positive	1 band is positive	no positive bands
The antigen band is positive	Positive	Positive	Positive
The antigen band is weakly positive	Positive	Positive	Negative
The antigen band is negative	Positive	Negative	Negative

Positive results were obtained in 47 (87.1%) patients, negative results in 7 (12.9%). No indeterminate results were found among those examined (Figure 10). It was established that among 28 foresters from Ternopil region with Lyme borreliosis, who tested positive for IgM antibodies to *B. burgdorferi s. l.* using the immunoblot method, 25 individuals had predominantly musculoskeletal system involvement and 3 had signs of intoxication syndrome. Among the 47 individuals whose serum showed positive IgG antibody results to *B. burgdorferi s. l.* using this method, 28 had musculoskeletal system involvement, 16 had signs of intoxication syndrome, and 3 had cardiovascular system involvement.

The EUROLINE-WB test systems contain strips with electrophoretically separated extracts of the same antigens for IgM and IgG antibodies. The etiological structure of LB was subsequently studied in 25 forestry workers from Ternopil region with predominantly musculoskeletal system involvement.

In serum samples from these 25 foresters, IgM antibodies were found to the following Borrelia antigens: p17 in 1 (4.0%) individual, p25 in 4 (16.0%), and p31 in 2 (8.0%).

Regarding the presence of IgG antibodies to various Borrelia antigens, antibodies of this class were found in the serum of the examined patients as follows: to VlsE in 22 (88.0%) foresters, to p39 in 21 (84.0%), and to p83 in 20 (80.0%) (Figure 11). IgG antibodies to other Borrelia antigens were detected less frequently: to p25 in 19 (76.0%), to p21 in 8 (32.0%), to p17 in 10 (40.0%), and to p19 in 7 (28.1%) individuals [41, 42].

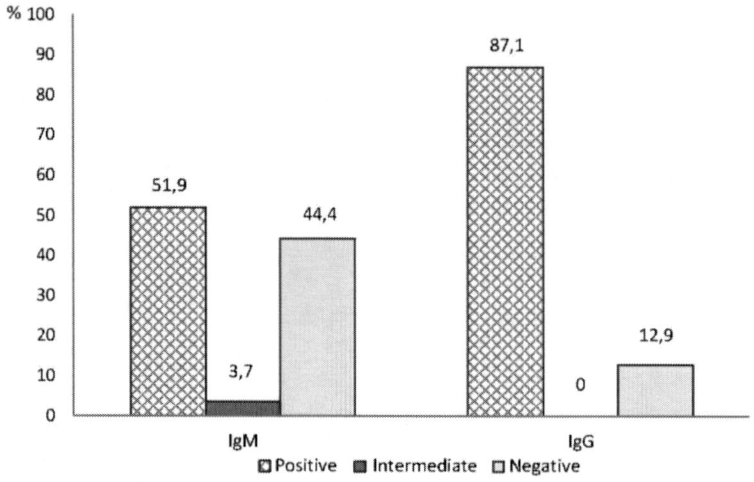

Figure 10. Results of serum samples from foresters in Ternopil region with NEM LB (n = 54) for the presence of IgM and IgG antibodies to *B. burgdorferi s. l.* (immunoblot test).

The investigations were conducted according to the manufacturer's recommendations [43, 44]. The results were evaluated using EURO Line Scan software, based on the colour intensity of the strips, where 0 indicated no colour and 256 indicated maximum black colour. Accordingly, strip colour intensity levels between 19 and 256 were considered positive, between 12 and 18 indeterminate, and between 0 and 11 negative (Figure 12).

The subsequent immunoblot used was EUROLINE Borrelia RN-AT, which combines the advantages of Western blot and line blot in a single test membrane. The Anti-Borrelia EUROLINE kit allows quantitative determination of human antibodies to Borrelia antigens in serum or plasma. For the determination of specific IgG antibodies, classic purified antigens (p83, p39) from Western blot, recombinant VlsE (variable-like sequence expressed), natural purified Osp C antigens from three Borrelia species (*B. burgdorferi s. s.*, *B. garinii*, and *B. afzelii*), immunoreactive lipids from Borrelia cytoplasmic membranes (Lipid Ba, Lipid Bb), and highly specific recombinant antigens p18, p19, p20, p21, and p58 were used.

Compared to the traditional WB system, EUROLINE Borrelia RN-AT offers significantly higher sensitivity (up to 89% depending on the antigen type) and higher specificity (at least 95%).

To detect IgM antibodies, a specific line in the RN-AT system is utilized, containing purified natural OspC antigens from three Borrelia species (*B. afzelii*, *B. burgdorferi s. s.*, and *B. garinii*), p39, VlsE, and the flagellar antigen (p41) (Figure 13). The specificity of the RN-AT system line ranges from 97% to 99%, with a sensitivity of 88%. The primary antigen for detecting IgG antibodies is VlsE, with a sensitivity of 89% and specificity of 99% [45].

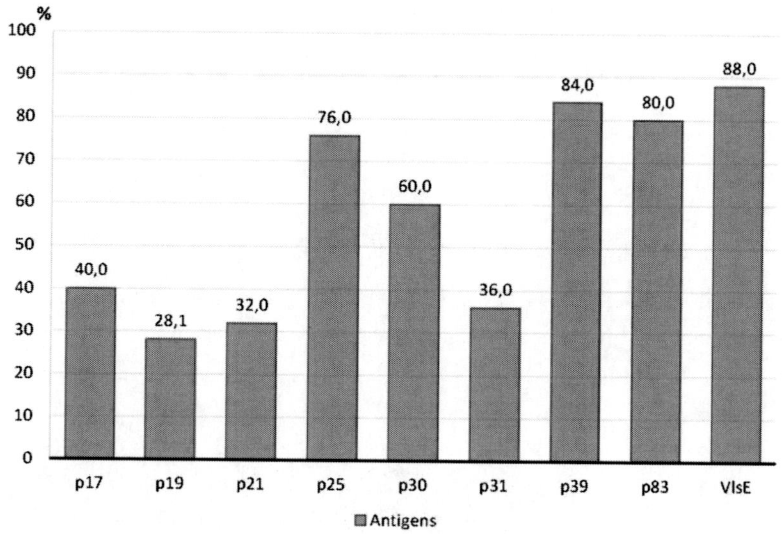

Figure 11. The presence of IgG antibodies to various antigens of *B. burgdorferi s. l.* in the serum of foresters with musculoskeletal involvement in the NEM LB (n = 25) (immunoblot test).

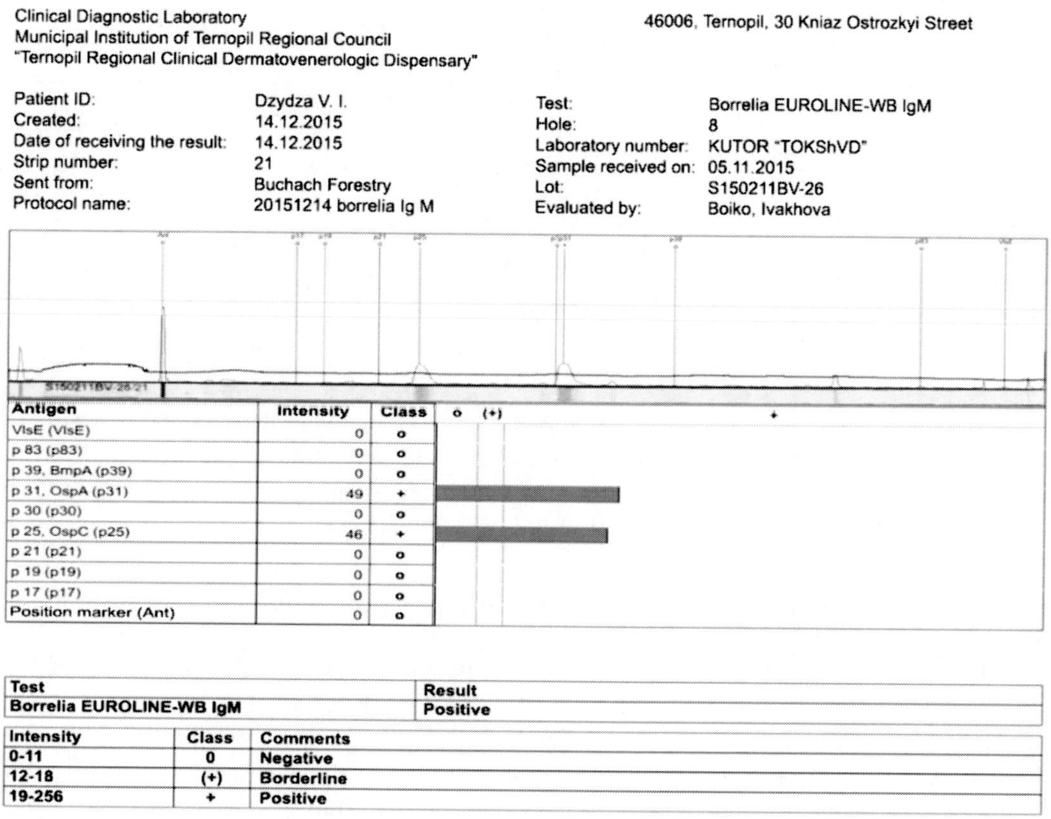

Clinical Diagnostic Laboratory
Municipal Institution of Ternopil Regional Council
"Ternopil Regional Clinical Dermatovenerologic Dispensary"

46006, Ternopil, 30 Kniaz Ostrozkyi Street

Patient ID:	Dzydza V. I.	Test:	Borrelia EUROLINE-WB IgM
Created:	14.12.2015	Hole:	8
Date of receiving the result:	14.12.2015	Laboratory number:	KUTOR "TOKShVD"
Strip number:	21	Sample received on:	05.11.2015
Sent from:	Buchach Forestry	Lot:	S150211BV-26
Protocol name:	20151214 borrelia Ig M	Evaluated by:	Boiko, Ivakhova

Antigen	Intensity	Class
VlsE (VlsE)	0	o
p 83 (p83)	0	o
p 39, BmpA (p39)	0	o
p 31, OspA (p31)	49	+
p 30 (p30)	0	o
p 25, OspC (p25)	46	+
p 21 (p21)	0	o
p 19 (p19)	0	o
p 17 (p17)	0	o
Position marker (Ant)	0	o

Test	Result
Borrelia EUROLINE-WB IgM	Positive

Intensity	Class	Comments
0-11	0	Negative
12-18	(+)	Borderline
19-256	+	Positive

Figure 12. Diagnostic band of *B. burgdorferi* antigens for determining IgM in the serum of forester D., 32 years old, using the EUROLINE-WB IgM test system.

This particular type of immunoblot was used to study the etiological structure of LB in 731 forestry workers from six regions of Ukraine who had positive and/or indeterminate results for specific IgM and IgG antibodies to *B. burgdorferi s. l.* using the ELISA.

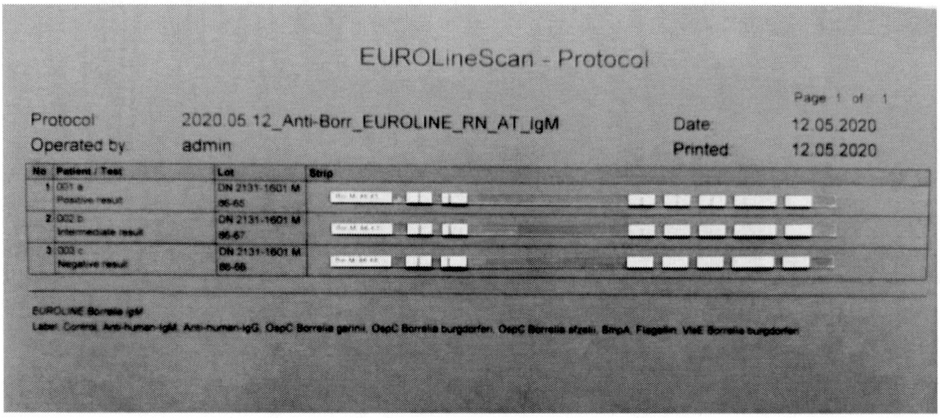

Figure 13. Example of the protocol for evaluating the obtained results of immunoblot (EUROLINE Borrelia RN-AT IgM) using EURO Line Scan software.

Table 8. Criteria for evaluating IgM class antibodies to antigens of the *B. burgdorferi s.* 1 *l* complex

OspC Ba or OspC Bb, or OspC Bg bands	Specific antigens bands: p39, VlsE Bb	
	1 band is positive	no positive bands
The antigen band is positive	Positive	Positive
OspC Ba or OspC Bg bands are weakly positive	Positive	Intermediate
The antigen band is negative	Positive	Negative

According to the manufacturer's recommendations of Euroimmun AG (Germany), the IgM indicator was considered positive, indeterminate, or negative depending on the combinations of OspC antigens from three Borrelia species (*B. afzelii*, *B. burgdorferi s. s.*, and *B. garinii*), p39, and VlsE Bb (Table 8).

According to the manufacturer's recommendations, the IgG test result was considered positive or negative depending on the combinations of VlsE antigens from three Borrelia species (*B. afzelii*, *B. burgdorferi s. s.*, and *B. garinii*), and other specific antigens: p18, p19, p20, p21, p58, OspC (p25), p39, p83, Lipid Ba, Lipid Bb (Table 9).

Serum samples from 190 forestry workers (123 positive and 67 indeterminate results) were analysed using the immunoblot method for IgM, and from 227 (187 positive and 40 indeterminate results) for IgG (Table 10).

Further verification of the presence of specific IgM antibodies in the blood serum of 123 forestry workers who had positive results in the ELISA test revealed the following by the immunoblot method: positive results were found in 77 individuals (62.6%), indeterminate in 20 (12.3%), and negative in 26 (21.1%). Analysing the blood samples of 67 individuals who had indeterminate results in the ELISA test for IgM antibodies to *B. burgdorferi s. l.*, it was determined that 12 (17.9%) had positive results, 18 (26.9%) had indeterminate results, and 37 (55.2%) had negative results. Therefore, positive results for the presence of IgM antibodies to *B. burgdorferi s. l.* by immunoblot were confirmed in 89 individuals (77 + 12) out of 190 forestry workers from Volyn, Zhytomyr, Transcarpathian, Khmelnytskyi, Chernivtsi, and Chernihiv regions, accounting for 46.8% of those who had positive and indeterminate results in the ELISA test.

The analysis of the presence of specific IgG antibodies in the blood serum of 187 forestry workers who initially tested positive in the ELISA test showed the following results by immunoblotting: positive results were obtained in 180 individuals (96.3%), and negative results in 7 individuals (3.7%). Examining the blood serum of 40 individuals who had indeterminate results in the ELISA test for IgG antibodies to *B. burgdorferi s. l.*, it was found that 27 (67.5%) had positive results and 13 (32.5%) had negative results. None of these individuals showed indeterminate results.

Table 9. Evaluation criteria for IgG class antibodies to antigens of the *B. burgdorferi s. l.* complex

VlsE Ba or VlsE Bb, or VlsE Bg bands	Specific antigens bands: p18, p19, p20, p21, p58, OspC (p25), p39, p83, Lipid Ba, Lipid Bb		
	2 or more bands are positive	1 band is positive	no positive bands
The antigen band is positive	Positive	Positive	Positive
The antigen band is weakly positive	Positive	Positive	Negative
The antigen band is negative	Positive	Negative	Negative

Table 10. Results of serum testing from forestry workers in six regions for the presence of IgM and IgG antibodies to *B. burgdorferi s. l.* (ELISA and EUROLINE Borrelia RN-AT tests) (n = 731)

IgM					
ELISA			EUROLINE Borrelia RN-AT		
Result	Total (n=731)		Result	Total (n = 190)	
	Absolute number	%		Absolute number	%
Positive	123	16,8	Positive	77	62,6
			Intermediate	20	12,3
			Negative	26	21,1
Intermediate	67	9,2	Positive	12	17,9
			Intermediate	18	26,9
			Negative	37	55,2
Negative	541	74,0	*		
			*		
			*		
IgG					
ELISA			EUROLINE Borrelia RN-AT		
Result	Total (n=731)		Result	Total (n = 227)	
	Absolute number	%		Absolute number	%
Positive	187	25,6	Positive	180	96,3
			Intermediate	0	0
			Negative	7	3,7
Intermediate	40	5,5	Positive	27	67,5
			Intermediate	0	0
			Negative	13	32,5
Negative	504	68,9	*		
			*		
			*		

Note. * – the test was not performed (the ELISA result was negative).

Therefore, the presence of IgG antibodies to *B. burgdorferi s. l.* by immunoblot was confirmed in 207 (180 + 27) forestry workers from Volyn, Zhytomyr, Transcarpathian, Khmelnytskyi, Chernivtsi, and Chernihiv regions, which accounted for 91.2% of the 227 individuals who had positive and indeterminate results in the ELISA test.

Further investigation focused on specific IgM antibodies to specific antigens in 89 forestry workers. It was found that the frequency of detecting IgM antibodies to OspC antigens of two types of Borrelia – *B. burgdorferi s. s.* and *B. garinii* – did not significantly differ in blood serum among forestry workers from different regions. However, IgM antibodies to OspC B. afzelii were least frequently detected in the blood serum of forestry workers from Transcarpathian (in 11 examined), and most frequently in Khmelnytskyi and Chernihiv regions (in 13 out of 17 and 18 examined, respectively) ($p < 0.05$).

Additionally, IgM antibodies to antigens p41, p39, and VlsE were assessed in the blood serum of these 89 forestry workers. It was found that IgM antibodies to p41 were detected in 70 (78.7%) individuals examined, whereas antibodies to p39 were not found in forestry workers from Volyn and Transcarpathian regions ($p < 0.05$). Positive results for IgM antibodies to p39 were found in only 9 (10.1%) individuals examined from the other four regions, with a nearly equal distribution among them ($p < 0.05$). IgM antibodies to VlsE were not detected in any of the individuals examined.

Table 11. Results of serum testing of forestry workers from each of the six regions (n = 89) for the presence of IgM antibodies to various antigens of B. burgdorferi s. l. (immunoblot method)

Antigen		Results											
		Volyn region (n = 16)		Zhytomyr region (n = 20)		Transcarpathian region (n = 11)		Khmelnytskyi region (n = 17)		Chernivtsi region (n = 7)		Chernihiv region (n = 18)	
		1		2		3		4		5		6	
		Absolute number	%	Absolute number	%	Absolute number	%	Absolute number	%	Absolute number	%	Absolute number	%
OspC	+	9	56,2	11	55,0	5	45,5	12	70,6	5	71,4	12	66,7
Bg	-	7	43,8	9	45,0	6	54,5	5	29,4	2	28,6	6	33,3
OspC	+	9	56,2	13	65,0	4	36,4	11	64,7	3	42,9	6	33,3
Bb	-	7	43,8	7	35,0	7	63,6	6	35,3	4	57,1	12	66,7
OspC	+	10	62,5	13	65,0	3	27,3	13	76,5	4	57,1	13	72,2
Ba	-	6	37,5	7	35,0	8	72,7	4	23,5	3	42,9	5	27,8
p39	+	0	0	3	15,0	0	0	2	11,8	1	14,3	3	16,7
	-	16	100,0	17	85,0	11	100,0	15	88,2	6	85,7	15	83,3
p41	+	12	75,0	18	90,0	8	72,7	16	94,1	5	71,4	11	61,1
	-	4	25,0	2	10,0	3	27,3	1	5,9	2	28,6	7	38,9

Note. OspC Bg, OspC Bb $p > 0.05$ for Pearson's chi-square test, OspC Ba $p < 0.05$ for Pearson's chi-square test; $p < 0.05$ compared to groups 1, 3; 2, 3; 3, 4; 3, 6; p39 $p < 0.05$ for Pearson's chi-square test; $p < 0.05$ compared to groups 1, 2; 1, 4; 1, 5; 1, 6; 2, 3; 3, 4; 3, 5; 3, 6; p41 $p < 0.05$ for Pearson's chi-square test; $p < 0.05$ compared to groups 1, 6; 2, 6; 3, 4; 4, 6.

Furthermore, the presence of IgG antibodies to various Borrelia antigens – VlsE (*B. burgdorferi s. s., B. garinii, B. afzelii*), p18, p19, p20, p21, p58, p39, p41, p83, LB (*B. burgdorferi s. s.* and *B. afzelii*) – was determined in the blood serum of 207 forestry workers from six regions: Volyn, Zhytomyr, Transcarpathian, Khmelnytskyi, Chernivtsi, and Chernihiv, who had specific IgG (positive) to *B. burgdorferi s. l.* detected by ELISA. The frequency of detecting IgG antibodies to immunoreactive lipids (Lipid Ba, Lipid Bb) did not vary significantly among forestry workers from all regions. The percentage of positive IgG detection to classic antigens p83, p39, and OspC in the blood serum of examined forestry workers also did not significantly differ across all regions (Table 11). However, IgG antibodies to p41 were present in all forestry workers from Volyn, Zhytomyr, Transcarpathian, Chernivtsi, and Chernihiv regions, while absent in 1 (2.2%) individual from Khmelnytskyi region. Positive IgG to p18 was found in the blood serum of 75 (36.2%) forestry workers, most frequently in Khmelnytskyi region – in 27 (58.7%) out of 46 ($p < 0.05$) (Table 12) [46-49].

Table 12. Results of serum testing of forestry workers from six regions (n=207) for the presence of IgG antibodies to various antigens of *B. burgdorferi s. l.* (immunoblot method)

Antigen		Results											
		Volyn region (n = 48)		Zhytomyr region (n=35)		Transcarpathian region (n = 32)		Khmelnytskyi region (n = 46)		Chernivtsi region (n = 11)		Chernihiv region (n = 35)	
		1		2		3		4		5		6	
		Absolute number	%	Absolute number	%	Absolute number	%	Absolute number	%	Absolute number	%	Absolute number	%
p18	+	14	29,2	17	48,6	6	18,7	27	58,7	4	36,4	7	20,0
	-	34	70,8	18	51,4	26	81,3	19	41,3	7	63,6	28	80,0
p19	+	12	25,0	10	28,6	2	6,3	14	30,4	5	45,5	5	14,3
	-	36	75,0	25	71,4	30	93,7	32	69,6	6	54,5	30	85,7
p20	+	4	8,3	3	8,6	2	6,3	3	6,5	0	0	3	8,6
	-	44	91,7	32	91,4	30	93,7	43	93,5	11	100,0	32	91,4
p21	+	7	14,6	2	5,7	3	9,4	8	17,4	1	9,1	5	14,3
	-	41	85,4	33	94,3	29	90,6	38	82,6	10	90,9	30	85,7
p58	+	9	18,8	5	14,3	5	15,6	6	13,1	3	27,3	10	28,6
	-	39	81,2	30	85,7	27	84,4	40	86,9	8	72,7	25	71,4
OspC	+	19	39,6	14	40,0	13	40,6	21	45,7	5	45,5	17	48,6
	-	29	60,4	21	60,0	19	59,4	25	54,3	6	54,5	18	51,4
p39	+	17	35,4	16	45,7	9	28,1	18	39,1	4	36,4	23	65,7
	-	31	64,6	19	54,3	23	71,9	28	60,9	7	63,6	12	34,3
P41	+	48	100,0	35	100,0	32	100,0	45	97,8	11	100,0	35	100,0
	-	0	0	0	0	0	0	1	2,2	0	0	0	0
p83	+	25	52,1	19	54,3	11	34,4	26	56,5	6	54,5	17	48,6
	-	23	47,9	16	45,7	21	65,6	20	43,5	5	45,5	18	51,4
LBb	+	5	10,4	12	34,3	8	25,0	18	39,1	2	18,2	5	14,3
	-	43	89,6	23	65,7	24	75,0	28	60,9	9	81,8	30	85,7
LBa	+	12	25,0	6	17,1	10	31,3	17	36,9	2	18,2	12	34,3
	-	36	75,0	29	82,9	22	68,7	29	63,1	9	81,8	23	65,7
VlsE-Bg	+	42	87,5	28	80,0	21	65,6	39	84,8	8	72,7	34	97,1
	-	6	12,5	7	20,0	11	34,4	7	15,2	3	27,3	1	2,9
VlsE-Bb	+	42	87,5	34	97,1	28	87,5	44	95,7	9	81,8	33	94,3
	-	6	12,5	1	2,9	4	12,5	2	4,3	2	18,2	2	5,7
VlsE-Ba	+	41	85,4	27	77,1	22	68,8	40	86,9	10	90,9	33	94,3
	-	7	14,6	8	22,9	10	31,2	6	13,1	1	9,1	2	5,7

Note. p18 $p < 0.05$ for Pearson's χ^2 test; $p<0.05$ compared to groups 1, 5; 2, 3; 2, 6; 3, 5; 4, 6; p19 $p < 0.05$ for Pearson's χ^2 test; $p<0.05$ compared to groups 1, 3; 2, 3; 3, 4; 3, 5; LBb $p < 0.05$ for Pearson's χ^2 test; $p<0.05$ compared to groups 1, 2; 1, 4; p20, p21, p58, OspC, p39, p41, p83, LBa, VlsE-Bg, VlsE-Bb, VlsE-Ba $p>0.05$ for Pearson's χ^2 test.

To detect only IgM antibodies against OspC antigens of four Borrelia species simultaneously – *B. burgdorferi s. s.*, *B. garinii*, *B. afzelii*, and *B. spielmanii* – the EUROLINE *Borrelia* RN-AT adv test system was used. According to the manufacturer's recommendations, the result was considered positive, indeterminate, or negative based on combinations of OspC antigens from the four Borrelia species: OspC Ba (*B. afzelii*), OspC Bb (*B. burgdorferi*), OspC Bg (*B. garinii*), OspC Bsp (*B. spielmanii*), p39, and VlsE Bb (Table 13) [50].

Under observation were 77 individuals aged 19 to 65 years with LB, who received outpatient and inpatient treatment between 2015 and 2020 at Ternopil Regional Clinical Dermatovenerologic Dispensary, the infectious diseases department of the Ternopil City Municipal Emergency Hospital, and the Ternopil University Hospital. Among them, there were 29 (37.7%) men and 48 (62.3%) women. The highest frequency of LB cases occurred in the age group of 30–39 years: 13 (28.2%) with EM and 12 (38.7%) with Bannwarth syndrome (BS).

Table 13. Criteria for evaluating IgM antibodies to antigens of the *B. burgdorferi s. l.* complex

OspC Ba or OspC Bb, or OspC Bg, or OspC Bs bands	Specific antigens bands: p39, VlsE Bb	
	1 band is positive	no positive bands
The antigen band is positive	Positive	Positive
OspC Ba, or OspC Bg, or OspC Bs band is weakly positive	Positive	Intermediate
The antigen band is negative	Positive	Negative

The diagnosis of LB was established based on characteristic epidemiological, anamnestic, and clinical data, confirmed by serological methods. Depending on the clinical manifestations of LB, patients were divided into two groups: Group 1 – 46 individuals with EM and Group 2 – 31 patients diagnosed with BS. Urban residents outnumbered rural residents numerically ($p < 0.05$), with slightly more individuals in urban areas presenting with EM compared to BS LB ($p > 0.05$).

Patients with BS LB exhibited diverse disease manifestations (Table 14); however, they predominantly presented with joint involvement over pathological changes in other organs and systems ($p < 0.05$).

According to the recommendations of the Centres for Disease Control and Prevention (CDC), a two-step serological scheme was used for the serological diagnosis of LB. In the first stage, antibodies to *B. burgdorferi s. l.* antigens in patients' serum were determined using an enzyme-linked immunosorbent assay (ELISA) method with test systems from Euroimmun AG (Germany): IgM antibodies were detected using the *Anti-Borrelia burgdorferi* ELISA (IgM), and IgG antibodies were detected using the *Anti-Borrelia* plus VlsE ELISA (IgG). According to the manufacturer's recommendations, a result ≥22 IU/mL was considered positive, 16–22 IU/mL was considered borderline, and ≤16 IU/mL was considered negative.

Using the ELISA test, specific IgM antibodies were found in 23 (50.0%) patients with EM LB, borderline results were found in 6 (13.1%), and negative results were found in 17 (36.9%). Specific IgG antibodies were detected in 9 (19.6%) examined individuals, borderline results in 3 (6.5%), and negative results in 34 (73.9%) (Figure 14).

A similar analysis of 31 patients with NEM LB showed specific IgM antibodies in 18 (58.1%) patients, borderline results in 4 (12.9%), and negative results in 9 (29.0%). Specific

IgG antibodies were also assessed in the serum samples, with positive results in 8 (25.8%) of those examined and negative results in 23 (74.2%) (Figure 15). No borderline results were observed in any of the examined cases.

Table 14. Clinical manifestations in patients with non-erythema migrans form of Lyme borreliosis (n=31)

Clinical manifestation	Absolute number	%
Joint involvement	24*	77,4
Cardiovascular system involvement	3	9,6
Nervous system involvement	2	6,5
Intoxication syndrome	2	6,5

Note. * – difference regarding other clinical manifestations, $p < 0.05$.

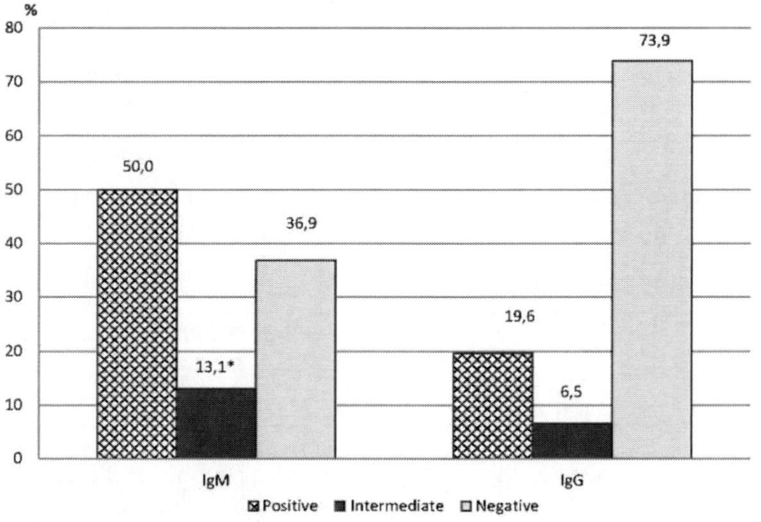

Note. * – significant difference between IgM and IgG, $p < 0.05$.

Figure 14. Results of serum testing of patients with erythema migrans Lyme borreliosis using the ELISA for the presence of IgM and IgG antibodies to *B. burgdorferi s. l.* (n=46).

Samples of blood with borderline and positive results from the first stage (ELISA test) were investigated using the EUROLINE Borrelia RN-AT adv immunoblot test system. Serum samples from two groups were studied: Group 1 included 29 individuals (23 positive and 6 borderline), and Group 2 included 22 individuals (18 positive and 4 borderline). Specifically, antibodies of the IgM class to OspC antigens of four Borrelia species – *B. burgdorferi s. s.*, *B. garinii*, *B. afzelii*, and *B. spielmanii* – were detected (Table 15).

Further verification of specific IgM antibody levels in the serum of 23 patients with EM LB who had positive results in the ELISA test revealed the following through immunoblotting: positive results were obtained in 18 (72.3%) individuals, borderline results in 4 (17.4%), and negative results in 1 (4.3%). Analysing the blood samples of 6 EM patients who had borderline results in the ELISA test for IgM antibodies to B. burgdorferi s. l., the results were as follows: positive results were found in 1 (16.7%), borderline in 3 (50.0%), and negative in 2 (33.3%) patients.

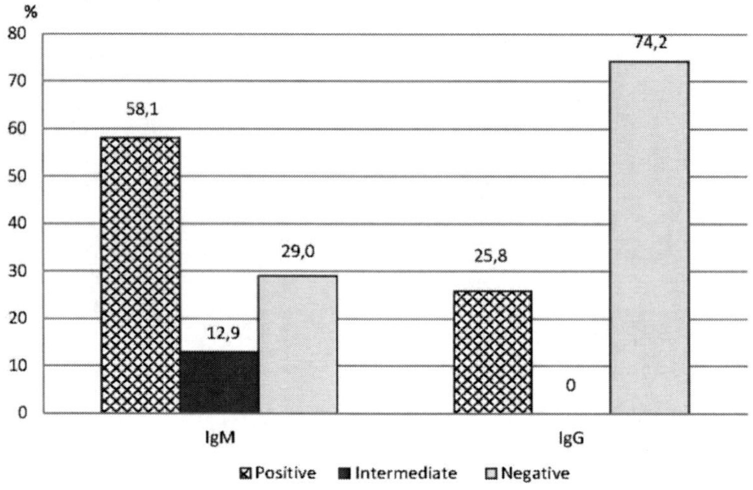

Figure 15. Results of serum testing of patients with non-erythema migrans form of Lyme borreliosis using the ELISA for the presence of IgM and IgG antibodies to *B. burgdorferi s. l.* (n = 31).

Table 15. Presence of IgM antibodies to *B. burgdorferi s. l.* in serum samples from patients with erythema migrans and non-erythema migrans forms of Lyme borreliosis (ELISA and EUROLINE *Borrelia* RN-AT adv tests) (n=77)

Patients with EM LB					
IgM (ELISA)			IgM (EUROLINE Borrelia RN-ATadv)		
Result	Total (n = 46)		Result	Total (n=29)	
	Absolute number	%		Absolute number	%
Positive	23	50,0	Positive	18	72,3
			Intermediate	4	17,4
			Negative	1	4,3
Intermediate	6	13,1	Positive	1	16,7
			Intermediate	3	50,0
			Negative	2	33,3
Negative	17	36,9	*		
			*		
			*		
Patients with NEM LB					
IgM (ELISA)			IgM (EUROLINE Borrelia RN-ATadv)		
Result	Total (n = 31)		Result	Total (n=22)	
	Absolute number	%		Absolute number	%
Positive	18	58,1	Positive	15	83,3
			Intermediate	1	5,6
			Negative	2	11,1
Intermediate	4	12,9	Positive	2	50,0
			Intermediate	2	50,0
			Negative	0	0
Negative	9	29,0	*		
			*		
			*		

Note: * – the test was not performed (the ELISA result was negative).

Thus, positive results for the presence of IgM antibodies to *B. burgdorferi s. l.* using the immunoblot method were confirmed in 19 (65.5%) out of 29 individuals with EM who had positive or borderline results in the ELISA test.

In the analysis of specific IgM antibody presence in the serum of 18 patients with NEM LB, who had positive results in the first stage (ELISA test), the immunoblot method showed the following: positive results were obtained in 15 (83.3%) individuals, borderline in 1 (5.6%), and negative in 2 (11.1%). When examining serum samples from 4 patients with NEM LB who had borderline results in the ELISA test for IgM antibodies to *B. burgdorferi s. l.*, positive results were found in 2 (50.0%) and borderline results in 2 (50.0%) patients. There were no negative results in the second stage of examination for any of these patients.

Therefore, the presence of IgM antibodies to *B. burgdorferi s. l.* by immunoblotting was confirmed in 17 (77.3%) out of 22 individuals with NEM LB who had positive or borderline results in the ELISA test.

The frequency of detection of IgM antibodies to antigens of the four Borrelia species separately in patients of both groups was also investigated. IgM antibodies to OspC *B. spielmanii* were found in the serum of 18 (94.7%) individuals in Group 1 and 16 (94.1%) in Group 2; to OspC *B. garinii* – in 18 (94.7%) and 14 (82.4%), respectively; to OspC *B. burgdorferi s. s.* – in 16 (84.2%) and 14 (84.2%); to OspC *B. afzelii* – in 17 (89.5%) and 12 (70.6%) patients, respectively. IgM antibodies to antigens p41, p39, and VlsE were also identified in the serum samples of examined patients. Specifically, IgM antibodies to p41 were detected in 11 (57.9%) patients of Group 1 and 8 (47.1%) of Group 2; to p39 – in 4 (21.1%) and 5 (29.4%), respectively; no antibodies to VlsE were found in any of the patients (Figure 16).

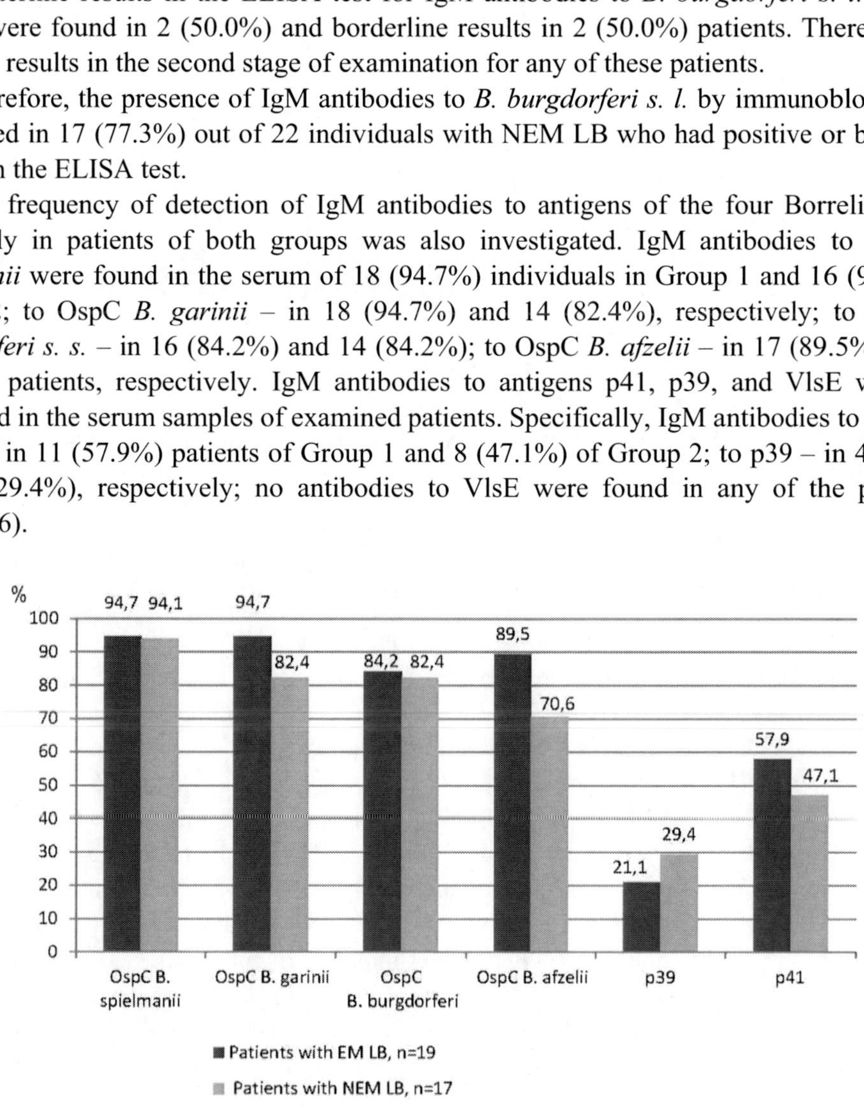

Figure 16. Frequency of detection of IgM (positive results) against OspC of *B. burgdorferi s. s.*, *B. garinii*, *B. afzelii*, and *B. spielmanii* in serum samples from patients with erythema migrans and non-erythema migrans forms of Lyme borreliosis using the EUROLINE *Borrelia* RN-AT adv test.

Variants combining IgM antibodies to different Borrelia OspC surface antigens were also studied. In many individuals with EM LB and NEM LB, antibodies to multiple pathogens were detected simultaneously (Figure 17).

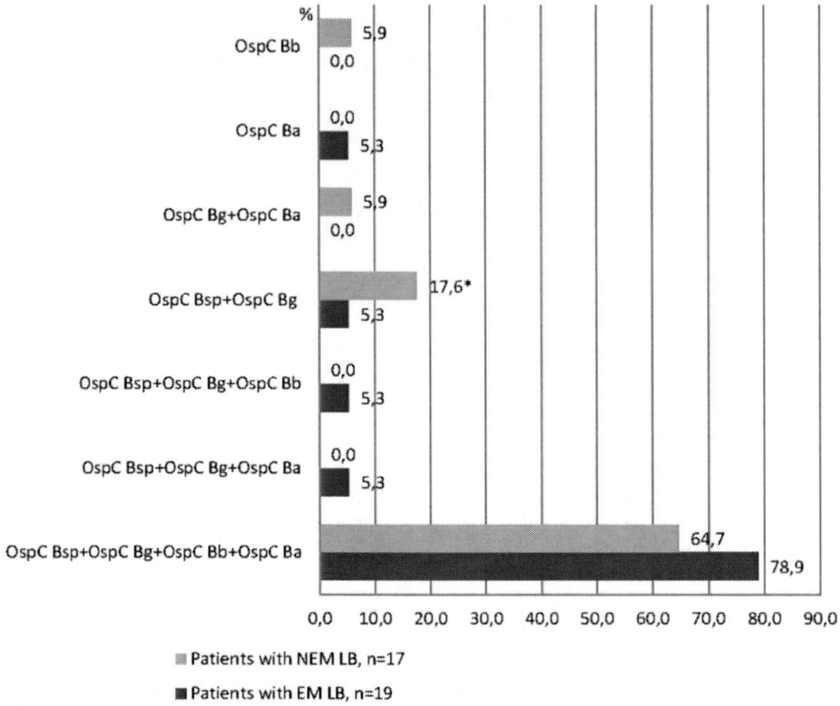

Note. * – significant difference regarding patients with non-erythema migrans form of Lyme borreliosis, $p < 0.05$.

Figure 17. Variants of simultaneous detection of IgM antibodies (positive results) to OspC antigens of *B. burgdorferi s. s.*, *B. garinii*, *B. afzelii*, and *B. spielmanii* in serum samples from patients with erythema migrans and non-erythema migrans forms of Lyme borreliosis using the EUROLINE Borrelia RN-AT adv test.

It is noteworthy that simultaneous IgM antibodies to OspC antigens of all four Borrelia species—*B. burgdorferi s. s.*, *B. garinii*, *B. afzelii*, and *B. spielmanii*—were detected in 15 (78.9%) EM patients and 11 (64.7%) NEM patients. Antibodies of this class to surface antigens of three pathogens (OspC Ba, OspC Bg, OspC Bsp) were found in only 1 (5.3%) individual with EM and none with NEM. Likewise, IgM antibodies to OspC antigens of three pathogens (OspC Bb, OspC Bg, OspC Bsp) were found in only 1 (5.3%) EM patient; antibodies to two antigens (OspC Bg and OspC Bsp) were diagnosed in 1 (5.3%) EM patient and 3 (17.6%) NEM patients; to OspC Bg and OspC Ba – only in 1 (5.9%) NEM patient. It is worth noting that antibodies to OspC Bg and OspC Bsp were more frequently detected concurrently in individuals with NEM compared to EM – 17.6% versus 5.3% ($p < 0.05$). Additionally, it was found that IgM antibodies only to *B. afzelii* were detected in only 1 (5.3%) EM patient and to B. burgdorferi s. l. in only 1 (5.9%) NEM patient. IgM antibodies solely to OspC *B. spielmanii* (mono-infection) were not found in any patient (Figure 17).

Therefore, the use of the EUROLINE Borrelia RN-AT adv IgM test system allowed expanding the spectrum of pathogens causing erythema migrans and non-erythema migrans forms of Lyme borreliosis in patients predominantly affected in the musculoskeletal system by detecting anti-IgM antibodies simultaneously to OspC *B. spielmanii*, *B. burgdorferi s. l.*, *B. garinii*, and *B. afzelii*. Specifically, these antibodies were detected in 78.9% of patients with erythema migrans and in 64.7% of those with non-erythema migrans forms [51, 52].

4. Methods of Instrumental Diagnostics

Ivan Klishch
and Inna Ishchuk

In LB, depending on the involvement of various organs and systems, instrumental diagnostic methods are applied. It is advisable for all patients, regardless of symptoms, to undergo electrocardiography to detect potential early asymptomatic heart involvement.

Patients with clinical symptoms of LB and focal neurological signs, seizures, or other signs of central or peripheral nervous system involvement undergo electroencephalography (EEG), magnetic resonance imaging (MRI), or computed tomography (CT) of the brain. In specific cases, electromyography (EMG) may also be performed. MRI is more informative than CT because it can detect inflammatory changes in the spinal cord, brainstem structures, white and grey matter of the brain, and vasculitis phenomena.

Individuals with LB who show signs of cardiovascular system involvement undergo echocardiography and Holter monitoring. Those with musculoskeletal system involvement undergo ultrasound examination of the joints, their X-ray examination, and scintigraphy. Ophthalmoscopy is performed in cases of ocular involvement. Ultrasound diagnostics of the abdominal organs are conducted when necessary.

For patients predominantly affected in specific organs and systems, consultation with relevant specialists is recommended [4, 53].

5. Thermographic Study of Lyme Borreliosis

Mykhaylo Andreychyn
Mariia Shkilna
and Vasyl Kopcha

For the diagnosis of LB, in addition to serological examination, we utilized one of the supplementary instrumental methods thermography, based on remote registration of infrared radiation emitted by the human body. This investigation is non-invasive for the patient since it involves no exposure or harm to the body. The capability to detect disease using thermography is grounded in the fact that various pathological conditions affect both the distribution and intensity of thermal (infrared) radiation. Skin temperature serves as an integral indicator influenced by several factors: vascular network, metabolic processes, thermal conductivity, and heat transfer. All these factors must be considered when analysing thermograms. Among them, vascular factors are paramount and define the principal thermovisual symptoms in clinical medicine [54].

Currently, there are numerous publications in Ukraine and worldwide dedicated to the thermographic method across various medical fields: oncology (detection and differential diagnosis of breast tumours, thyroid gland diseases, skin melanoma, etc.), angiology (in Raynaud's disease, endarteritis, angiopathy, varicose veins), obstetrics and gynaecology (early thermographic pregnancy markers, mastitis, benign and malignant tumours, postoperative purulent complications), surgery (acute pancreatitis, appendicitis, infected wounds), urology (nephritis, cystitis, orchitis), orthopaedics and traumatology (osteochondrosis, arthritis, osteomyelitis), burn care (graft survival, determination of burn or frostbite limits), ophthalmology (intraorbital tumours, conjunctivitis), neurology (autonomic nervous system disorders, paresis and paralysis), dermatology (collagen diseases, dermatitis, acne, etc.), and many other fields [55–57]. Thermographic studies are widely applied in infectology as well. For instance, researchers from the Department of Infectious Diseases, Epidemiology, Skin, and Venereal Diseases at I. Horbachevsky Ternopil National Medical University of Ukraine have developed thermosymiotics for viral hepatitis, acute respiratory viral infections (ARVI), scabies, erysipeloid, leptospirosis, and other gastrointestinal infections [1]. Therefore, we decided to utilize this diagnostic method in patients with EM and NEM LB.

Preparation for thermography and the examination itself were conducted in accordance with the recommendations of the Chinese company "ULIRvision" [58]: patients were instructed to abstain from all types of physiotherapy, massage, intake of vasoactive drugs, application of therapeutic ointments, and gels on the area of interest 24 hours before the examination, and refrain from smoking and eating 40-60 minutes prior to the examination. The temperature in the thermography room was maintained at a constant range of 18–22°C. During a 10-15 minute period, patients acclimated to the air temperature of the thermographic chamber to establish stable temperature relationships between the human body and the environment.

Thermal imaging of the area of interest was performed with the patient in a sitting or standing position, focusing the device at a distance of 40-50 cm in frontal projection. Areas of interest included the tick bite site, erythema, and surrounding tissues, and in the case of bilateral involvement (limbs, lateral surfaces of the trunk), the symmetrical part of the body was also assessed.

To determine the characteristics of infrared radiation within normal limits, 42 healthy volunteers with normal body temperature, without organic skin or internal organ pathologies, aged 19 to 57 years (mean age: 34.4 ±6.5 years), were examined. Among them, 24 were male, comprising 57.1%, and 18 were female, comprising 42.9%. The average age was approximately equal between genders, with (34.9 ± 7.2) years for males and (33.7 ± 7.8) years for females.

Thermal imaging was evaluated visually by comparing the colour palette with the surrounding areas, and in the presence of thermosymmetry, thermograms were described according to the following algorithm: thermosymmetry; localization of areas with increased and decreased intensity of infrared radiation; temperature values and their difference from the symmetric area. The temperature values at all points of the image were automatically recorded by the program. For greater informativeness, thermographs and histograms were used. This methodology is precise and allows for the representation of temperature distribution not only in the general region but also in specific points.

When analysing the zone of interest, the shape of the thermally active area (focal, diffuse), its structure by uniformity (homogeneous, heterogeneous), contour features (distinct, indistinct), topographical correspondence of the zone of interest, and localization of pathological foci were considered. The system can simultaneously process up to 20-point objects, 10 lines, 20 fields, 10 polygonal, and 10 elliptical objects.

To compare symmetric areas or areas of heating focus with surrounding tissues, options such as points, horizontal lines, and rectangular fields were primarily used. In this case, the temperature of designated points was recorded, allowing for the subsequent calculation of temperature difference (ΔT) across the entire line of interest with automatic indication of extreme values (maximum and minimum temperatures). The selected rectangular field ensured automatic construction of a histogram, visually demonstrating the distribution of temperature array from minimum to maximum (Figure 18).

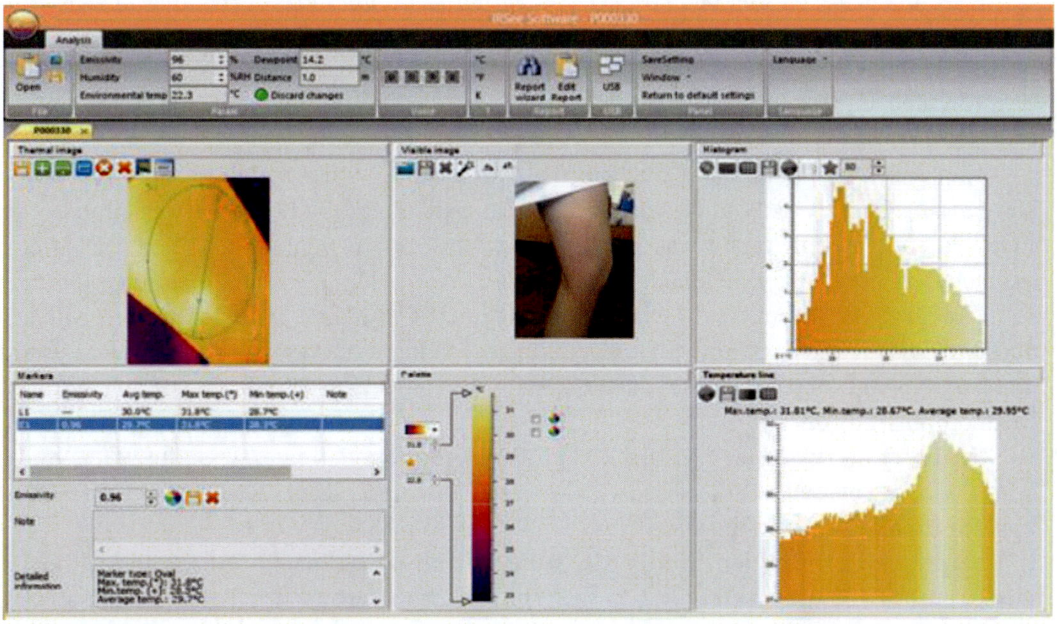

Note: In the upper left corner – infrared image with highlighted line L1 and region of interest e1; in the upper right corner – histogram of the selected region e1, showing temperature distribution in percentages ranging from 28.3 to 31.8°C; in the lower left corner – objects and palette indicating average, maximum, and minimum temperatures of oval e1 (Tmax = 31.8°C, Tmin = 28.3°C, ΔT = 3.5°C); in the lower right corner – temperature of line of interest L1 with temperature fluctuations ranging from 28.67 to 31.81°C.

Figure 18. Analysis of the thermogram of the left thigh of patient B. with erythema migrans in Lyme borreliosis using the "IRSee Software" program.

Processed thermograms were stored in an electronic archive for subsequent comparison during patient observation in dynamics.

The remote thermography method was used to study the indicators of temperature difference (ΔT) between the affected and healthy skin areas in patients with the erythema migrans form of Lyme borreliosis before and after etiological treatment, including consideration of process dissemination.

A total of 31 patients with EM LB were observed, of which 17 (54.8%) were men and 14 (45.2%) were women. The average age of the patients was (44.19 ± 12.68) years. The diagnosis of LB was established according to ICD-10. Patients with chronic vascular diseases were excluded from the study.

All patients responded to a standardized questionnaire developed by scientists from I. Horbachevsky Ternopil National Medical University, Ukraine, and Pope John Paul II State School of Higher Education (Biała Podlaska, Poland).

For serological confirmation of LB, a two-stage diagnostic process was used. In the first stage, specific IgM and/or IgG antibodies to the B. burgdorferi s.l. complex antigens were determined in the patients' blood serum using an enzyme immunoassay with test kits from Euroimmun AG (Germany): IgM antibodies with the *Anti-Borrelia burgdorferi* ELISA (IgM) test system and IgG antibodies with the *Anti-Borrelia* plus VIsE ELISA (IgG). In the second stage, positive and intermediate results from the ELISA were confirmed by immunoblotting using the EUROLINE *Borrelia* RN-AT test system, Euroimmun AG (Germany). The results were evaluated according to the manufacturer's recommendations.

All patients received the following treatment: doxycycline hydrochloride at 200 mg per day (divided into two 100 mg doses) for 14 days, along with Carsil and Hilak drops in therapeutic doses.

The areas of interest for the thermographic study were the zone of erythema and surrounding tissues, as well as the symmetrical part of the body in cases of limb or torso involvement. Thermography was performed twice: upon patient presentation and after the visible erythema on the skin had disappeared.

The shape, topographical location, and degree of erythema coloration were taken into account. The Glamorgan Protocol (atlas of healthy skin thermographic patterns) was used for comparison and objectification of the data [59]. The skin emission coefficient on the thermograms was 0.96.

Of the 31 patients with EM LB, 22 (71.0%) reported a tick bite, while 9 (29.0%) did not recall one but associated the disease with frequent forest visits. The average time of EM appearance after the tick bite was (21.00 ± 8.87) days.

Based on dissemination, 20 (64.5%) patients with disseminated EM LB formed the first group, and 11 (35.5%) with only EM were in the second group. Erythema was uniform and evenly coloured in 18 (58.1%) patients, while 13 (41.9%) had ring-shaped erythema. The erythema lasted (23.13 ± 9.61) days and disappeared (7.61 ± 5.40) days after the start of etiological therapy.

Two-stage serological testing (ELISA and immunoblot) revealed specific IgM and/or IgG antibodies to *B. burgdorferi s. l.* in the blood serum of 23 (74.2%) patients with EM LB.

ΔT of erythema foci in patients with EM LB was compared before and after treatment. A significant reduction in temperature was observed in all patients after treatment ($p < 0.001$, Table 16). This trend was noted in both localized and disseminated EM LB ($p < 0.05$), with no difference between groups.

It was found that the temperature difference between affected and healthy areas was not the same before and after treatment. All patients were divided into three groups: Group 1 – ΔT >0.5°C before treatment, ≤ 0.5°C after treatment; Group 2 – ΔT > 0.5°C before and after treatment; Group 3 – ΔT ≤ 0.5°C before and after treatment (Table 17).

The duration of erythema in each group was analysed. It was longer in Group 3 patients compared to Group 1: (31.56 ± 6.89) vs. (22.83 ± 9.58) days ($p < 0.05$) and compared to Group 2: (31.56 ± 6.89) vs. (15.90 ± 4.93) days ($p < 0.001$). However, the time for erythema to disappear after treatment did not significantly differ (Table 18).

Table 16. Temperature difference (ΔT) indicators of patients with erythema migrans form of Lyme borreliosis before and after treatment

Group	ΔT °C		p
	before treatment	after treatment	
Total (n = 31)	1,10 (0,40; 1,70)	0,40 (0,30; 0,90)	<0,001*
EM LB with dissemination (n = 20)	0,85 (0,40; 1,35)	0,45 (0,30; 1,00)	<0,001*
EM LB without dissemination (n = 11)	1,40 (0,80; 2,00)	0,40 (0,20; 0,50)	<0,05*
p	>0,05	>0,05	

Table 17. Groups of patients with erythema migrans form of Lyme borreliosis depending on the temperature difference (ΔT) between affected and healthy areas, before and after treatment, n = 31

Group	n	%	Confidential interval (95% CI)
Group 1 (before treatment ΔT >0,5°C, after treatment ≤0,5°C)	12	38,7	20,00; 67,62
Group 2 (before treatment ΔT >0,5°C, after treatment >0,5°C)	10	32,4	15,47; 59,32
Group 3 (before treatment ΔT ≤0,5°C, after treatment ≤0,5°C)	9	29,0	13,28; 55,11

Table 18. Duration of erythema migrans form of Lyme borreliosis and the time of its disappearance after the use of antibiotics in different groups

Indicator	Group 1 (n = 12)	Group 2 (n = 10)	Group 3 (n = 9)	Tukey's test
Duration of erythema, days	22,83 ± 9,58	15,90 ± 4,93	31,56 ± 6,89	pI-II => 0,05; pI-III =< 0,05*; pII-III < 0,001*
Time for erythema to disappear after taking antibiotics, days	6,42 ± 4,85	6,80 ± 3,01	10,11 ± 7,54	pI-II => 0,05; pI-III => 0,05; pII-III => 0,05

The relationship between the duration of erythema migrans and the ΔT of affected and healthy skin areas before and after treatment was investigated. Significant inverse correlations were established (Figures 19, 20).

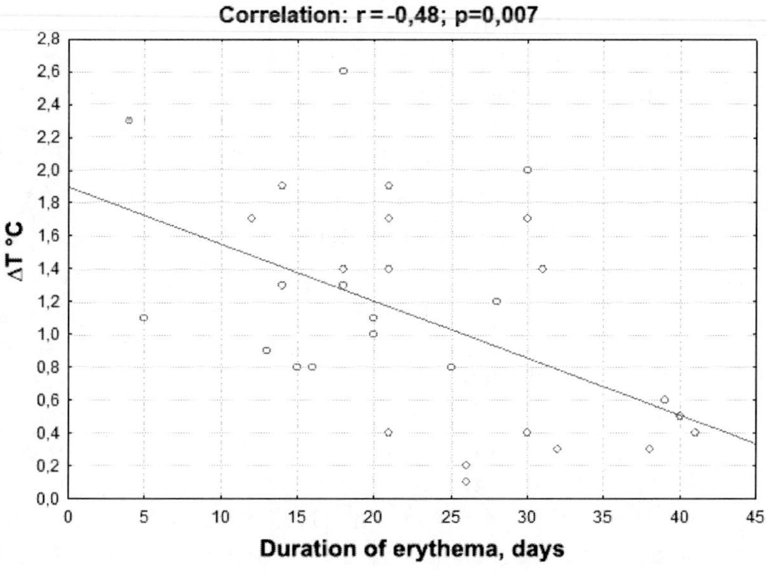

Figure 19. Relationship between the duration of erythema migrans form of Lyme borreliosis and ΔT before treatment.

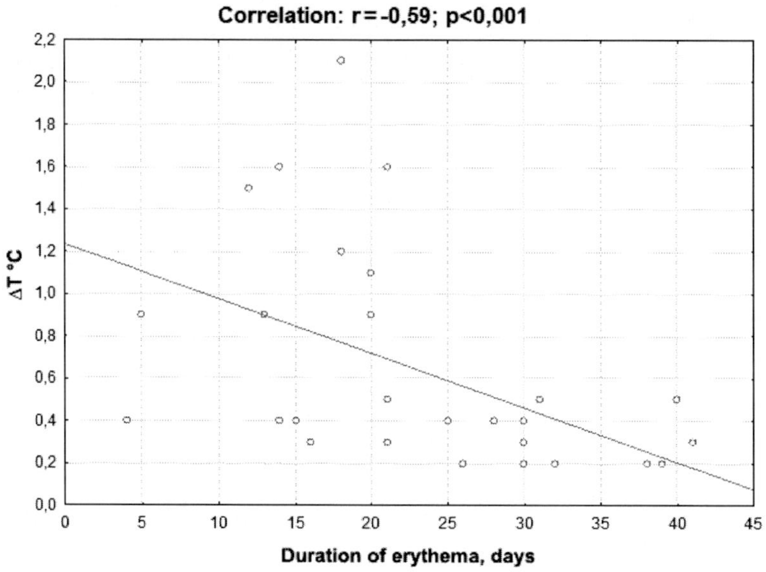

Figure 20. Relationship between the duration of erythema migrans form of Lyme borreliosis and ΔT after treatment.

A statistically significant inverse correlation between the duration of EM and ΔT before and after treatment was established, explained by the reduction of local inflammation in the affected skin area caused by the presence of *B. burgdorferi s. l.* [60, 61]. Similar results were obtained by scientists from the Department of Biochemistry and Molecular Biology and the Infectious Diseases Department of New York Medical College, USA, which identified an inverse correlation between the number of detected Borrelia in skin biopsies and the duration and size of EM ($p < 0.05$) [62].

Thus, under the influence of complex antibiotic treatment for LB, the temperature difference of both solitary and disseminated erythema decreases. The longest erythema duration was observed in patients without significant local heating ($\Delta T \leq 0.5°C$) before treatment (Group 3), compared to patients with a significant temperature difference ($\Delta T > 0.5°C$) before treatment (Groups 1 and 2), $p < 0.05$ and<0.001, respectively. An inverse correlation between the duration of EM and the temperature difference in affected and healthy skin areas was established both before ($r = -0.48$; $p < 0.05$) and after ($r = -0.59$; $p < 0.001$) etiological treatment.

Thirty-three patients with LB were observed: 12 individuals with an non-erythema-migrans and mildly symptomatic form, who were receiving outpatient and inpatient treatment at the infectious diseases department of the Ternopil City Municipal Emergency Hospital and Ternopil University Hospital; and 21 with erythema migrans (skin form), treated at Ternopil Regional Clinical Dermatovenerologic Dispensary.

The patients ranged in age from 24 to 49 years, with a mean age of (34.3 ± 1.5) years. Among those examined, there were 15 (45.5%) males and 18 (54.5%) females. The majority of the patients (28; 84.8%) were of active working age (up to 60 years).

The diagnosis of LB was established based on characteristic complaints, medical history, clinical data, and confirmed by the detection of specific antibodies. Antibodies to antigens of the *B. burgdorferi s. l.* complex in serum were determined using enzyme-linked immunosorbent assay (ELISA) methods with Euroimmun AG test systems (Germany): IgM antibodies – *Anti-Borrelia burgdorferi* ELISA (IgM), IgG antibodies – *Anti-Borrelia* plus VIsE ELISA (IgG).

It was considered that Borrelia, entering the skin due to tick bite, causes minimal local inflammation, which, even in the absence of visible erythema, is accompanied by local body temperature elevation ("heating"). Such local hyperthermia can be detected by thermography.

After collecting anamnestic data, the site of tick attachment was determined.

An analysis of the responses from patients, both overall and within each group, revealed that the most frequent attachment site for ticks was the legs – found in 39.1% of individuals with the non-erythema migrans form and 26.1% with erythema migrans. The most common attachment sites following the legs in individuals with the non-erythema migrans form of Lyme borreliosis were the anterior torso and abdomen (30.4% and 21.7%, respectively), while in patients with erythema migrans, the arms were the most common ($p < 0.05$) (Figure 21).

Further investigation involved studying the thermal image of the skin using remote thermometry at the tick attachment site, and the conclusion about the presence of skin lesions in the form of subclinical erythema migrans was made based on the detection of local "heating."

It was noted that under normal conditions, the thermographic image of human skin is characterized by symmetry and homogeneity (ΔT – temperature difference between adjacent or symmetrical body areas does not exceed 0.3°C). In the case of local inflammation of the skin, local "heating" (ΔT greater than 0.5°C) would be detected.

The diagnosis of non-erythema migrans form of LB was established based on the presence of local skin inflammation at the tick attachment site, manifested as slight hyperthermia (ΔT = 0.6-1.1°C), persisting for two weeks or more.

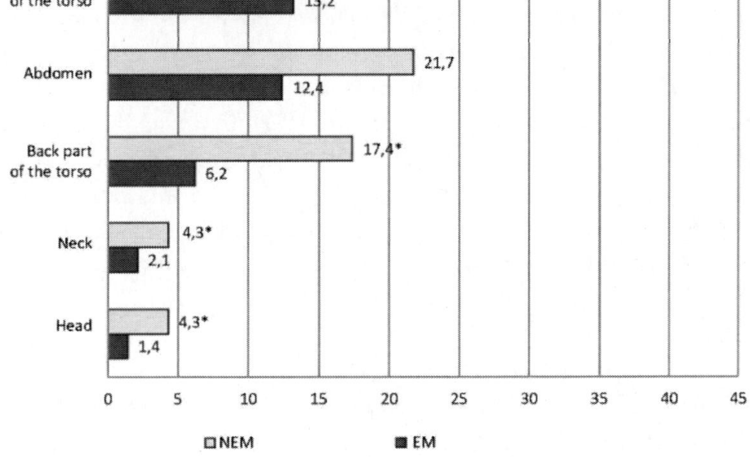

Note. * – significance compared to patients with another form of the disease at the same localization.

Figure 21. Attachment sites of ticks in patients with erythema migrans (n = 21) and suberythematous (n = 12) forms of Lyme borreliosis.

Table 19. Results of thermographic examination of tick bite sites in patients with erythema migrans form of Lyme borreliosis and non-erythema migrans form of Lyme borreliosis

Presence of hyperthermia (ΔT °C)	EM	Patients with localized "skin warming" at the site of a tick bite	
		Absolute number	%
0–0,5 (normal)	Present (n = 12)	0	0,0
	No (n = 21)	0	0,0
0,6–1,1	Present (n = 12)	5	23,7
	No (n = 21)	4	33,3
1,2–1,6	Present (n = 12)	10	47,6
	No (n = 21)	6	50,0
>1,6	Present (n = 12)	6	28,6
	No (n = 21)	2	16,7

In all patients with clinically manifest skin form of Lyme borreliosis (erythema migrans), hyperthermia at the tick bite site was detected, with ΔT exceeding 0.6°C. In nearly half of the patients, it ranged from 1.2 to 1.6°C, and in every fourth patient, it even exceeded 1.6°C (Table 19). Thermograms of the attachment areas in patients with suberythematous form of Lyme borreliosis always showed local "heating." In almost every fourth person with this form, ΔT ranged from 0.6 to 1.1°C, in half it was between 1.2 and 1.6°C, and only in 16.7% did it exceed 1.6°C. Local "heating" of attachment areas exceeding 1.6°C was observed almost twice as often in patients with erythema migrans compared to those with suberythematous form.

Hereby presenting a clinical observation.

Patient S. O., 32 years old, was hospitalized with a diagnosis of acute infectious-allergic myocarditis. Proximal third-degree AV block with episodes of ventricular fibrillation was noted. Stage 2a heart failure was diagnosed based on clinical manifestations and ECG findings. Additionally, it was added to the medical history that approximately 1 month ago, she found an attached Ixodes tick on her back, which she managed to remove without seeking medical attention. There were no signs of local skin involvement such as erythema migrans. Treatment with antiarrhythmic, hormonal, and other therapies proved effective, and the patient was discharged with recovery after 3 weeks. Antibiotics were not administered. Subsequent serological testing (ELISA and immunoblot) revealed IgM and IgG antibodies against B. burgdorferi s. l., confirming the diagnosis of Lyme carditis.

Thermography of the back, performed 1 month after discharge from the hospital, showed local rounded hyperthermia with a diameter of up to 8 cm in the left scapular region (ΔT=1.5°C). The prolonged presence of local "heating" of the skin at the tick bite site (approximately 3 months) excluded the possibility of a physiological skin reaction to the tick bite in favour of pathological hyperthermia. Considering that Lyme borreliosis affects not only the heart but also other organs, including the skin, a diagnosis of suberythematous Lyme borreliosis was made.

One month after initiating specific etiotropic therapy for the skin form of Lyme borreliosis with doxycycline hydrochloride 200 mg per day (in 2 doses of 100 mg), administered for 21 days, the local hyperthermia disappeared (Figures 22–24).

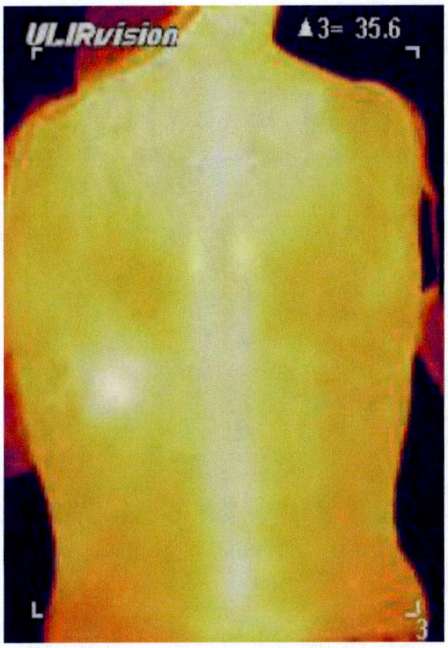

Figure 22. Thermographic image of patient S. O. with suberythematous Lyme borreliosis form (localized "warmth" focus in the left axillary region).

Therefore, the method of remote thermometry of the tick attachment site to human skin, which we first applied, allowed us to diagnose the suberitemal skin form of Lyme borreliosis, justify the necessity of etiotropic therapy to prevent the development of adverse long-term consequences of the disease. This method is advisable to recommend to general practitioners as a non-invasive, safe, and highly informative diagnostic method for the suberitemal form of Lyme borreliosis, with no absolute contraindications to its use [59-62].

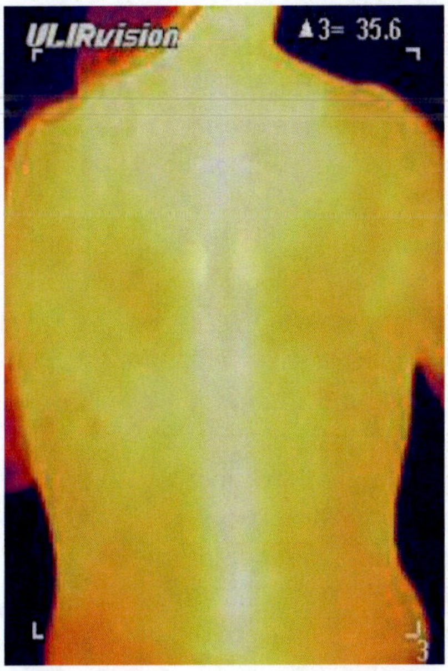

Figure 23. Thermographic image of patient S. O. one month after specific treatment (no pathological changes detected).

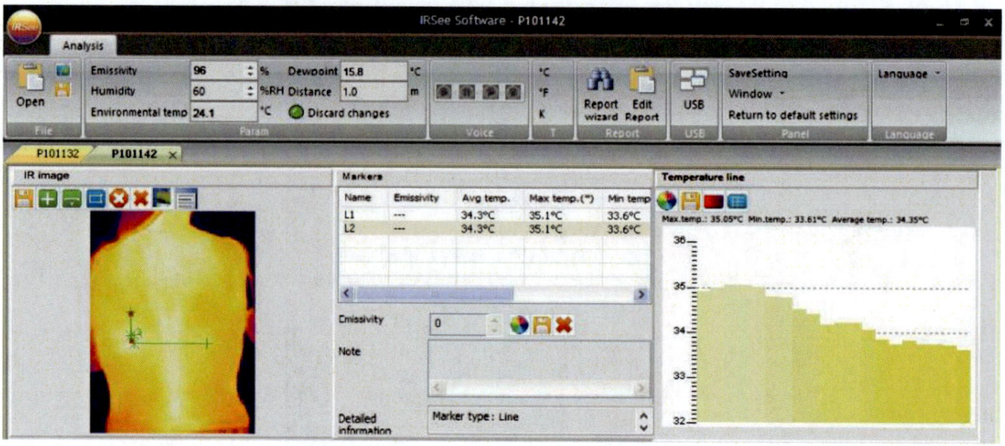

Note: 1 – in the left half – infrared image with highlighted lines of interest L1 (centre of "heating" and surrounding area) and L2 (centre of "heating" and symmetric area of the torso); 2 – in the right half – histogram of the highlighted line L2, connecting symmetric points on opposite areas of the torso, showing temperature distribution in percentages in the range from 33.6 to 35.1°C; in the middle – temperature of lines of interest L1 and L2 with temperature fluctuations from 33.6 to 35.1°C.

Figure 24. Analysis of the thermogram of patient S. O. with suberythematous Lyme borreliosis using the "IRSee Software" program.

Conclusion

Specific laboratory diagnostic methods for Lyme borreliosis are based on the detection of the pathogen itself (via bacterioscopic and bacteriological methods) or its DNA, as well as the identification of antibodies against it (serological methods).

In blood samples from pregnant women, DNA of *B. burgdorferi s. l.* was found in 11.6% of cases, *A. phagocytophilum* in 6.9%, and *Babesia sp.* in 4.7%. Notably, in 9.3% of these women, both antibodies and B. burgdorferi DNA were simultaneously detected, which supports a positive diagnosis. Therefore, pregnant women with adverse obstetric histories should be additionally tested for Lyme borreliosis and other tick-borne infections that may contribute to pregnancy complications.

Serological methods detect antibodies in serum, cerebrospinal fluid (intrathecal), and synovial fluid. Screening is typically performed using ELISA, complement fixation, passive hemagglutination, or indirect immunofluorescence assays. These are crucial for the routine diagnosis of Lyme borreliosis, especially in non-erythema, latent, and chronic forms. A promising approach is the multiplex indirect immunofluorescence assay with BIOCHIP technology, which enables the simultaneous detection of IgM and/or IgG antibodies to multiple infectious and parasitic agents in a single blood sample. This method proved informative in patients with joint involvement and lymphadenopathy and should be more broadly implemented in clinical practice. Immunoblotting detects antibodies to specific pathogen proteins and offers greater sensitivity and specificity compared to other techniques. It is used to confirm positive or equivocal screening results.

Using the two-tiered serological approach (ELISA), IgM and/or IgG antibodies to *B. burgdorferi s. l.* were detected in 73.9% of patients with erythema migrans form of Lyme borreliosis, 63.3% of hospital patients in Ternopil, and 65.6% of forestry workers with non-erythema migrans form of Lyme borreliosis. Immunoblot confirmed the presence of anti-IgM antibodies in 62.7% of erythema migrans patients, 50.0% of non-erythema migrans form of Lyme borreliosis hospital patients, and 57.9% of forestry workers. Anti-IgG antibodies were found in 54.4%, 82.5%, and 87.9%, respectively. Anti-IgG to the VlsE antigen of *B. afzelii* was present in all forestry workers with signs of intoxication syndrome and only 45.5% of patients with morphea; antibodies to VlsE of *B. burgdorferi s. s.* were detected in all patients with cardiovascular involvement and 54.5% with morphea; to VlsE of *B. garinii* – in 94.7% of forestry workers with intoxication syndrome and only 41.9% of patients with erythema migrans form of Lyme borreliosis. Serological confirmation of Lyme arthritis and neuroborreliosis was also obtained in forestry workers from Ternopil region, with highly specific anti-IgG antibodies to p39 and p83 antigens found in 80.0% of cases. The use of the EUROLINE Borrelia RN-AT adv IgM test system expanded the spectrum of detectable pathogens in erythema and non-erythema migrans forms of Lyme borreliosis among patients with predominantly musculoskeletal involvement by simultaneously identifying anti-IgM antibodies to OspC of B. spielmanii, *B. burgdorferi s. s.*, *B. garinii*, and *B. afzelii*, in 78.9% of erythema migrans cases and 64.7% of non-erythema cases.

All listed specific diagnostic methods can yield both false-positive and false-negative results. Therefore, in questionable cases, patient evaluation should be comprehensive and repeated over the course of the illness.

The use of remote thermometry at the site of tick attachment made it possible to diagnose sub-erythema forms of Lyme borreliosis and justify the need for etiotropic therapy to prevent adverse long-term outcomes.

References

[1] Andreychyn, M. A., Kopcha, V. S., Shkilna, M. I., Klishch, I. M., Korda, M. M., Nykytyuk, S. O., Zavidnyuk, N. G., Nychyk, N. A., eds. *Lyme Borreliosis. Diagnostic criteria, treatment, and prevention.* Ternopil: TSMU, "Ukrmedknyga"; 2018. 42 p. [in Ukrainian].

[2] Popovych, O. Lyme borreliosis: current problem of infectiology (Clinical Lecture). *Actual Infectology.* 2022;(3.12):114-22. doi: 10.22141/2312-413x.3.12.2016.81725. [in Ukrainian].

[3] Svintsitskyi, A. S. Lyme disease as a current integrated problem of modern internal medicine. *Health of Ukraine* [Internet]. Thematic issue "Cardiology. Rheumatology. Cardiac Surgery" 2012 [cited 2025 Feb 3];(5):84-87. Available from: http://ir.librarynmu.com/handle/123456789/4113. [in Ukrainian].

[4] Stanek, G., Strle, F. Lyme borreliosis-from tick bite to diagnosis and treatment. *FEMS Microbiol Rev.* 2018;42(3):233-258. doi: 10.1093/femsre/fux047.

[5] Guérin, M., Shawky, M., Zedan, A., Octave, S., Avalle, B., Maffucci, I., Padiolleau-Lefèvre, S. Lyme borreliosis diagnosis: state of the art of improvements and innovations. *BMC Microbiol.* 2023 Aug 1;23(1):204. doi: 10.1186/s12866-023-02935-5.

[6] Kulias, S. M. Current opinion on peculiarities of specific diagnostics, treatment and prevention of Lyme borreliosis [Internet]. *Biomedical and biosocial anthropology.* 2013 [cited 2025 Feb 3];(20):245-251. Available from: http://nbuv.gov.ua/UJRN/bba_2013_20_62. [in Ukrainian].

[7] MacDonald, A. B. Borrelia burgdorferi tissue morphologies and imaging methodologies. *Eur J Clin Microbiol Infect Dis.* 2013;32(8):1077-82. doi: 10.1007/s10096-013-1853-5.

[8] Kuchynka, P., Palecek, T., Grus, T., Schramlova, J., Krsek, D., Vitkova, I., Rohn, V., Lindner, J., Wicks, E., Nemecek, E., Dostalova, G., Podzimkova, J., Linhart, A. A high frequency of viral agents yet absence of Borrelia burgdorferi is seen within the myocardium of subjects with normal left ventricular systolic function: an electron microscopy study. *Folia Microbiol* (Praha). 2016;61(2):129-35. doi: 10.1007/s12223-015-0417-8.

[9] Lindsay, L. R., Bernat, K., Dibernardo, A. Laboratory diagnostics for Lyme disease. *Can Commun Dis Rep*. 2014;40(11):209-217. doi: 10.14745/ccdr.v40i11a02.

[10] Tylewska-Wierzbanowska, S., Chmielewski, T. Tick-borne bacterial diseases in Poland. *Health Problems of Civilization*. 2017;11(2):56-65. doi: 10.5114/hpc.2017.69017.

[11] Lacout, A., Mone, Y., Franck, M., Marcy, P. Y., Mas, M., Veas, F., Perronne, C. Blood cell disruption to significantly improve the Borrelia PCR detection sensitivity in borreliosis in humans. *Med Hypotheses*. 2018;116:1-3. doi: 10.1016/j.mehy.2018.04.012.

[12] Nolte, O. Nucleic Acid Amplification Based Diagnostic of Lyme (Neuro-) borreliosis – Lost in the Jungle of Methods, Targets, and Assays? *Open Neurol J*. 2012;6:129-39. doi: 10.2174/1874205X01206010129.

[13] Dunaj, J., Moniuszko, A., Zajkowska, J., Pancewicz, S. The importance of PCR in the diagnosis of Lyme borreliosis. *Epidemiological Review* [Internet]. 2013 [cited 2025 Feb 3];67(1):119-23. Available from: https://www.przeglepidemiol.pzh.gov.pl/Znaczenie-metody-PCR-w-diagnostyce-boreliozy-z-Lyme,180168,0,2.html.

[14] Ružić-Sabljić, E., Cerar, T. Progress in the molecular diagnosis of Lyme disease. *Expert Rev Mol Diagn*. 2017;17(1):19-30. doi: 10.1080/14737159.2016.1246959.

[15] Li, X., McHugh, G. A., Damle, N., Sikand, V. K., Glickstein, L., Steere, A. C. Burden and viability of Borrelia burgdorferi in skin and joints of patients with erythema migrans or lyme arthritis. *Arthritis Rheum*. 2011;63(8):2238-47. doi: 10.1002/art.30384.

[16] Reagent Kit (D1499) for Detection of *Borrelia burgdorferi s. l.* DNA Complex by Real-Time Polymerase Chain Reaction. RealBest DNA Borrelia burgdorferi s.l (Kit 2). URL: https://diavector.com/tick-borne-infections.htm. [in Ukrainian].

[17] Reagent Kit (D5399) for Detection of *Anaplasma phagocytophilum/Ehrlichia muris*, *Ehrlichia chaffeensis* DNA Complex by Real-Time Polymerase Chain Reaction. RealBest DNA *Anaplasma phagocytophilum/Ehrlichia muris*, *Ehrlichia chaffeensis* (Kit 2). URL: https://diavector.com/tick-borne-infections.htm. [in Ukrainian].

[18] Reagent Kit (D1496) for Detection of *Borrelia miyamotoi* DNA Complex by Real-Time Polymerase Chain Reaction. RealBest DNA *Borrelia miyamotoi* (Kit 2). URL: https://vector-best.kiev.ua/drupalcon/uploads/2019/11/nabory-plr-diagnostyky-kompaniyi-vektor-best-ukrayina.pdf. [in Ukrainian].

[19] Reagent Kit (D5390) for Detection of *Babesia species* DNA by Real-Time Polymerase Chain Reaction. RealBest DNA *Babesia species* (Kit 2). URL: https://vector-best.kiev.ua/drupalcon/uploads/2019/11/nabory-plr-diagnostyky-kompaniyi-vektor-best-ukrayina.pdf. [in Ukrainian].

[20] Andreychyn, M. A., Shkilna, M. I., Ivakhiv, O. L., Huk, M. T., Nychyk, N. A. Anaplasmosis in the Residents of Ternopil Region. In: *Modern Diagnostic, Treatment, and Preventive Technologies in the Practice of Infectiologist*; Oct 4-5 2018; Chernivtsi. Chernivtsi; 2018. pp. 3-4. [in Ukrainian].

[21] Korda, M. M., Shkilna, M. I., Andreychyn, M. A., Boychuk, A. V., Yakymchuk, Y. U., Huk, M. T. Application of the Polymerase Chain Reaction Method for Diagnosing Transmissible Infections in the Residents of Ternopil Region. *Medical and Clinical Chemistry*. 2019;21(3):197-8. [in Ukrainian].

[22] Boychuk, A. V., Yakymchuk, Y. B., Andreychyn, M. A., Skilna, M. I., Ivakhiv, O. L., Klishch, I. M., Korda, M. M, Zaporozhanm S, Yo., Huk, M. T., Sydorenko, I. H. Diagnosis of tick-borne infections in pregnant women. *Actual Problems of Pediatrics, Obstetrics and Gynecology*. 2020;(2):50-5. doi: 10.11603/24116-4944.2020.2.11837. [in Ukrainian].

[23] Volokha, A. P. Lyme Disease (Tick-Borne Borreliosis) in Children. *Infectious Diseases*. 2014;(1):80–87. doi: 10.11603/1681-2727.2014.1.4739 [in Ukrainian].

[24] Ružić-Sabljić, E., Maraspin, V., Cimperman, J., Strle, F., Lotrič-Furlan, S., Stupica, D., Cerar, T. Comparison of isolation rate of Borrelia burgdorferi sensu lato in two different culture media, MKP and BSK-H. *Clin Microbiol Infect*. 2014;20(7):636-41. doi: 10.1111/1469-0691.12457.

[25] Stanek, G., Lusa, L., Ogrinc, K., Markowicz, M., Strle, F. Intrathecally produced IgG and IgM antibodies to recombinant VlsE, VlsE peptide, recombinant OspC and whole cell extracts in the diagnosis of Lyme neuroborreliosis. *Med Microbiol Immunol*. 2014;203(2):125-32. doi: 10.1007/s00430-013-0322-1.

[26] Matuszek, P., Herbst, V., Woźniak, M. The role of laboratory diagnostic of boreliose in the environment of forest workers [Internet]. *Environmental Medicine.* 2013 [cited 2025 Feb 3];16(4):16-25. Available from: https://www.environmed.pl/Diagnostyka-laboratoryjna-boreliozy-w-srodowisku-pracownikow-lesnych,113489,0,2.html.

[27] Halperin, J. J. Nervous system Lyme disease. *Handb Clin Neurol.* 2014;121:1473-83. doi: 10.1016/B 978-0-7020-4088-7.00099-7.

[28] Hauser, U. Modified interpretation criteria significantly improve performance of commercially available confirmatory assays for the serodiagnosis of Lyme borreliosis: a case-control study with clinically defined serum samples. *Eur J Clin Microbiol Infect Dis.* 2019;38(3):529-539. doi: 10.1007/s10096-018-03455-1.

[29] Tokarska-Rodak, M., Kozioł-Montewka, M., Pańczuk, A., Paszkiewicz, J., Szepeluk, A., Plewik, D. The assessment of the level of antibodies against specific antigenic Proteins Borrelia Burgdorferi s.l. in the group of persons occupationally exposed to tick stings in the North-Eastern region of Lubelskie Voivodeship. *Human and Health.* 2013;2(7):26-32. [in Polish].

[30] Reagent Kit for Immunoenzymatic Detection of IgM Immunoglobulins to the Pathogens of Ixodes Tick-Borne Borrelia. *Anti-Borrelia* ELISA (IgM) (Catalogue Number: EI 2132-9601 M). URL: https://www.euroimmun.us/fda-cleared/elisa. [in Ukrainian].

[31] Reagent Kit for Immunoenzymatic Detection of IgG Immunoglobulins to the Pathogens of Ixodes Tick-Borne Borrelia. *Anti-Borrelia* plus VlsE ELISA (IgG) (Catalogue Number: EI 2132-9601-2 G). URL: https://www.euroimmun.com/documents/Indications/Infections/Borrelia/HI_2132_I_UK_C.pdf. [in Ukrainian].

[32] Shkilna, M., Andreychyn, M., Ivakhiv, O., Ischuk, I., Nychyk, N., Vyshnevska, N., Korda, M., Klishch, I. Increasing of informational content of serological diagnosis of acute Lyme- borreliosis. *Acta Medica Leopoliensia.* 2020;26(1):35-9. doi: 10.25040/aml2020.01.035 [in Ukrainian].

[33] Seriburi, V., Ndukwe, N., Chang, Z., Cox, M. E., Wormser, G. P. High frequency of false positive IgM immunoblots for *Borrelia burgdorferi* in clinical practice. *Clin Microbiol Infect.* 2012;18(12):1236-40. doi: 10.1111/j.1469-0691.2011.03749.x.

[34] Bušová, A., Dorko, E., Feketeová, E., Rimárová, K., Diabelková, J., Rovenská, T., Csank, T. Association of seroprevalence and risk factors in Lyme disease. *Cent Eur J Public Health.* 2018;26 Suppl:S61-S66. doi: 10.21101/cejph.a5274.

[35] Centers for Disease Control and Prevention (CDC). Recommendations for test performance and interpretation from the Second National Conference on Serologic Diagnosis of Lyme Disease. *MMWR Morb Mortal Wkly Rep.* 1995;44(31):590-1.

[36] Cerar, T., Strle, F., Stupica, D., Ruzic-Sabljic, E., McHugh, G., Steere, A. C., Strle, K. Differences in Genotype, Clinical Features, and Inflammatory Potential of Borrelia burgdorferi sensu stricto Strains from Europe and the United States. *Emerg Infect Dis.* 2016;22(5):818-27. doi: 10.3201/eid2205.151806.

[37] Branda, J. A., Strle, F., Strle, K., Sikand, N., Ferraro, M. J., Steere, A. C. Performance of United States serologic assays in the diagnosis of Lyme borreliosis acquired in Europe. *Clin Infect Dis.* 2013;57(3):333-40. doi: 10.1093/cid/cit235.

[38] Molins, C. R., Delorey, M. J., Sexton, C., Schriefer, M. E. Lyme Borreliosis Serology: Performance of Several Commonly Used Laboratory Diagnostic Tests and a Large Resource Panel of Well-Characterized Patient Samples. *J Clin Microbiol.* 2016;54(11):2726-34. doi: 10.1128/JCM.00874-16.

[39] Kodym, P., Kurzová, Z., Berenová, D., Pícha, D., Smíšková, D., Moravcová, L., Malý, M. Serological Diagnostics of Lyme Borreliosis: Comparison of Universal and Borrelia Species-Specific Tests Based on Whole-Cell and Recombinant Antigens. *J Clin Microbiol.* 2018;56(11):e00601-18. doi: 10.1128/ JCM.00601-18.

[40] Branda, J. A., Strle, K., Nigrovic, L. E., Lantos, P. M., Lepore, T. J., Damle, N. S., Ferraro, M. J., Steere, A. C. Evaluation of Modified 2-Tiered Serodiagnostic Testing Algorithms for Early Lyme Disease. *Clin Infect Dis.* 2017;64(8):1074-80. doi: 10.1093/cid/cix043.

[41] Shkilna, M. I. Lime borreliosis in fores try wor kers of terno pil region. *Infectious Diseases.* 2016;(1):36-40. doi: 10.11603/1681-2727.2016.1.5957 [in Ukrainian].

[42] Tokarska-Rodak, M., Shkilna, M., Plewik, D., Pańczuk, A., Korda, M., Klishch, I., Paszkiewicz, J., Andreychyn, M. Serological research towards lyme borreliosis in hunters and forestry workers in

selected areas of Poland and Ukraine. *Health Problems of Civilization.* 2017;11(4):287-92. doi: 10.5114/hpc.2017.69024.

[43] Reagent Kit for Detection of IgM Antibodies to Antigens (p17, p19, p21, p25, p30, p31, p39, p41, p83, VlsE) by Western Blot Method. *Anti-Borrelia* EUROLINE-WB IgM (Catalog Number: DY 2131-1601-1 M). URL: tinyteria.com. [in Ukrainian].

[44] Reagent Kit for Detection of IgG Antibodies to Antigens (p17, p19, p21, p25, p30, p31, p39, p41, p83, VlsE) by Western Blot Method. *Anti-Borrelia* EUROLINE-WB IgG (Catalog Number: DY 2131-1601-1 G). URL: tinyteria.com. [in Ukrainian].

[45] Nebogatkin, I., Shulhan, A. Epidemiological and epizootic features of Lyme disease in 2019 in Ukraine. *Actual Infectology.* 2020;8(5-6):44-8. doi: 10.22141/2312-413x.8.5-6.2020.217959. [in Ukrainian].

[46] Andreychyn, M., Pańczuk, A., Shkilna, M., Tokarska-Rodak, M., Korda, M., Kozioł-Montewka, M. Epidemiological situation of lyme borreliosis and diagnosis standards in Poland and Ukraine. *Health Problems of Civilization.* 2017;11(3):190-194. doi: 10.5114/hpc.2017.69020.

[47] Shkilna, M. I., Andreychyn, M. A., Korda, M. M., Klishch, I. M., Zaporozhan, S. Y., Morochkovskyi, R. S. The frequency of seropositive individuals to the complex b. burgdorferi sensu lato among forestry workers of Zhytomyr, Khmelnytskyi and Volyn region. *Infectious Diseases.* 2018;(3):18-25. doi: 10.11603/1681-2727.2018.3.9408 [in Ukrainian].

[48] Andreychyn, M. A., Shkilna, M. I., Korda, M. M., Klishch, I. M., Zaporozhan, S. Y. Two-stage diagnosis of Lyme borreliosis in forestry workers [Internet]. *Journal of the National Academy of Medical Sciences of Ukraine.* 2019 [cited 2025 Feb 3];(1):73-8. Available from: http://journal.amnu.gov.ua/images/pdf/2019-25-1/11.pdf [in Ukrainian].

[49] Shkilna, M. I., Andreychyn, M. A., Vasylieva, N. A. Evaluation of immunoblot results for detecting antibodies to Lyme disease pathogens in workers from some forestry enterprises in Ukraine. In: *Pharmacotherapy in Infectious Diseases*; April 12-13 2018; Kyiv. Kyiv; 2018. pp. 81-3. [in Ukrainian].

[50] Reagent kit for detecting human class M antibodies to antigens of *Borrelia burgdorferi* s. l. (OspC-adv Bsp, OspC-adv Bg, OspC-adv Bb, OspC-adv Ba, p39, p41, and VlsE Bb) in blood serum using immunoblotting *Anti-Borrelia* EUROLINE-RN-AT adv, reagent catalog number: DN 2131-3201-2 M. URL: http://shop.tinyteria.com/index.php?route=extension/module/free_downloads/download&did=275. [in Ukrainian].

[51] Shkilna, M. I., Andreychyn, M. A., Ivakhiv, O. L. Borrelia spielmanii in residents of Ternopil region. *Modern Diagnostic, Treatment, and Preventive Technologies in the Practice of Infectious Disease Specialists: materials of the All-Ukrainian scientific-practical conference and Plenary Session of the NGO In: Ukrainian Association of Infectious Disease Specialists; Oct 4-5 2018; Chernivtsi.* Chernivtsi; 2018. pp. 124–126. [in Ukrainian].

[52] Shkilna, M. I. Etiological structure of acute lyme borreliosis by types of pathogen. *Infectious Diseases.* 2019;(1):43-9. doi: 10.11603/1681-2727.2019.1.9942 [in Ukrainian].

[53] Chemych, M., Lutai, I. Lyme disease. Modern issue condition. *East Ukr Med J.* 2020;8(2):230-41. doi: 10.21272/eumj.2020;8(2):230-41. [in Ukrainian].

[54] Choi, M. S., Seong, G. H., Park, M. J., Park, M., Hong, S. P., Park, B. C., Kim, M. H. Rapidly Progressing Generalized Morphea with High Lyme Disease Titer. *Indian J Dermatol.* 2020;65(5):432-434. doi: 10.4103/ijd.IJD_279_18.

[55] Panteleeva, O. H. Computer thermography in the diagnosis of malignant tumors of the eye and orbit. *Clinical Ophthalmology.* 2011;42(1): 36-42. [in Russian].

[56] Andreychyn, M. A., Kopcha, Y. V. Distance thermography and it value at diagnostics of acute tonsillitis. *Infectious Diseases.* 2016;1(3):82-8. doi: 10.11603/1681-2727.2016.3.6897 [in Ukrainian].

[57] Ata, M. A. Remote thermometric study of altered skin coverings in patients with focal scleroderma. *Dermatology and Venereology.* 2018;(2):50-3. [in Russian].

[58] Brom.ua [Internet]. Thermal Imager Xintest HT-18; 2023 [cited 5 Feb. 2025]. Available from: https://brom.ua/index.php?route=product/product&product_id=18190 [in Ukrainian].

[59] Shkilna, M. I., Vasylieva, N. A. Erythema migrans in Lyme borreliosis: thermographic changes. In: *Epidemiological and Clinical*; Oct 5-6 2017; Zhytomyr. Zhytomyr; 2017. pp. 165-7. [in Ukrainian].

[60] Shkilna, M. I., Andreychyn, M. A., Korda, M. M., Klishch, I. M., Huk, M. T. Thermosemiotics of the skin form of Lyme borreliosis. In: *Achievements in Clinical and Experimental Medicine; June 13 2019*; Ternopil. Ternopil; 2019. pp. 31-2. [in Ukrainian].

[61] Andreychyn, M. A., Korda, M. M., Kopcha, V. S., Shkilna, M. I. Method for diagnosing the erythema-free form of Lyme disease. *Infectious Diseases*. 2020;(1):16-9. doi: 10.11603/1681-2727.2020.1.11092 [in Ukrainian].

[62] Andreychyn, M. A., Korda, M. M., Kopcha, V. S., Shkilna, M. I., inventors. Method for diagnosing the erythema-free form of Lyme disease: *Utility model. Patent Ukraine 133091*. May 25, 2018. [in Ukrainian].

Chapter 5

Treatment of Patients with Lyme Borreliosis

Mykhaylo Andreychyn[1]
Mariia Shkilna[2]
Oleh Ivakhiv[3]
Mariana Huk[4]
Svitlana Marchyshyn[5]
Oksana Shevchuk[6]
Nataliya Vyshnevska[7]
and Tetiana Yuzkiv[8]

[1]Academician of the National Academy of Medical Sciences of Ukraine,
Honoured Master of Sciences and Technologies of Ukraine, DSc in Medicine, Professor,
Head of the Department of Infectious Diseases with Epidemiology, Dermatology and Venerology,
I. Horbachevsky Ternopil National Medical University, Ternopil, Ukraine
[2]DSc in Medicine, Professor, Department of Infectious Diseases with Epidemiology,
Dermatology and Venerology, I. Horbachevsky Ternopil National Medical University, Ternopil, Ukraine
[3]Honoured Doctor of Ukraine, PhD in Medicine, Associate Professor,
Department of Infectious Diseases with Epidemiology, Dermatology and Venerology,
I. Horbachevsky Ternopil National Medical University, Ternopil, Ukraine
[4]PhD in Medicine, Assistant Professor, Department of Infectious Diseases with Epidemiology,
Dermatology and Venerology, I. Horbachevsky Ternopil National Medical University, Ternopil, Ukraine
[5]DSc in Pharmacy, Professor, Head of the Department of Pharmacognosy and Medical Botany,
I. Horbachevsky Ternopil National Medical University, Ternopil, Ukraine
[6]DSc in Medicine, Professor, Department of Pharmacology and Clinical Pharmacology,
I. Horbachevsky Ternopil National Medical University, Ternopil, Ukraine
[7]PhD in Medicine, Associate Professor, Department of Infectious Diseases with Epidemiology,
Dermatology and Venerology, I. Horbachevsky Ternopil National Medical University, Ternopil, Ukraine
[8]PhD Student, Department of Infectious Diseases with Epidemiology, Dermatology and Venerology,
I. Horbachevsky Ternopil National Medical University, Ternopil, Ukraine

Abstract

Patients with Lyme borreliosis are treated using both etiological and pathogenetic therapeutic agents. Antibiotics from four groups – tetracyclines, penicillins, cephalosporins, and macrolides – to which Borrelia are sensitive, are commonly employed.

In: Lyme Borreliosis
Editors: Mykhaylo Andreychyn, Mykhaylo Korda, Maria Shkilna and Oleh Ivakhiv
ISBN: 979-8-89530-657-4

The most effective agents include doxycycline, amoxicillin, and azithromycin. The choice of antibiotic, its dosage, and duration of administration depend on the clinical form and stage of the disease. Current treatment protocols recommend the use of first- and second-line antibacterial drugs, as well as alternative agents, taking into account the patient's age. In cases of neuroborreliosis, treatment may include immunocorrective and neurotropic agents alongside antibiotics.
A combined treatment regimen for adults and children with erythema migrans due to Lyme borreliosis – using doxycycline hydrochloride and an infusion of Stevia rebaudiana – resulted in clinical recovery in a significantly higher proportion of patients compared to antibiotic monotherapy: 87.1% vs. 38.2% ($p < 0.05$). It also helped reduce the incidence of doxycycline-associated phototoxic drug reactions ($p < 0.05$). This treatment was accompanied by a decrease in the level of pro-inflammatory interleukin-18 and an increase in anti-inflammatory interleukin-10 in the patients' blood serum.
It has been demonstrated that concurrent chronic Epstein-Barr virus infection and vitamin D deficiency adversely affect the course of Lyme borreliosis. Therefore, patients with such combined pathologies benefit from comprehensive treatment involving oral administration of doxycycline hydrochloride and ergocalciferol, which not only leads to remission of arthritis and full elimination of vitamin D deficiency but also reduces the proportion of individuals with active Epstein-Barr virus infection.

Keywords: Lyme borreliosis, treatment, antibiotics, doxycycline, Stevia rebaudiana infusion, ergocalciferol

1. Introduction

To date, relatively effective treatment protocols have been developed for Lyme borreliosis using antibiotics to which Borrelia species are susceptible. When necessary, immunosuppressive agents and other pathogenetic therapies may be added. However, during prolonged disease progression, Borrelia may shift to L-forms and produce biofilms that are poorly responsive to antibiotic therapy. Additionally, antibiotic-resistant strains of the pathogen have already been identified, and their prevalence is gradually increasing. When the pathological process extends to the joints or central nervous system (brain and spinal cord), antibiotic penetration into inflamed tissues becomes limited.

These and other factors may reduce the effectiveness of antibiotic therapy and often prompt an increase in daily dosage or treatment duration – measures that, in turn, raise the risk of complications such as dysbiosis, allergic reactions, and drug toxicity. Comorbid conditions such as pulmonary tuberculosis, Epstein-Barr virus infection, or vitamin D deficiency must also be taken into account. For these reasons, the search for more rational treatment strategies tailored to the specific course of Lyme borreliosis in individual patients is ongoing.

2. Etiotropic Therapy

Mykhaylo Andreychyn
Mariia Shkilna
Oleh Ivakhiv
Nataliya Vyshnevska
and Oksana Shevchuk

Currently, there are no universally accepted standards for etiotropic treatment of LB [1]. Results from numerous randomized clinical trials have demonstrated the efficacy of antibiotic therapy in patients with early localized LB with erythema, showing equivalent effectiveness of antibiotics such as Doxycycline hydrochloride, Amoxicillin, and Cefuroxime axetil [2, 3]. Doxycycline is commonly used and has proven effective against tick-borne infections caused by *A. phagocytophilum*, *B. miyamotoi*, and *Babesia sp.* [4].

Patients with mild Lyme borreliosis (localized infection with erythema without severe systemic symptoms) can be managed on an outpatient basis under the supervision of an infectious disease specialist. Hospitalization in infectious disease wards is reserved for patients with moderate to severe disease or suspicion of co-infection with other tick-borne pathogens (for differential diagnosis). Patients with severe involvement of the cardiovascular, nervous, musculoskeletal systems, or atypical skin manifestations that not pose epidemiological risks to others may require treatment in specialized units [5].

Treatment of Lyme borreliosis involves comprehensive therapy with both etiotropic and pathogenetic agents. The main principles of antibiotic therapy for LB are as follows.

Use of antibiotics from 4 groups to which Borrelia are sensitive:

- Tetracyclines, including Doxycycline and its hydrate [6, 7].
- Broad-spectrum beta-lactam antibiotics, such as Amoxicillin.
- Second and third-generation cephalosporins, particularly effective when administered parenterally, including Cefotaxime and Ceftriaxone [8].
- Macrolides [9].

Treatment of patients with Lyme disease is carried out considering the stage of the disease, individual characteristics, contraindications, and the results of sensitivity testing to medications. Based on these factors, different treatment methods will be required (Table 1) [5].

Early initiation of etiotropic therapy is crucial, ideally starting within 3 days to 4 weeks after the manifestation of the disease onset to minimize the risk of treatment ineffectiveness later on [10].

Selection of antibiotics considers their ability to penetrate relevant organs and tissues and achieve concentrations sufficient to eliminate the pathogen:

- Tetracyclines accumulate well in bone tissue, eye tissues, liver, kidneys, lungs, pancreas, lymph nodes, but poorly in cerebrospinal fluid [11].
- Doxycycline and Azithromycin penetrate cells effectively, which is important due to the intracellular localization of the pathogen [11].

- Second and third-generation cephalosporins rapidly penetrate blood and reach various organs and tissues, including bone marrow, joints, and prostate [12].

Table 1. Antibiotic treatment for adults and young people aged 12 and over according to symptoms of Lyme borreliosis

Form of the Disease	Treatment	First Alternative	Second Alternative
Lyme Disease without Focal Symptoms but with erythema migrans and/or Non-Focal Symptoms	Oral Doxycycline: 100 mg twice daily or 200 mg once daily for 21 days	Oral Amoxicillin: 1 g three times daily for 21 days	Oral Azithromycin: 500 mg daily for 17 days Note: Do not use Azithromycin to treat patients with cardiac complications related to Lyme disease due to its effect on the QT interval.
Lyme Disease Affecting Cranial Nerves or the Peripheral Nervous System	Oral Doxycycline: 100 mg twice daily or 200 mg once daily for 21 days	Oral Amoxicillin: 1 g three times daily for 21 days	-
Lyme Disease Affecting the Central Nervous System	Intravenous Ceftriaxone: 2 g twice daily or 4 g once daily for 21 days (if considering transition to oral treatment, use Doxycycline)	Oral Doxycycline: 200 mg twice daily or 400 mg once daily for 21 days	-
Lyme Arthritis	Oral Doxycycline: 100 mg twice daily or 200 mg once daily for 28 days	Oral Amoxicillin: 1 g three times daily for 28 days	Intravenous Ceftriaxone: 2 g once daily for 28 days
Lyme Disease with Chronic Atrophic Acrodermatitis	Oral Doxycycline: 100 mg twice daily or 200 mg once daily for 28 days	Oral Amoxicillin: 1 g three times daily for 28 days	Intravenous Ceftriaxone: 2 g once daily for 28 days
Lyme Carditis	Oral Doxycycline: 100 mg twice daily or 200 mg once daily for 21 days	Intravenous Ceftriaxone: 2 g once daily for 21 days	-
Lyme Carditis with Hemodynamic Disturbance	Intravenous Ceftriaxone: 2 g once daily for 21 days (if considering transition to oral treatment, use Doxycycline)	-	-

Note: Azithromycin should not be used for treating patients with cardiac complications related to Lyme disease due to its impact on the QT interval. For patients with symptomatic bradycardia resulting from pharmacotherapy-resistant Lyme carditis, temporary pacing measures are recommended instead of implanting a permanent pacemaker.

Before offering antibiotic treatment for Lyme borreliosis to women, it is essential to confirm whether they are pregnant. If symptoms worsen during Lyme disease treatment, it is important to check for an allergic reaction to the antibiotic. It should be noted that a Jarisch-Herxheimer reaction may cause a worsening of symptoms but usually does not require discontinuation of treatment.

Treatment of children with Lyme disease involves the use of antibacterial medications, the list of which is provided in Tables 2, 3, and 4, taking into account the stage of the disease, individual characteristics, contraindications, and the results of sensitivity testing to medications.

Table 2. Recommended doses of antibacterial agents for the treatment of children under 12 with Lyme borreliosis

Medication	Dose
Oral Administration	
Amoxicillin	50 g/kg per day in 3 equal doses (maximum 500 mg per dose)
Cefuroxime Axetil	30 mg/kg per day in 2 equal doses (maximum 500 mg per dose)
Azithromycin	10 mg/kg per day as a single daily dose (maximum 500 mg per dose)*
Intravenous Therapy	
Ceftriaxone	50-75 mg/kg per day as a single dose (maximum 2.0 g per day)
Penicillin G	200,000–400,000 units/kg per day in 6 equal doses (maximum 24 million units per day)

Note: * – Due to concerns about the lower effectiveness of macrolide antibiotics, including Azithromycin, they are considered second-line agents and should be prescribed to patients for whom other classes of antibiotics are contraindicated.

Table 3. Treatment regimen for specific manifestations of Lyme borreliosis in children

Form of the Disease	Route of Administration	Antibiotic	Duration of Treatment (days, range)
Erythema Migrans	Oral	Doxycycline*	10
		Amoxicillin or Cefuroxime Axetil	14
		Azithromycin	7 (range: 5–10)
Meningitis or Radiculopathy	Oral	Doxycycline*	14–21
	IV	Ceftriaxone	14–21
Cranial Nerve Paralysis	Oral	Doxycycline*	14–21
Carditis	Oral	Doxycycline*, Amoxicillin or Cefuroxime Axetil	14–21
	IV	Ceftriaxone	14–21
Arthritis			
Initial Treatment	Oral	Doxycycline*, Amoxicillin or Cefuroxime Axetil	28
Recurrent or Refractory Arthritis	Oral	Doxycycline*, Amoxicillin or Cefuroxime Axetil	28
	IV	Ceftriaxone	14
Chronic Atrophic Acrodermatitis	Oral	Doxycycline*, Amoxicillin or Cefuroxime Axetil	21–28
Lymphocytoma	Oral	Doxycycline*, Amoxicillin pr Cefuroxime Axetil	14

Note: * – In Ukraine, the administration of Doxycycline to children is carried out according to the drug's medical use instructions approved by the Ministry of Health of Ukraine.

2.1. Treatment of Children with Erythema Migrans

Initial intravenous therapy is administered to patients with Lyme carditis who require hospitalization, while children who do not need hospitalization are treated with an oral antibacterial agent. Treatment of patients with erythema migrans leads to the disappearance of the rash within a few days after starting antibiotic use and almost always prevents the development of late stages of the disease.

Table 4. Antibiotic treatment for children under 12 according to symptoms of Lyme borreliosis

Form of the Disease	Age	Treatment	First Alternative	Second Alternative
Lyme disease without focal symptoms but with erythema migrans and/or non-focal symptoms	9-12 years	Oral Doxycycline for children weighing up to 45 kg: 5 mg/kg, divided into 2 doses on the 1st day, then 2.5 mg/kg once daily or divided into 2 doses for 21 days. For severe infections, up to 5 mg/kg daily for 21 days (clinical judgment should be used to determine the doxycycline dose for children under 12 years with severe infections)*.	Oral Amoxicillin for children weighing 33 kg or less: 30 mg/kg 3 times daily for 21 days	Oral Azithromycin for children weighing 50 kg or less: 10 mg/kg daily for 17 days**
Lyme disease without focal symptoms but with erythema migrans and/or non-focal symptoms	Up to 9 years	Oral Amoxicillin for children weighing 33 kg or less: 30 mg/kg 3 times a day for 21 days	Oral Azithromycin for children weighing 50 kg or less: 10 mg/kg daily for 17 days**	-
Lyme disease affecting cranial nerves or the peripheral nervous system	9-12 years	Oral Doxycycline for children weighing up to 45 kg: 5 mg/kg, divided into 2 doses on the 1st day, then 2.5 mg/kg once daily or divided into 2 doses for 21 days. For severe infections, up to 5 mg/kg daily for 21 days*.	Oral Amoxicillin for children weighing 33 kg or less: 30 mg/kg 3 times daily for 21 days	-
Lyme disease affecting cranial nerves or the peripheral nervous system	Up to 9 years	Oral Amoxicillin for children weighing 33 kg or less: 30 mg/kg 3 times a day for 21 days	-	-
Lyme disease affecting the central nervous system	9-12 years	Intravenous Ceftriaxone for children weighing up to 50 kg: 80 mg/kg (up to 4 g) once daily for 21 days	Oral Doxycycline for children weighing up to 45 kg: 5 mg/kg, divided into 2 doses on the 1st day, and then 2.5 mg/kg daily, either as a single dose or divided into 2 doses for 21 days. For severe infections – up to 5 mg/kg daily for 21 days*.	-
Lyme disease affecting the central nervous system	Up to 9 years	Intravenous Ceftriaxone for children weighing up to 50 kg: 80 mg/kg (up to 4 g) once daily for 21 days	-	-
Lyme disease with arthritis or chronic atrophic acrodermatitis	9-12 years	Oral Doxycycline for children weighing up to 45 kg: 5 mg/kg, divided into 2 doses on the 1st day, then 2.5 mg/kg once daily or divided into 2 doses for 28 days. For severe infections, up to 5 mg/kg daily for 28 days*.	Oral Amoxicillin for children weighing 33 kg or less: 30 mg/kg three times a day for 28 days	Intravenous Ceftriaxone for children weighing up to 50 kg: 80 mg/kg (up to 2 g) once daily for 28 days
Lyme disease with Lyme arthritis or chronic atrophic acrodermatitis	Up to 9 years	Oral Amoxicillin for children weighing 33 kg or less: 30 mg/kg 3 times a day for 28 days	Intravenous Ceftriaxone for children weighing up to 50 kg: 80 mg/kg (up to 2 g) once daily for 28 days	-
Lyme disease with Lyme carditis and stable hemodynamics	9-12 years	Oral Doxycycline for children weighing up to 45 kg: 5 mg/kg, divided into 2 doses on the 1st day, then 2.5 mg/kg once daily or divided into 2 doses for 21 days. For severe infections, up to 5 mg/kg daily for 21 days*.	Intravenous Ceftriaxone for children weighing up to 50 kg: 80 mg/kg (up to 2 g) once daily for 21 days	-

Table 4. (Continued)

Form of the Disease	Age	Treatment	First Alternative	Second Alternative
Lyme disease with Lyme carditis and stable hemodynamics	Up to 9 years	Intravenous Ceftriaxone for children weighing up to 50 kg: 80 mg/kg (up to 2 g) once daily for 21 days	-	-
Lyme disease with Lyme carditis and unstable hemodynamics	9-12 years	Intravenous Ceftriaxone for children weighing up to 50 kg: 80 mg/kg (up to 2 g) once daily for 21 days	Oral Doxycycline for children weighing up to 45 kg: 5 mg/kg, divided into 2 doses on the 1st day, and then 2.5 mg/kg daily, either as a single dose or divided into 2 doses for 21 days. For severe infections – up to 5 mg/kg daily for 21 days*.	-
Lyme carditis with unstable hemodynamics	Up to 9 years	Intravenous Ceftriaxone for children weighing up to 50 kg: 80 mg/kg (up to 2 g) once daily for 21 days	-	-

Notes:

* – In Ukraine, according to the medical instructions approved by the Ministry of Health of Ukraine, doxycycline is not prescribed to children under 12 years old. However, according to NICE guidelines on drug prescriptions, doxycycline may be used for this age group in cases of severe infections based on clinical considerations.

** – For children under 12, azithromycin was contraindicated until April 2018. Azithromycin should not be used for treating patients with cardiac complications related to Lyme disease due to its effect on the QT interval.

2.2. Treatment of Children with Lyme Arthritis

Patients with possible Lyme arthritis should be tested for specific antibodies in the blood serum or PCR of the synovial fluid. Patients with Lyme arthritis are recommended to receive oral antibiotic therapy for 28 days. As with erythema migrans, children under 8 years old are usually treated with oral amoxicillin, while children over 8 years old are treated with oral doxycycline*. Patients with Lyme arthritis who have a minimal response or no response at all to the initial course of oral antibiotic therapy are recommended to undergo a 2-4-week course of intravenous ceftriaxone instead of a repeat course of oral antibiotics. Post-infectious proliferative synovitis, although rare, especially in prepubertal children, can develop after both oral and intravenous therapy. Such children should be referred to a rheumatologist to consider treatment with anti-rheumatic drugs.

2.3. Treatment of Children with Lyme Carditis

An electrocardiogram is recommended for patients with signs or symptoms consistent with Lyme carditis, such as shortness of breath, swelling, palpitations, dizziness, chest pain, or syncope. Patients with PR interval prolongation >300 milliseconds or other arrhythmias, or signs of myopericarditis should be hospitalized for continuous electrocardiographic monitoring. Hospitalized patients with Lyme carditis should be treated with intravenous ceftriaxone and then, if clinical improvement is evident, transitioned to oral antibiotics. An outpatient with Lyme carditis can receive oral antibiotics instead of intravenous antibiotics.

2.4. Management of Children and Adolescents with Neurological Involvement in Lyme Borreliosis

Treatment of neuroborreliosis is often similar regardless of the presence of meningitis, so decisions regarding the need for lumbar puncture should be individualized. Analysis of cerebrospinal fluid (CSF) in patients with suspected neurological disease is indicated to rule out bacterial, viral, or other aetiologies of inflammation. Additionally, children with neuroborreliosis may exhibit a pseudotumor-like syndrome, which can be diagnosed based on elevated intracranial pressure. Routine testing for Lyme disease in children with developmental, behavioural, or psychiatric disorders is not recommended, as infection with *B. burgdorferi* is unlikely to cause such disorders. For patients with meningitis related to Lyme disease or cranial neuropathy, oral doxycycline therapy is generally recommended over intravenous treatment due to ease of administration, lower risk of side effects, and evidence of equivalent outcomes in European studies. For the very rare condition of encephalomyelitis in Lyme disease (parenchymal involvement of the brain or spinal cord), intravenous ceftriaxone is recommended instead of oral antibiotic therapy. Routine corticosteroid therapy for children under 16 with cranial neuropathy is not recommended based on the lack of evidence of benefit.

If symptoms that may be related to Lyme disease do not resolve or change despite antibiotic therapy, the following causes should be considered:

- Alternative diagnosis
- Possibility of re-infection
- Incomplete prior continuous course of antibiotics
- Organ damage caused by Lyme disease, such as neurological paralysis.

If there are historical indications of re-infection, antibiotic treatment should be administered according to the symptoms. In cases of a definitive diagnosis but unsuccessful prior treatment, an alternative antibiotic may be prescribed. For example, an adult with Lyme borreliosis of the arthritic form who has not responded to an initial course of doxycycline may be offered amoxicillin.

However, if symptoms persist after two completed courses of antibiotic therapy, further antibiotic treatment is not warranted. In such cases, it is necessary to re-evaluate for an alternative diagnosis or consider that persistent symptoms do not always indicate ongoing active infection. They may be the result of irreversible damage caused by Lyme borreliosis. In such instances, serological tests are of limited value due to their retrospective nature [13].

3. Pathogenetic Therapy

Mykhaylo Andreychyn
and Mariia Shkilna

In LB, autoimmune mechanisms play an important role with predominant disruption of the humoral response (intrathecal synthesis of anti-Borrelia monoclonal antibodies, some of which are similar to myelin), leading to myelin breakdown and secondary axonal damage in the nervous system akin to a "molecular mimicry" mechanism [14-15]. There are hypotheses suggesting possible involvement of Borrelia in initiating autoimmune processes through activation of myelin-specific T-cells and detection of auto-reactive antibodies to myelin and its components in LB [16].

Ignoring the significance of autoimmune and other intimate mechanisms in the pathogenesis of LB has led some researchers to overemphasize the role of antibiotics in LB treatment and even propose their prolonged use (up to several months according to some recommendations). Such an approach is considered formal and unsubstantiated, as Borrelia species are highly sensitive to certain antibiotics. However, the frequent presence of L-forms of pathogens and other antibiotic-resistant strains selected under prolonged etiotropic therapy typically diminishes the impact of these medications. Other inevitable side effects of prolonged antibiotic therapy such as dysbiosis, vitamin K deficiency associated with it, toxic and allergic effects, and cephalosporin cholelithiasis should also be taken into account.

Optimal treatment outcomes for patients with neuroborreliosis are achieved not only with antibiotics but also with immunomodulators and neurotropic bioregulators. Corticosteroids should not be overused in neuroborreliosis. They are primarily recommended in cases of significant radicular pain syndrome that persists despite antibiotics and analgesics. Immunosuppressive therapy (corticosteroids, cyclophosphamide) is also indicated in neuroborreliosis-associated vasculitis confirmed by pronounced angiographic changes [17].

Since prolonged courses of antibiotic treatment cause intestinal dysbiosis, it is advisable to concurrently administer bioenteroseptics naturally resistant to antibiotic action such as *Saccharomyces boulardii*, and others.

4. Optimization of Complex Treatment of Patients with Erythematous Form of Lyme Borreliosis Using Doxycycline Hydrochloride and Stevia Rebaudiana Bertoni

Mariia Shkilna
Svitlana Marchyshyn
and Oleh Ivakhiv

It is known that individuals living in regions endemic for LB, during attacks by Ixodes ticks, may become infected with agents of other tick-borne infections spread by ticks. According to the results of our research conducted at the laboratory of Centre for Lyme Borreliosis and Other Tick-Borne Diseases Research, functioning at the I. Horbachevsky Ternopil National Medical University, the infection rate of Ixodes ricinus ticks removed from humans was as follows: B. burgdorferi s. l. – 19.2% of specimens, *A. phagocytophilum* – 14.7%, *B. miyamotoi* – 1.7%, *Babesia sp.* – 0.3%, with multiple pathogens concurrently in 3.8% of cases.

Using PCR methods, we examined the serum of pregnant women with complicated obstetric histories. It was found that DNA of *B. burgdorferi s. l.* was detected in 9.3% of women, DNA of *A. phagocytophilum* in 6.9%, and DNA of *Babesia sp.* in 4.7%.

Taking the above into account, for the treatment of patients with EM LB, we chose doxycycline hydrochloride. The optimal duration of therapy for EM LB has been determined by researchers from various European countries. Most consider etiotropic treatment of individuals with EM LB using doxycycline hydrochloride to be 10-21 days, and with amoxicillin or cefuroxime axetil to be 14-21 days [18]. Within this range, some specialists prefer shorter treatment durations, for example, 10 days with doxycycline hydrochloride and 14 days with amoxicillin or cefuroxime [19].

Borrelia of the *B. burgdorferi s. l.* species are pleomorphic microorganisms (bacteria) capable of changing their morphological form in response to adverse conditions (nutrient deficiency, high pH of the environment, or unfavourable temperature) [20]. They transform from their active spirochaetal form into latent round forms (cysts) and biofilm [21, 22].

Latent round forms are live forms with low metabolism. Unlike spirochetes, they are non-motile; however, like spirochetes, they can be transmissive and capable of causing infection. Morphologically, these bacteria disperse into granular forms (pointed spirochetes), forms lacking a cell wall (spheroplast, L-form, bubble-like spirochete), or cystic forms (round body/shape) [23]. They are considered responsible for the persistence of the disease manifestations [24–27].

In contrast, biofilm is a thin-layered agglomerate of bacteria covered with a self-formed extracellular polysaccharide substance formed for protection against harsh conditions [28]. Biofilm may contain a heterogeneous population of spirochetes and round forms with different genetic and protein profiles. Borrelia inside biofilm are much more difficult to eliminate, and they can be up to 1000 times more resistant to antibiotics [28, 29]. Moreover, it has been established that antibiotics themselves can provoke the formation of atypical bacterial forms.

Therefore, in some cases, the treatment of patients with EM LB is insufficiently effective.

We observed 146 patients with EM LB, including 63 males (43.2%) and 83 females (56.8%). The patients were aged between 19 and 79 years, with a mean age of (43.09 ± 14.29) years. Of these, 108 (73.9%) patients lived in urban areas, and 38 (26.1%) in rural areas. Among them, 96 (65.8%) individuals had no signs of infection dissemination, and 50 (34.2%) had organ involvement in the early period. Acute disease course was observed in 112 examined individuals, including 89 with EM and 33 with EM with early organ involvement, subacute course in 34 patients, including 7 without dissemination and 27 with dissemination (Table 5). None of the patients had a chronic course of the disease.

Table 5. Distribution of patients with erythema migrans form of Lyme borreliosis by course (M ± m)

Course of the disease	Patients with EM LB					
	without dissemination (n = 96)		with dissemination (n = 50)		Total (n = 146)	
	Absolute number	%	Absolute number	%	Absolute number	%
Acute	89	92,7	33	66,0	112	76,7
Subacute	7	7,3	27	34,0	34	23,3
Total	96	100,0	50	100,0	146	100,0

The severity of the pathological process was assessed on a scale: from 1 to 3 points – mild; from 4 to 6 – moderate severity; 7 points and more – severe. Severe disease course was registered in only 8 individuals with EM with dissemination, moderate severity in 8 (8.3%) patients from the group with EM only and 20 (40.0%) with EM with dissemination, mild in 88

(91.7%) and 22 (44.0%) individuals respectively. Thus, patients with severe disease course and moderate severity predominated in the group of patients with EM, who also had early organ involvement, while mild course was more common in patients with EM only – respectively, 91.7 versus 44.0% ($p < 0.05$). It should be noted that the moderate severity in 8 patients with EM only was caused by multiple (from 3 to 6 foci) erythemas (Table 6).

Table 6. Distribution of patients with erythema migrans form of Lyme borreliosis by severity (M ± m)

Degree of severity:	Patients with EM LB					
	without dissemination (n = 96)		with dissemination (n = 50)		Total (n = 146)	
	Absolute number	%	Absolute number	%	Absolute number	%
Severe	–	–	8	16,0*	8	5,5
Moderate	8	8,3	20	40,0*	28	19,2
Mild	88	91,7*	22	44,0	110	75,3
Total	96	100,0	50	100,0	146	100,0

Note. * – significant difference between groups, $p < 0.05$.

During the treatment process, the following therapy regimen was applied to patients: oral administration of doxycycline hydrochloride at 100 mg twice daily for 21 days, along with a dry extract from the fruits of milk thistle (Silybum marianum) and an aqueous substrate of metabolites from Escherichia coli (DSM 4087), Enterococcus faecalis (DSM), and Lactobacillus acidophilus (DSM 414, DSM 4183) in average therapeutic doses for the same duration. In total, 76 patients received this treatment, including 50 individuals with only EM and 26 with EM and signs of early disseminated infection.

The evaluation of treatment effectiveness in the examined patients was based on several criteria: clinical effectiveness, reduction in severity of LB, disappearance of EM, presence/absence of side effects from doxycycline hydrochloride (phototoxic drug reaction), dynamics of pro-inflammatory (IL-18) and anti-inflammatory (IL-10) cytokines, as well as presence and concentration of specific IgM and IgG antibodies in serum.

Clinical effectiveness of treatment for patients with EM LB was assessed on the 30th day from the start of therapy, with the following possible outcomes: clinical recovery, significant improvement, and improvement. Clinical recovery was defined as the disappearance of EM and all clinical manifestations of LB; significant improvement as disappearance of EM and reduction of LB symptoms by at least 2 points in severity; improvement as disappearance of EM and one other LB symptom, or reduction of severity by at least 1 point.

Table 7. Clinical efficacy of treatment in patients with erythema migrans form of Lyme borreliosis with doxycycline hydrochloride for 21 days (on the 30th day, n = 76)

Clinical effectiveness	Patients with EM LB					
	without dissemination (n = 50)		with dissemination (n = 26)		Total (n = 76)	
	Absolute number	%	Absolute number	%	Absolute number	%
Clinical recovery	20	40,0	9	34,6	29	38,2
Significant improvement	12	24,0	10	38,5	22	28,9
Improvement	18	36,0	7	26,9	25	32,9

Table 8. Levels of IL-10 and IL-18 in the serum of patients with erythema migrans form of Lyme borreliosis before treatment (Me (Lq; Uq))

Interleukin	Healthy individuals (n = 33)	Patients with EM LB (n = 76)
IL-10, pg/mL	0,15 (0,00; 1,50)	4,10 (3,10; 10,40)
IL-18, pg/mL	110,35 (75,30; 165,40)	211,45 (163,25; 264,15)

After completing the treatment, positive treatment dynamics in terms of improvement, significant improvement, and clinical recovery were achieved in patients with EM LB, both with and without dissemination. However, the groups predominantly consisted of patients showing improvement and significant improvement – where EM disappeared but signs of borrelia dissemination persisted (expressed in severity points) compared to those with clinical recovery (no clinical manifestations of LB): among patients without dissemination – 60.0% vs. 40.0% and with dissemination – 65.4% vs. 34.6% (Table 7).

Next, the dynamics of disease severity were investigated in patients with EM LB. Under the influence of monotherapy with doxycycline hydrochloride, a tendency towards reduction in disease severity was noted in patients on the 10th day, and by the 30th day, it had decreased significantly. Specifically, the severity of the pathological process by summing up the scores before therapy was (4.37 ± 0.42) points, and by the 30th day, it was (0.85 ± 0.43) points ($p < 0.05$).

The dynamics of these cytokines were studied because IL-10 is one of the most important anti-inflammatory interleukins with anti-cytokine action, an inhibitor of the hypersensitive response of Th1 cells, which mediates enhanced production of IgG antibodies, synthesis of Th1 cytokines, chemokines, adhesive molecules, and suppresses the formation of monocyte-macrophage TNF-α, IL-1, IL-6, IL-12. This mediator enhances the growth of suppressor cells, B-cell proliferation, and secretion of immunoglobulins. Thus, the main function of IL-10 is to limit and eliminate the inflammatory process [30–33]. At the same time, IL-18 has a pleiotropic effect on various types of cells and affects the secretion of various mediators [34]. There is data indicating both pro-inflammatory and anti-inflammatory effects [35]. IL-18 stimulates the production of pro-inflammatory cytokines such as IFN-γ, TNF-α, IL-2, IL-5, IL-6, IL-8, IL-1β, prostaglandin E2 [36–39], and anti-inflammatory IL-4, IL-13 [40], playing a key role in the resolution of infectious diseases [41]. Its primary effect is the induction of IFN-γ production by T lymphocytes and natural killer cells, which is why IL-18 was initially termed IFN-γ-inducing factor [34, 36].

Primary determination of these cytokine data showed that their concentration in blood was elevated compared to donors but remained within reference values (Table 8).

Elevated levels of the anti-inflammatory IL-10 against high levels of the pro-inflammatory cytokine IL-18 may indicate the need for immediate initiation of etiotropic treatment or switching antibiotics to prevent further dissemination of the pathogen in the body. Therefore, we used the levels of these cytokines to monitor the effectiveness of treatment [42].

Before treatment, the concentration of IL-10 in the serum of patients was four times higher than in healthy individuals (control group), but remained within the reference range (Table 9). By the 60th day, the level of this cytokine had increased twofold compared to the initial content and eightfold compared to the control group ($p < 0.05$), but still did not exceed physiological norms. Prior to treatment, the levels of the pro-inflammatory IL-18 in the serum of patients were not elevated. In the dynamics by the 60th day of treatment, the concentration of this cytokine in the serum of patients decreased but did not differ from the levels observed in healthy individuals.

At the same time, in 8 (10.5%) patients undergoing treatment with doxycycline hydrochloride, skin changes unrelated to tick attachment occurred, along with several subjective complaints. These manifestations appeared after prolonged sun exposure. Specifically, in 5.3% of individuals, photodermatosis manifested as erythema, while 2.6% reported various subjective sensations.

The persistence of certain clinical signs of Lyme borreliosis (improvement and significant improvement, but not clinical recovery) after the disappearance of erythema migrans, as well as the occurrence of phototoxic drug reactions during prolonged treatment with doxycycline hydrochloride, prompted us to search for an alternative treatment regimen.

Considering the possibility of prescribing doxycycline hydrochloride for 10 to 21 days, we proposed the following treatment regimen (Scheme II) for patients with erythema migrans in Lyme borreliosis: doxycycline hydrochloride 100 mg twice daily for 14 days together with a dry extract from the fruits of milk thistle (*Silybum marianum*) and an aqueous substrate of metabolites from *Escherichia coli* (DSM 4087), *Enterococcus faecalis* (DSM), and *Lactobacillus acidophilus* (DSM 414, DSM 4183) in average therapeutic doses over the same period, followed by a decoction of stevia leaves 1 glass twice daily for 14 days.

In choosing this treatment regimen, we took into account, as mentioned earlier, that *B. burgdorferi s. l.* belongs to pleomorphic bacteria capable of transforming their active spirochaetal form into latent forms, specifically round bodies and biofilm [20]. This transformation occurs in response to a range of adverse factors (nutritional deficiency, high environmental pH, or unfavourable temperature) [30, 43]. *In vitro* studies have demonstrated high activity of doxycycline hydrochloride against the motile form of *Borrelia sp.*, moderate activity against biofilms, and inefficacy against atypical forms of these bacteria [43]. Therefore, in our opinion, in some cases, treatment of patients with Lyme borreliosis is insufficiently effective.

To mitigate these negative effects, several studies have already been conducted on the effectiveness of doxycycline hydrochloride in combination with various natural antimicrobial agents, including Baikal skullcap, yellow bedstraw, rosemary, and vitamins D3 and C, which mitigate or complement the detrimental effects of antibiotics on Borrelia [43]. It is known that several plants are valuable sources of natural compounds that demonstrate efficacy against various infectious agents, including Lyme borreliosis [44, 45].

Table 9. Dynamics of IL-10 and IL-18 levels in the serum of patients with erythema migrans form of Lyme borreliosis before and after treatment with doxycycline hydrochloride for 21 days (Me (Lq; Uq))

Interleukin	Healthy individuals (n = 33)	Patients with EM LB (n = 76)	
		before treatment	on the 60th day
IL-10, pg/mL	0,15 (0,00; 1,50)	4,10 (3,10; 10,40)	8,35 (4,30; 14,20)*
IL-18, pg/mL	110,35 (75,30; 165,40)	211,45 (163,25; 264,15)	190,65 (158,80; 220,70)

One of such plants is honey leaf stevia (Stevia rebaudiana (Bertoni) Hemsley) – a perennial herbaceous plant found in the wild only in Paraguay and Southern Brazil. It is cultivated in Paraguay, Japan, the USA, Israel, Argentina, and in southern Ukraine [46]. It has found wide application in medical practice in the treatment of conditions such as diabetes, obesity, and hypertension [47].

The antimicrobial action of honey leaf stevia against a range of infectious agents, including LB, is provided by bioactive compounds: terpenes and flavonoids, as well as a number of so-called phytochemicals – austroinulin, β-carotene, riboflavin, thiamine, and others, of which it possesses over 100 [45, 47]. Stevia contains ferulic, rosmarinic, chlorogenic, and caffeic acids and their derivatives; flavonoids such as kaempferol, rutin, catechin, luteolin, quercetin; derivatives of benzoic and salicylic acids; epicatechin. The plant's leaves contain a significant amount of protocatechuic acid, which provides antioxidant and anti-inflammatory activities [48–50].

According to research from the University of New Haven (USA), honey leaf stevia demonstrates pronounced activity against various morphological forms of *B. burgdorferi* [44]. Specifically, to address the aforementioned limitations of doxycycline hydrochloride by reducing its duration of use in the comprehensive treatment of patients with erythema migrans in Lyme borreliosis, we decided to incorporate honey leaf stevia leaves in the form of a decoction.

In Scheme II, 70 individuals were treated: 46 patients solely with erythema migrans and 24 with erythema migrans and other manifestations of LB. It was found that with the use of Scheme II, by the 30th day of treatment, there were significantly more patients with clinical recovery among those with erythema migrans alone and among those with signs of organ involvement – 42 (91.3%) and 19 (79.2%) respectively ($p < 0.05$) (Table 5.10). Comparing the treatment results of patients receiving Scheme II with those receiving Scheme I, it was determined that among the former, there were significantly more individuals with clinical recovery, particularly in cases of erythema migrans without dissemination – 42 (91.3%) versus 20 (40.0%) in the comparison group, and among patients with erythema migrans with organ involvement – 19 (79.2%) versus 9 (34.6%) ($p < 0.001$).

Table 10. Clinical effectiveness of different treatment regimens for patients with erythema migrans in Lyme borreliosis (on the 30th day)

Clinical effectiveness	Patients with EM LB																	
	without dissemination (n = 96)						with dissemination (n = 50)						without dissemination and with dissemination Total (n = 146)					
	Treatment regimen																	
	I (n = 50)		II (n = 46)		Total (n = 96)		I (n = 26)		II (n = 24)		Total (n = 50)		I (n = 76)		II (n = 70)		Total (n = 146)	
Clinical recovery	20	40,0	42	91,3*,**	62	64,6	9	34,6	19	79,2*,**	28	56,0*	29	38,2	61	87,1*,**	90	61,6
Significant improvement	12	24,0	3	6,5	15	15,6	10	38,5	4	16,7	14	28,0	22	28,9	7	10,0	29	19,9
Improvement	18	36,0	1	2,2	19	19,8	7	26,9	1	4,1	8	16,0	25	32,9	2	2,9	27	18,5

Notes: 1. * – the difference is significant within the limits of one treatment regimen, $p < 0.05$.
2. ** – the difference is significant between different treatment regimens, $p < 0.05$.

Table 11. Dynamics of the severity of pathological process in patients with erythema migrans form of Lyme borreliosis using different treatment regimens, scores (M ± m)

Treatment regimen	Examination date		
	Before treatment	Day 10	Day 30
I (n = 76)	4,37 ± 0,42	3,68 ± 0,52	0,85 ± 0,43*
II (n = 70)	4,06 ± 0,40	2,46 ± 0,37	0,26 ± 0,15*,**

Notes: 1. * – the difference is significant with the indicator before treatment, $p < 0.05$.
2. ** – the difference is significant between groups in the same term, $p < 0.05$.

Regarding patients whose treatment led to significant improvement or improvement only, the percentage was significantly higher among patients treated with Scheme I compared to Scheme II, both among individuals with disseminated disease – 17 (65.4%) versus 5 (20.8%) ($p < 0.001$), and among those with erythema migrans alone – 30 (60.0%) versus 4 (8.7%) ($p < 0.001$) (Table 10).

Next, the dynamics of disease severity were compared in patients with EM LB depending on the treatment scheme. Prior to treatment, groups of patients receiving different treatments did not significantly differ in terms of the severity of the pathological process, expressed in scores ($p > 0.05$). Under the influence of Scheme II therapy, disease severity scores decreased only by the 10th day and were significantly lower by the 30th day compared to pre-treatment levels ($p < 0.05$) (see Table 7). At the same time, it is worth noting that by the 30th day, individuals treated under Scheme II had significantly lower severity of the pathological process compared to patients in the Scheme I group ($p < 0.05$) (Table 11).

Thus, in patients with EM LB who received comprehensive treatment including a decoction of Stevia rebaudiana leaves, the severity of the disease decreased more rapidly, and by the 30th day, it was significantly lower compared to individuals who did not receive phytonasties.

Simultaneously, the time to disappearance of EM, which is one of the indicators of clinical effectiveness of treatment, was assessed. It was found that this time during treatment in 146 patients averaged 11 (7; 15) days and did not depend on the proposed therapy schemes. Additionally, no correlation was found between the disappearance time of EM and factors such as gender, age of the patients, season, location of tick bites, number of bites, and the time of their removal. Analysing the disappearance time of EM in relation to antibiotic administration, differences were noted based on the location of tick attachment to different body areas: upper and lower limbs and abdomen ($p = 0.014$; $p = 0.026$).

It is noteworthy that the results of the conducted correlation analysis showed that the time to disappearance of EM during antibiotic therapy significantly depends on the duration of its existence. This confirms a positive correlation of moderate strength between these indicators (Spearman's correlation coefficient, $r=0.38$, $p < 0.001$) (Figure 1). Therefore, etiotropic therapy for EM LB should be initiated as early as possible.

The effectiveness of the tested Scheme II in patients with EM LB, like the previous Scheme I, was also evaluated based on the dynamics of cytokine levels in the patients' serum: pro-inflammatory IL-18 and anti-inflammatory IL-10. Interleukins were determined twice—before treatment and at 60 days. Reference concentrations of cytokines were as follows: IL-10 – up to 31 pg/mL; IL-18 – from 104 to 650 pg/mL.

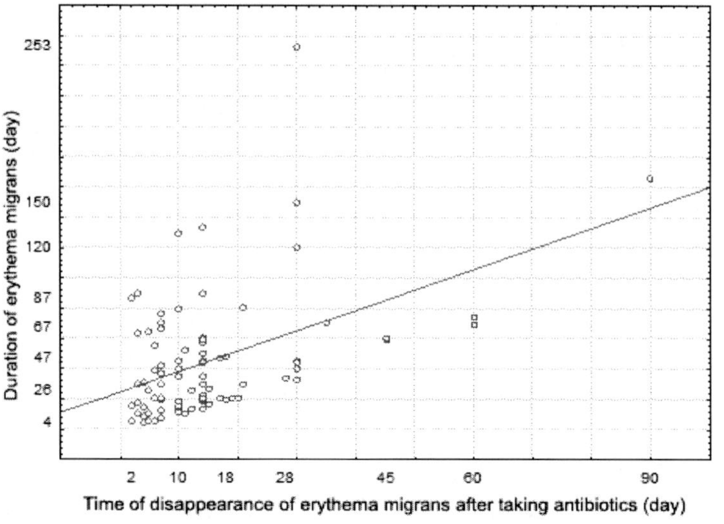

Figure 1. The relationship between the time of disappearance of erythema migrans and its duration in 137 patients with erythema migrans form of Lyme borreliosis. Spearman's correlation coefficient, r = 0.38 ($p < 0.001$).

Before treatment, the concentration of IL-10 in the serum of patients was nearly 4 times higher than in healthy individuals, but remained within the reference range. By the 60th day, the level of this cytokine increased nearly 3 times compared to the initial content and 18 times compared to healthy individuals ($p < 0.05$), although it remained within normal limits (Table 12). Before therapy, the level of pro-inflammatory IL-18 in the serum of patients and healthy individuals was within the physiological norm. During the dynamics on the 60th day from the start of treatment, the content of this cytokine in the serum of patients decreased by half compared to the initial level, remaining within the physiological norm.

Therefore, treatment of patients using a decoction of Stevia rebaudiana leaves contributed to an increase in the concentration of anti-inflammatory IL-10 in their serum. By the 60th day, it was three times higher than the initial level and 18 times higher than in the control group, and twice as high as in individuals who received therapy without phytonasties.

Table 12. Dynamics of IL-10 and IL-18 levels in the serum of patients with erythema migrans form of Lyme borreliosis using different treatment regimens (Me (Lq; Uq))

Interleukin	Healthy individuals	Examination date			
		I (n = 76)		II (n = 70)	
		Before treatment	Day 60	Before treatment	Day 60
IL-10, pg/mL	0,15	4,10	8,35	3,85	18,55
	(0,00;	(3,10;	(4,30;	(1,25;	(12,40;
	1,50)	10,40)	14,20)*	17,08)	26,00)
IL-18, pg/mL	110,35	211,45	190,65	276,35	128,70
	(75,30;	(163,25;	(158,80;	(174,60;	(134,40;
	165,40)	264,15)	220,70)	314,40)	221,10)*

Notes:

1. * – the difference is significant between groups in one term, $p < 0.05$.
2. ** – the difference is significant regarding the start of treatment, $p < 0.05$.

The application of Stevia rebaudiana leaf decoction in patients with EM LB led to a two-fold decrease in the content of pro-inflammatory IL-18 in serum compared to the initial level in individuals receiving only traditional antibiotic treatment (Table 12) [51].

Table 13. Dynamics of IgM and IgG antibody levels to *B. burgdorferi s. l.* in serum samples from patients with erythema migrans form of Lyme borreliosis, receiving different treatments, U/ml (M ± m)

Treatment regimen	Examination date					
	Before treatment (n = 146)		Day 60 (n = 146)		Day 120 (n = 146)	
	IgM	IgG	IgM	IgG	IgM	IgG
I (n = 76)	54,42 ± 8,95*	37,15 ± 6,86	62,18 ± 8,79	21,27 ± 3,77	16,40 ± 2,43**	16,00 ± 2,45**
II (n = 70)	27,20 ± 3,12	27,56 ± 3,99	36,83 ± 3,98	18,17 ± 2,47	12,61 ± 1,26**	13,14 ± 1,74**

Notes:
1. * – the difference is significant between groups in one term, $p < 0.05$.
2. ** – the difference is significant regarding the start of treatment, $p < 0.05$.

A peculiar feature of LB is a relatively slow and weak specific humoral immune response, which involves the formation of anti-Borrelia antibodies, predominantly of classes IgM and IgG, and a small amount of antibodies of other classes such as IgA and IgE. These antibodies typically appear no earlier than 2-3 weeks from the onset of the disease, complicating early diagnosis [52]. The level of specific IgM gradually decreases by the 8-10th week of LB, but in the case of dissemination, their formation may be prolonged. IgG levels (mainly G1, G3, which are complement-activating isotypes) begin to rise by 4-6 weeks from the onset of the disease, reaching peak levels at 4-6 months [53, 54].

B-cell responses may be suppressed by early administration of antibacterial therapy at the initial stage of the disease. In cases of localized manifestations of the disease, early antibiotic administration may not result in specific antibodies [55].

We also studied the dynamics of the concentration (quantitative determination) of specific IgM and IgG antibodies to *B. burgdorferi s. l.* in the serum of patients with EM LB depending on the treatment schemes. Specific antibodies were determined three times: before treatment, at 60 days, and 120 days. It was found that before treatment, the concentration of IgM antibodies was higher in patients treated with Scheme I compared to those treated with Scheme II ($p < 0.01$), while the concentration of anti-IgG did not differ significantly (Table 10). At 60 days, the content of specific anti-IgM antibodies slightly increased: in patients treated with Scheme II, it increased by 1.35 times, and with Scheme I by 1.14 times, while the concentration of anti-IgG antibodies decreased by 1.52 and 1.75 times, respectively ($p > 0.05$). On the 120th day, a significant decrease in the concentration of specific antibodies of both classes was observed ($p < 0.01$): the level of IgM antibodies was lower compared to their content on the 60th day and before treatment. Their concentration decreased by 2.15 times in patients treated only with doxycycline hydrochloride, and by 3.31 times in patients who also received a decoction of Stevia rebaudiana leaves. Considering the manufacturer's recommendations, according to which the antibody level of 16-22 AU/mL in serum is considered intermediate, and ≤ 16 AU/mL is negative, it can be concluded that antibodies of both classes to *B. burgdorferi s. l.* disappeared only in patients treated with Scheme II (IgM (12.61 ± 1.26) and IgG (13.14 ± 1.74) AU/mL), while in those treated with Scheme I, they remained intermediate (Table 13).

Therefore, a significant reduction in the concentration of specific IgM and IgG antibodies on the 120th day of observation indicates the effectiveness of the tested treatment regimen for patients with EM in Lyme borreliosis and the possible elimination of *B. burgdorferi s. l.* Additionally, in individuals treated with Scheme II, the frequency of photodermatoses and subjective complaints related to the use of doxycycline hydrochloride was investigated (Table 14).

It was found that reducing the duration of antibiotic administration from 21 to 14 days decreased the frequency of the aforementioned negative effects. For instance, erythema on exposed skin areas remote from tick attachment sites was present in only 1.4% of patients compared to 5.3% in the group treated with Scheme I, and subjective sensations were reported by 1.4% versus 2.6% of individuals ($p < 0.05$) (see Table 14).

Therefore, treatment of patients with doxycycline hydrochloride and a stevia leaf decoction contributed to a nearly 3.8-fold reduction ($p < 0.05$) in the frequency of occurrence of phototoxic drug reactions associated with doxycycline hydrochloride.

In a follow-up examination after 8–10 months post-treatment, 44 patients with EM in Lyme borreliosis were examined. Of these, 21 individuals received oral doxycycline hydrochloride 100 mg twice daily for 21 days along with silymarin and hilak (Group 1), while 23 patients received doxycycline hydrochloride 100 mg twice daily for only 14 days along with silymarin and hilak, followed by stevia leaf decoction 1 glass twice daily for 14 days (Group 2). Throughout the post-treatment period, the examined individuals did not experience tick attacks (Figure 2).

Patients treated only with antibiotics (Group 1) more frequently reported worsening of condition in the form of new LB symptoms (arthralgia, decreased vision, facial nerve paresis) compared to those in Group 2 – 9.5% versus 4.3% ($p < 0.05$). Likewise, remission of the disease was more common among Group 2 patients compared to Group 1 – 82.6% versus 71.4% (Figure 2).

Thus, the results of the study demonstrated that among 146 patients with EM in Lyme borreliosis, 96 (65.8%) had disease without signs of Borrelia dissemination, while 50 (34.2%) had early-stage organ involvement. Severe and moderate disease courses were more prevalent among patients with early-stage organ involvement, whereas mild disease courses were more common among patients with only EM – 91.7% versus 44.0% ($p < 0.05$). The degree of moderate severity in 8 patients with only EM was characterized by multiple (3 to 6) erythemas.

Table 14. Frequency of photodermatoses occurrence in patients with non-erythema migrans form of Lyme borreliosis under different treatments (n = 26)

Symptoms	Treatment regimen			
	I (n = 76)		II (n = 70)	
	Absolute number	%	Absolute number	%
Erythema on exposed areas of skin, away from tick attachment sites	4	5,3	1	1,4
Skin swelling	1	1,3	1	1,4
Vesicles	1	1,3	0	0
Subjective sensations: tingling, itching, general weakness	2	2,6	1	1,4
Total	8	10,5	3	4,3

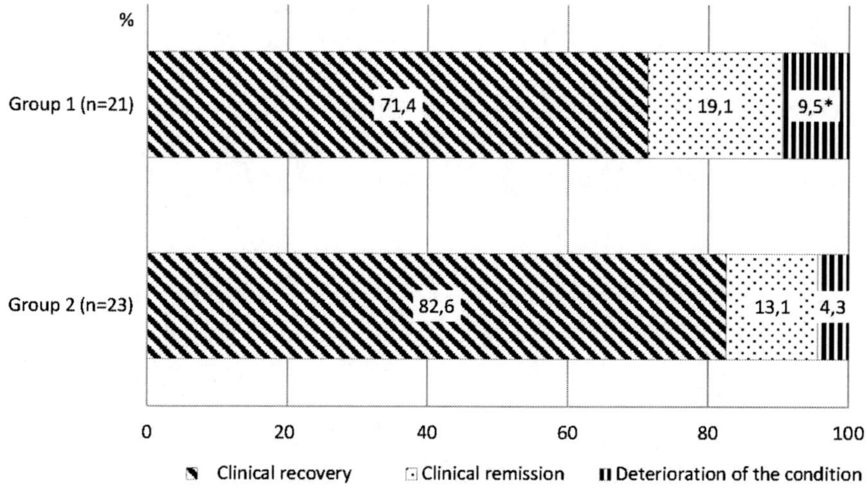

Note. * – significant difference between groups, $p < 0.05$.

Figure 2. Follow-up of patients depending on the treatment regimens received (n = 44).

76 patients with EM in Lyme borreliosis, including 50 individuals with only EM and 26 with EM and signs of early organ dissemination, received the following treatment: oral doxycycline hydrochloride 100 mg twice daily for 21 days, along with a dry extract from the fruits of milk thistle (Silybum marianum) and an aqueous substrate of metabolites from Escherichia coli (DSM 4087), Enterococcus faecalis (DSM), and Lactobacillus acidophilus (DSM 414, DSM 4183) at moderate therapeutic doses.

After the treatment, patients with and without Borrelia dissemination showed positive dynamics in terms of improvement, significant improvement, and clinical recovery. However, both groups predominantly had patients showing improvement and significant improvement – those where erythema migrans disappeared but signs of Borrelia dissemination (expressed in scores) persisted, compared to individuals with clinical recovery (no clinical signs of LB): in patients without dissemination – 60.0% versus 40.0%, and with dissemination – 65.4% versus 34.6%.

Some patients experienced skin changes not related to tick attachment and various subjective complaints during the prescribed treatment with doxycycline hydrochloride. These adverse reactions appeared after prolonged exposure to sunlight. Specifically, photodermatosis manifested as erythema in 5.3% of individuals and various subjective sensations in 2.6%.

The presence of certain clinical signs of LB in some patients after the disappearance of erythema migrans (improvement and significant improvement, but not clinical recovery), as well as the occurrence of phototoxic drug reactions during prolonged treatment with doxycycline hydrochloride, prompted us to seek an alternative treatment regimen. It was decided to shorten the duration of doxycycline hydrochloride treatment to 14 days and incorporate a stevia leaf decoction afterward. According to literature data, this medicinal plant has shown effectiveness against all morphological forms of Borrelia, even those resistant to doxycycline hydrochloride. Therefore, the treatment scheme II for patients with EM in Lyme borreliosis looked as follows: doxycycline hydrochloride 100 mg twice daily for 14 days along with a dry extract from the fruits of milk thistle (Silybum marianum) and an aqueous substrate of metabolites from Escherichia coli (DSM 4087), Enterococcus faecalis (DSM), and

Lactobacillus acidophilus (DSM 414, DSM 4183) at the same doses, followed by stevia leaf decoction 1 glass twice daily for 14 days. 70 individuals received this treatment: 46 patients with only EM and 24 with EM and other manifestations of LB.

The developed comprehensive treatment of patients with EM in Lyme borreliosis using doxycycline hydrochloride and stevia leaf decoction ensured clinical recovery in a greater number of individuals compared to therapy with antibiotics alone – 87.1% versus 38.2% ($p < 0.05$).

It was established that the time of disappearance of erythema migrans during antibiotic treatment significantly depends on the localization of tick attachment and its duration, confirmed by a positive, moderately strong correlation between these indicators.

The use of stevia leaf decoction in the comprehensive treatment of patients with EM in Lyme borreliosis also significantly contributed to the reduction in the level of pro-inflammatory IL-18 and increase in the concentration of anti-inflammatory IL-10 in the patients' blood serum ($p < 0.05$), which promotes an early inflammatory response, formation of cellular and humoral immunity, and consequently, contributes to the elimination of Borrelia and patient recovery.

In the comprehensive treatment of patients with EM in Lyme borreliosis, the prescription of doxycycline hydrochloride together with stevia leaf decoction led to a nearly 3.8-fold reduction in the frequency of occurrence of doxycycline hydrochloride's phototoxic drug reaction ($p < 0.05$).

5. Optimization of Treatment for Patients with Lyme Borreliosis Combined with Epstein-Barr Virus Infection and Vitamin D Deficiency

Mariia Shkilna
Mykhaylo Andreychyn
Oleh Ivakhiv
Mariana Huk
and Tetiana Yuzkiv

The objective of the study was to develop optimal comprehensive treatment for patients with Lyme borreliosis combined with chronic Epstein-Barr virus infection (CEBVI) in the active phase, against the backdrop of vitamin D deficiency.

Vitamin D is a fat-soluble vitamin. The two main precursors of its active forms are ergocalciferol (vitamin D2) and cholecalciferol (vitamin D3). These are obtained from dietary sources (in small amounts) and synthesized in the skin (the primary source of vitamin D).

This unique vitamin is essential not only for regulating calcium and phosphorus levels in blood and tissues but also plays a crucial role in ensuring an adequate immune response. Numerous scientific studies have demonstrated a correlation between serum vitamin D levels and the frequency and severity of various infectious diseases of viral, bacterial, and fungal aetiology. Furthermore, the effectiveness of therapeutic and preventive measures for these diseases also depends on the serum concentration of vitamin D [56, 57].

The mechanisms of vitamin D's antiviral activity are not fully understood. It is believed that vitamin D directly inhibits viral replication, may significantly modulate viral gene transcription, and has immunomodulatory and anti-inflammatory effects [58].

Globally, about 1 billion people across all ethnic and age groups have low serum vitamin D levels [56, 59].

To prevent and treat VDD and insufficiency, two forms of the vitamin are most commonly used: vitamin D2 and D3. International researchers note that vitamin D3 has a lower affinity for plasma vitamin D-binding protein, a higher discrimination coefficient (predominance of activity), and greater rate of 25-hydroxylation in the liver and subsequent hydroxylation in the kidneys to form active metabolites [95-98]. Recent randomized clinical trials and meta-analyses have shown higher clinical efficacy of vitamin D3 compared to vitamin D2 [64, 65].

Treatment of patients with VDD should be carried out over 4-12 weeks, depending on the degree of deficiency and other risk factors, until a target level of 30-50 ng/ml (75-125 nmol/L) is achieved. For individuals with conditions affecting vitamin D metabolism, higher doses (up to 10,000 IU/day) are recommended. Subsequently, to maintain optimal vitamin D status, doses of 800-2,000 IU/day are used [66].

Currently, vitamin D in Ukraine is available in the form of capsules, tablets, and oral solutions for daily or weekly intake [66].

We observed 67 patients aged 28 to 65 years with LB affecting the joints. There were 22 men (32.8%) and 45 women (67.2%).

Among the 67 patients examined, 31 (44.3%) had both LB and CEBVI. Depending on the presence of this viral disease, all patients were divided into two groups: Group 1 consisted of 36 individuals with LB without CEBVI (LB only), and Group 2 comprised 31 patients with LB combined with CEBVI (LB + CEBVI).

Vitamin D status was assessed according to the recommendations of the First Ukrainian Consensus on Vitamin D Management by measuring serum total 25(OH)D levels [66]: <20 ng/mL (< 50 nmol/L) – VDD; ≥ 20 ng/mL (≥ 50 nmol/L) and < 30 ng/mL (< 75 nmol/L) – vitamin D insufficiency; 30-50 ng/mL (75-125 nmol/L) – adequate vitamin D level; > 50-60 ng/mL (> 125-150 nmol/L) – safe but not target level; > 60-100 ng/mL (> 150-250 nmol/L) – uncertainty zone with potential benefits or risks; > 100 ng/mL (>250 nmol/L) – excess/toxicity zone of vitamin D.

Inclusion criteria for the study were the following individuals aged 28 to 65 years; residence in an endemic area for LB and/or tick bite history; clinical signs of LB, CEBVI; known vitamin D status determined from September to May; individuals without acute infections or other chronic diseases in an exacerbation stage (primarily osteoarthritis); patients not taking immunotropic drugs or receiving vaccinations in the last 30 days before blood sampling; positive laboratory results for LB (via two-stage serological testing: ELISA and immunoblot), and for CEBVI in the active phase –IIFR and PCR.

Patients reported joint pain and swelling in their arms and legs. To assess the activity of the pathological process in the affected joints, the DAS (disease activity score) index was used, specifically the DAS28 modification. This was calculated using a special calculator, considering the number of swollen and painful out of 28 joints: hand joints – from the first to the fifth metacarpophalangeal joints, the interphalangeal joint of the thumb, and from the second to the fifth proximal interphalangeal joints; elbow, shoulder, and knee joints; as well as the erythrocyte sedimentation rate, and the patient's overall assessment of joint pain intensity, measured using a visual analogue scale. A DAS28 score exceeding 5.1 indicates high disease activity in the affected joints; > 3.2 and ≤ 5.1 – moderate activity, ≥ 2.6 and ≤ 3.2 – low activity, and less than 2.6 – remission [102].

In addition to joint involvement, patients in both groups reported muscle pain, sleep disturbances (insomnia and/or chronic lack of sleep), enlarged lymph nodes, fever, increased fatigue/general weakness, memory and cognitive impairment, especially with mental tasks, and reduced ability to perform precise actions. The frequency of these complaints was assessed separately for each group of patients.

Statistical analysis was performed using Microsoft Office Excel and STATISTICA computer programs. Non-parametric Mann-Whitney test was used for comparing non-normally distributed values. Results were considered statistically significant at $p < 0.05$.

When analysing the results of assessing the activity of the pathological process in affected joints using the DAS28 index before the start of treatment, it was established that there were no patients with arthritis remission in any of the examined groups.

It was found that individuals with low arthritis activity were significantly more common in Group 1 (LB only) compared to Group 2 (LB + CEBVI): 12 (33.3%) vs. 4 (12.9%), $p < 0.05$. The number of individuals with medium and high degrees of joint activity did not differ significantly between the groups – in Group 1, there were 10 (27.8%) and 14 (38.9%) vs. 15 (48.4%) and 12 (38.7%) in Group 2, $p > 0.05$.

Apart from joint pain, patients in both groups had other complaints. For instance, patients with combined LB + CEBVI (Group 2) significantly more frequently complained of muscle pain, fever, and enlarged lymph nodes compared to those with only LB (Group 1) – 12 (38.7%) vs. 6 (16.7%), 14 (45.2%) vs. 8 (22.2%), and 16 (51.6%) vs. 10 (27.7%) respectively, $p < 0.05$. The frequency of complaints such as sleep disturbances, increased fatigue/general weakness, and cognitive impairment did not differ statistically significantly between the groups – in patients with LB only (Group 1) it was 13 (36.1%), 12 (33.3%), and 10 (27.7%) vs. 12 (38.7%), 11 (35.5%), and 10 (32.3%) in Group 2, $p > 0.05$.

Subsequently, the 25(OH)D levels in the serum of all patients were determined. It was found that there were no patients with safe levels of Vitamin D in either group. However, patients with sufficient level of Vitamin D were significantly more common in Group 1 (LB only) compared to Group 2 (LB + CEBVI): 13 (36.1%) vs. 4 (12.9%), $p < 0.05$. Patients with VDD were somewhat more prevalent in Group 2 – 16 (51.6%) vs. 11 (30.6%) in Group 1, but without significant difference, $p > 0.05$. The percentage of individuals with VDI did not differ significantly between the groups – 33.3% in Group 1 and 35.5% in Group 2.

For treating LB, patients in both groups were prescribed doxycycline hydrochloride orally at 100 mg twice daily for 28 days. In addition to etiotropic therapy, patients also received Enterol 250 (lyophilized Saccharomyces boulardii CNCM I-745, 250 mg) 1 sachet twice daily and Carsil 2 tablets three times daily per os for the same duration as the antibiotic.

The existing deficiency and insufficiency of 25(OH)D levels in serum led to an additional prescription of cholecalciferol (vitamin D3) at 5,600 IU, 1 tablet weekly per os for 4 weeks (28 days) to all patients in both groups. Vitamin D was used in doses recommended by the Consensus of Ukrainian Experts: "Diagnosis, Prevention, and Treatment of Vitamin D Deficiency in Adults" (2023).

The effectiveness of treatment for Lyme disease patients in both groups was analysed on the 29th day of combined therapy. The criteria for assessment included the dynamics of clinical manifestations of the disease, the activity of the pathological process in the affected joints (according to DAS28), and the levels of 25(OH)D in patients' serum.

It was found that on the 29th day from the start of combined therapy, remission of the pathological process in the affected joints was achieved in some patients in both groups.

However, this was significantly more frequent in Group 1 (LD only) compared to Group 2 (LD + CEBVI) – 23 (63.9%) versus 9 (29.0%), $p < 0.05$ (Table 15). It should be noted that none of the patients had remission of arthritis before treatment.

After treatment, the number of patients with low activity of arthritis significantly increased only in Group 2 (LD + EBV) – from 4 (12.9%) to 12 (38.7%), $p < 0.05$. In contrast, the number of such patients in Group 1 (LD only) did not change significantly – from 10 (27.8%) to 11 (30.6%). This is likely due to some patients in Group 2 achieving remission of the pathological process in the affected joints, while patients with reduced activity from moderate and high levels transitioned into this group.

It is worth noting that the number of patients with moderate activity of the pathological process in the affected joints significantly decreased in both groups – from 10 (27.8%) to 2 (5.5%) in Group 1 (LD only) and from 15 (48.4%) to 7 (22.6%) in Group 2 (LD + CEBVI), $p < 0.05$. At the same time, patients with this level of arthritis activity were fewer in Group 1 (LD only) compared to Group 2 (LD + CEBVI) – 5.5% versus 22.6%, $p < 0.05$. Regarding patients with high arthritis activity, only 3 (9.7%) remained in Group 2 (LD + CEBVI). Meanwhile, their number decreased more than fourfold compared to the start of treatment – from 38.7% to 9.7%, $p < 0.05$. However, in Group 1 (LD only), no patients with such high arthritis activity were detected at this time (Table 15).

Table 15. Dynamics of the frequency of various levels of pathological process activity in affected joints (according to DAS28) in patients from the examined groups after 28 days of combined treatment, %

Activity according to DAS28, score	Group of patients							
	1, n = 36				2, n = 31			
	Day of treatment							
	Before treatment		29		Before treatment		29	
	Absolute number	%	Absolute number	%	Absolute number	%	Absolute number	%
Remission, ≤2,6	-	-	23	63,9**	-	-	9	29,0
Low, ≥2,6 i ≤3,2	12	33,3*	11	30,6	4	12,9	12	38,7***
Moderate, >3,2 i ≤5,1	10	27,8	2	5,5***	15	48,4	7	22,6**,***
High, >5,1	14	38,9	-	-	12	38,7	3	9,7***
Total	36	100	36	100,0	31	100	31	100

Notes:

* – The difference is significant between groups before treatment within the same activity level, $p < 0.05$;

** – The difference is significant between groups after treatment within the same activity level, $p < 0.05$;

*** – The difference is significant within the same group before and after treatment within the same activity level, $p < 0.05$.

The effectiveness of treatment for patients in both groups on the 29th day of therapy was also assessed based on the dynamics of other clinical signs of the disease. It was found that among patients in Group 1 (only with Lyme borreliosis), after treatment, there was a significant reduction in the number of individuals suffering from sleep disturbances (insomnia and/or chronic sleep deprivation), increased fatigue/general weakness, impaired memory and cognitive function, muscle pain, fever, and swollen lymph nodes, $p < 0.05$ (Table 16).

In contrast, among patients in Group 2 (LB + CEBVI), the positive dynamics of clinical symptoms were less pronounced. After treatment, there was a significant reduction only in the percentage of individuals troubled by sleep disturbances (insomnia and/or chronic sleep deprivation), increased fatigue/general weakness, and memory and cognitive impairments, p <

0.05. However, the number of patients in this group who reported muscle pain, fever, and swollen lymph nodes did not significantly decrease after treatment, $p > 0.05$ (Table 16).

Table 16. Dynamics of the frequency of other clinical manifestations of the illness in patients of the examined groups after 28 days of combined treatment, %

Complaints	Group of patients							
	1, n = 36				2, n = 31			
	Day of treatment							
	Before treatment		29		Before treatment		29	
	Absolute number	%	Absolute number	%	Absolute number	%	Absolute number	%
Sleep disturbances (insomnia and/or chronic sleep deprivation)	13	36,1	4	11,1***	12	38,7	5	16,1***
Increased fatigue/general weakness	12	33,3	3	8,3***	11	35,5	4	12,9***
Impaired memory and cognitive function	10	27,7	3	8,3***	10	32,3	3	9,6***
Muscle pain	6	16,7	1	2,8***	12	38,7*	7	22,6**
Fever	8	22,2	2	5,6***	14	45,2*	9	29,0**
Swollen lymph nodes	10	27,7	3	8,3***	16	51,6*	12	38,7**

Notes:
* – The difference is significant between groups before treatment within a given complaint, $p < 0.05$;
** – The difference is significant between groups after treatment within a given complaint, $p < 0.05$;
*** – The difference is significant within the same group before and after treatment within a given complaint, $p < 0.05$.

Moreover, it is worth noting that after combined treatment, there were significantly fewer patients in Group 1 (only LB) who complained of muscle pain, fever, and swollen lymph nodes compared to patients in Group 2 (LB + CEBVI) – specifically, 1 (2.8%), 2 (5.6%), and 3 (8.3%) versus 7 (22.6%), 9 (29.0%), and 12 (38.7%), $p < 0.05$. Only the number of individuals with sleep disturbances (insomnia and/or chronic sleep deprivation), increased fatigue/general weakness, and memory and cognitive impairments did not differ significantly after the combined treatment course (Table 16).

At the same time, after the complex treatment involving cholecalciferol (vitamin D3), the dynamics of the frequency of different levels of 25(OH)D in the serum of patients from both groups were analysed. It was found that there were only 6 (19.4%) patients with vitamin D deficiency in group 2 (Lyme borreliosis + CEBVI), although this number had significantly decreased compared to the start of therapy – from 16 (51.6%), $p < 0.05$ (Figure 3). In contrast, no patients with severe VDD were found in Group 1 (only LB), although there were 11 (30.6%) before treatment. The proportion of patients with VDI in the serum slightly decreased in both Group 1 (only LB) and Group 2 (LB + CEBVI) – from 33.3% to 25.0% and from 35.5% to 29.0%, respectively, $p > 0.05$. The number of patients with adequate vitamin D levels significantly increased in both groups – by 2.1 times (from 36.1% to 75.0%) in Group 1 and by 4.0 times (from 12.9% to 51.6%) in Group 2, $p < 0.05$.

Thus, patients in both groups showed a positive trend in the frequency of different levels of 25(OH)D in the serum, but this improvement was more significant in individuals with only LB (Group 1) compared to patients with combined pathology (LB + CEBVI, Group 2). This difference can likely be explained by the fact that EBV contributes to a more significant reduction in vitamin D levels in patients with combined infection. Other researchers have noted this pattern as well. For instance, a reverse correlation was established between the amount of EBV in the blood of patients and the level of 25(OH)D3 – viral load was significantly higher with lower levels of vitamin D3 [68]. Therefore, in cases of vitamin D deficiency in patients, EBV replication occurs more intensively.

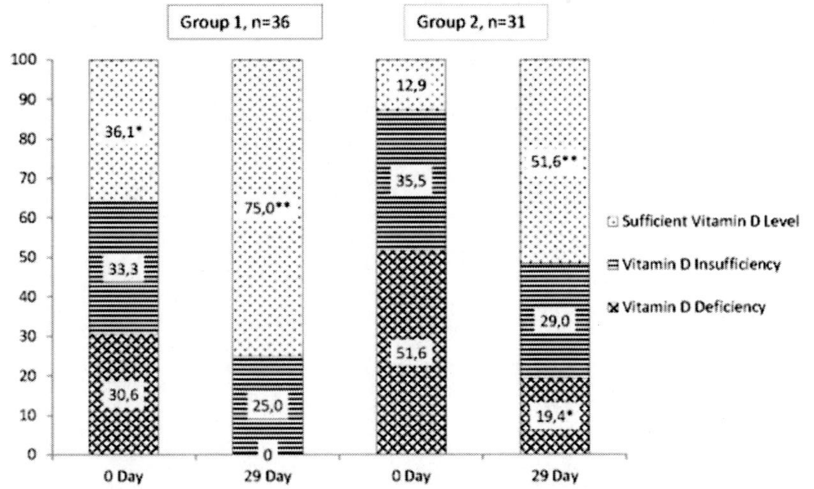

Notes:
* – The difference is significant between groups for the same vitamin D level before treatment, $p < 0.05$;
** – The difference is significant within the same vitamin D level in one group before and after treatment, $p < 0.05$.

Figure 3. Dynamics of the Frequency of Detection of Different Levels of 25(OH)D in Serum of Patients from the Examined Groups After 28 Days of Combined Treatment, %.

Since in Group 1 (only LB) 75.0% of patients achieved sufficient vitamin D levels after 28 days of combined therapy with doxycycline hydrochloride and cholecalciferol, and only 25.0% had VDI in their serum, it was decided to use a therapeutic diet to correct the vitamin D levels. The diet consisted of consuming vitamin D-rich foods, specifically fish and other seafood (rainbow trout, cod liver oil, etc.), eggs and organ meats (beef liver), and mushrooms (chanterelles, shiitake, porcini) [66]. Patients were recommended to follow this diet for 4 weeks (28 days).

Meanwhile, considering that almost every second patient in Group 2 (LB + CEBVI) had vitamin D deficiency in their serum, specifically 19.4% with vitamin D deficiency and 29.0% with vitamin D insufficiency, it was decided to continue the therapy with cholecalciferol for these patients at the same therapeutic dose (1 tablet of 5,600 IU weekly) for an additional 4 weeks (28 days).

After the four-week (28 days) dietary therapy course, 97.2% of patients in Group 1 (only LB) achieved adequate vitamin D levels, with only 1 (2.8%) patient having a vitamin level in their serum slightly lower, corresponding to vitamin D insufficiency (Figure 4).

The dynamics of the frequency of different levels of 25(OH)D in the blood of patients in Group 2 (LB + CEBVI) after 8 weeks of combined treatment using cholecalciferol were analysed (Figure 4). It was found that this course of therapy was quite effective – 90.3% of individuals achieved adequate vitamin D levels, and only 3 (9.7%) were diagnosed with vitamin D insufficiency.

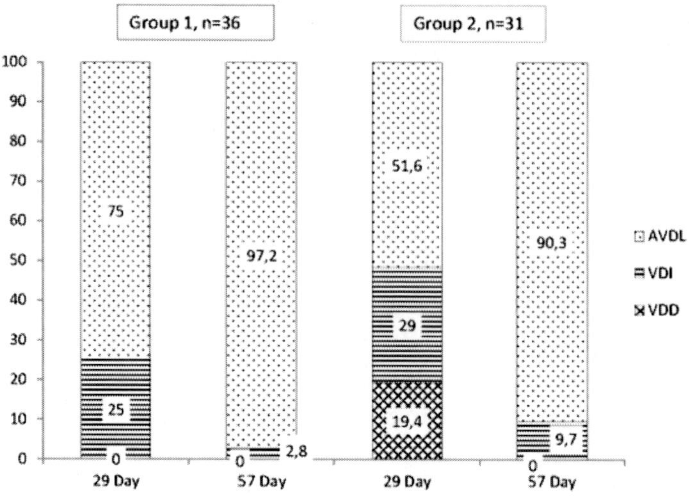

Notes:

* – The difference is significant for vitamin D insufficiency before and after extended treatment within the same group, $p < 0,05$;

** – The difference is significant for adequate vitamin D levels before and after extended treatment within the same group, $p < 0,05$.

Figure 4. Dynamics of the Frequency of Detection of Different Levels of 25(OH)D in Serum of Patients from the Examined Groups After 56 Days of Combined Treatment, %.

Considering the results of foreign studies indicating some antiviral activity of vitamin D, including against EBV, we analysed the dynamics of the number of patients with LB + CEBVI (Group 2) and high EBV DNA levels (10^3-10^7 copies/mL) in their serum and/or saliva depending on the duration of cholecalciferol treatment at a dose of 5,600 IU weekly.

It was established that using cholecalciferol at 5,600 IU weekly to correct the low vitamin D levels in the serum of patients also contributed to a decrease in the number of individuals with active EBVI already by the 29th day of therapy, reducing it by 2.8 times – from 31 (100.0%) to 11 (35.5%), $p < 0.05$. Continuing cholecalciferol treatment at the same therapeutic dose for an additional 28 days led to a reduction in the number of individuals with high EBV viral load by 5.5 times compared to the 29th day of treatment and by 15.5 times relative to the start of treatment, $p < 0.05$. Only 2 (6.5%) patients had laboratory signs of active EBVI – high EBV DNA levels in serum and/or saliva.

Further analysis was conducted on the dynamics of the pathological process activity in affected joints in both groups on the 57th day of different treatment regimens (Table 17).

Complex treatment of patients in Group 1 (only LB) with doxycycline and cholecalciferol for 28 days led to remission of the pathological process in affected joints in 23 (63.9%) individuals. Low arthritis activity was present in 11 (30.6%) patients, and medium activity was found in only 2 (5.5%). The subsequent four-week (28 days) dietary therapy with vitamin D-containing products resulted in remission in 32 (88.9%) patients, with low arthritis activity reported in only 4 (11.1%) patients.

Table 17. Dynamics of the frequency of different levels of pathological process activity in affected joints (according to DAS28) in patients from the examined groups depending on the treatment regimen, %

Activity according to DAS28	Group of patients											
	1, n = 36						2, n = 31					
	Course of treatment											
	Doxycycline + Vitamin D3				Dietary therapy		Doxycycline + Vitamin D3				Vitamin D3	
	Day of treatment											
	Before treatment		29		57		Before treatment		29		57-ий	
	Absolute number	%	Absolute number	%	Absolute number	%	Absolute number	%	Absolute number	%	Absolute number	%
Remission	-	-	23	63,9****	32	88,9***	-	-	9	29,0	27	87,2***
Low	12	33,3	11	30,6	4	11,1**,***	4	12,9	12	38,7*	2	6,4***
Moderate	10	27,8	2	5,5*	-	-	15	48,4	7	22,6*,****	2	6,4**
High	14	38,9	-	-	-	-	12	38,7	3	9,7*	-	-
Total	36	100	36	100,0	36	100,0	31	100	31	100	31	100

Notes:
* – The difference is significant within the same activity in the group before and on the 29th day of treatment, $p < 0.05$;
** – The difference is significant within the same activity in the group before and on the 57th day of treatment, $p < 0.05$;
*** – The difference is significant within the same activity in the group on the 29th and 57th day of treatment, $p < 0.05$;
**** – The difference is significant between groups on the same day after treatment, $p < 0.05$.

In contrast, in patients of Group 2 (LB + CEBVI) after the same initial 28-day treatment, remission of arthritis developed in only 9 (29.0%) individuals, which is significantly fewer than in the comparison group. Low arthritis activity was found in 12 (38.7%) patients, medium activity in 7 (22.6%), and high activity in 3 (9.7%) individuals. Continuing treatment with cholecalciferol for another 28 days (a total of 56 days) achieved remission in 27 (87.2%) patients, with 2 (6.4%) having medium arthritis activity, and the remaining 2 (6.4%) having low activity.

The weaker dynamics of the pathological process activity in affected joints in patients with LB combined with active phase of CEBVI, compared to those with only LB after a 4-week (28 days) treatment with doxycycline and cholecalciferol, is likely related to the fact that the presence of EBV in high concentrations maintains both low vitamin D levels in serum and arthritis activity. Continuing treatment with cholecalciferol (for an additional 28 days) resulted in the suppression of EBV replication and, consequently, the reduction or disappearance of the pathological process activity in the affected joints.

We also assessed the dynamics of other clinical manifestations of the diseases in the examined groups on the 57th day from the start of treatment (Table 18). It was found that at this time, no patient with only LB (Group 1) reported muscle pain, and only 1 (2.8%) patient from this group complained of sleep disturbances (insomnia and/or chronic sleep deprivation), increased fatigue/general weakness, impaired memory and thinking, fever, and swollen lymph nodes.

Meanwhile, among patients with combined infection (LB + CEBVI) receiving ergocalciferol, the percentage of individuals complaining of muscle pain, fever, and swollen lymph nodes significantly decreased compared to the 29th day, $p < 0.05$. At the same time, on the 57th day of therapy, there was no significant difference in the frequency of complaints regarding these issues, as well as sleep disturbances (insomnia and/or chronic sleep deprivation), increased fatigue/general weakness, and impaired memory and thinking between the groups, $p > 0.05$.

Table 18. Dynamics of other clinical manifestations of diseases in the examined groups depending on the treatment regimen, %

Criterion	Group of patients											
	1, n = 36						2, n = 31					
	Course of treatment											
	Doxycycline + Vitamin D3			Dietary therapy			Doxycycline + Vitamin D3			Vitamin D3		
	Day of treatment											
	Before treatment		29		57		Before treatment		29		57	
	Absolute number	%	Absolute number	%	Absolute number	%	Absolute number	%	Absolute number	%	Absolute number	%
Sleep disturbances (insomnia and/or chronic sleep deprivation)	13	36,1	4	11,1*	1	2,8**	12	38,7	5	16,1*	1	3,2**
Increased fatigue/general weakness	12	33,3	3	8,3*	1	2,8**	11	35,5	4	12,9*	1	3,2**
Deterioration of memory and cognition	10	27,7	3	8,3*	1	2,8**	10	32,3	3	9,6*	1	3,2**
Muscle pain	6	16,7	1	2,8*	-	-	12	38,7	7	22,6****	1	3,2**,***
Fever	8	22,2	2	5,6*	1	2,8**	14	45,2	9	29,0****	2	6,5**,***
Enlargement of lymph nodes	10	27,7	3	8,3*	1	2,8**	16	51,6	12	38,7****	4	12,9**,***

Notes:
* – The difference is significant within the same activity in the group before and on the 29th day of treatment, $p < 0.05$;
** – The difference is significant within the same activity in the group before and on the 57th day of treatment, $p < 0.05$;
*** – The difference is significant within the same activity in the group on the 29th and 57th day of treatment, $p < 0.05$;
**** – The difference is significant between groups on the same day after treatment, $p < 0.05$.

Thus, for patients with Lyme borreliosis combined with chronic Epstein-Barr virus infection and vitamin D deficiency, it is advisable to prescribe a combined treatment with doxycycline hydrochloride and ergocalciferol (vitamin D2) orally. This approach not only achieves remission of arthritis and complete correction of vitamin D deficiency but also reduces the percentage of individuals with active Epstein-Barr virus infection.

Conclusion

The primary etiological treatments for Lyme borreliosis include tetracyclines (doxycycline), penicillins (amoxicillin), and cephalosporins (cefuroxime or ceftriaxone). Macrolides (azithromycin, clarithromycin) serve as reserve agents. The selection of antibiotic, its dosage, and duration depend on the patient's age (adult or child), as well as the clinical form and stage of the disease. For patients with Lyme arthritis who show insufficient improvement, a second 2-4-week course of intravenous ceftriaxone should be considered.

Combined treatment using doxycycline hydrochloride and Stevia rebaudiana infusion for adult and paediatric patients with erythema migrans led to a significantly higher clinical recovery rate compared to antibiotic monotherapy and also helped reduce the incidence of doxycycline-induced phototoxic reactions ($p < 0.05$).

Chronic Epstein-Barr virus infection and vitamin D deficiency negatively affect the course of Lyme borreliosis. In such cases, comprehensive treatment that includes doxycycline hydrochloride and ergocalciferol is advisable. This approach results not only in remission of Lyme arthritis and normalization of vitamin D levels, but also in a reduced percentage of individuals with active-phase Epstein-Barr virus infection.

References

[1] Shostakovych-Koretska, L., Budayeva, I., Cherginets, A., Mavrutenkov, V., Marchenko, N. Lyme Borreliosis: Diagnosis and Treatment Issues. *Actual Infectology*. 2014;(2.03):34–8. doi: 10.22141/2312-413x.2.03.2014.82346. [in Ukrainian].

[2] Lindblom, P., Wilhelmsson, P., Fryland, L., Sjöwall, J., Haglund, M., Matussek, A., Ernerudh, J., Vene, S., Nyman, D., Andreassen, A., Forsberg, P., Lindgren, P. E. Tick-borne encephalitis virus in ticks detached from humans and follow-up of serological and clinical response. *Ticks Tick Borne Dis.* 2014;5(1):21–8. doi: 10.1016/j.ttbdis.2013.07.009.

[3] Rollend, L., Fish, D., Childs, J. E. Transovarial transmission of *Borrelia* spirochetes by *Ixodes scapularis*: a summary of the literature and recent observations. *Ticks Tick Borne Dis.* 2013;4(1–2):46–51. doi: 10.1016/j.ttbdis.2012.06.008.

[4] Sanchez, E., Vannier, E., Wormser, G. P., Hu, L. T. Diagnosis, Treatment, and Prevention of Lyme Disease, Human Granulocytic Anaplasmosis, and Babesiosis: A Review. *JAMA*. 2016;315(16):1767–77. doi: 10.1001/jama.2016.2884.

[5] Dubrov, S. O., Andreychyn, M. A., Andreychyn, S. M., Boychuk, A. V., Velychko, V. I., Huk, M. T., Ivakhiv, O. L., Kopcha, V. S., Korda, M. M., Kramariov, S. O., Lahoda, D. O., Putiyenko, O. O., Smiyan, S. I., Chopiak, V. V., Shkilna, M. I., Shkrobot, S. I., Denysiuk, L. I. Standard of medical care. Lyme disease. *Infectious Diseases*. 2024;(4):73–86. doi: 10.11603/1681-2727.2024.4.15009. [in Ukrainian].

[6] Shapiro, E. D. Clinical practice. Lyme disease. *N Engl J Med*. 2014;370(18):1724–31. doi: 10.1056/NEJMcp1314325.

[7] Cameron, D. J., Johnson, L. B., Maloney, E. L. Evidence assessments and guideline recommendations in Lyme disease: the clinical management of known tick bites, erythema migrans rashes and persistent disease. *Expert Rev Anti Infect Ther*. 2014;12(9):1103–35. doi: 10.1586/14787210.2014.940900.

[8] Pothineni, V. R., Parekh, M. B., Babar, M. M., Ambati, A., Maguire, P., Inayathullah, M., Kim, K. M., Tayebi, L., Potula, H. S., Rajadas, J. *In vitro* and *in vivo* evaluation of cephalosporins for the treatment of Lyme disease. *Drug Des Devel Ther*. 2018;12:2915–2921. doi: 10.2147/DDDT.S164966.

[9] Arnež, M., Ružić-Sabljić, E. Azithromycin Is Equally Effective as Amoxicillin in Children with Solitary Erythema Migrans. *Pediatr Infect Dis J*. 2015;34(10):1045–8. doi: 10.1097/INF.0000000000000804.

[10] Feng, J., Auwaerter, P. G., Zhang, Y. Drug combinations against *Borrelia burgdorferi* persisters *in vitro:* eradication achieved by using daptomycin, cefoperazone and doxycycline. *PLoS One.* 2015;10(3):e0117207. doi: 10.1371/journal.pone.0117207.

[11] Cross, R., Ling, C., Day, N. P., McGready, R., Paris, D. H. Revisiting doxycycline in pregnancy and early childhood –time to rebuild its reputation? *Expert Opin Drug Saf.* 2016;15(3):367–82. doi: 10.1517/14740338.2016.1133584.

[12] Klempner, M. S., Baker, P. J., Shapiro, E. D., Marques, A., Dattwyler, R. J., Halperin, J. J., Wormser, G. P. Treatment trials for post-Lyme disease symptoms revisited. *Am J Med.* 2013;126(8):665–9. doi: 10.1016/j.amjmed.2013.02.014.

[13] National Institute for Health and Care Excellence [Internet]. *Lyme disease. NICE guideline [NG95]*; April 11, 2018 [cited 5 February 2025]. Available at: https://www.nice.org.uk/guidance/NG95

[14] Rupprecht, T. A., Koedel, U., Fingerle, V., Pfister, H. W. The pathogenesis of Lyme neuroborreliosis: from infection to inflammation. *Mol Med.* 2008;14(3–4):205–12. doi: 10.2119/2007-00091.

[15] Stricker, R. B., Winger, E. E. Natural killer cells in chronic Lyme disease. *Clin Vaccine Immunol.* 2009;16(11):1704; author reply 1704–6. doi: 10.1128/CVI.00260-09.

[16] Kesteman, T., Rossi, C., Bastien, P., Brouillard, J., Avesani, V., Olive, N., Martin, P., Delmée, M. Prevalence and genetic heterogeneity of *Borrelia burgdorferi* sensu lato in *Ixodes* ticks in Belgium. *Acta Clin Belg.* 2010;65(5):319–22. doi: 10.1179/acb.2010.069.

[17] Zinchuk, O. M. Etiotropic therapy of Lyme borreliosis [Internet]. *News of Medicine and Pharmacy.* 2010;330 [cited 4 Feb 2025]. Available from: http://www.mif-ua.com/archive/article/13590. [in Ukrainian].

[18] Kozlovska, A. Lyme borreliosis: modern principles of treatment from A to Z [Internet]. *Clinical Immunology. Allergology. Infectology.* 2020 [cited 4 Feb 2025];5:34–39. Available from: https://kiai.com.ua/ua/archive/2020/5%28126%29/pages-34-39/laym-borelioz-suchasni-principi-likuvannya-vid-a-do-ya. [in Ukrainian].

[19] Stupica, D., Maraspin, V., Bogovic, P., Ogrinc, K., Blagus, R., Cerar, T., Strle, F. Comparison of Clinical Course and Treatment Outcome for Patients With Early Disseminated or Early Localized Lyme Borreliosis. *JAMA Dermatol.* 2018;154(9):1050–1056. doi: 10.1001/jamadermatol.2018.2306.

[20] Berndtson, K. Review of evidence for immune evasion and persistent infection in Lyme disease. *Int J Gen Med.* 2013;6:291–306. doi: 10.2147/IJGM.S44114.

[21] Timmaraju, V. A., Theophilus, P. A., Balasubramanian, K., Shakih, S., Luecke, D. F., Sapi, E. Biofilm formation by *Borrelia burgdorferi* sensu lato. *FEMS Microbiol Lett.* 2015;362(15):fnv120. doi: 10.1093/femsle/fnv120.

[22] Sapi, E., Balasubramanian, K., Poruri, A., Maghsoudlou, J. S., Socarras, K. M., Timmaraju, A. V., Filush, K. R., Gupta, K., Shaikh, S., Theophilus, P. A., Luecke, D. F., MacDonald, A., Zelger, B. Evidence of *in vivo* existence of *Borrelia* biofilm in borrelial lymphocytomas. *Eur J Microbiol Immunol (Bp).* 2016;6(1):9–24. doi: 10.1556/1886.2015.00049.

[23] Di Domenico, E. G., Cavallo, I., Bordignon, V., D'Agosto, G., Pontone, M., Trento, E., Gallo, M. T., Prignano, G., Pimpinelli, F., Toma, L., Ensoli, F. The emerging role of microbial biofilm in Lyme neuroborreliosis. *Front Neurol.* 2018;9:1048. doi: 10.3389/fneur.2018.01048.

[24] Sapi, E., Gupta, K., Wawrzeniak, K., Gaur, G., Torres, J., Filush, K., Melillo, A., Zelger, B. *Borrelia* and *Chlamydia* can form mixed biofilms in infected human skin tissues. *Eur J Microbiol Immunol (Bp).* 2019;9(2):46–55. doi: 10.1556/1886.2019.00003.

[25] Embers, M. E., Barthold, S. W., Borda, J. T., Bowers, L., Doyle, L., Hodzic, E., Jacobs, M. B., Hasenkampf, N. R., Martin, D. S., Narasimhan, S., Phillippi-Falkenstein, K. M., Purcell, J. E., Ratterree, M. S., Philipp, M. T. Persistence of *Borrelia burgdorferi* in rhesus macaques following antibiotic treatment of disseminated infection. *PLoS One.* 2012;7(1):e29914. doi: 10.1371/journal.pone.0029914.

[26] Stricker, R. B., Johnson, L. *Borrelia burgdorferi* aggrecanase activity: more evidence for persistent infection in Lyme disease. *Front Cell Infect Microbiol.* 2013;3:40. doi: 10.3389/fcimb.2013.00040.

[27] Hodzic, E. Lyme borreliosis: Is there a preexisting (natural) variation in antimicrobial susceptibility among *Borrelia burgdorferi* strains? *Bosn J Basic Med Sci.* 2015;15(3):1–13. doi: 10.17305/bjbms.2015.594.

[28] Bezrodnyi, B. H., Petrenko, O. M. Biofilms of pathogenic bacteria and their role in the chronicization of infectious processes. *Health of Ukraine*. 2014;(3):25–9. [in Ukrainian].

[29] Algburi, A., Comito, N., Kashtanov, D., Dicks, L. M. T., Chikindas, M. L. Control of biofilm formation: antibiotics and beyond. *Appl Environ Microbiol*. 2017;83(3):e02508-16. doi: 10.1128/AEM.02508-16.

[30] Berndtson, K. Review of evidence for immune evasion and persistent infection in Lyme disease. *Int J Gen Med*. 2013;6:291–306. doi: 10.2147/IJGM.S44114.

[31] Kulias, S. M. Current opinion on peculiarities of specific diagnostics, treatment and prevention of Lyme borreliosis [Internet]. *Biomed Biosoc Anthropol*. 2013 [cited 2025 Feb 3];(20):245–51. Available from: http://nbuv.gov.ua/UJRN/bba_2013_20_62. [in Ukrainian].

[32] Steere, A. C., Strle, F., Wormser, G. P., Hu, L. T., Branda, J. A., Hovius, J. W., Li, X., Mead, P. S. Lyme borreliosis. *Nat Rev Dis Primers*. 2016;2:16090. doi: 10.1038/nrdp.2016.90.

[33] Fallahi, P., Elia, G., Bonatti, A. Interferon-γ-induced protein 10 in Lyme disease. *Clin Ter*. 2017;168(2):e146–e150. doi: 10.7417/CT.2017.1997.

[34] Nakanishi, K. Unique action of interleukin-18 on T cells and other immune cells. *Front Immunol*. 2018;9:763. doi: 10.3389/fimmu.2018.00763.

[35] Marques-Rocha, J. L., Samblas, M., Milagro, F. I., Bressan, J., Martínez, J. A., Marti, A. Noncoding RNAs, cytokines, and inflammation-related diseases. *FASEB J*. 2015;29(9):3595–611. doi: 10.1096/fj.14-260323.

[36] Yasuda, K., Nakanishi, K., Tsutsui, H. Interleukin-18 in health and disease. *Int J Mol Sci*. 2019 Feb 2;20(3):649. doi: 10.3390/ijms20030649.

[37] Vuolo, F., Petronilho, F., Sonai, B., Ritter, C., Hallak, J. E., Zuardi, A. W., Crippa, J. A., Dal-Pizzol, F. Evaluation of serum cytokines levels and the role of cannabidiol treatment in animal model of asthma. *Mediators Inflamm*. 2015;2015:538670. doi: 10.1155/2015/538670.

[38] Pages, M., Atard, C. T., Galan, M. B3-integrin sequence variation and rodent susceptibility to hantaviruses. In: *HFRS, HPS and Hantaviruses; 2010 May; Athens, Greece*. Athens; 2010. p. 205.

[39] Paragas, N., Qiu, A., Zhang, Q., Samstein, B., Deng, S. X., Schmidt-Ott, K. M., Viltard, M., Yu, W., Forster, C. S., Gong, G., Liu, Y., Kulkarni, R., Mori, K., Kalandadze, A., Ratner, A. J., Devarajan, P., Landry, D. W., D'Agati, V., Lin, C. S., Barasch, J. The Ngal reporter mouse detects the response of the kidney to injury in real time. *Nat Med*. 2011;17(2):216–22. doi: 10.1038/nm.2290.

[40] Maraspin, V., Lusa, L., Blejec, T., Ružić-Sabljić, E., Pohar Perme, M., Strle, F. Course and outcome of erythema migrans in pregnant women. *J Clin Med*. 2020;9(8):2364. doi: 10.3390/jcm9082364.

[41] Piper, S. C., Ferguson, J., Kay, L., Parker, L. C., Sabroe, I., Sleeman, M. A., Briend, E., Finch, D. K. The role of interleukin-1 and interleukin-18 in pro-inflammatory and anti-viral responses to rhinovirus in primary bronchial epithelial cells. *PLoS One*. 2013;8(5):e63365. doi: 10.1371/journal.pone.0063365.

[42] Shkilna, M. I., Andreychyn, M. A., Ivakhiv, O. L., Iosyk, I. I., Zavidniuk, N. H., Tvorko, M. S. Interleukins dynamic in patients with Lyme borreliosis. *Med Clin Chem*. 2020;(1):17–22. doi: https://doi.org/10.11603/mcch.2410-681X.2020.v.i1.11051. [in Ukrainian].

[43] Sapi, E., Kaur, N., Anyanwu, S., Luecke, D. F., Datar, A., Patel, S., Rossi, M., Stricker, R. B. Evaluation of in-vitro antibiotic susceptibility of different morphological forms of *Borrelia burgdorferi*. *Infect Drug Resist*. 2011;4:97–113. doi: 10.2147/IDR.S19201.

[44] Theophilus, P. A., Victoria, M. J., Socarras, K. M., Filush, K. R., Gupta, K., Luecke, D. F., Sapi, E. Effectiveness of *Stevia rebaudiana* whole leaf extract against the various morphological forms of *Borrelia burgdorferi in vitro*. *Eur J Microbiol Immunol (Bp)*. 2015;5(4):268–80. doi: 10.1556/1886.2015.00031.

[45] Goc, A., Rath, M. The anti-borreliae efficacy of phytochemicals and micronutrients: an update. *Ther Adv Infect Dis*. 2016;3(3–4):75–82. doi: 10.1177/2049936116655502.

[46] Popova, N. V., Litvinenko, V. I., Kutsanyan, A. S. Medicinal plants of the world flora. Kharkiv: Dika Plus; 2016. 405 p. [in Russian].

[47] Siddique, A. B., Rahman, S. M. M., Hossain, M. A., Hossain, M. A., Rashid, M. A. Phytochemical screening and comparative antimicrobial potential of different extract of *Stevia rebaudiana* Bertoni leaves. *Asian Pac J Trop Biomed*. 2014;4:275–80. doi: 10.1016/S2222-1808(14)60572-7.

[48] Muanda, F. N., Soulimani, R., Diop, B., Dico, A. Study on chemical composition and biological activities of essential oil and extracts from *Stevia rebaudiana* Bertoni leaves. *Food Sci Technol.* 2011;44:1865–72. doi: 10.1016/j.lwt.2010.12.002.

[49] Kakkar, S., Bais, S. A review on protocatechuic acid and its pharmacological potential. *ISRN Pharmacol.* 2014 Mar 26;2014:952943. doi: 10.1155/2014/952943.

[50] Gaweł-Bęben, K., Bujak, T., Nizioł-Łukaszewska, Z., Antosiewicz, B., Jakubczyk, A., Karaś, M., Rybczyńska, K. *Stevia rebaudiana* Bert. leaf extracts as a multifunctional source of natural antioxidants. *Molecules.* 2015;20(4):5468–86. doi: 10.3390/molecules20045468.

[51] Shkilna, M. I., Marchyshyn, S. M., Andreychyn, M. A., Ivakhiv, O. L., Korda, M. M., Zaporozhan, S. Y., et al., Increasing efficiency of complex treatment of patients with Lyme borreliosis using *Stevia rebaudiana. Achiev Clin Exp Med.* 2020;(1):195–201. doi: 10.11603/1811-2471.2020.v.i1.11087. [in Ukrainian].

[52] Leeflang, M. M., Ang, C. W., Berkhout, J., Bijlmer, H. A., Van Bortel, W., Brandenburg, A. H., et al., The diagnostic accuracy of serological tests for Lyme borreliosis in Europe: a systematic review and meta-analysis. *BMC Infect Dis.* 2016;16:140. doi: 10.1186/s12879-016-1468-4.

[53] Eldin, C., Raffetin, A., Bouiller, K., Hansmann, Y., Roblot, F., Raoult, D., Parola, P. Review of European and American guidelines for the diagnosis of Lyme borreliosis. *Med Mal Infect.* 2019;49(2):121–32. doi: 10.1016/j.medmal.2018.11.011.

[54] Volokha, A. P. Lyme disease (tick-borne borreliosis) in children. *Infect Dis (Ukr).* 2014;(1):80–7. doi: 10.11603/1681-2727.2014.1.4739. [in Ukrainian].

[55] Kvashnina, L. V., Maidan, I. S. The influence of vitamin D on the immune system during the COVID-19 pandemic (recent data) [Internet]. *Clin Immunol Allergol Infectol.* 2020 [cited 2025 Feb 3];(7):22–30. Available from: https://kiai.com.ua/ua/archive/2020/7%28128%29/pages-22-30/vpliv-vitaminu-d-na-stan-imunnoyi-sistemi-v-period-pandemiyi-covid-novitni-dani-. [in Ukrainian].

[56] Charoenngam, N., Shirvani, A., Holick, M. F. Vitamin D for skeletal and non-skeletal health: what we should know. *J Clin Orthop Trauma.* 2019;10(6):1082–93. doi: 10.1016/j.jcot.2019.07.004.

[57] Teymoori-Rad, M., Shokri, F., Salimi, V., Marashi, S. M. The interplay between vitamin D and viral infections. *Rev Med Virol.* 2019;29(2):e2032. doi: 10.1002/rmv.2032.

[58] Palacios, C., Gonzalez, L. Is vitamin D deficiency a major global public health problem? *J Steroid Biochem Mol Biol.* 2014;144 Pt A:138–45. doi: 10.1016/j.jsbmb.2013.11.003.

[59] Alonso, N., Zelzer, S., Eibinger, G., Herrmann, M. Vitamin D metabolites: analytical challenges and clinical relevance. *Calcif Tissue Int.* 2023;112(2):158–77. doi: 10.1007/s00223-022-00961-5.

[60] Bikle, D. D. Vitamin D: newer concepts of its metabolism and function at the basic and clinical level. *J Endocr Soc.* 2020;4(2):bvz038. doi: 10.1210/jendso/bvz038.

[61] Tuckey, R. C., Cheng, C. Y. S., Slominski, A. T. The serum vitamin D metabolome: what we know and what is still to discover. *J Steroid Biochem Mol Biol.* 2019;186:4–21. doi: 10.1016/j.jsbmb.2018.09.003.

[62] Araújo, J., Santos, A., Ramos, E. Vitamin D – from the pro-hormone to the biological actions. *Acta Port Nutr.* 2019;19:50–4. doi: 10.21011/apn.2019.1909.

[63] Hammami, M. M., Yusuf, A. Differential effects of vitamin D2 and D3 supplements on 25-hydroxyvitamin D level are dose, sex, and time dependent: a randomized controlled trial. *BMC Endocr Disord.* 2017;17(1):12. doi: 10.1186/s12902-017-0163-9.

[64] Tripkovic, L., Lambert, H., Hart, K., Smith, C. P., Bucca, G., Penson, S. Comparison of vitamin D2 and vitamin D3 supplementation in raising serum 25-hydroxyvitamin D status: a systematic review and meta-analysis. *Am J Clin Nutr.* 2012;95(6):1357–64. doi: 10.3945/ajcn.111.031070.

[65] Grygorieva, N., Tronko, M., Kovalenko, V., Komisarenko, S., Tatarchuk, T., Dedukh, N. Diagnosis, prevention and treatment of vitamin D deficiency in adults: Ukrainian experts consensus statement. *Pain Joints Spine.* 2023;13(2):60–76. doi: 10.22141/pjs.13.2.2023.368.

[66] DAS28 [Internet]. *DAS28 calculator.* (n.d.) [cited 2025 Feb 5]. Available from: https://www.das-score.nl/das28/DAScalculators/dasculators.html

[67] Pérez-Pérez, S., Domínguez-Mozo, M. I., García-Martínez, M. Á., Aladro, Y., Martínez-Ginés, M., García-Domínguez, J. M., et al., Study of the possible link of 25-hydroxyvitamin D with Epstein-Barr virus and human herpesvirus 6 in patients with multiple sclerosis. *Eur J Neurol.* 2018;25(12):1446–53. doi: 10.1111/ene.13749.

Chapter 6

Prevention of Lyme Borreliosis

Mykhaylo Andreychyn[1]
Mariia Shkilna[2],
Oleh Ivakhiv[3]
Ihor Rogalskyi[4]
and Stepan Zaporozhan[5]

[1]Academician of the National Academy of Medical Sciences of Ukraine,
Honoured Master of Sciences and Technologies of Ukraine, DSc in Medicine, Professor,
Head of the Department of Infectious Diseases with Epidemiology, Dermatology and Venerology,
I. Horbachevsky Ternopil National Medical University, Ternopil, Ukraine
[2]DSc in Medicine, Professor, Department of Infectious Diseases with Epidemiology,
Dermatology and Venerology, I. Horbachevsky Ternopil National Medical University, Ternopil, Ukraine
[3]Honoured Doctor of Ukraine, PhD in Medicine, Associate Professor,
Department of Infectious Diseases with Epidemiology, Dermatology and Venerology,
I. Horbachevsky Ternopil National Medical University, Ternopil, Ukraine
[4]Honoured Doctor of Ukraine, PhD in Medicine, Associate Professor,
Department of Paediatrics of the Postgraduate Education Faculty,
I. Horbachevsky Ternopil National Medical University, Ternopil, Ukraine
[5]Honoured Health Worker of Ukraine, DSc in Medicine, Professor,
Department of General Surgery, I. Horbachevsky Ternopil National Medical University, Ternopil, Ukraine

Abstract

The chapter presents data on primary prevention of Lyme borreliosis, specifically regarding appropriate attire when visiting endemic areas. It outlines key modern repellents, their mechanisms of action, application methods, duration of protective effect, and age categories for which they are suitable. A classification of repellents by dosage form is provided. The importance of self- and mutual body examination to detect attached ticks is emphasized. Guidelines for tick removal using micro-forceps or tick-twisters are discussed. The chapter also presents primary and alternative schemes for emergency antibiotic prophylaxis of Lyme borreliosis and a physician's algorithm for justifying secondary (post-contact) prevention.

Keywords: Lyme borreliosis, primary and secondary prevention, repellents, acaricides, antibiotic prophylaxis, vaccines

In: Lyme Borreliosis
Editors: Mykhaylo Andreychyn, Mykhaylo Korda, Maria Shkilna and Oleh Ivakhiv
ISBN: 979-8-89530-657-4

1. Introduction

Prevention plays a crucial role in combating Lyme borreliosis. Both primary and secondary (post-contact) prevention methods are employed. Currently, several repellents are available; however, the general public is often unaware of how to correctly and frequently apply them to the body or clothing, the duration of their protective effect, which products are suitable for children, and whether repellents can be combined with other creams or sprays. Post-contact prevention requires particular attention. It involves the emergency use of antibiotics to which Borrelia are sensitive, with a shorter course than the treatment of the disease. Often, physicians prescribe antibiotics unnecessarily and for prolonged periods, which can negatively impact the human body.

1. Primary Prophylaxis

Mariia Shkilna
Stepan Zaporozhan
and Ihor Rogalskyi

To avoid Lyme borreliosis, it is recommended not to visit places where ticks may be present. If unavoidable, it is necessary to take the following steps: wear protective clothing such as long pants tucked into socks and a shirt with long sleeves to maximize skin isolation from tick attacks. It is preferable to wear light-coloured clothing, as ticks are more visible on such clothing [1].

Before visiting forests or other areas populated by ticks, it is advisable to treat clothing and exposed skin with repellents. Repellents (Latin repellentia, repellere – to repel, drive away) are substances that deter arthropods (insects, ticks). They are used to protect humans and animals from arthropod attacks for the prevention of vector-borne diseases (Lyme borreliosis, anaplasmosis, tick-borne encephalitis, leishmaniasis, malaria, mosquito-borne fever, etc.). Repellents typically include synthetic compounds of varying chemical structure with different durations of repellent action. By their mechanism of action, repellents are classified as follows: olfactory, or fumigants (volatile substances that act at a distance on the nervous endings of arthropods' olfactory organs), contact (act upon contact of arthropods with the treated surface), deodorizing, or masking (neutralize or destroy odours that attract arthropods) [2, 3].

Modern repellents that exhibit both olfactory and contact actions simultaneously are the most effective. These include diethyltoluamide, benzimidazole, carboxylic acid, ethylamide of phenoxyacetic acid, benzoylpyridine, and oxyimine. They are used in the form of solutions, water emulsions, and aerosols for treating clothing, protective nets, and tents at a rate of 20-30 grams of the preparation per 1 square meter of fabric. A single application of repellent to the skin provides protection against blood-sucking arthropods for 2-5 hours; clothing impregnated with repellent retains protective properties for 2-3 weeks without washing, and when treated with an aerosol can, for 1-2 days. The duration of protective action depends on the dosage of the substance, the number and type of blood-sucking arthropods, meteorological factors, and working conditions. Formulations of universal action have been developed that combine repellent properties with insecticidal ones. Repellents are available in the form of sprays, sticks, and lotions. The most common form is spray, which allows for quick and even treatment of large surfaces of clothing or the body.

Rules for applying repellents:

1. Apply a very thin layer only on exposed skin areas, but not under clothing.
2. Before applying to the face, distribute a small amount of repellent between the palms, then apply to the face.
3. After application, thoroughly wash hands with soap to prevent residue from getting into the eyes, mouth, or mucous membranes.
4. Do not apply to damaged skin (burns, wounds).
5. Avoid contact with mucous membranes of the eyes, lips, and nose.
6. Do not apply repellents in aerosols and sprays in enclosed spaces or near food products.
7. Do not apply to the hands of small children (they may suck fingers or rub their eyes).
8. Reapply according to the manufacturer's recommendations.
9. Do not combine products: sunscreen + repellent, as sunscreen needs to be reapplied more frequently than repellent.
10. Wash off with water immediately upon skin irritation.

The most common repellents are products containing:

1. N,N-Diethyl-meta-toluamide (DEET) – the "gold standard" among repellents, effective against mosquitoes, ticks, flies, and gnats. It is used in concentrations ranging from 10 to 30%. The duration of protection depends on the concentration of the active ingredient: at 10% concentration, protection lasts for 2 hours, and at over 24%, it lasts for up to 5 hours. The American Academy of Paediatrics allows the use of DEET in children from 2 months of age when all safety rules are followed.
2. Picaridin – odourless, non-irritating to the skin, effective at concentrations of 20% and higher. It is less toxic than DEET and approved for use in children older than 2 months.
3. Oil of lemon eucalyptus – a plant-based compound, less effective than DEET and picaridin. It is used in concentrations of at least 30% and can cause eye irritation. Approved for use in children older than 3 years.

Ticks spend a long time searching for a spot to attach (they latch onto the body for up to 2 hours). To promptly detect them, it's necessary to conduct self-examinations and mutual inspections every 2 hours while in forests or other tick-infested areas, and after leaving them [4].

When performing self and mutual body inspections to detect attached parasites, special attention should be paid to the neck, armpits, groin areas, and ear shells – as these areas have particularly delicate and thin skin, ticks most commonly attach there [5]. If a tick is found, it should be immediately removed using fine-tipped tweezers or a special tool called a tick twister (Figures 1, 2), avoiding crushing the parasite itself. It is strongly recommended not to treat an attached tick with any ointments or alcohol that could interfere with its breathing. Such actions can cause the tick to release saliva into the skin more intensely, increasing the risk of infection with Lyme disease bacteria in humans.

Measures aimed at reducing the tick population in their habitats include mowing tall grass and acaricide treatment of the area, among others.

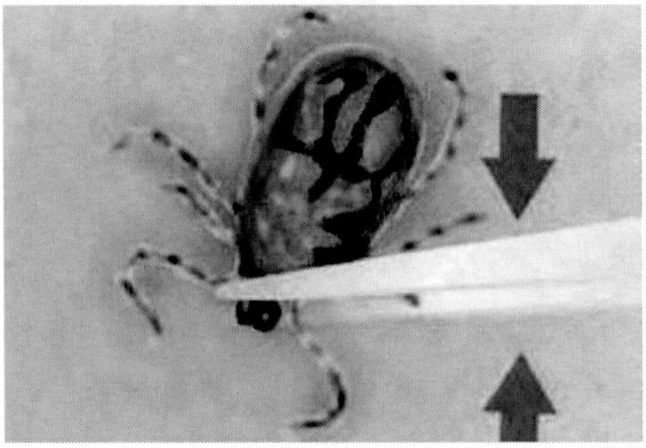

Figure 1. Tick removal using fine-tipped forceps.

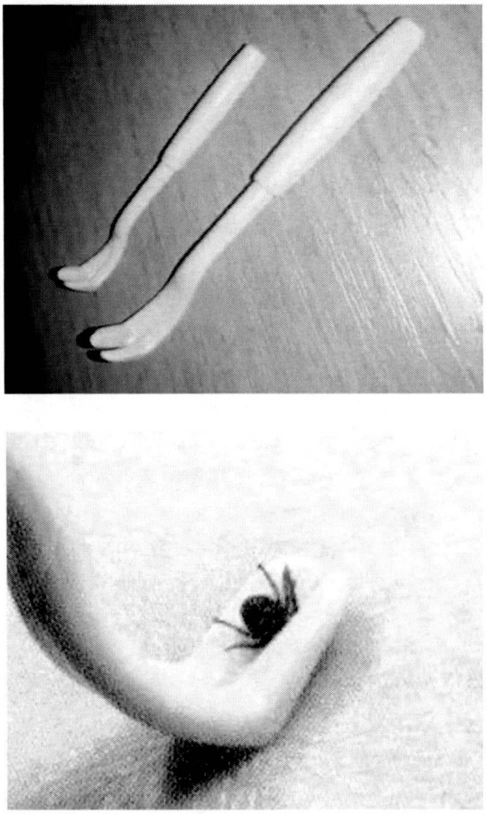

Figure 2. Tick twisters for tick removal and the process of performing such an operation.

Vaccination is currently not available. In the USA, a corresponding vaccine was developed, and it even underwent clinical trials [6]. Its effectiveness reached 80%. However, due to weak demand, the vaccine was removed from the market. Currently, the search continues for a more effective and affordable vaccine for populations in hyperendemic areas and high-risk groups (foresters, hunters, mushroom and berry pickers, park and recreational workers, etc.) [7].

2. Secondary (Post-Exposure) Prophylaxis

Mykhaylo Andreychyn
and Oleh Ivakhiv

Emergency antibiotic prophylaxis for LB involves administering antibiotics during the incubation period when Borrelia bacteria are present in relatively low quantities. This approach allows for using lower doses of antibiotics for a shorter duration compared to treatment during active disease.

Emergency prophylaxis for LB is strictly individualized in cases where it is precisely determined that the tick was infected with Borrelia or when the tick bite occurred in an area with a high risk of infection, typically where more than 20% of ticks are infected. Ticks are tested for Borrelia infection using methods such as dark-field microscopy or PCR, which is more sensitive.

One of the key requirements for the use of antibiotics from various pharmacological groups in emergency prophylaxis is their effective penetration and accumulation in the skin – the site of pathogen persistence during the incubation period of Lyme borreliosis. In the past, various classes of antibiotics (penicillins, tetracyclines, macrolides), which are also indicated for the treatment of manifest forms of the disease, were used for this type of Lyme borreliosis prophylaxis. The recommended duration of antibiotic prophylaxis typically ranged from 5 to 10 days. However, prolonged courses of antibiotic prophylaxis have not demonstrated high efficacy, while the risk of adverse reactions remains significant.

Therefore, new recommendations for emergency antibiotic prophylaxis of Lyme borreliosis have now been proposed. An evidence-based post-contact prevention scheme includes the administration of oral doxycycline hydrochloride (0.2 g for adults and 4.4 mg/kg body weight for children over 8 years old) as a single dose [8]. When prescribing post-contact prophylaxis, the following indications must be strictly adhered to:

- The bite occurred in an area with a tick infection rate of B. burgdorferi s. l. of 20.0% or more;
- The tick belongs to the Ixodidae family;
- The duration of tick attachment was ≥ 36 hours;
- Post-contact prophylaxis is initiated no later than 72 hours after tick removal;
- The patient has no contraindications to the use of doxycycline hydrochloride (the drug is contraindicated in pregnant women, breastfeeding mothers, children under 8 years old, and in cases of allergy).

Antibiotic prophylaxis is not indicated if the tick attachment time was less than 36 hours.

Antibiotic therapy in the early stages (up to 5 days after tick attachment) is capable of interrupting the infectious process in practically all patients, with the effectiveness quite high (67-87%). The use of antibiotic prophylaxis later may likely have lower effectiveness.

According to the guidelines of the Polish Society of Epidemiologists and Infectious Diseases Specialists, the sole indication for prophylactic use of a single dose of doxycycline (200 mg) could be multiple tick bites in an endemic region on an adult who has arrived from another locality [9].

The use of a single dose of doxycycline for the prophylaxis of Lyme disease following a tick bite is debated for several reasons: the low risk of Borrelia transmission, the contraindication of the antibiotic for children under eight years of age and pregnant women, and the lack of convincing evidence regarding the clinical effectiveness of such prophylaxis. Given that the risk of infection remains low even in regions endemic for Lyme borreliosis, and that the disease is generally responsive to treatment after symptom onset, a watchful waiting approach is preferred over prophylaxis – particularly in paediatric cases [10]. It is recommended that individuals who have experienced a tick bite be observed for 30 days for monitoring purposes. Should clinical manifestations such as erythema migrans, fever, or arthralgia occur, appropriate treatment is administered.

Therefore, the decision to prescribe antibiotic prophylaxis should be made on a case-by-case basis. Further research in this area is warranted.

Conclusion and Future Prospects

The authors advocate for a comprehensive approach to addressing current issues in Lyme borreliosis prevention. Numerous acaricidal agents have been developed to reduce tick populations in the environment; however, their rational use in specific field conditions requires additional scientific and practical efforts. Special preventive protection is needed for at-risk groups, including professionals such as foresters. Public health education plays a vital role in preventing tick bites and the onset of the disease. Timely antibiotic prophylaxis significantly reduces the likelihood of developing Lyme borreliosis.

The use of new vaccines against Lyme borreliosis, which are currently in the stages of development and testing, should decrease the incidence of this infection. At the same time, the modern trend of Lyme borreliosis and other tick-borne infections spreading necessitates the study and development of new methods to combat arthropods. One such method is biological control of tick populations in nature [11]. This is implemented through natural tick antagonists, such as birds, insects, microscopic fungi, helminths, etc. Scientific research in this direction is at an early stage. The introduction of new types of vaccines in the future may potentially reduce the incidence of tick-borne infections in humans. Currently, promising anti-Borrelia vaccines are being developed. Researchers are also working on creating reservoir-oriented vaccines to be administered to rodents (the primary reservoir of the infection), which will help reduce pathogen transmission by ticks [12]. Another new and promising approach is the creation of Borrelia-refractory ticks with modified genomes; however, this area requires thorough research.

References

[1] Andreychyn, M. A., Kopcha, V. S., Shkilna, M. I., Klishch, I. M., Korda, M. M., Nykytyuk, S. O., Zavidnyuk, N. G., Nychyk, N. A., eds. *Lyme Borreliosis. Diagnostic criteria, treatment, and prevention.* Ternopil: TSMU, Ukrmedknyga; 2018. 42 p. [in Ukrainian].

[2] Aenishaenslin, C., Michel, P., Ravel, A., Gern, L., Milord, F., Waaub, J. P., Bélanger, D. Factors associated with preventive behaviors regarding Lyme disease in Canada and Switzerland: a comparative study. *BMC Public Health.* 2015;15:185. doi: 10.1186/s12889-015-1539-2.

[3] Vynohrad, N. O., Vasylyshyn, Z. P., Kozak, L. P. General epidemiology. Kyiv: Medicine; 2017. 200 p. [in Ukrainian].

[4] Valente, S. L., Wemple, D., Ramos, S., Cashman, S. B., Savageau, J. A. Preventive behaviors and knowledge of tick-borne illnesses: results of a survey from an endemic area. *J Public Health Manag Pract*. 2015;21(3):E16-23. doi: 10.1097/PHH.0000000000000098.

[5] Stjernberg L., Berglund J. Risk of acquiring tick bites in south-eastern Sweden. *Scand J Infect Dis*. 2002;34(11):840-4. doi: 10.1080/0036554021000026955.

[6] Slunge, D., Boman, A. Learning to live with ticks? The role of exposure and risk perceptions in protective behaviour against tick-borne diseases. *PLoS One*. 2018;13(6):e0198286. doi: 10.1371/journal.pone.0198286.

[7] Kullberg, B. J., Vrijmoeth, H. D., van de Schoor, F., Hovius, J. W. Lyme borreliosis: diagnosis and management. *BMJ*. 2020;369:m1041. doi: 10.1136/bmj.m1041.

[8] Harms, M. G., Hofhuis, A., Sprong, H., Bennema, S. C., Ferreira, J. A., Fonville, M., Docters van Leeuwen, A., Assendelft, W. J. J., Van Weert, H. C. P. M., Van Pelt, W., Van den Wijngaard, C. C. A single dose of doxycycline after an ixodes ricinus tick bite to prevent Lyme borreliosis: An open-label randomized controlled trial. *J Infect*. 2021 Jan;82(1):98-104. doi: 10.1016/j.jinf.2020.06.032.

[9] Flisiak, R. Boreliosa of Lyme. In: Cianciara, J., Juszczyk, J., editors. *Infectious and parasitic diseases*. Vol.2. Lublin: Czelej Publishing House; 2012. 621 p.

[10] Sutton D, Spry C. One Dose of Doxycycline for the Prevention of Lyme Disease: A Review of Clinical Effectiveness and Guidelines [Internet]. *Ottawa (ON): Canadian Agency for Drugs and Technologies in Health; 2019 May 21*. Available from: https://www.ncbi.nlm.nih.gov/books/NBK545493/.

[11] Hunfeld, K., Gray, J. eds. Lyme Borreliosis. *Cham: Springer International Publishing, 2022*. http://dx.doi.org/10.1007/978-3-030-93680-8.

[12] Kern, A., Zhou, C. W., Jia, F., Xu, Q., Hu, L. T. Live-vaccinia virus encapsulation in pH-sensitive polymer increases safety of a reservoir-targeted Lyme disease vaccine by targeting gastrointestinal release. *Vaccine*. 2016. 34(38), 4507–4513. https://doi.org/10.1016/j.vaccine.2016.07.059.

Chapter 7

Results and Suggestions

Mykhaylo Andreychyn[1]
Mykhaylo Korda[2]
Mariia Shkilna[3]
and Oleh Ivakhiv[4]

[1]Academician of the National Academy of Medical Sciences of Ukraine,
Honoured Master of Sciences and Technologies of Ukraine, DSc in Medicine, Professor,
Head of the Department of Infectious Diseases with Epidemiology, Dermatology and Venerology,
I. Horbachevsky Ternopil National Medical University, Ternopil, Ukraine
[2]Corresponding Member of the National Academy of Medical Sciences of Ukraine,
Honoured Master of Sciences and Technologies of Ukraine, DSc in Medicine, Professor,
Department of Medical Biochemistry, I. Horbachevsky Ternopil National Medical University,
Ternopil, Ukraine
[3]DSc in Medicine, Professor, Department of Infectious Diseases with Epidemiology,
Dermatology and Venerology, I. Horbachevsky Ternopil National Medical University, Ternopil, Ukraine
[4]Honoured Doctor of Ukraine, PhD in Medicine, Associate Professor,
Department of Infectious Diseases with Epidemiology, Dermatology and Venerology,
I. Horbachevsky Ternopil National Medical University, Ternopil, Ukraine

Lyme borreliosis (LB) is the most common natural focal infection from the group of bacterial zoonoses, which is caused by *Borrelia* spp., is transmitted mainly by ticks and affects the skin, musculoskeletal, cardiovascular and nervous systems. In recent years, the geographical range of disease registration has significantly expanded, with a substantial increase in incidence. WHO experts believe that the number of reported cases is at least five times less than the actual incidence. Ticks are already being detected in more than 80 countries, and by 2050 they could affect 35% of the world's population.

In Ukraine, Lyme borreliosis has been officially classified as a group of particularly dangerous infectious diseases, with official registration starting in 2000. There is a trend of increasing Lyme borreliosis incidence in all regions, with the highest number of cases registered in the forest-steppe landscape-geographical zone. There are reasons to believe that current official statistics regarding Lyme borreliosis are significantly underestimated. The underreporting is due, on one hand, to insufficient public awareness regarding Lyme borreliosis and, consequently, neglect of preventive measures, delayed seeking of medical help after tick

In: Lyme Borreliosis
Editors: Mykhaylo Andreychyn, Mykhaylo Korda, Maria Shkilna and Oleh Ivakhiv
ISBN: 979-8-89530-657-4

bites, and on the other hand, low suspicion among doctors regarding this disease, frequent misdiagnoses, and imperfect laboratory diagnostics.

Obviously, there are no isolated natural foci of individual blood infections. In Europe, there are associated foci in which up to seven pathogens circulate, that can be transmitted to humans during the tick bites. It was found that 84.4% of LB cases occur as a mixed infection with tick-borne encephalitis, human granulocytic anaplasmosis and/or monocytic ehrlichiosis. In addition, ticks are also carriers or reservoirs of pathogens of tularaemia, tick-borne viral and spring-summer encephalitis, Crimea-Congo haemorrhagic fever, rickettsioses, babesiosis, Q fever and others. In recent years, the epidemic situation is often complicated by an increase in the number of tick attacks in urban areas. The formation of urban endemic foci is a recognized problem.

The results of our research confirmed the possibility of LB in the population of Ukraine in the form of both mono- and mixed infections in connection with the proven infection of 36.0% of ticks selected from humans by pathogens of tick-borne infections. Thus, *B. burgdorferi s. l.* was found in 19.2% of ticks, *A. phagocytophilum* – in 14.7%, *B. miyamotoi* – in 1.7%, *Babesia sp.* – in 0.3%. At the same time, 3.8% of ticks removed from humans were infected with several pathogens simultaneously.

Lyme borreliosis is caused by a heterogeneous population of different species of bacteria of the Borrelia genus. The general list of *Borrelia spp.* includes not only pathogenic for humans bacteria that are factors of LB, tick-borne fever, louse typhus, but also a large group of spirochetes of this genus, whose role in the pathology of humans is proven only in certain areas or not yet clarified, as well as non-pathogenic microbes. At present, Borrelia of the LB group (more than 50 species) form the *B. burgdorferi s. l.* complex. Of the spirochetes of the group of tick-borne relapsing fever, *B. miyamotoi, B. lonestari*, and *B. theileri* are mostly found in humans. Thus, cases of *B. miyamotoi* disease have been reported in Europe and the United States, including foresters. We established the involvement of *B. miyamotoi* in the occurrence of intoxication syndrome and lesions of the musculoskeletal system in 29.8% of foresters of Ternopil region on the basis of detection of IgM antibodies and/or IgG (immunoblot) simultaneously to *B. miyamotoi* and *B. burgdorferi s. l.*

The performed studies allowed us to expand the range of pathogens for EF (erythematous form) and NEF (non-erythematous form) LB in patients with predominant lesions of the musculoskeletal system. In some of such patients, anti-IgM was detected simultaneously to OspC of *B. spielmanii, B. burgdorferi s. l., B. garinii* and *B. afzelii*, in particular in 78.9% of patients with EF and in 64.7% – with NEF, using the method of immunoblot EUROLINE *Borrelia* RN-AT adv.

In addition to the typical form of *Borrelia* spp., other morphologically altered variants are described, which are called "forms of unbalanced growth". It has been proven that cystic and granular forms retain the ability to reproduce, and under certain conditions can reverse into normal spiral forms, while retaining pathogenic properties. It is assumed that the formation of atypical forms contributes to the survival of spirochetes and the development of chronic forms of LB.

Not all *Borrelia* spp. from *B. burgdorferi s. l.* complex are pathogenic to humans. In Europe, the pathogenicity of five gene species – *B. burgdorferi s. l., B. garinii, B. afzelii, B. spielmanii* and *B. bavariensis*, is proven. Some scientists note that in the western regions of Ukraine pathogenic to humans are *B. burgdorferi s. l., B. garinii, B. afzelii, B. lusitaniae* and *B. valaisiana*; other scientists note that besides *B. burgdorferi s. l., B. garinii, B. afzelii*, also *B. valaisiana* and *B. spielmanii* are considered. The prevalence of these *Borrelia* spp. in different countries is different, as well as other members of the *B. burgdorferi s. l.* complex.

More than 100 proteins (lipoproteins) have been found in *B. burgdorferi*, the biological significance of most of them is unknown. The quantitative ratio of individual surface proteins, even in Borrelia of one species, varies widely. Particularly variable content of surface proteins OspA and OspC was noted. The greatest heterogeneity of protein composition is found in *B. garinii* (for OspA – 7, OspC – 13 variants) and *B. afzelii* (for OspA – 2, OspC – 8 variants).

Borrelia of the *B. burgdorferi s. l.* complex use hard ticks of the genus *Ixodes* as vectors, with the main role played by four species of ticks of the complex *I. ricinus*: *I. ricinus L* (Europe), *I. persulcatus Schulze* (Asia), *I. scapularis Say* (Atlantic coast of the USA) and *I. pacificus Cooley & Kohls* (Pacific Coast of the USA). It has been proved that the ticks *I. pavlovskyi* (taiga tick), common in the Altai and the Far East, are also carriers of *Borrelia* spp.

Borrelia-infected ticks infect animals through feeding through saliva, and uninfected ticks become infected from animals with Borrelia in their blood. The population of vertebrates, which are the sources and reservoirs of LB pathogens, includes more than 200 species, including small mammals (voles, rats, squirrels, hares, hedgehogs, etc.), other wild and domestic animals, and more than 170 species of birds (mostly those nesting on the ground). Migratory birds probably play a significant role in the spread of Borrelia, as they are not only reservoirs and hosts for species such as *B. burgdorferi, B. garinii, B. valaisiana*, but also carry infected ticks over long distances.

Borrelia are transmitted to humans during the bites of *Ixodes* ticks, which are not only vectors, but also the main reservoirs of *Borrelia* spp, as they retain them throughout their lives and can be transmitted transovarially to offspring. Due to transphase, transovarian and transmissible transmission of the pathogen, ticks become infected at any stage of their development and are able to retain Borrelia when the seasons change for more than 4 years.

It was found that one *I. ricinus* tick can simultaneously carry up to seven pathogens of viral and bacterial aetiology. Mixed infection mostly causes an atypical course of the disease, complicates diagnosis and, as a consequence, treatment. According to the literature review, the infestation of ticks with several pathogens simultaneously in different European countries ranges from 3.2 to 45.0% of the tick population.

Ticks attach to humans most often to the neck, chest, armpits and other skin folds, i.e. in areas with thin skin and heavy blood supply. Initially, the tick transmits Borrelia, which are located in the salivary glands. If they are only in the intestines of the tick, their transmission is carried out in the second phase of nutrition (1–2 days after the bite). Therefore, early removal of ticks prevents in some cases human infection. There is a possibility for the transmission of the pathogens through the feces of ticks when they get on the skin followed by their subsequent rubbing and incorporation into the skin microcracks when scratching. Cases of mechanical transmission of Borrelia during accidental crushing of ticks during their removal from animals (dogs, cats), when the contents of the tick intestine get into the microcracks of the skin or conjunctiva of the eyes, are also likely. There is also an alimentary way of infection (i.e., eating contaminated raw goat's milk or dairy pro- ducts without prior heat treatment). Borrelia can also be transmitted transplacentally during pregnancy from mother to foetus.

To collect ticks, we have developed tools that are more effective than the traditional "flag" method, including a flag on an L-shaped holder and a flag on 2 parallel metal rods. On the traditional flag after its application, the average number of ticks per flag-kilometre was 3.9 pieces, on the flag on a L-shaped holder – 12.7 pieces, while on the flag on 2 parallel metal rods – 13.4 pieces. Therefore, the proposed modified flags have significant advantages over the traditional flag for collecting ticks in natural habitats.

To assess epidemic threats, predict the activity of natural foci of tick infections, the stability of the parasitic system, traditionally the so-called zooparasitological indices are used, namely: abundance, dominance, detection and others. However, in our opinion, the main objective indicator of the number of ticks on territories can be the population index, or the settlement index, i.e. the number of ticks per unit area. Estimation of the number of ticks in the terms of area allows us to talk about the population density of ticks and has a perspective on the standardization of indicators. This indicator in combination with others (for example, tick infestation and the degree of infection with pathogenic microorganisms) allows to develop criteria for assessing epidemic risks.

During 2017–2019, acarological surveys of various forest biotopes of Ternopil region were conducted: 8 biotopes, 5 forestries, 3 climatic and weather zones (Small Polissia, Cold and Warm Podilia (Dniester Canyon)) and 5 parks in Ternopil. When analysing the obtained results using the coefficient of oscillation, it was found that when using our method, compared to the conventional one, it is smaller, so it allows you to more accurately calculate and estimate the population of habitats or surveyed areas by ticks.

During the observation period, the lowest average level of tick abundance index was established in the area of Small Polissia (7.3). In the zone of Cold Podilia it was 11.1 with fluctuations from 3.7 to 19.1, in the zone of Warm Podilia – 11.2 with fluctuations from 8.0 to 13.1. Thus, this index increases from north to south, from the zone of coniferous forests (Small Polissia) to mixed (forest-steppe) and in the direction of increasing average annual air temperatures.

Among the collected ticks, 96.2% were of the species *I. ricinus*, of which 33.2% were females and 30.4% were males, and 36.4% were nymphs. The share of *D. reticulatus* was 3.7% of all collected ticks, of which 65.6% were females and 34.4% – males.

The surveyed habitats and natural-geographical areas differ in the number and species composition of murine rodents. The most common are forest mice and yellow-breasted mice. Their numbers are growing in the direction from north to south. The number of bank voles is the highest in Small Polissia. The area of Warm Podilia, especially the southern biotope with oak-hornbeam forest and undergrowth, has the highest number of rodents and the largest species composition.

According to PCR tick studies, DNA of *B. burgdorferi s. l., B. miyamotoi, A. phagocytophilum* and *Babesia sp.*, were found in Ternopil region. At the same time, no DNA of pathogens monocytic ehrlichiosis – *E. muris* and *E. chaffeensis* – were found in ticks. Share of *B. burgdorferi s. l.* amounted up to 53.6% of all detected pathogens: in the area of Small Polissia their percentage was 66.7%, Cold Podilia – 60.9%, and Warm Podilia – 44.5%. That is, the share of these Borrelia in the sum of positive findings decreased in the direction from north to south. At the same time, the percentage of positive results in general and the findings of *Babesia sp., B. miyamotoi* had the opposite trend. Obviously, the peculiarities of flora and fauna, geographical remoteness, weather conditions contributed to the formation of various natural foci of tick infections in Ternopil region.

Among ticks, males and females accounted for 72.5% of all pathogens detected, of which 80% were *A. phagocytophilum*, 70% – *B. burgdorferi s. l.*, and 67% – *B. miyamotoi*. The simplest *Babesia sp.* was more often found in pools of larvae and nymphs (62.5%). The higher infestation of adults with pathogenic bacteria is obviously due to the changes in a larger number of hosts, as *I. ricinus* and *D. reticulatus* belong to ticks with a three-year development cycle.

Between 2018 and 2019, 358 ticks were collected from five recreational parks of Ternopil, which were divided into 63 pools. Two pools were *D. reticulatus* (female and nymph), the rest (61) – *I. ricinus* (111 females, 130 males, 115 larvae and nymphs). The most common pathogens were *B. burgdorferi s. l.* (found in 46.8% of pools), less often – *A. phagocytophilum*, even less often – *Babesia sp.* In general, infestation with pathogens other than *Babesia sp.*, of imago ticks is higher than ticks of preimaginal stages of development. No significant difference was found between the infection of male and female pools, with the exception of *B. miyamotoi* infection. In pools, where DNA fragments of several pathogenic microorganisms were detected simultaneously, *B. burgdorferi s. l.* (72.7%) and *A. phagocytophilum* (66.6%), were the most common. Thus, in the parks of Ternopil, there are combined anthropurgical foci of transmissible infections, which maintain the circulation of *B. burgdorferi s. l., B. miyamotoi, A. phagocytophilum*, and *Babesia sp.* The dominant vector is *I. ricinus*. The existing risks of human infection are exacerbated by the recreational function of parks. These studies are used during a set of anti-epidemic measures and in clinical practice. An important scientific task is to identify the circulation on the territory of various landscape-geographical zones of Ukraine of unexplored species and genotypes of Borrelia and pathogens of other tick infections.

During 2017–2019, we studied 1226 ticks removed from humans, of which 1179 were obtained from residents of Ternopil and the region, 47 – from residents of other regions of Ukraine. According to the interviews of bitten humans, almost one in five of them was attacked by ticks in the cities and villages of Ternopil region, except for the city of Ternopil. One in three Ternopil residents has been attacked by ticks in park areas, one in five – in the suburban areas of the city and surrounding villages, and one in seven – even in places outside the parks. Tick attacks were recorded from February to November with peaks in May – June.

Among the identified ticks, 98.9% were *I. ricinus*, 0.9% – *D. reticulatus*, and 0.2% – *R. sanguineus*. When identifying ticks of the species *I. ricinus* by sex and stage of development, it was noted that females were 32.3%, males – 0.9%, larvae – 2.6%, most (53.5%) were nymphs; in 10.6% of ticks we failed to establish the stage of development and sex. DNA of only one of the pathogens (*B. burgdorferi s. l., B. miyamotoi, A. phagocytophilum and Babesia sp.*) was found in a third of the studied ticks, simultaneous presence of several pathogens – in 3.8%. There are 6 types of different combinations: two pathogens were found in 45 ticks, three – in 2 ticks, *B. burgdorferi s. l.* was present in all 6 combinations, *A. phagocytophilum* – in 84.4% of all mixed infections.

For the first time, we conducted a survey of 1,070 forestry workers in Volyn, Zhytomyr, Transcarpathian, Ternopil, Khmelnytskyi, Chernivtsi and Chernihiv regions to find out their knowledge of LB and to identify the risks of infecting foresters with Borrelia while performing their professional duties. Also, 723 students of Ternopil National Universities were interviewed, including two non-medical and one medical, namely, 119 students from Ternopil Volodymyr Hnatiuk National Pedagogical University, 133 – from Ternopil Ivan Puluj National Technical University, and 471 – from I. Horbachevsky Ternopil National Medical University.

This survey was conducted in the framework of research projects of the European Union. To achieve this goal, a unified questionnaire was used, developed by scientists from I. Horbachevsky Ternopil National Medical together with colleagues from the State Higher School named after Pope John Paul II (Biala Podlaska, Poland).

All respondents answered the questions of the unified International Questionnaire, in which they noted the number of ticks and locations of their bites, described methods of removal, informed about the use of repellents before entering the forest areas, and about self-examination of skin after returning from such areas. In addition, forest workers and patients reported complaints that plagued them after the tick attacks. Based on the results of the survey, an analysis of the awareness of forestry workers in some regions of Ukraine and students of Ternopil about LB was conducted, as well as we suggested new ways to improve their knowledge about this problem.

The survey revealed insufficient awareness of respondents about the prevention of LB: 57.7% of foresters and 65.4% of students did not know methods of removing ticks, only 4.6% of foresters and 10.0% of students used the help of health workers; 56.7% of foresters (in Chernivtsi region – 90.4%) and 42.2% of students did not use protection before the entrance to the forest area, only 18.0% of foresters and 8.9% of students conducted a self-examination of the skin after returning from the forest areas.

It follows from the above data, that in order to prevent LB and other tick-borne infections, it is necessary to provide foresters with appropriate means of protection (clothing and footwear), repellents, special individual devices (tick twisters) to remove ticks and to oblige them to use them. It is necessary to systematically increase the level of sanitary education about LB among not only foresters, but also among the general population with the help of forest safety engineers, family doctors, research and teaching staff of the departments of infectious diseases and epidemiology, regional and national media.

A number of epidemiological features of LB in patients with EM and NEM have been elucidated. Among patients with EM LB, more than three tick attacks were noted by 41.8% of people, almost every fourth patient did not remember the tick bites, but the appearance of EM was associated with visits to forests, parks, or village cottages. Most often, the subjects pulled out the tick after the bite (21.9%), 12.3% of the subjects twisted it out with tweezers, almost every tenth removed with simple movements or lubricated with oil, and only 8.2% of subjects sought medical help. More than a third of the patients removed the tick within one day after the bite, and almost half could not indicate the time of removal. Ticks attacked most often when a person was in the forest (31%) or in the backyard (23%), less often in a park area (17%), 29% of the respondents did not remember the event. Tick bites were recorded from March to November with peaks between May – July or September in different years. The majority of patients reported ticks biting to the lower extremities ($p < 0.05$), and one in five could not clearly indicate the site of tick attack. The risk of EM LB was established: the risk of developing EM is significantly higher when ticks are biting to one area compared to ticks attacking several locations (OR = 0.28; 95% CI 0.09-0.89; $p = 0.031$); tick attack in autumn reduces the risk of EM compared to attacks which occurred in spring and summer (OR = 0.31; 95% CI 0.10-0.98; $p = 0.046$).

We have created an interactive medical map (based on a geographic information system) that allows an interested person to get information online. It is expedient to use it for the development and carrying out of a complex of actions for diagnostics and prevention of tick infections, forecasting of epidemic danger in the inspected territories, in practical activity of infectiologists, employees of service of sanitary and epidemiological supervision, public health centres.

Lyme borreliosis as a multisystem disease is often called the “new great simulator” for the variety of clinical manifestations. In the course of the disease, there is a period of early infection, which distinguishes between stages of localized and disseminated infections, and the period of late infection. The stage definition and differentiation are quite conditional and is largely based on clinical manifestations, as well as on temporal characteristics from the moment of infection. The disease can sequentially move from one stage to another or skip any of them, as well as appear for the first time in any stage without a previous one.

For the most part, Lyme borreliosis manifests itself as a skin disease, while lesions of other organs and systems are noted much less frequently. At the site of the pathogen penetration, there is a primary affect in the form of EM, which is a pathognomonic sign of LB. The frequency of its occurrence varies from 27 to 90%. There are typical and atypical variants of EM. We found out some clinical features of EM LB: single foci of erythema (94.5%) prevail over the multiple ones; typical forms (64.4%) – over atypical ones ($p < 0.05$); from atypical forms, a continuous hyperaemic spot is observed more often; erythema is localized mainly in the areas of tick bites

(82.8%), most commonly – in the lower extremities, less often – remotely ($p < 0.001$); the average duration of EM was 30 days (95% CI 19; 59); the risk of developing other clinical signs of LB during EM is higher if it occurs up to 30 days from the time of tick bite (OR = 0.12; 95% CI 0.01-0.95; $p = 0.04$); EM with dissemination of Borrelia was registered in 34.2% of patients with lesions mainly of the musculoskeletal system (10.9%), cardiovascular (5.5%) and nervous (6.2%) systems and intoxication syndrome (11.6%).

Skin lesions in LB can also manifest themselves in the form of benign lymphocytoma of the skin, acrodermatitis chronica atrophicans (ACA), localized scleroderma. A number of clinical features of localized scleroderma of the skin in NEM LB were revealed, in particular: multiple foci occur mainly on the abdomen, in places of tick bite ($p < 0.05$) in contrast to single superficial atrophies mostly on the legs of patients with localized scleroderma without LB; significantly lower degree of skin induration (according to a modified skin score by G. P. Rodnan).

Skin lesions in NEM LB may be less common in the form of urticaria, pityriasis rosea rash, Weber-Christian panniculitis, Lichen ruber planus, Pasini-Pierini atrophoderma, which develops 6 months (or up to 4 years) after Borrelia infection.

The problem of LB is becoming increasingly important for rheumatological practice, as the disease is often manifested by lesions of the musculoskeletal system which are difficult to diagnose. A mysterious feature of LB is the slow increase in the pathological symptoms of the musculoskeletal system, which may not disappear after a full course of treatment, and some patients develop chronic inflammatory arthritis, resistant to antibiotic therapy.

Lyme arthritis is the most common and serious joint disease in LB. It is suggested that spirochetes usually enter the joints long before the onset of clinical symptoms. In some patients, episodes of arthralgia may precede clinical arthritis. Lyme arthritis is a monoarticular or oligoarticular arthritis of the large joints, characterized by episodes of inflammation with swelling, large effusions and slight pain. The knee joint is most often affected, but other large and small joints, such as the ankle (the second most frequently involved joint), shoulder, elbow or wrist, may also be involved in the pathological process; isolated lesions of small joints are atypical.

Arthritis associated with *B. burgdorferi* is prone to chronicity, can lead to long- term disability and disablement. The common symptoms of Lyme arthritis with inflammatory diseases of the joints contribute to masking each other. It is often necessary to differentiate from RA in its atypical course.

Lyme arthritis can have an isolated course, and in other cases it can trigger the mechanisms of other forms of arthritis and aggravate the course of the latter. Inflammatory arthritis, such as RA, reactive or psoriatic arthritis, osteoarthritis, can develop within a few months after LB, as if triggered by a spirochete infection. In the case of inflammatory arthritis on the background of LB, there are three options: patients with active infection in the joints; patients with post-infectious Lyme arthritis; patients with other form of inflammatory arthritis that occurs after LB.

Rheumatic joint disease can mask the course of Lyme arthritis, so we analysed the clinical course of isolated RA and RA associated with *B. burgdorferi*. It was found that among the examined patients, RA associated with *B. burgdorferi* was diagnosed in 53.97% of people, and this condition was accompanied by more intense pain with high visual analogue pain scale (VAS) score, greater activity of the inflammatory syndrome, the presence of hypertrophic synovitis, mainly of the knee joint, with synovial cysts of popliteal space, also known as Baker's cysts, which together contribute to the progression of arthritis and lead to a more severe course of the disease compared with isolated RA. We believe that early detection of Borrelia presence and their elimination will contribute to a less aggressive course of RA.

The stratification of factors influencing the quality of life of patients with RA associated with *B. burgdorferi* and with isolated RA was also investigated on the basis of the Health Assessment Questionnaire-Disability Index (HAQ-DI) and the Short Form Medical Outcomes Study (SF-36). The data obtained indicated a negative impact of arthritis on all indicators of quality of life of patients based on SF-36 scale and the HAQ-DI index. Decreased physical functioning in patients of both groups was observed against the background of increased activity of the inflammatory process according to the DAS 28. However, differences were found: in patients with RA associated with *B. burgdorferi*, significantly lower psychological component of health was observed, which can be explained by difficult psychological adaptation to their own disease, given the prevalence of LB and its tendency to chronicity. Factors that affect the quality of life of patients in both groups are the physical activity and duration of the disease.

The study of the dynamics of the activity of pro-inflammatory and anti- inflammatory cytokines allows us to elucidate new links in the immunopathogenesis of LB. In patients with Lyme arthritis, the content of anti-inflammatory cytokines (IL-10 and IL-4) was significantly higher than in patients with RA associated with *B. burgdorferi* and with isolated RA. This suggests that the onset of joint inflammation in Borrelia infection is accompanied by the formation of an adequate immune response. The high level of these anti-inflammatory cytokines reduces the activity of macrophages, the synthesis of TNF-α, IL-1, IL-6, creating conditions for the transition of the disease to a stage of limited inflammation and rapid termination of the pathological process.

Fibromyalgia is the second most common "rheumatic" disease (after osteo- arthritis), occurring in 2 to 8% of the general population. One of its probable triggers is LB. The disease can also induce complex dermatological conditions that lead to autoimmune inflammatory dermatomyopathies, including dermatopolymyositis. Prolonged persistence of *B. burgdorferi* is thought to cause systemic scleroderma.

It should be noted that while most patients who receive adequate treatment for LB recover, some individuals develop unexplained chronic conditions in the form of persistent or recurrent symptoms after treatment that cannot be explained. Moreover, the phenotype of symptoms is similar to the recently described "long-COVID-19". The most common manifestations are fatigue, pain in the musculo-skeletal system and cognitive dysfunction. The term "post-Lyme disease" (PLD) has been proposed for this condition. However, patients with PLD often also report other, extremely diverse neurological symptoms: sleep disturbances, mood disorders, eye damage, and so on. PLD requires further research to develop clear diagnostic criteria, elucidation of factors that contribute to and prevent its development, and adequate therapeutic measures.

We also observed other systemic manifestations of LB, namely: lymphadenopathy, muscle pain (VAS score 90 mm), localized scleroderma, Sjogren's syndrome, leukocytoclastic vasculitis, Pfeifer – Weber – Christian panniculitis, systemic lupus erythematosus-like conditions, antiphospholipid syndrome, polyneuropathy (systemic vasculitis was suspected) with signs of inflammatory syndrome.

Thus, the rheumatological aspects of LB and PLD are currently imperfectly studied, which encourages further research.

Lesions of the cardiovascular system in LB also have signs of systemic inflammatory response of the body with a possible autoimmune component, which causes damage to both heart tissue and vascular wall. Lyme carditis usually occurs in the early disseminated stage, often with cardiac arrhythmias and conduction deviation, usually not alone, but in combination with joint damage manifestations or symptoms of lymphatic and nervous system damage, although cardiac lesions may dominate. Dissemination of the pathogen without previous EM is observed in about 20 to 45% of cases.

Heart lesions can be manifested by myocarditis both with circulatory failure, as well as without it (mostly the left ventricle suffers), less often – pericarditis with pericardial friction noise or with the appearance of effusion. Endocarditis with the formation of heart defects is extremely rare.

Atrioventricular block is one of the most severe, sometimes fatal, complications of LB. It is characterized by an intermittent nature: the degree changes rapidly from smaller to larger and back within a few hours. In addition to conduction disturbances, the electrocardiogram often records attacks of supraventricular and ventricular tachycardia, extrasystoles from various parts of the heart, up to bigeminy, episodes of atrial fibrillation, migration of the pacemaker in the atria.

It is necessary to purposefully identify complaints from the patients with suspected LB about cardiovascular system and, conversely, to ask patients with acute unexplained cardiac symptoms about facts of a possible tick attack and the presence of other manifestations of Lyme disease. As carditis usually develops within 2 months of the onset of infection, it often occurs in the same period as erythema migrans or neurological lesions, making it easier to diagnose.

It is advisable to conduct a serological examination for LB detection for all patients living in endemic regions of LB with dilatation of the chambers of the heart of unknown or ischemic origin, regardless of the presence of a history of tick bite. The same applies to people from endemic regions who have progressive coronary heart disease, or have suffered several myocardial infarctions. If diagnostic titres of antibodies to Borrelia are detected, an infectious disease specialist should be consulted to choose further treatment tactics.

In the absence of EM, the clinical manifestations of Lyme carditis are not very specific. It is necessary to determine the presence of specific antibodies to Borrelia for diagnosis. Most patients with cardiac manifestations of LB are seropositive at the time of cardiac symptoms.

Hospitalization of patients and continuous monitoring are appropriate in the presence of symptoms of cardiovascular disease, such as syncope, shortness of breath or chest pain, as well as atrioventricular block (the second or the third degree), and even the first degree, if the PR interval is greater than 30 ms. It is important to perform ECG examinations of patients for each suspected disease. In doubtful diagnostic cases, magnetic resonance imaging of the heart is the method of choice for verification of myocarditis in patients with LB.

In the period of chronic LB, endothelial and myocardial damage causes both diastolic dysfunction of the left ventricle and vascular disorders, which necessitates blood pressure monitoring, dynamic ECG monitoring, and preventive measures for the development of atherosclerosis. In patients with acute and chronic LB in the presence of concomitant hypertension, one should consider the possibility of worsening of its course.

In persons who were treated for LB, the list of mandatory tests at the posthospital stage should include the determination of acute inflammation markers, myocardial enzyme activity, ECG and echocardiography, if necessary – daily ECG monitoring; if myocarditis is detected, the tactics of further management of patients should be developed by a cardiologist. Determination of HLA phenotypes – markers for the formation of risk groups for chronic disease, specific heart tissue damage, cardiosclerosis, if possible, may be useful for stratification of the risk of cardio- vascular complications caused by LB in endemic areas.

Lesions of the nervous system (NS) or neuroborreliosis are noted quite often in LB. They are mostly associated with *B. garinii*, although Borrelia of other species can cause such pathology. NS lesions, depending on the geographical area, were observed in 10 to 60% of patients with LB. Such significant fluctuations in the frequency of NS damage are associated with the variety of the Borrelia species and genotypes, as well as with the insufficient study of this problem in a number of regions.

Elements of parenchyma of central nervous system (CNS) are damaged both in the early, as well as in the late periods, during the course of LB. The acute form of neuroborreliosis, according to our data, is manifested mainly by unilateral lesions of the cranial nerves: facial – in 80.0% of patients, and ocular – in 20.0% of patients. The structure of chronic LB with NS lesions is dominated by the syndromes of encephalopathy (50.0%), radiculopathy (45.2%), polyneuropathy (19.0%) and encephalomyelitis (7.1%). There are combined lesions of the peripheral and central nervous systems in 21.4% of patients. The acute period of LB precedes the development of chronic forms of neuroborreliosis in only 59.5% of patients, while there is a primary-chronic course of the disease in other cases (40.5%). Risk factors for chronic LB are multiple episodes of tick bites, absence of primary EM in patients, early development of signs of dissemination, delayed and/or incomplete course of antibacterial therapy in the acute period of the disease.

Chronic LB is characterized by a gradual progression of the NS lesions, which is accompanied by a general infectious syndrome in 45.2% of cases, by lymphadenopathy in 14.3% of cases, and in 57.1% of cases – is combined with extraneural syndromes, among which myalgias predominate (in 50.0% of cases), as well as arthralgia/arthritis. Radiculopathy in chronic LB is characterized by multilevel damage (in 63.2% of patients), moderate persistent pain, independent of changes in body position and physical exercise, a combination of nerve root and polyneuritic disorders (82.8%), mainly with bilateral irradiation of pain (52.4% of cases), mild vertebral syndrome, weak response to non-steroid antiinflammatory drugs (NSAIDs).

The main manifestations of encephalopathy in chronic LB are mild or moderate cognitive impairment (90.5%) in combination with atactic syndrome (71.4%) and pyramidal insufficiency (80.9%). Chronic Borrelia encephalomyelitis, in contrast to multiple sclerosis, is characterized by primary-progressive course, lesions of peripheral NS with nerve root pathology, lack of damage to the optic, vestibulocochlear, facial and trigeminal nerves, multiorgan manifestations. In 20.0% of cases, a combination of MS and LB was noted, which is manifested by frequent polysymptomatic onset, severe sensory disturbances, the development of polyneuropathy and arthralgia.

Serum anti-IgM and anti-IgG titres to *B. burgdorferi* in the blood of patients with chronic LB are significantly reduced during the course of antibacterial therapy. In 17.9% of patients, the titre of antibodies to Borrelia remains above normal in the absence of clinical signs of disease progression. In chronic LB, inflammatory changes in the cerebrospinal fluid are detected mainly in the case of combined lesions of the peripheral and central nervous systems in the form of increased protein levels (27.2%) and lymphocytic pleocytosis (18.2%).

It is known that the prevalence of tuberculosis remains high in the world and in Ukraine in particular, including regions that are endemic for tick-borne and parasitic infections, such as LB and giardiasis. The influence of LB, giardiasis and their combination on the course of newly diagnosed pulmonary tuberculosis was studied. The aggravating effect of LB and giardiasis on the clinical course of pulmonary tuberculosis was established: in the case of concomitant giardiasis – more frequent clinical manifestations of digestive system disorders ($p < 0.05$); combination of LB and giardiasis caused intoxication syndrome, disorders of the musculoskeletal system ($p < 0.05$), cardiovascular system ($p < 0.05$). Destructive changes in the lungs and mycobacterial excretion in concomitant LB and giardiasis were significantly more common in patients with tuberculosis than in their absence. The effectiveness of treatment of patients with newly diagnosed pulmonary tuberculosis, in terms of cessation of mycobacterial excretion and healing of the cavities of pulmonary destruction, was higher compared to patients with tuberculosis and concomitant LB and giardiasis ($p < 0.05$).

It has been established that concomitant chronic Epstein-Barr virus infection affects the course of Lyme borreliosis. Specifically, such patients more frequently reported joint pain, insomnia and/or chronic sleep deprivation, enlarged lymph nodes, periodic fever, and increased fatigue/general weakness.

A low level of vitamin D (deficiency and insufficiency combined) was more commonly observed in the blood serum of patients with chronic EBV infection in the active phase, both with and without LB, compared to patients with this viral infection alone in the latent phase ($p < 0.05$) or in combination with LB.

A safe, but not target, level of vitamin D was noted only in the blood serum of patients with chronic EBV infection in the latent phase, either alone or in combination with LB. AVDL (sufficient and safe, but not target levels combined) in the blood serum were mostly seen in patients with only chronic EBV infection in the latent phase or in combination with LB, compared to those with the viral disease in the active phase, either with LB or alone ($p < 0.05$). In patients with chronic EBV infection in the latent phase, the average level of 25 (OH) D in the blood serum was significantly higher than in individuals with the same disease in the active phase, both with and without LB ($p < 0.05$). At the same time, the vitamin D content in the blood serum of patients with chronic EBV infection in the latent phase in combination with LB was also higher than in individuals with only the active phase of the viral infection ($p < 0.05$).

Therefore, for patients with Lyme borreliosis combined with chronic EBV infection and vitamin D deficiency, it is advisable to prescribe comprehensive treatment using both doxycycline hydrochloride and ergocalciferol per os. This approach not only achieves remission of arthritis and complete elimination of vitamin D deficiency but also reduces the percentage of individuals with the active phase of EBV infection.

Specific methods of laboratory diagnosis of LB are based on the detection of the pathogen itself (bacterioscopic and bacteriological methods) or its DNA, as wells as antibodies to it (serological).

The pathogen can be detected in various biological materials by direct microscopic methods. Pathogens in the form of a spiral are visible in a dark field of a microscope or at a phase contrast. Fluorescence and electron microscopy can be used as well. Direct dark field microscopy is used to establish the fact of tick infestation and its degree. However, it does not allow to determine the species of Borrelia and assess their pathogenicity to humans.

Serological methods detect antibodies to pathogen antigens in blood serum, cerebrospinal fluid (intrathecal) and intra-articular fluid. Screening studies are performed using ELISA, complement fixation test (CF), indirect hemagglutination test (IHA), indirect immunofluorescence assay (IIFA). These methods are not interchangeable in the routine diagnosis of LB, especially NEM LB, latent and chronic forms. Seroconversion is observed in 20 to 50% of patients with acute LB. The titre of specific anti-IgM becomes the highest at 4 to 6 weeks from the onset of the disease, and in the presence of clinical manifestations, these antibodies are detected even up to one year. However, there can be both false-negative and false-positive results. The dynamics of antibody titre in the patient should be assessed in 3 to 4 weeks. After effective treatment of the disease and elimination of the pathogen, the level of antibodies decreases rapidly, which is a positive prognostic sign.

Quite promising now is a multiplex IIFA using BIOCHIP technology, which allows to detect specific IgM and/or IgG antibodies simultaneously to many pathogens of infectious and parasitic diseases in one sample. The first results which we obtained during examination of patients with joint damage and patients with lymphadenopathy were quite informative. Therefore, this method should be more widely implemented in practical medicine.

Immunoblot allows us to detect antibodies to certain proteins of the pathogen, it has a higher sensitivity and specificity compared to other methods. It is used to confirm positive and intermediate results of serological screening tests. There are several types of immunoblot reactions: Western blot (WB), EUROLINE-WB, EUROLINE Borrelia RN-AT. They differ in the number of available antigens and, accordingly, the interpretation of the results. Anti-Borrelia EUROLINE-WB allows the detection of anti-IgM and anti-IgG against different antigens of the same Borrelia species/genotype. The next used immunoblot, namely, EUROLINE *Borrelia* RN-AT, combines the advantages of Western blot and linear blot in one test membrane. Western blot antigens, recombinant VlsE, natural purified OspC antigens of Borrelia species (*B. burgdorferi ss, B. garinii,* and *B. afzelii*), immunoreactive lipids from the cytoplasmic membrane of Borrelia (Lipb Ba, Lipid Bb), and the most specific recombinant antigens p18, p19, p20, p21, p58, all were used to detect specific IgG. Compared to the traditional WB system, EUROLINE *Borrelia* RN-AT is much more sensitive and specific.

Using the ELISA, we surveyed serum samples of 1,070 forestry workers from seven regions – Volyn, Zhytomyr, Transcarpathian, Ternopil, Khmelnytskyi, Chernivtsi and Chernihiv. Frequency of seropositive individuals for *B. burgdorferi s. l.* among foresters in different regions of Ukraine ranged from 22.8% in Chernivtsi region to 58.0% in Zhytomyr region. The presence of IgM and IgG antibodies to *B. burgdorferi s. s., B. garinii, B. afzelii* (alone or in combination) was confirmed by immunoblotting in 84.1% of surveyed foresters; the frequency of anti-IgM detection to OspC of *B. burgdorferi s. l.* and *B. garinii* did not differ significantly between regions, while anti-IgM to OspC of *B. afzelii* was most often detected in the serum of foresters from Khmelnytskyi and Chernihiv regions, least often – from Transcarpathian ($p < 0.05$); frequency of anti-IgG detection to VlsE of *B. burgdorferi s. l., B. garinii, B. afzelii* did not differ significantly in foresters of the surveyed regions ($p > 0.05$).

The obtained results give grounds to classify the forestry workers of Ukraine as a high-risk group for LB, and this infectious disease should be considered as an occupational disease of foresters.

The use of a two-stage serological method for the diagnosis of LB allowed the ELISA test to detect IgM and/or IgG antibodies to *B. burgdorferi s. l.* in 73.9% of patients with EM LB, 63.3% of patients in hospitals in Ternopil and 65.6% of foresters with NEM LB. By immunoblotting, the presence of anti-IgM to *B. burgdorferi s. l.* was confirmed in 62.7% of patients with EM LB, with NEF – in 50.0% of hospital patients and 57.9% of foresters, anti-IgG – in 54.4, 82.5 and 87.9% of persons, respectively. Anti-IgG to VlsE antigen of *B. afzelii* was found in 100.0% of foresters with signs of intoxication syndrome and only in 45.5% of patients with morphea; to VlsE of *B. burgdorferi s. l.* – in 100.0% of patients with cardiovascular lesions and 54.5% of patients with morphea; to VlsE of *B. garinii* – in 94.7% of foresters with intoxication syndrome and only in 41.9% of patients with EM LB. Serological confirmation of Lyme arthritis and neuroborreliosis was also shown in foresters of Ternopil region, in the blood serum of which in 80.0% of cases highly specific anti-IgG to p39 and p83 antigens were detected.

The use of the EUROLINE *Borrelia* RN-AT adv IgM test system allowed us to expand the range of detected pathogens of EF and NEM LB in patients with lesions mainly of the musculoskeletal system by detecting anti-IgM simultaneously to OspC of *B. spielmanii, B.*

burgdorferi s. l., B. garinii and *B. afzelii*, in particular in 78.9% of patients with EF and 64.7% of patients with NEF.

Linear blotting in the laboratory of IGeneX Inc., Milpitas, California, USA, revealed IgM and/or IgG antibodies simultaneously to *B. miyamotoi* and *B. burgdorferi s. l.* in 29.8% of foresters from Ternopil region with NEM LB with intoxication syndrome and musculoskeletal disorders, which proved the involvement of *B. miyamotoi* in the occurrence of this pathology. Therefore, patients with EF and NEM LB in the absence of specific anti-IgM to *B. burgdorferi s. l., B. garinii, B. afzelii* and *B. spielmanii* should be advised to examine for the presence of other species of Borrelia and pathogens of tick-borne infections. It is very important to expand the study of the etiological structure of LB and confirm it in patients.

The most promising method for the diagnosis of LB is PCR, which allows to detect fragments of Borrelia DNA and identify their species in different biological material. The sensitivity of the method varies from 20 to 80%; it can establish human infection as early as 7 to 14 days after the removal of the tick, even during the incubation period of the disease. PCR is used in meningitis, meningoencephalitis, atypical erythema, arthritis. This method can diagnose Borrelia mixed infections, recurrent diseases, monitor the effectiveness of treatment. The use of several diagnostic systems allows to obtain more reliable results.

We observed pregnant women in whom ultrasound revealed a number of pathological changes. While examining their blood, DNA of *B. burgdorferi s. l.* was found in 11.6% of subjects, DNA of *A. phagocytophilum* – in 6.9%, RNA of *Babesia sp.* – in 4.7%. It should be noted that in 9.3% of pregnant women both antibodies to Borrelia and *B. burgdorferi s. l.* DNA were detected simultaneously, so the result can be considered positive. Therefore, pregnant women with a burdensome obstetric history should be further examined for the presence of LB pathogens and other blood infections that can lead to pregnancy pathology.

Therefore, laboratory examination of patients with LB should be performed in two stages: the first – screening using IIFA or ELISA; the second – confirmation of the results of the first stage and determination of specific antibodies to certain antigens of pathogens by immune blotting, or by detecting the DNA of the pathogen by PCR. Unfortunately, at present, all the above specific research methods do not prevent obtaining both false-positive and false-negative results, so in doubtful cases, the patient's examination should be comprehensive, long-lasting, and it should be carried out in dynamics.

To diagnose EM and also the sub-erythema form of LB, in addition to serological examination, we performed thermography, which is based on remote registration of infrared radiation from the human body. Normally, the thermographic picture of human skin is characterized by symmetry and homogeneity (ΔT does not exceed 0.3 °C). In the case of local damage (inflammation) of the skin, local "heating" (ΔT over 0.5 °C) was observed.

Under the influence of comprehensive treatment for LB using antibiotics, there is a reduction in the temperature difference in both single and disseminated migrating erythema, as well as in symmetrical areas.

The longest duration of erythema was observed in patients without localized heating in the area of migrating erythema ($\Delta T \leq 0.5$ °C) before treatment, compared to those with diagnostically significant temperature differences ($\Delta T > 0.5$ °C) before treatment, with $p < 0.05$ and < 0.001, respectively. A reverse correlation was found between the duration of EM and the temperature difference between the affected and healthy areas of skin, both before ($r = -0.48$; $p < 0.05$) and after ($r = -0.59$; $p < 0.001$) etiotropic treatment.

All patients with EM LB had hyperthermia at the site of the tick attack, and ΔT exceeded 0.6 °C, almost half of the patients had it in the range of 1.2–1.6 °C, and in every fourth patient it was even greater than 1.6 °C. The diagnosis of sub-erythema form of LB was established by the presence of local inflammation of the skin at the site of tick bite in the form of its slight hyperthermia (ΔT = 0.6–1.1 °C), which lasted for 2 weeks or more.

The method of remote thermometry of the place of tick attachment to human skin, which we used for the first time, allowed to diagnose sub-erythema form of LB, to justify the need for etiotropic therapy to prevent the development of adverse long-term consequences of the disease. This method should be used by general practitioners as non-invasive, safe, without absolute contraindications and, at the same time, highly informative.

At present, public health care does not have uniform standards of etiotropic treatment of patients with LB. Antibiotics of four groups, to which Borrelia are sensitive, are used: tetracyclines, in particular doxycycline; beta-lactam antibiotics, broad-spectrum penicillins, mostly amoxicillin; cephalosporins of the second and the third generations (cefotaxime, ceftriaxone); macrolides. Etiotropic therapy should be prescribed as early as possible. It is optimal to start it from three days to four weeks from the moment of the disease, as later there is a risk factor for its ineffectiveness. Doxycycline is one of the most commonly used drugs in the treatment of patients with LB, it is quite effective in tick-borne infections caused by *A. phagocytophilum, B. miyamoto* and *Babesia sp.*

Treatment should be long and adequate in the methods of medicine administration and doses, in order to eliminate the pathogen and prevent recurrence. In acute local infection, the course of antibiotic therapy lasts 10 to 21 days; in the dissemination stage, its duration should be increased, or the drug should be administered parenterally, or the dose of antibiotic should be increased. In the stage of chronic infection, long courses of antibiotic therapy are used (at least 3 to 4 weeks).

In LB, according to the indications, detoxification therapy, NSAIDs, drugs that improve microcirculation, antioxidants, immunomodulatory, antihistamines and other symptomatic agents are used.

In some patients with EM LB on the background of prescribed treatment with doxycycline hydrochloride, there are phenomena of photodermatosis and no clinical recovery. Therefore, we decided to reduce the duration of doxycycline hydrochloride therapy (100 mg twice a day) to 14 days, then apply an infusion of stevia plant (Stevia rebaudiana Bertoni), which is effective against all morphological forms of Borrelia, even resistant to doxycycline, 1 cup twice a day for 14 days. This treatment provided a clinical recovery of more patients compared with antibiotic therapy alone – in 87.1% versus 38.2% ($p < 0.05$), and also contributed to a significant reduction in the level of pro-inflammatory IL-18 and an increase in the concentration of anti-inflammatory IL-10 in patient blood serum ($p < 0.05$), which caused an early inflammatory reaction, the formation of cellular and humoral immunity, and thus helped to eliminate Borrelia and accelerate complete recovery of the patient. In addition, in patients treated according to our scheme, the incidence of phototoxic drug reaction to doxycycline hydrochloride decreased by almost 3.8 times ($p < 0.05$).

Therefore, to accelerate clinical recovery, to reduce the duration of antibiotic use and decrease the likelihood of phototoxic drug response to doxycycline hydrochloride in the treatment of patients with EM LB, it is advisable to use the scheme of complex therapy, which we proposed. At the same time, it is necessary to continue the work aimed at further optimization of complex therapy of patients in order to prevent the formation of a chronic process and achieve better treatment results in its presence.

A number of effective methods of primary and secondary prevention have been developed to prevent the occurrence of LB. Vaccination is not currently available. Although a vaccine has been developed in the United States, demand for it is weak and it has been eliminated from the market. The search for a more effective and cheaper vaccine for the population of hyperendemic areas and groups at high risk of Borrelia infection is ongoing.

In recent years, significant progress has been made in studying the problem of Lyme borreliosis, recommendations were developed for practical medicine to improve the diagnosis of the disease, increase the effectiveness of treatment of patients, improve preventive measures. However, a number of issues need in-depth research and quick solutions.

Index

A

B

C

D

E

V

W